Clinical Surgery in General:
RCS Course Manual

For Churchill Livingstone
Project Editor: Deborah Russell
Copy editor: Julie Gorman
Indexer: Nina Boyd
Project Controller: Anita Sekhri

Clinical Surgery in General:
RCS Course Manual

Edited by

R. M. Kirk MS FRCS
Honorary Consulting Surgeon, Royal Free Hospital, London, UK

Averil O. Mansfield ChM FRCS
Professor, Director of Academic Surgical Unit;
St Mary's Hospital and Medical School, London, UK

John Cochrane MS FRCS
Penrose May Tutor, Royal College of Surgeons of England, London;
Consultant Surgeon, Whittington Hospital, London, UK

SECOND EDITION

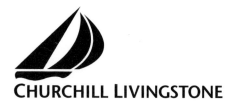

CHURCHILL LIVINGSTONE

NEW YORK EDINBURGH LONDON MADRID MELBOURNE SAN FRANCISCO TOKYO 1996

CHURCHILL LIVINGSTONE
Medical Division of Pearson Professional Limited

Distributed in the United States of America by Churchill
Livingstone Inc., 650 Avenue of the Americas, New York,
N.Y. 10011, and by associated companies, branches and
representatives throughout the world.

First Published 1996

ISBN 0 443 05461 4

British Library Cataloguing in Publication Data
A catalogue record for this book is available from the British
Library.

Library of Congress Cataloging in Publication Data
A catalogue record for this book is available from the library
of Congress.

Medical knowledge is constantly changing. As new
information becomes available, changes in treatment,
procedures, equipment and the use of drugs become necessary.
The editors/authors/contributors and the publishers have, as
far as it is possible, taken care to ensure that the information
given in this text is accurate and up to date. However, readers
are strongly advised to confirm that the information, especially
with regard to drug usage, complies with the latest legislation
and standards of practice.

Printed at Butler & Tanner Ltd, Somerset, UK

Contents

Contributors

Wynne Aveling MB BChir FRCA
Consultant anaesthetist, University College Hospital,
London, UK

Tom Bates FRCS
Consultant Surgeon, The William Harvey Hospital,
Ashford, Kent, UK

Laura J. Buist MD FRCS
Consultant Renal Surgeon, University Hospital
Birmingham NHS Trust, Queen Elizabeth Hospital,
Birmingham, UK

R. Carpenter BDS FRCS
Director of Breast Unit, Consultant Surgeon,
Surgical Oncologist, St Bartholomew's Hospital,
London, UK

John Cochrane MS FRCS
Consultant Surgeon, Whittington Hospital, London,
UK

Carmel Coulter FRCP FRCR
Consultant in Clinical Oncology, St Mary's Hospital
and the Middlesex Hospital, London, UK

Richard Cowie MB ChB FRCSE(SN)
Senior Consultant Neurosurgeon, Hope Hospital,
Salford and Royal Manchester's Children's Hospital,
Manchester, UK

M. K. H. Crumplin MB FRCS
Consultant Surgeon, Wrexham Maelor Hospital,
Wrexham, Wales, UK

Ara Darzi MD FRCS FRCSI
Consultant Surgeon St Mary's Hospital, London,
UK

Brian R. Davidson MB ChB MD FRCS
Consultant Senior Lecturer, Department of Surgery,
Royal Free Hospital, and Medical School, London,
UK

Dai Davies FRCS
Consultant Plastic Surgeon, Charing Cross Hospital,
London, UK

John Dawson MS FRCS
Former Consultant Surgeon, Kings College Hospital,
London, UK

Len Doyal BA MSc
Professor of Medical Ethics, St Bartholomew's and The
Royal London Hospital School of Medicine and
Dentistry, London, UK

Peter Driscoll BSc MD FRCS(Ed) FFAEM
Senior Lecturer in Emergency Medicine, Hope
Hospital, Salford, UK

Hugh Dudley CBE ChM FRCS(E) FRACS FRCS
Emeritus Professor, University of London, UK

Brian V. Ellis FRCS
Consultant Surgeon, Ashford Hospital, Ashford,
Middlesex, UK

Michael Emmerson MB BSc FRC Path FRCP(G)
Professor and Head of Microbiology, University
Hospital, Queen's Medical Centre, Nottingham, UK

Roshan Fernando MB BCh FRCA
Consultant Anaesthetist, Royal Free Hospital, London,
UK

Jane Fothergill FRCP FRCS(Ed) FFAEM
Consultant in Accident and Emergency Medicine, St
Mary's Hospital, London, UK

C. G. Fowler MRCP FRCS FRCS(UROL)
Consultant Urological Surgeon, Royal London
Hospital, London, UK

Charles Galasko MSc ChM FRCS
Professor of Orthopaedic Surgery, University of
Manchester; Clinical Director, Dept of Orthopaedic
Surgery, Salford Hospital, Salford, Manchester, UK

Pierre J. Guillou BSc, MD, FRCS
Professor of Surgery, St James' University Hospital, University of Leeds, UK

Colin Hamilton-Davis MB BS FRCA
Senior Registrar, Charing Cross Hospital, London, UK

R. W. Hoile MS FRCS
Consultant General Surgeon and Director of Surgery, Medway NHS Trust, Gillingham, Kent, UK

Robert Huddart MA MB BS MRCP FRCR
Senior Lecturer in Clinical Oncology, Royal Marsden Hospital, Surrey, UK

Jennifer Jones BSc FRCP FRCA
Consultant Anaesthetist and Director, Intensive Care Unit, St Mary's Hospital, London, UK

R. M. Jones MD FRCA
Professor of Anaesthetics, Imperial College School of Medicine, St Mary's Hospital, London, UK

R. M. Kirk MS FRCS
Consulting Surgeon, Royal Free Hospital, London, UK

Roop Kishen MBBS DA MD FFARCS
Consultant in Intensive Care Medicine and Anaesthesia, Hope Hosptial, Salford, Manchester; Honorary Lecturer in Anaesthesia, University of Manchester, Manchester, UK

Anna Kurowska BSc, BA FRCP
Consultant in Palliative Medicine, Whittington Hospital, London; Deputy Medical Director, Edenhall, Marie Curie Centre, London, UK

David Leaper MD ChM FRCS(Ed)
Professor of Surgery, Professorial Unit of Surgery, University of Newcastle, North Tees Hospital, Cleveland, UK

Roderick Little PhD MRCPath
Professor of Surgical Science, Head of MRC Trauma Group; Director, North Western Injury Research Centre, University of Manchester, Manchester, UK

J. Ludbrook MD BSc ChM BMedSc FRCS FRACS
Dept of Surgery, University of Melbourne, Royal Melbourne Hospital, Victoria, Australia

Kevin Mackway-Jones MA MRCP FRCS
Senior Registrar in Accident and Emergency Medicine, University Department of Accident and Emergency Medicine, University of Manchester, Hope Hospital, Salford, Manchester, UK

Kay MacDermot MPhil FRCP
Senior Lecturer and Consultant in Clinical Genetics, Royal Free Hospital School of Medicine, London, UK

David Marsh MD FRCS
Senior Lecturer and Honorary Consultant in Orthopaedic Surgery, Clinical Sciences Building, Hope Hospital, Salford, Manchester, UK

Geraldine C. McMahon BSc(Hons) Anatomy MRCGP BAO FRCS(Ed)
Lecturer in Emergency Medicine, Hope Hospital, Salford, UK

Paul McMaster MA MB ChM FRCS
Hepatobiliary and Transplant Surgeon, The Queen Elizabeth Hospital, Edgbaston, Birmingham, UK

Atulkumar Mehta MA MB BChir MD FRCP FRCP FRCPath
Consultant Haematologist, Royal Free Hospital, London, UK

Hugh Mitchell BSc
Deputy Director Supraregional Assay Laboratory, Charing Cross Hospital, London, UK

John Moorhead MB FRCP
Professor of Urological Medicine, Royal Free Hospital and School of Medicine, Hampstead, London, UK

Jason Payne-James MB FRCS (Edin & Eng) LLM
Honorary Senior Research Fellow, Department of Gastroentrology and Nutrition, Central Middlesex Hospital, London, UK

A. Peel MChir MA MBchir FRCS FRCS(Ed)
Consultant Surgeon, North Tees Hospital, Stockton on Tees, UK

Michael Pietroni MB BS FRCS
Consultant Surgeon, Whipps Cross Hospital, Associate Dean of Postgraduate Medicine, University of London, UK

Michael Platt MB BS FRCA
Consultant in Pain and Anaesthetics, Honorary Senior Lecturer, St Mary's Hospital, London, UK

Mohamed Rady MB BChir MA(Cantab) MD(Cantab) MRCP(UK) FRCS(Ed) FRCS(Eng)
Lecturer in Accident and Emergency Medicine, University of Manchester, UK

P. M. Robbins FRCA
Specialist Registrar, Department of Anaesthesia, Royal Free Hospital, Hampstead, London, UK

Gordon Rustin MD MSc FRCP
Director of Medical Oncology, Mount Vernon Hospital, Northwood, UK

Michael Schachter BSc MB BS MRCP
Senior Research Fellow, Department of Clinical Pharmacology, Imperial College School of Medicine, St Mary's Hospital, London, UK

J. E. Scoble MA MD MB BS MRCP FRCP
Consultant Renal Physician, Guys Hospital, London, UK

Jean Simpson BSc MSc
Public Health Specialist, Ealing Hammersmith &
Hounslow Health Authority, Middlesex, UK

J. Smith MB ChB PhD FRCS(Eng) FRCS(Ed)
Consultant Surgeon, Northern General NHS Trust,
Sheffield, UK

Jeremy Tate MS FRCS
Consultant in Gastrointestinal and Laparoscopic
Surgery, Royal United Hospital, Bath, UK

Adrian Tookman MB BS MRCP
Medical Director, Edenhall, Marie Curie Centre,
Consultant in Palliative Medicine, Royal Free Hospital
Trust, London UK

Robin Touquet MD FRCS FFAEM
Consultant in Accident and Emergency Medicine,
St Mary's Hospital, London, UK

C. Wastell MS FRCS
Professor of Surgery and Honorary Consultant,
Chelsea Westminister Hospital, London UK

Stewart Watson FRCS MRCP
Consultant in Plastic and Hand Surgery, Plastic
Surgery and Burns Unit, Withington Hospital,
Manchester, UK

David Whitby MB BS FRCS
Senior Lecturer, Department of Plastic and
Reconstructive Surgery, Honorary Clinical Research
Fellow, Department of Cell and Structural Biology,
University of Manchester, Manchester, UK

Marc Winslet MB MS FRCS (Eng) FRCS(Ed)
Senior Lecturer and Consultant Surgeon, Royal Free
Hospital, London, UK

Neville Woolf MB ChB MMed(Path) PhD FRCPath
Vice Dean, Faculty of Clinical Sciences, University
College, London, UK

John Yarnold MRCP FRCR
Reader and Honorary Consultant in Clinical Oncology,
Royal Marsden Hospital, Sutton, UK

Preface to the 2nd Edition

We have elected to produce a new edition rather than reprint the first one because of the continuing change in the curriculum and examinations taken at the end of basic surgical training. The four Royal Colleges of Surgeons in the British Isles have continued their cooperation towards agreement on what knowledge and skills an aspiring surgeon should acquire before embarking on higher specialist training in surgery.

An important change is the merging of Applied Basic Sciences and Clinical Surgery in General. For the present the texts in anatomy, physiology, pathology, clinical surgery and operative surgery remain separate. This book continues to cover areas that do not properly fit into the other established specialist books and we think that the original title properly describes our aims.

This break with the long established two part examination is signalled by a change in title given to diplomates of the different Royal Colleges – Member (MRCS), or Associate FRCS. The 'full' Fellowship diploma is awarded at the end of higher surgical training.

In the past a candidate for the Primary FRCS and Final FRCS examinations could, in theory, be questioned over a wide, and largely unspecified area. Tales of unusual questions were circulated and entered the realms of an unofficial curriculum.

For the first time an attempt has been made to lay down a core curriculum and a list of skills that trainees are expected to have acquired, and examiners no longer have the freedom to ask idiosyncratic, irrelevant questions.

Attempts to shorten the period of surgical training make it imperative to ensure that young surgeons are given a more structured training, rather than, as formerly, pick up their knowledge haphazardly, often over a long period.

Assessment in the traditional Final FRCS was directed particularly at clinical ability and other aspects of surgical competence were largely ignored. Now, other areas are included, such as safety of equipment in the operating theatre, genetic aspects of surgery, and economic considerations. In the new examination it is likely that interpersonal relationships with patients will be assessed during discussion of problems with them.

Be assured that the curriculum and examinations are not static. There is world-wide co-operation in attempting to devise better methods of assessment that test not only factual knowledge and psychomotor skills but the even more elusive and important affective aptitudes that a safe, skilled and compassionate surgeon requires.

1996

R. M. K.
A. O. M.
J. C.

Acknowledgements

We are grateful to our contributors for foregoing financial reward, in order that the royalties are passed on to the Royal College of Surgeons of England for the Audiovisual Unit.

Special thanks are also due to Mrs Angela Christie for producing new illustrations and also to the team at Churchill Livingstone for their cooperation and support.

Introduction

R. M. Kirk   A. O. Manfield   J. Cochrane

The purpose of this manual is to help you to apply the knowledge of the basic sciences to clinical practice. Of course, even if you are able to do this you will still not have a complete grasp of surgery. The reason is that much practice is still based not on science but on empiricism – that is, as a result of the accumulated experience of your predecessors who have observed the effects of their actions, and compared different methods. You will, during your own practice, add to and modify the pool of knowledge. The methods of determining the effectiveness of, for example, various treatments, have been refined by the careful application of statistical methods and the neutralization of bias. Nevertheless, many treatments remain unproven. Our profession is under pressure to correct this deficiency and practise what is termed, 'evidence-based medicine.'

It is not our intention to produce a definitive textbook of surgery. We wish to introduce you to some of the areas of knowledge with which you must be familiar, in whatever branch of surgery you intend to practice. At the end of most chapters, are lists of references for further reading.

Expand your knowledge from clinical textbooks which offer generally accepted knowledge and practices, but remember that they cannot be completely up to date because of delays in preparing, publishing and distributing them. Critically read surgical journals. Original articles offer you not only more up-to-date knowledge but also the opportunity to judge if the authors have planned and carried out investigations logically, measured the results accurately, and drawn valid conclusions from them. Authoritative reviews provide a digest of current thinking but do not rely too heavily upon them, because it is valuable for you to read the literature and make up your own mind, rather than act on received wisdom.

The best time to read up a subject is when you are about to see, or have just seen, a relevant clinical problem. Your knowledge of the patient provides a 'peg' on which to hang the new information you acquire, so that you avoid the need to learn a list of facts. Notes read in a clinical vacuum, and taken at lectures, that you may never read again, do not remain in your memory. Listen carefully to your seniors, ask questions when a suitable opportunity occurs, and watch the development of events, noting the outcome of the action taken. At frequent intervals review and organize your knowledge. it is valueless unless it is accessible and usable. The prospect of examinations serves a valuable purpose quite apart from the assessment by the examiners: it drives you to identify gaps in your knowledge, complete it and organize it.

In addition to acquiring knowledge on which you can draw, you must develop attitudes which enable you to use it effectively. You are not training to become a mere technical wizard, who, placed before a patient, can carry out an operation with panache. Of course you wish to become a surgeon for personal satisfaction, enjoyment of the skilful use of techniques and so on. However, the successful practice of surgery is expressed in the American aphorism, 'Choose well, cut well, get well'. It must be the correct operation, on the correct patient, who is brought to surgery in the best possible condition and will be carefully monitored thereafter. 'Choose well' is, therefore, as important as 'Cut well'.

Our satisfaction as surgeons also depends upon our confidence that we are serving our patients sympathetically as well as effectively. We are immensely privileged that we are trusted by people who often have no previous knowledge of us, to make good decisions on their behalf and carry out the necessary actions with skill and care. We require a wide range of qualities to fulfil all these functions. There have been many attempts to list the unique characteristics that together make a good surgeon. Apart from technical competence, we need stamina, good interpersonal and communications skills, 'common sense', decisiveness, ability to withstand stress, leadership, the humility to admit error, self-motivation and, perhaps above all, integrity. This last, elusive quality is important. None of us has all the required attributes in full measure: we need to recognize the deficiencies and determine to compensate for them to the best of our ability.

Patient assessment and emergency

1. Clinical history and examination

R. M. Kirk

Should you read this chapter? Maybe you think you are already too experienced to need instruction. If you think so, then you are definitely lacking self-knowledge. Of all the skills you require in surgery and in medicine generally, taking a history, examining the patient and interpreting your findings are paramount. They form the base from which you work. If you take the wrong diagnostic path all the rest of your activities are misdirected.

HISTORY

Traditionally, surgeons have prided themselves on their ability to elicit physical signs and make accurate 'spot diagnoses'. We have, perhaps, not always sufficiently developed the skills of history-taking. Do not be in any doubt that a good history is vital. Many surgical diseases produce no physical signs. If you embark on surgical treatment after concentrating on a localized lesion you will be unprepared if complications develop.

As you first encounter the patient, take in every aspect of gender, age, dress, speech, gait and attitude. This prejudices your interpretation of what you are told. 'Prejudice' is often considered a pejorative term; it is reprehensible only if it is rigidly maintained against the evidence. By sensibly incorporating their impressions of the patient with the history, experienced clinicians often make a provisional diagnosis within a few seconds (Fig.

Young child	Appendicitis
Young woman	Gynaecological
Young man	Hernia, appendicitis
Middle-aged woman	Gynaecological, diverticulosis coli
Middle-aged man	Diverticulosis coli
Elderly woman	Gynaecological, cancer colon
Elderly man	Cancer colon

Fig. 1.1 The presenting patient prejudices the clinician. If you are seeing a patient with lower abdominal pain, the diagnoses that you first consider are influenced by the type of patient.

1.1). Treat such a diagnosis merely as a working hypothesis, useful for the present, to be tested and abandoned at once if it is refuted.

The next time you sit before a new patient, try to analyse the sequence of your questions, your motivation in asking them in that manner, and your interpretation of the answers. It is sometimes valuable to place a tape recorder on the table so that you can subsequently analyse the progression of your questions. Listen to others while they take a history. Can you differentiate between the skilled and the unskilled? What is the difference?

There are two parts to taking the history – determining the cause of the complaint that has brought the patient to you, and determining the general state and feeling of the patient.

Presenting complaint

Do not passively listen and record the patient's words. The danger of this is that it leaves the direction of the discussion to the patient; you must control and lead the interview. This entails asking a question, letting the patient answer it, then cutting in at the correct moment to ask for clarification, ask a supplementary question, or change tack. Too early an interruption causes resentment but if the opportunity is missed the patient is likely to go off at a tangent and resist being brought back to your line of thought.

The object of questions about the presenting symptom is to determine the anatomical site of the lesion causing it. Does function of the suspect system affect the symptom, does the symptom affect the function of the system? The same line of questioning must be applied to all suspect systems. Your intention is that one system may be confidently implicated and the others exonerated (Fig. 1.2).

Supplementary questions are intended to reveal a pattern of a group of features that 'run' together and form a syndrome (Greek: *syn* = together, *dromos* = a course). As a likely diagnosis enters your mind you will ask about other features that are usually associated with it.

As the origin of the presenting symptom is localized, its severity, duration, mode of onset and general effects must be determined.

General assessment

Having reached a provisional explanation for the presenting complaint, carefully assess each body system by means of questions about its function now and in the past. There are sets of fairly standard questions that may reveal malfunctions. If the patient answers 'Yes' to the question, 'Are you short of breath when climbing stairs?' the possibilities of cardiorespiratory disease and anaemia immediately spring to mind.

Ask what the patient thinks about the cause of the symptoms. The answers provide guidance in deciding how to explain the problem and give reassurance.

EXAMINATION

Where is the local lesion?

If there is a localized lesion, first determine exactly where it is. Remember the standardized progression: *look, feel, percuss, listen*. Review the structures in the area and carry out tests to find out whether they lie over or under the lesion and whether it is attached to them. Examples are upward movement of a structure attached to the trachea when the patient swallows, and intra-abdominal tenderness to palpation that is allayed when the patient is asked to perform a manoeuvre that tenses the overlying abdominal muscles. If you know where the lesion is and know the structures you can usually deduce the likely diagnosis in the patient. Do not distress the patient by clumsy, painful palpation; except in some emergencies it is never necessary and is counterproductive because the patient guards against your examination, preventing you from gaining vital information.

What are the characteristics of a lump? You should already know the site. Now determine the size, shape, surface, consistency and special characteristics. For example, is it tender, hot, pulsatile, reducible, bilateral, fluctuant, coloured, translucent? Is there a cough impulse, overlying inflammation, oedema or vascularity? What is the effect of movement or function of the part?

Do not forget the simple principles of examination. For example, when you discover an enlarged lymph node in the neck you should automatically remember to examine the drainage area of the gland and the remainder of the reticuloendothelial system.

Remarkably, we all miss diagnoses not because they are obscure but because we do not assiduously follow the routines which we learned at the beginning of clinical training.

General examination

Develop the skill to carry out a rapid but thorough examination of the patient. In this way you familiarize yourself with the range of normality and can quickly and confidently detect abnormalities.

Thoughtless, repeated observation, palpation and other examinations are a waste of time and may be distressing for the patient. Try to examine everything once only, concentrating on the findings. A common fault is to 'go through the motions' of, for example, palpating lymph nodes, rather than to obtain accurate, crucial information at a single examination. However, if a single examination is equivocal, be willing to repeat it after an interval. Physical signs often change rapidly in acute conditions.

When you have completed the physical examination, ask yourself if there is anything you missed out and why you forgot it.

DIAGNOSIS

The mechanism of diagnosis is complex. Do not make your task more difficult by uncritically gathering vast amounts of irrelevant information. Medical students are often taught that if they listen to what the patient tells them then a diagnosis will emerge. This is not so. The clinician cannot then pick out the relevant, dis-

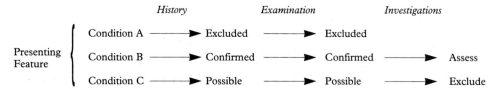

Fig. 1.2 The presenting feature may suggest a number of diagnoses. Each step is intended to exclude or confirm each diagnosis. You hope to end with only one diagnosis, with the others confidently excluded.

criminating features from the confusing mass of accumulated facts. Medical and surgical diagnosis resembles scientific investigation. You must ask the right questions to obtain the correct answer.

You do not carry a ranked list of causes for each presenting feature in your head. In some cases it is pattern recognition. From your accumulated experience, reading, and listening to others, you develop associations in your mind. The overweight multiparous lady with postprandial upper abdominal symptoms forms a pattern which triggers the possibility of gallstones or reflux oesophagitis. However, the discovery of an unexpected feature should warn you of the possibility of another diagnosis. Remember that young, slim males may also develop gallstones.

You now hope to have a reasonably confident diagnosis, have eliminated other causes for the presenting features, and have made an assessment of the physical and mental state of the patient.

Suitable investigations can now be ordered, to corroborate the working diagnosis, to exclude others more certainly, and to assess the severity or anatomical site of an identified condition.

A firm diagnosis may not always be possible, but sufficient information may be gained to plan a course of action. In a patient with an 'acute abdomen', the information often allows you to make a clinical decision to perform exploratory laparotomy, further investigation, medical treatment, to ask a specialist in another field, or to observe the patient for a limited period and reassess the clinical features.

If you are still in doubt after taking a history and examining the patient, do not necessarily rush to order investigations in the hope that 'something will turn up'. Of course, intelligently selected investigations may be invaluable in confusing cases. All too often they are instruments for vacillation. It is frequently more profitable and less time consuming to go back to the beginning and retake the history, repeat the examination, or ask a colleague to do so with an open mind.

On many occasions the newly given history may differ markedly from the first, perhaps because you have misinterpreted what the patient has said, or allowed the patient to take charge and been led astray.

Some questions and signs have a high discriminatory value, others do not. A clinical feature or test may give a falsely positive prediction of the diagnosis. Two or three points that suggest one diagnosis may be of less value than one that has a high discriminatory capacity. For example, the diagnosis of acute, uncomplicated appendicitis is often mistakenly made because the pain is in the right iliac fossa, the patient has gastrointestinal symptoms and is tender in the right iliac fossa. However, if there is also tenderness in the left iliac fossa, this must either be complicated (i.e. perforated) appendicitis or another diagnosis must be considered.

When in doubt between the likely, i.e. the most common, diagnosis and a less frequent but important diagnosis, do not lightly pass over the important one. It is dangerous to miss a rarer but serious condition.

RECORD

All the effort you have put into elucidating the problem may be lost if you do not make a careful record that can be read and understood by others – and by yourself. Although various devices for recording are available, they sometimes fail. Even if you have dictated into a recording machine, write the details as well.

Having recorded the findings in the history and the examination, state your conclusions, your policy and what emerged from your discussion with the patient. If you intend to arrange investigations, state what you have in mind. If you arrange treatment, state what monitoring procedures should be carried out.

THINK

Have you missed anything? Have you rushed to the wrong conclusion? Is there a vital question that you could ask, or a physical sign to test your provisional diagnosis?

Remember your obligations to the patient, not just to make a correct diagnosis but also to give reassurance that you have excluded a serious alternative condition. For example, the confident discovery that minimal haemorrhoids, which may not even warrant any treatment, are the cause of rectal bleeding, does not absolve you from carrying out sigmoidoscopy and any other tests to exclude large bowel cancer.

DISCUSS

In the past, informing the patient, and discussing and explaining possible actions and their consequences were often casually performed. This is no longer tolerable. Listen to the patient and, if necessary, change your policy of management. Do not forget to inform relatives in appropriate circumstances.

EMERGENCY

You cannot stick obsessively to a routine in some situations. A patient may have airway obstruction, calamitous bleeding, be in excruciating pain, be mentally disarranged, violent or unconscious. In each case you must quickly and accurately determine the cause of the emergency state, correct it and deal with lesser conditions as the opportunities occur. It is particularly important to record everything, otherwise some vital consideration may be missed when routines are broken. When the emergency condition is under control, meticulously carry out a thorough assessment.

We would all prefer to see patients one by one and complete our examination before seeing the next patient. Sometimes a number of patients present simultaneously or in rapid sequence. Do not obsessively continue examining a patient with a trivial complaint while keeping others waiting who have life-threatening or painful conditions.

When a number of emergencies present at the same time you must apply triage (French: *trier* = to pick out). In principle, this recognizes that loss of life is more important than loss of a limb.

2. Resuscitation

R. Touquet   J. Fothergill   M. W. Platt

The cause of the collapse or coma (a symptom of a broad spectrum of life-threatening conditions that depress or injure the central nervous system) precipitating a patient's arrival in the resuscitation room is often unknown. Furthermore, there may be more than one pathology, for example the patient with hypoglycaemia who has fallen striking his head.

When a patient is brought into an accident and emergency (A&E) department with an altered level of consciousness, the resuscitation sequence described in the American College of Surgeons' Advanced Trauma Life Support Course is appropriate whether the cause is a medical or a surgical emergency. The initial sequence is known as the primary survey (ABCDE, see below). This is a systematic form of assessment that is carried out at the same time that any resuscitative procedures are undertaken. There is ongoing monitoring of the vital signs and, in particular, monitoring of the vital signs in response to any procedure undertaken, such as the immediate infusion of 2 litres of crystalloid for the adult in hypovolaemic shock.

The standard sequence of the initial primary survey is as follows:

Airway, with cervical spine control
Breathing
Circulation
Disability – a brief neurological assessment
Exposure – undress the patient completely.

Due notice must be taken of the history from the ambulance crew. The ambulance transfer form must be signed by a member of the A&E staff. It is prudent to involve the ambulance crew in the initial resuscitation and to have that crew immediately available to give any further details about the history.

When the patient has stabilized, with clinically acceptable vital signs, the patient is examined from head to toe in order to prevent any pathology being missed. It is not infrequent that the A&E doctor is the last doctor to examine the patient in their totality. This systematic methodical examination is known as the secondary survey. However, if the patient has to be taken to theatre urgently then this secondary survey will have to be carried out later on the ward by the responsible admitting team.

PART 1: PRIMARY SURVEY WITH INITIAL RESUSCITATION

Greet the conscious patient from the ambulance by talking to him and reassuring him that he is in the right place and that you know what to do. Do not treat the patient as an inanimate object.

Airway

In all trauma victims apply an appropriately sized head cervical collar. Steady the head – in-line cervical spine immobilization – to prevent those with unsuspected neck injury from sustaining an iatrogenic injury to the cervical spinal cord during manoeuvres on the airway. The neck is at particular risk during orotracheal intubation, when extreme vigilance is mandatory in those in whom a cervical spine injury has not been ruled out.

Assessment

Assess the patency of the airway by talking to the patient, looking for signs of confusion or agitation which may indicate cerebral hypoxia. Listen for stridor or gurgling sounds from a compromised airway. Feel for warm air against your hand in a patient who is breathing. Following smoke inhalation there may be carbon deposits in the mouth or nostrils, raising the possibility of upper airway burns and associated carbon monoxide poisoning. In this situation call an anaesthetist, as early tracheal intubation will be required.

Look to see whether chest movements are adequate.

Management

Keep the airway open and clear it. Remove any foreign bodies such as sweets, or vomit which must be sucked out. Lift the chin forwards to bring the tongue off the back of the nasopharynx, and if the gag reflex is diminished insert an oral (Guedel) airway. If a Guedel airway is not tolerated, but obstruction is still present, consider gently inserting a well-lubricated nasopharyngeal airway, ensuring that this is done automatically. Once the airway is secured deliver 10–15 l min^{-1} of oxygen via a face mask with a reservoir device, providing 95% oxygen.

None of these basic airway manoeuvres protects the lungs from aspiration of gastric contents or blood. In those unable to protect their own airway (absent gag reflex) a cuffed tracheal tube must be inserted via the oral or nasal route, both to facilitate efficient ventilation and to protect the lungs.

If the airway cannot be secured by any of the above methods, urgently carry out a needle cricothyroidotomy followed, if necessary, by a surgical cricothyroidotomy.

Breathing

Assessment

Note any degree of cyanosis. Assess the neck veins and if they are engorged consider the possibility of a tension pneumothorax, cardiac tamponade, air embolus, pulmonary embolus or myocardial contusion. Feel for the position of the trachea, and if it is deviated to one side decide whether it has been pushed over by a tension pneumothorax on the other side. Count the respiratory rate (normally 12–20 per minute) and expose, inspect and palpate the anterior chest wall. Assess air entry or the lack of it by auscultation. A severe asthmatic may prevent with collapse and have a silent chest because with extreme airway narrowing no air can move in or out of the lungs. In a flail chest there are three or more consecutive ribs, each fractured in two or more places, with a segment of paradoxical chest wall motion, the underlying pulmonary contusion may cause acute respiratory failure. If there is any doubt about the adequacy of a patient's airway or breathing, urgently obtain expert help from physicians and anaesthetists.

Management: control of ventilation

Preventing hypoventilation, hypercarbia, cerebral vasodilatation and a resultant increase in intracerebral pressure is vital in trauma patients, especially if they have suffered a head injury. Both adults and children have a normal tidal volume of 7 ml/kg. If the patient is obviously unable to sustain a normal tidal volume (with obvious shallow respirations, often associated with tachypnoea, signs of fatigue and distress), then respiration must be assisted, initially by bag–valve–mask positive pressure ventilation. An arterial blood sample will demonstrate a high arterial carbon dioxide tension ($P_a$co$_2$) level if the patient is breathing inadequately. Ventilate and oxygenate the hypoxic or apnoeic patient if possible for at least 3 minutes prior to attempted intubation, and do not prolong any attempt for more than 60 seconds before returning to bag–valve–mask ventilation. Any patient who is apnoeic obviously needs ventilation urgently.

The aim of assisted ventilation is to keep the arterial blood oxygen above 10 kPa (80 mmHg) and the carbon dioxide below 5.5 kPa (40 mmHg). A reduction of the $P_a$co$_2$ to about 4 kPa (30 mmHg) will reduce cerebral oedema and intracerebral acidosis in a patient with a head injury and a decreased level of consciousness.

In those who are breathing spontaneously, assume that agitation, aggression or depressed level of consciousness is due to hypoxia, demonstrating how all collapsed patients who are not likely to recover immediately must have arterial blood samples taken urgently for measurement of oxygen, carbon dioxide and acid–base balance. (Also consider, where appropriate, a full bladder or tight plaster of Paris as causes of restlessness.) Aspirate arterial blood into a heparinized syringe (a 2-ml syringe whose dead-space has been filled with heparin 1000 units/ml) from the radial artery or, failing this, the femoral artery.

The arterial oxygen tension (P_ao$_2$) should be maintained above 10 kPa (80 mmHg) with added inspired oxygen, for tissue viability. The exception is the patient with chronic obstructive airways disease (COAD), who depends on hypoxic drive rather than $P_a$co$_2$ to breathe, and will tend to hypoventilate when given added oxygen of more than 35%. The only way to diagnose this problem is by the arterial blood gas, which will show a high $P_a$co$_2$ with a normal pH. All collapsed patients should initially be given 85% oxygen, as the problem of the patient whose respiration is dependent on hypoxic drive is uncommonly encountered in A&E.

Oxygen administration may also be necessary to produce a higher than normal P_ao$_2$. This is indicated to correct a pathological state the treatment of which is with an elevated P_ao$_2$; some examples are carbon monoxide poisoning, elevated pulmonary vascular resistance, sickle cell crisis and anaerobic infections.

Circulation

This is the third priority after **A**irway with cervical spine control, and **B**reathing.

Assessment

Assessment of the patient for shock requires skill. Remember that the earliest signs of shock are anxiety, a tachycardia of 100–120 beats per minute, tachypnoea of 20–30 breaths per minute, skin mottling and a prolonged capillary refill time of more than 2 s, and postural hypotension. If there is postural hypotension with a fall of systolic blood pressure of 20 mmHg, a fall of diastolic blood pressure of 10 mmHg and a rise of pulse of 20 beats per minute (20:10:20 rule), diagnose hypovolaemia due to an occult bleeding until proved otherwise. Supine systolic blood pressure does not drop until an adult has lost around 1500–2000 ml of blood, or 30–40% of the blood volume of 70 ml kg^{-1} body weight; by this time the patient is ashen in colour because of blood-drained extremities.

The level of consciousness is also decreased because of inadequate cerebral circulation, particularly if blood loss was rapid. As a guide, a palpable peripheral pulse indicates a systemic blood pressure of at least 60 mmHg. If the carotid pulse is absent, initiate immediate basic cardiopulmonary resuscitation (CPR see below).

Management

Control haemorrhage from any external bleeding points by direct pressure, with limb elevation where appropriate.

Intravenous access. Poiseuille's law states that the rate of flow of fluid through a pipe is proportional to the fourth power of the radius, and inversely proportional to the length. In a severely traumatized or hypovolaemic patient, never fail to insert two short wide-bore cannulae of 14 gauge or larger, sited in peripheral veins, whether introduced percutaneously or by surgical cutdown.

Preferred sites for cutdown are the long saphenous vein anterior to the medial malleolus, or the basilic vein in the elbow crease. Cutdown is a safe, simple and quick procedure in which every surgical trainee should be skilled.

Technique for venous cutdown. Make a transverse 2 cm incision anterior to the medial malleolus or to the medial epicondyle of the humerus. By blunt dissection delineate the long saphenous vein or basilic vein. Ligate the vein distally with 2/0 black silk. Control the vein proximally with a similar loose ligature. Make a transverse incision for one-third of the circumference of the vein, such that it is possible to insert a 14- to 12-gauge cannula into the vein. Secure the cannula in place by tightening the proximal suture. This technique is applicable for collapsed infants.

Intraosseous infusion. An even simpler technique for children is to use an intraosseous trocar and cannula: these are specially designed to be inserted through the cortex of bone into the bone marrow. The site for introduction of the needle is two fingers distal to the tibial tuberosity on the anteromedial surface of the tibia. Clean the area thoroughly as osteomyelitis is a possible complication of the technique. Crystalloid and colloid may slowly be injected into the marrow (20 ml kg^{-1} initially for the collapsed child) together with drugs used in resuscitation, with the exception of sodium bicarbonate and bretylium. The circulation time from here to the heart is only 20 seconds.

Central venous cannulation may be dangerous, even in experienced hands, for the trauma patient, who is often restless. Such patients may not survive an iatrogenic pneumothorax or cervical spinal cord injury caused by the turning of an unsuspected neck injury, and as the above routes of access avoid the possibility of these complications they are to be preferred. Central venous pressure monitoring is useful in the stabilized patient, but these lines are not for resuscitation other than in patients with cardiac arrest, when drugs should be administered centrally.

Correct hypovolaemia with the rapid intravenous infusion of warmed crystalloid or colloid solution followed by blood. Rapid loss of greater than 40% of a patient's blood volume produces electromechanical dissociation leading to circulatory standstill unless immediate resuscitation is carried out. It is not possible to measure the blood volume of a patient in the resuscitation room. Therefore you must monitor the vital signs (delineated in Part 2) especially in response to treatment such as fluid replacement, and tailor your treatment accordingly.

If the carotid pulse is impalpable, the heart has become an ineffective pump, and irreversible brain damage results unless immediate action is taken to correct the specific causes of electromechanical dissociation such as massive blood loss, tension pneumothorax or cardiac tamponade. If there is no improvement or these conditions are not present, commence cardiac massage for cardiac arrest (Fig 2.1A). Check the heart's electrical rhythm on the monitor. Place the leads in the correct positions as quickly as possible. If no rhythm shows, ensure that the gain knob is turned up on the monitor and check for a rhythm in two different ECG leads; alternatively, monitor through the paddles of a defibrillator, one placed just to the left of the expected position of the apex beat and one inferior to the right clavicle.

External chest compression. When the carotid pulse is not palpable after you have controlled ventilation, place one hand over the other on the sternum,

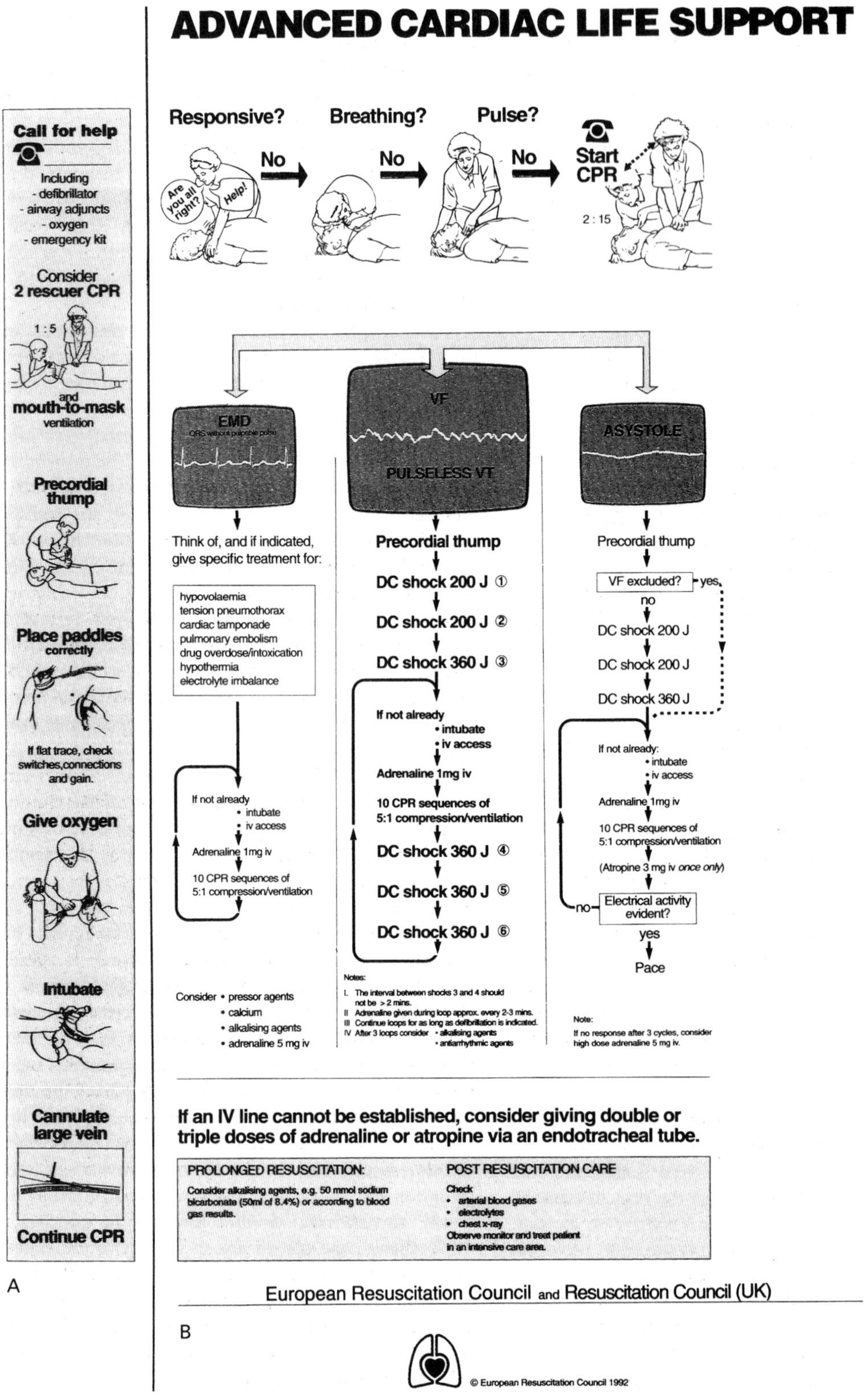

ADVANCED CARDIAC LIFE SUPPORT

Call for help

Including
- defibrillator
- airway adjuncts
- oxygen
- emergency kit

**Consider
2 rescuer CPR**

1:5

and
mouth-to-mask ventilation

Precordial thump

Place paddles correctly

If flat trace, check switches, connections and gain.

Give oxygen

Intubate

Cannulate large vein

Continue CPR

A

Responsive? — No → Breathing? — No → Pulse? — No → Start CPR

2:15

Are you all right? Help!

EMD
QRS without palpable pulse

VF

PULSELESS VT

ASYSTOLE

EMD

Think of, and if indicated, give specific treatment for:

hypovolaemia
tension pneumothorax
cardiac tamponade
pulmonary embolism
drug overdose/intoxication
hypothermia
electrolyte imbalance

If not already
• intubate
• iv access

Adrenaline 1mg iv

10 CPR sequences of
5:1 compression/ventilation

Consider • pressor agents
• calcium
• alkalising agents
• adrenaline 5 mg iv

VF / PULSELESS VT

Precordial thump

DC shock 200 J ①

DC shock 200 J ②

DC shock 360 J ③

If not already
• intubate
• iv access

Adrenaline 1mg iv

**10 CPR sequences of
5:1 compression/ventilation**

DC shock 360 J ④

DC shock 360 J ⑤

DC shock 360 J ⑥

Notes:
I. The interval between shocks 3 and 4 should not be > 2 mins.
II. Adrenaline given during loop approx. every 2-3 mins.
III. Continue loops for as long as defibrillation is indicated.
IV. After 3 loops consider • alkalising agents • antiarrhythmic agents

ASYSTOLE

Precordial thump

VF excluded? — yes

no

DC shock 200 J

DC shock 200 J

DC shock 360 J

If not already:
• intubate
• iv access

Adrenaline 1mg iv

10 CPR sequences of
5:1 compression/ventilation

(Atropine 3 mg iv once only)

Electrical activity evident? — no

yes

Pace

Note:
If no response after 3 cycles, consider high dose adrenaline 5 mg iv.

If an IV line cannot be established, consider giving double or triple doses of adrenaline or atropine via an endotracheal tube.

PROLONGED RESUSCITATION:
Consider alkalising agents, e.g. 50 mmol sodium bicarbonate (50ml of 8.4%) or according to blood gas results.

POST RESUSCITATION CARE
Check
• arterial blood gases
• electrolytes
• chest x-ray
Observe monitor and treat patient in an intensive care area.

European Resuscitation Council and Resuscitation Council (UK)

B

© European Resuscitation Council 1992

Fig. 2.1 (A) Cardiopulmonary resuscitation. (B) Protocol for the treatment of cardiac arrest cases in hospitals. The Resuscitation Council (UK).

the lower border of the hands being two fingers above the xiphisternal–sternal junction. If the hands are lower there is risk of damage to the liver. Keep the arms straight with the shoulders in a direct line over the hands in order that you do not tire. Depress the sternum smoothly for 4–5 cm, at a rate of 80 per minute, with a ratio of one ventilation to about five compressions, both actions being carried out synchronously. Keep the compression rate regular so that the ventilation between compression five and the next compression runs from the fifth compression into the next compression. In this way the pressure is increased generally in the chest both during part of compression five and compression one by that ventilation. In addition, the expanding lungs drive the diaphragm down, leading to compression of the vena cava. This further facilitates blood being forced up the carotid arteries (the thoracic pump effect); feel for the carotid or femoral pulse every 2 minutes.

The correct cardiac rhythm must be diagnosed quickly. In a non-traumatic cardiac arrest patient the rhythm is ventricular fibrillation in 70% of cases, and the chances of a successful resuscitation are directly proportional to the speed of applying DC shock in the correct manner and sequence (Fig. 2.1B). Therefore there must be no delays from the time of arrest, and this is why ambulance crews are now being trained to use, and are issued with, defibrillators.

Internal cardiac massage. External chest compression does not effectively resuscitate an empty heart in cardiac arrest due to hypovolaemic shock. When there is not an appropriate response to prompt rapid transfusion, you should consider internal cardiac massage. This is the only indication for an emergency thoracotomy for internal cardiac massage in the A& E department by trained personnel. Internal cardiac massage is, in the hands of those with appropriate training, both safe and haemodynamically superior to external cardiac massage, although the latter can be initiated without delay and performed by non-surgeons. Open-chest cardiopulmonary resuscitation (CPR) enables direct palpation and observation of the heart and direct electric defibrillation.

The technique for internal cardiac massage (by trained personnel) is as follows: make a left-sided thoracotomy through the fourth or fifth intercostal space once the patient is receiving intermittent positive pressure ventilation through a tracheal tube. Immediately compress the heart using the left hand, without at first opening the pericardial sac, by placing the thumb over the left ventricle posteriorly and the fingers anteriorly in front of the heart. The heart is compressed at the rate of 80 per minute, adjusting the compression force and rate to the filling of the heart. Open the pericardium,

avoiding the phrenic and vagus nerves. Adrenaline, atropine and lignocaine, but not sodium bicarbonate, may be injected directly into the left ventricle, avoiding the coronary arteries. For internal defibrillation use internal 6 cm paddle electrodes with saline-soaked gauze pads and insulated handles. Place one paddle posteriorly over the left ventricle and one over the anterior surface of the heart (10–20 J).

Drugs. In a patient with cardiac arrest, drugs such as adrenaline should, if possible, be given centrally, and for this reason you must be proficient in at least one method of central venous cannulation. You should use the approach with which you are most familiar; however, the infraclavicular approach is often the most convenient and practicable means of access for the surgeon.

Technique for subclavian vein cannulation

1. Preparation: clean the area with surgical antiseptic solution.
2. Position: use a 20° head-down tilt (in patients without head injury) to fill the vein and to reduce the risk of air embolus. For access to the right subclavian vein pull the right arm caudally, to place the vein in the most convenient position to the clavicle for cannulation. If the shoulder is obstructing access, place a sand bag below the upper thoracic spine so that the shoulders lie more posteriorly, unless there is any possibility of spinal injury.
3. Access: introduce the needle through the skin 2 cm inferior to the junction of the lateral and middle thirds of the clavicle. Advance the needle, aspirating continuously and snugging the inferior bony surface of the clavicle, aiming at the superior aspect of the right sternoclavicular joint for not more than 6 cm.
4. Technique: aspirate until blood freely appears, ensure the bevel of the needle is now directed caudally, remove the syringe and immediately insert the Seldinger wire, flexible end first, through the needle. Remove the needle, railroad the plastic cannula over the Seldinger wire, then remove the wire. Check that the cannula is in the central vein by briefly allowing retrograde blood flow into the attached intravenous giving set.
5. Aftercare: secure the line with a black silk suture through the skin and dress with sterile dressing. Return the patient to the horizontal position and obtain a chest X-ray to check the position of the central venous cannula and exclude a pneumothorax. Note that absence of a pneumothorax on this film does not exclude the possibility of one developing subsequently, possibly under tension. If there is trauma to only one side of the chest, then use this side for cannulation because there is already a risk of pneumothorax there.

If this direct venous access is not obtained during CPR for immediate drug therapy to the heart muscle, then drugs should be given via a peripheral venous line, with an infusion of 5% dextrose solution running after each drug to flush it into the central circulation. Certain drugs such as adrenaline, atropine, lignocaine and naloxone may be given via the tracheal tube route, in double the intravenous dosage diluted to 10 ml.

Disability

This term is used to signify a brief neurological assessment which must be carried out at this stage of the initial examination. The mnemonic used in the Advanced Trauma Life Support Course is useful:

A = **A**lert
V = responds to **V**erbal stimuli
P = responds to **P**ainful stimuli
U = **U**nresponsive

In addition, now assess the presence or absence of orientation in time (knows day and month), space (knows where he is) and person (knows who he is). These perceptions are usually lost in this sequence with lessening of consciousness. Defer delineation of the Glasgow Coma Scale until a more detailed head-to-toe examination can be carried out after the initial assessment is completed and resuscitation is underway.

Record the pupil size and response to light (Table 2.1).

Bilateral small pupils denote opiate poisoning unless disproved by failure of naloxone to reverse the constriction. If necessary, up to 2 mg of naloxone (i.e. five vials of 0.4 mg) are given.

If there is a response, more may have to be given because it has a short half-life; it may be given via an endotracheal tube if you do not have intravenous access. The other common cause of bilateral small pupils is a pontine haemorrhage, for which there is no specific treatment.

Exposure

In a severely traumatized patient always carry out a complete examination of all the skin. This necessitates the removal of every scrap of clothing, being careful to protect the spine. Full examination includes log-rolling with a minimum of four trained personnel to examine the back. Perform this earlier if there is a specific indication (e.g. trauma to the posterior chest wall) or at the latest at the end of the secondary survey.

Consider inserting a nasogastric tube or, if there is a suspicion of a cribriform plate fracture, an orogastric tube. Insert a urinary catheter after inspecting the perineum for bruising, and carrying out a rectal examination in an injured patient (see Ch. 3).

Table 2.1   Pupil size and response to light in comatose patients

	One pupil	Both pupils

Dilated	Atropine in eye
	3rd nerve lesion normal
	consensual light reflex, e.g. posterior communicating artery aneurysm
	Enlarging mass lesion above the tentorium, causing a pressure cone
	
	Optic nerve lesion:
	Old: pale disc and afferent pupil
	New: afferent pupil with normal disc, loss of direct light reflex, loss of consensual reflex in other eye – both constrict with light in other eye
		Cerebral anoxia
		Very poor outlook if increasing supratentorial pressure – if dilated pupils preceded by unilateral dilation or if due to diffuse cerebral damage
		
		Overdose: e.g. amphetamines
		                carbon monoxide
		                phenothiazines
		                cocaine
		                glutethimide
		                antidepressants
		Hypothermia

Constricted	Pilocarpine in eye Horner's, e.g. brachial plexus lesion Acute stroke uncommonly (brain stem occlusion or carotid artery ischaemia: small pupil opposite side to weakness)	Pilocarpine in both eyes (glaucoma treatment) Opiates, organophosphate insecticides and trichloroethanol (chloral) Pontine haemorrhage or ischaemia (brisk tendon reflexes, and temperature increased: poor prognostic sign)

If pupils normal in size, and reacting to light, consider metabolic, systemic non-cerebral causes
(N.B. Normal pupils do not exclude an overdose)

PART 2: MONITORING

Throughout this initial assessment, resuscitation proceeds with constant ongoing monitoring of vital signs and simple clinical measurements. You must constantly tailor your resuscitation according to results of your monitoring and keep an open mind to possible diagnoses and, therefore, appropriate treatment.

Pulse

Remember that in an elderly or even middle-aged person a rate of more than 140 per minute is very unlikely to be sinus tachycardia as this is too fast for someone of that age. Atria flutter runs at around 300 beats per minute, and therefore if there is 2–1 atrioventricular block the ventricular rate is 150 per minute. The rate of supraventricular tachycardia is usually 160–220 beats per minute.

Respiratory rate

The importance of this is all too easily forgotten. The normal range is 12–20 breaths per minute. It rises early with blood loss or hypoxia, and as well as being a very useful indication of the patient's clinical state it is one of the physiological parameters that is mandatory for the calculation of the Revised Trauma Score.

Blood pressure

With hypovolaemia this drops when the blood loss is greater than 1500–2000 ml. Fit young adults, and especially children, maintain their blood pressure resiliently, but then it falls precipitously when compensatory mechanisms are overwhelmed.

Pulse pressure

This is the difference between systolic pressure and diastolic pressure. Initially, with haemorrhage the diastolic pressure rises due to vasoconstriction from circulating catecholamines, while the systolic stays constant. Therefore the pulse pressure decreases. This is followed by a greater decrease in the pulse pressure as the systolic blood pressure falls once 30% of the patient's blood volume has been lost.

Capillary refill time

This is the time it takes for blood to return to a compressed nail bed on release of pressure – the time can be longer because of hypothermia, peripheral micro-vascular disease and collagen diseases as well as in hypovolaemia. The normal value is 2 seconds, but this time increases early in shock, following a 15% loss of blood volume.

Temperature

Quite apart from primary hypothermia, in a hypovolaemic patient a decreased temperature is an indication of the degree of blood loss. Blood volume must be restored adequately, because if the hypovolaemic patient is simply warmed the blood pressure falls further by virtue of the resulting vasodilation. The patient with primary hypothermia is usually hypovolaemic as well, which is why rapid rewarming results in a drop in blood pressure unless blood volume is replaced. Every resuscitation room should have a warming cabinet so that intravenous fluid can be immediately infused at 37°C to the hypovolaemic or hypothermic patient.

Urinary output

The minimal normal obligatory output is 30 ml h^{-1}. In a child it is easily remembered as 1 ml kg^{-1} h^{-1}.

Central venous pressure (CVP)

This is measured in centimetres of water by positioning the manometer on a stand such that the zero point is level with the patient's right atrium. The normal pressure is around 5 cmH$_2$O from the angle of Louis, with the patient at 45° to the horizontal.

With a normally functioning heart the measurement of CVP is an indirect indicator of the preload to the left ventricle (left ventricular end-diastolic pressure, LVEDP) or the state of filling of the systemic circulation. It does not give a direct measurement of LVEDP.

The CVP is low if the patient is hypovolaemic, and rises to normal with correction. The CVP is raised if the circulating volume is too large, as might happen with renal failure or with overtransfusion. Overtransfusion not only precipitates heart failure, but in a patient with a head injury the resultant rise in intracranial pressure may cause irreversible damage to the already bruised brain. Monitoring the CVP in these circumstances is therefore crucial.

The CVP also rises if the right side of the heart is malfunctioning. The CVP cannot then be used as an indication of the filling of the systemic circulation. It may be raised for mechanical reasons such as a tension pneumothorax or cardiac tamponade. It is raised in the presence of pulmonary embolism, or when the heart is

Table 2.2 Production and elimination of hydrogen ions

Class		Daily production (mol)	Source	Excreted in breath	Metabolic removal possible	Normal organ of elimination
I	CO_2	15	Tissue respiration	+	−	Lungs
II	*Organic acids and urea synthesis*					
	Lactic	1.2	Muscle, brain erythrocytes, skin, etc.	−	+	Liver (50%), kidneys, heart Many tissues (not liver)
	Hydroxybutyric and acetoacetic	0.6*	Liver	−	+	
	Fatty free acids (FFA)	0.7	Adipose tissue	−	+	Most tissues
	H^+ generated during urea synthesis	1.1†	Liver	−	+	Most tissues (see text), small fraction in urine
III	*'Fixed acids'* Sulphuric	0.1	Dietary sulphur-containing amino acids	−	−	Urinary excretion (partly)
	Phosphoric		Organic phosphate metabolism			

The daily production rates for the organic acids are calculated from results obtained in resting 70 kg man after an overnight fast, and are proportioned up to 24-hour values.
*Because of ingestion of food during daytime and consequent suppression of FFA and ketone body production, the values for these acids may be considerable overestimates.
†On 100 g protein diet.

failing for lack of muscular power due to contusion or infarction.

Arterial blood gases

Normal values for P_aO_2 and P_aCO_2 are described above (see Breathing – Management). Arterial blood pH is normally between 7.36 and 7.42. This is dependent upon the arterial PCO_2 being 4.7–5.7 kPa and the plasma bicarbonate being 24–30 mmol l^{-1}. Carbon dioxide is the largest generator of H^+ ions, ten times more than the production from lactic and other organic acid production or from urea synthesis (Table 2.2).

Patients in early hypovolaemic shock have a respiratory alkalosis due to tachypnoea. Respiratory alkalosis gives way to a mild metabolic acidosis which then becomes more severe if the inadequate organ perfusion is not successfully treated.

Most acid–base abnormalities are the result of an imbalance between the production and removal of H^+ ions, as demonstrated in Table 2.2. When the primary disturbance is due to abnormal carbon dioxide elimination it is respiratory, while all other primary disturbance – classes II and III – are termed metabolic. Interpretation of pH results may be facilitated by an acid–base diagram with pH on the y axis and PCO_2 on the x axis, as in Figure 2.2. The bands shown demonstrate the expected response to uncomplicated disorders of acid–base balance.

The central shaded area shows the normal limits. Thus the patient with uncomplicated metabolic acidosis has values above and to the left of the shaded area, while the patient with uncomplicated respiratory acidosis lies in the band above and to the right. A patient with a result in sector A or C probably has a combination of two primary conditions, while one in sectors B or D would be the result of compensation of a primary abnormality. The diagram facilitates the plotting of response to treatment.

Treatment with sodium bicarbonate has in the past been overenthusiastic and there are definite hazards in its uses (see Table 2.3). It is now recognized that bicarbonate should not be given during the first 15 minutes of a cardiac arrest in a previously healthy patient. The principal method of controlling acid–base status during a cardiorespiratory arrest is adequate ventilation. At 15 minutes give either 50 ml of 8.4% sodium bicarbonate (1 ml = 1 mmol) or calculate the amount of bicarbonate needed to correct the metabolic acidosis from the blood gas result. Multiply the base deficit by the estimated extracellular volume, i.e. divide the product of the patient's weight in kilograms and their base deficit by 3.

Table 2.3   Hazards of bicarbonate therapy

1. Inactivates simultaneously administered catecholamines
2. Shifts the oxyhaemoglobin dissociation curve to the left, inhibiting the release of oxygen to the tissues
3. Exacerbates central venous acidosis and may, by production of carbon dioxide, produce a paradoxical acidosis
4. Induces hypernatraemia, hyperosmolarity and an extracellular alkalosis; the latter causes an acute intracellular shift of potassium and a decreased plasma ionized calcium

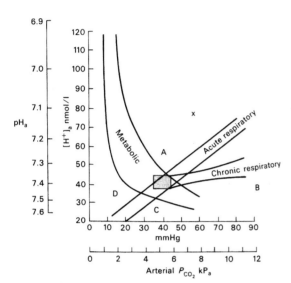

Fig. 2.2   Blood gases. Reproduced from Cohen & Woods (1987), with permission.

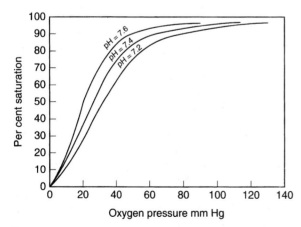

Fig. 2.3   Effect of pH on the oxyhaemoglobin dissociation curve of human blood at 38°C. From Roughton (1964).

Base deficit is defined as the millimoles of alkali required to restore the pH of 1 litre of the patient's blood to normal at P_{CO_2} = 5.33 kPa. In practice, the initial amount to be given should seldom exceed 1 mmol kg^{-1}. In the traumatized patient, what is of paramount importance, in addition to ventilation, is restoration of blood volume.

Acidosis increases ease of unloading oxygen from the blood into tissues ('Bohr effect' of pH on the oxygen dissociation curve (Fig. 2.3)). Increasing temperature and increasing partial pressure of carbon dioxide have the same effect, the latter not just because of an associated acidosis but also because carbon dioxide combines directly with haemoglobin to form carbamino compounds.

In summary, in cardiac arrest a lowered pH is desirable provided that it does not fall below 7.2. Below this, further acidosis lowers the threshold of the heart to ventricular fibrillation and inhibits normal cell metabolism, and should therefore be corrected.

Blood sugar

Order an immediate blood glucose estimation using a reagent strip on every patient who has an altered level of consciousness, otherwise hypoglycaemia will be missed. This is followed by a laboratory estimation.

PART 3: THE SECONDARY SURVEY: DETERMINING THE CAUSE OF THE PATIENT'S COLLAPSE

After carrying out the initial assessment (primary survey) and resuscitation of a collapsed patient presenting to the A&E department with no history, a deceptively incomplete history or, worse, an incorrect history, you must now go on to make a full head-to-toe examination. This is the secondary survey, during which you aim to gain a clearer picture of the cause of the patient's collapse. Ensure that there is no occult injury. Examine all the skin, including the mouth and throat, the external auditory meati and the perineum. Always remember the possibility of non-accidental injury in children, and in the elderly. Consider all the forensic possibilities, noting needle marks, pressure blisters and the presence of any visible soft tissue injuries. Remember that bruising may appear at a distance from the site of injury.

You must:

1. Keep an open mind to all diagnostic possibilities while both collecting the clinical evidence and monitoring the response of the vital signs to treatment.

2. Actively consider the common causes of collapse. This is especially important when there is a problem of communication, perhaps because of language, or when obvious initial clinical signs deflect you from finding the hidden life-threatening pathology. An example is a patient found by the police smelling of alcohol but developing an acute intracranial haematoma after a relatively trivial head injury. Beware!

It is wise to leave on the cervical collar in all trauma patients while they are in the resuscitation room. This is mandatory for all patients who have evidence of trauma above the level of the clavicle and have any decrease in their level of consciousness, whether it be from the trauma itself or from drugs, especially alcohol.

A synopsis of the main causes of collapse is best considered under systems in order that sins of omission are not committed in the frenetic atmosphere of the resuscitation room of the A&E department (Table 2.4). The synopsis is not comprehensive, but does include the common causes, together with less common causes that are easily missed, with dire consequences for the patient (Table 2.5).

If the gag reflex is depressed the patient cannot protect his own airway. Provided he is breathing spontaneously, place the patient in the recovery position on his side (ensure first there is no evidence whatever of a spinal injury). Otherwise intubate the trachea in order to protect the lungs. This applies if the patient is to receive gastric lavage and cannot protect his own airway with complete certainty. If gastric contents are aspirated into the lungs they must be promptly sucked out because they produce a chemical pneumonitis and bacterial pneumonia. The clinical picture may well develop into adult respiratory distress syndrome.

Rhabdomyolysis and myoglobinuria may develop in any comatose patient after prolonged tissue pressure and muscle ischaemia, which is then relieved. Local swelling of muscles may be evident and compartment syndromes can develop because of positional obstruction of the circulation. Muscle death starts after 4 hours of complete ischaemia.

Look for the early symptoms and signs of pain and paraesthesiae in a pallid, cool weak limb. Passively extend the fingers or flex the foot to test for a developing compartment syndrome (anterior tibial compartment

syndrome is the commonest). Losses of distal pulses, numbness, paralysis and development of a flexion contracture are all late signs.

With myoglobinuria ensure that the urinary output is maintained at over 100 ml h^{-1} in an adult, or 2 ml kg^{-1} h^{-1} in a child. Alkalinization of the urine increases the excretion of myoglobin, and will help prevent renal failure.

The basics of how to read arterial blood gases

1. pH (normal range 7.35–7.45)

Does the patient have an acidosis, alkalosis or neither?

2. P_aCO_2 (normal range 35–45 mmHg, 4.5–5.5 kPa)

PCO_2 is high: suggests a respiratory acidosis (if pH is low); or a compensated metabolic alkalosis (see below). PCO_2 is low: suggests a respiratory alkalosis (if pH is high); or a compensated metabolic acidosis (see below).

3. Base excess (or deficit) (normal range − 3 to + 3)

High negative value: (e.g. − 10) always means metabolic acidosis. pH will try to normalize as there is normally an attempt to compensate by hyperventilation to reduce P_aCO_2, producing a compensatory 'respiratory alkalosis'. High positive value: (e.g. + 10) always means metabolic alkalosis. Similarly, hypoventilation to increase P_aCO_2 will compensate somewhat to try to normalize the pH.

Chronic respiratory acidosis, with normal pH. Chronic lung disease associated with chronic hypercarbia, results in the kidneys retaining bicarbonate ion, causing an increase in plasma bicarbonate concentration and a normalizing of blood pH, despite the hypercarbia (metabolic compensation). These changes take several days to occur, but will identify those patients who normally run high P_aCO_2 levels, and not those with just acute changes.

4. P_aO_2 and oxygen saturation

The partial pressure of oxygen in the arterial blood (also called the *oxygen tension*) is that pressure which oxygen gas would produce if it was in a gaseous phase (e.g. if the blood was in a glass vessel with a gaseous phase immediately above it). Gases move down pressure gradients, and so oxygen in the body will always move from an area of higher partial pressure to an area of lower pressure (e.g. from lung alveoli to mixed venous blood

Table 2.4 Synopsis of causes of collapse to be considered during secondary survey

System	Diagnosis	Notes
Respiratory	Upper airway obstruction	Inhaled foreign body (try Heimlich manoeuvre)
		Infection such as epiglottitis (occurs in adults although commoner in children)
		Call help urgently
		Trauma including respiratory burns
	Ventilatory failure	Asthma
		Chest trauma such as sucking open wound
		Paralysis such as in Guillain–Barré syndrome
	Failure of alveolar gas exchange	Pneumonia
		Pulmonary contusions
		Cardiogenic pulmonary oedema
		Adult respiratory distress syndrome
	Tension pneumothorax	From trauma (including iatrogenic)
		ruptured emphysematous bulla
Cardiac	Ventricular fibrillation	Follow Resuscitation Council (UK) guidelines for treatment of
	Asystole	cardiac arrest
	Electromechanical dissociation	Look for treatable cause: tension pneumothorax, cardiac tamponade, hypoxia or hypovolaemia, drug overdose
	Cardiogenic shock or failure	Acute myocardial infarct
		Arrhythmia
		Pulmonary embolism
		Cardiac contusions after blunt chest trauma
		Valve rupture
Vascular	Hypovolaemic shock	Revealed or concealed haemorrhage
		Diarrhoea and vomiting
		Fistulae
		Heat exhaustion
	Anaphylactic shock	From stings and bites, drugs or iodine-containing contrast used for radiological investigation
	Dissecting thoracic aorta	Usually in previously hypertensive patients, pain radiates to back
	Leaking abdominal aortic aneurysm	Always check femoral pulses so that you consider aortic pathology (although pulses may not be lost)
	Septic shock	Initially massive peripheral vasodilation: 'warm shock'. Temperature may be normal
	Neurogenic shock	From loss of sympathetic vascular tone in cervical or high thoracic spinal cord injury
Gastrointestinal	Haemorrhage	
	Perforated peptic ulcer	
	Pancreatitis	Always check serum amylase
	Mesenteric embolism	Abdominal signs may be absent initially
Gynaecological	Ruptured ectopic pregnancy	Usually at 4–6 weeks' gestation. Always think of diagnosis in collapsed young woman
Obstetric	Supine hypotension	The gravid uterus obstructs venous return from the vena cava unless the pregnant woman is turned onto her left side
	Eclampsia	
	Pulmonary embolism	
	Amniotic fluid embolism	
Neurological	Head injury	Isolated head injuries do not cause shock in adults. Look for sites of blood loss elsewhere
	Infection	Meningitis in children (often meningococcal in UK), tetanus, botulism, poliomyelitis, rabies
	Cerebrovascular	Intracranial embolism or haemorrhage
		Subarachnoid haemorrhage may present solely as a severe headache
	Epilepsy	Including the postictal state
	Poisoning	see Table 2.5
Haematological	Sickle cell crisis	May lead to respiratory failure
	Malaria	Cerebral malaria causes coma
	Coagulopathy	Thrombocytopenia may present with bleeding

Table 2.4   *(contd)*

System	Diagnosis	Notes
Metabolic	Hypoglycaemia	Check blood glucose in *every* patient
	Hyperglycaemia	Coma may be first presentation of diabetes melitus
	Hyponatraemia	May be Addisonian crisis
	Hypocalcaemia	May present with fits
	Hepatic failure	Precipitated by paracetamol overdose in previously fit people, and by intestinal haemorrhage, drugs, or high-protein diet in those with chronic liver disease
	Renal failure	Pre-renal from dehydration
		Renal, e.g. from crush syndrome and myoglobinuria
		Post-renal from ureteric obstruction (dangerous hyperkalaemia causes tall tented T waves and widening of the QRS complexes)
	Hypothermia	Resuscitation may include passive or active core rewarming
		Sepsis and hypovolaemia often coexist
Endocrine	Addisonian crisis	Give 200 mg hydrocortisone i.v. (hypotension, low serum sodium, raised serum potassium)
	Myxoedemia	Always consider in hypothermic patients

Table 2.5   Common drugs and poisons

Drug	Symptoms and signs	Treatment
Paracetamol	Liver and renal failure, hypoglycaemia May be asymptomatic initially	Lavage charcoal or methionine Acetylcysteine
Salicylates	Tinnitus, abdominal pain Vomiting, hypoglycaemia, hyperthermia, sweating Acid–base disturbances	Lavage and charcoal Rehydration Diuresis
Tricyclic antidepressants	Arrhythmias and hypotension Dilated pupils, convulsions Coma	Lavage and charcoal Cardiopulmonary support
Benzodiazepines	Respiratory depression	Flumazenil if acute iatrogenic
Opiates	Pinpoint pupils Loss of consciousness Respiratory depression Needle marks	Naloxone
Phenothiazines	Dyskinesia, torticollis	Procyclidine
Lignocaine	Tingling tongue Perioral paraesthesia Ventricular fibrillation Convulsions	Cardiopulmonary support Diazepam
Carbon monoxide	33% of fatal poisoning in UK insidious from inefficient gas fires Nausea and vomiting Headache, drowsiness Hallucinations, convulsions	100% or hyperbaric oxygen
Cyanide	Headache, vomiting, weakness Tachypnoea, convulsions Coma	Dicobalt edetate
Iron	Hypotension, vasodilatation Gastric haemorrhage	Lavage Desferrioxamine
Organophosphates (pesticides, nerve gases)	Nausea, vomiting, diarrhoea Salivation, pulmonary oedema Pinpoint pupils, convulsions, coma	Lavage Atropine

in the pulmonary artery). The P_aO_2 gives some idea of the amount of oxygen reaching the arterial blood from the lungs, or if there is some dilution with venous blood (shunting).

Oxygen saturation is that amount of the haemoglobin concentration which is bound to oxygen, expressed as a percentage. Oxygen carriage is dependent on haemoglobin and it is the haemoglobin-bound oxygen that is the main supply for the tissues. The amount of oxygen in solution in the blood is tiny, only becoming significant at ambient pressures which are multiples of atmospheric pressure. This is demonstrated in the oxygen flux equation, which gives the amount of oxygen flowing to the tissues per minute:

$$O_2 \text{ Flux} = CO \: [(S_aO_2 \times Hb \times 1.34) + F]$$

where CO is the cardiac output, S_aO_2 is the arterial oxygen saturation, 1.34 is Hoeffner's constant (the amount of oxygen that is capable of combining to Hb) and F is the small amount of oxygen dissolved in the blood. The values are converted to give ml/minute: normal oxygen flux is 1000 ml/min; the minimum flux compatible with life is 400 ml/min.

Oxygen saturation is now routinely measured non-invasively by shining several infra-red wavelengths of light across a finger or nose or other piece of skin. A sensor detects those waves not absorbed by haemoglobin. Oxyhaemoglobin and deoxyhaemoglobin have different infra-red absorption spectra, and so the machine can calculate the mean oxygen saturation of blood reaching the part with each pulse, compensating for tissue absorption by an algorithm.

The relationship between Po_2 and So_2 is shown in the oxygen dissociation curve (Fig. 2.3). Note how the curve becomes steep below 90% saturation – the situation that many patients with lung disease are in.

This curve is calculated for HbA, with normal characteristics. Other haemoglobins produce curves in different positions – e.g. sickle cell anaemia shows a marked shift to the right, and fetal haemoglobin is shifted to the left.

CONCLUSION

Patients are often brought into the resuscitation room in a physical condition which is very alarming to the inexperienced trainee. Unless the patient is rapidly transported to the operating theatre, adhere to the methodical sequence of Primary Survey with Initial Resuscitation (see Part 1), Monitoring (see Part 2), Secondary Survey (see Part 3) while the patient is in the resuscitation room of the A&E department. By having a known sequence of procedures to go through you and the nurse

will gain confidence as the resuscitation continues, and you will not miss pathology. The patient then has the best chance of survival and also the least chance of morbidity.

Keep an open mind as to the cause of the clinical signs. Monitor the vital signs and level of consciousness, and do not jump to preconceived conclusions – this is all too easy to do under pressure. If there is any clinical deterioration return to the basic initial sequence of the primary survey and recheck AIRWAY, BREATHING, CIRCULATION yet again.

Do not allow the patient to leave the A&E department without stable vital signs, appropriate intravenous lines in place, and having been thoroughly examined, unless there is an acceptable reason. A patient may all too easily deteriorate clinically in the X-ray room or, even more dangerously by reasons of secluded space, in the computed tomography (CT) scanner.

Patients with a diminished level of consciousness must be seen by an anaesthetist, at the very latest before they leave the A&E department. Patients must be in the best possible clinically supported condition for transportation, whether their journey is to the CT scanner, a ward or to another hospital. If necessary the patient must be ventilated, depending on the length of journey and vehicle employed, and must be accompanied by appropriate attendants such as an anaesthetist.

Strictly adhere to standard guidelines for protection of medical and nursing staff from contamination with body fluids: wear gloves, waterproof gowns and masks with visors. Staff must be immunized against hepatitis B virus.

Keep clear, precise medical records of any resuscitation sequence, remembering that from 1 November 1991 patients or their relatives have the legal right to see medical records. This record keeping is the responsibility of the senior doctor present. Take appropriate care with forensic evidence, especially from terrorist incidents – anything removed from victims must be removed by a named person and be handed to a named person who personally seals the item in a labelled bag.

There must be at the very least a doctor of registrar grade in command of the resuscitation team. For an A&E department to receive patients who need immediate resuscitation from a 'blue-light' ambulance, the hospital must have a minimum of an anaesthetic registrar, medical registrar and surgical registrar 'living in' on site 24 hours a day. Even if the patient does not survive you will be able to tell the relatives truthfully that everything possible was done.

Both medical audit and medicolegal considerations dictate the above minimal adequate standards of care.

All doctors who are expected to resuscitate the collapsed patient as part of their work practice are expected to be trained in the above. This is your responsibility, but more especially of the supervising consultant and above all of the employing authority.

FURTHER READING

Advanced Trauma Life Support Course Manual 1993. American College of Surgeons

Cohen R D, Woods H F 1987 Disturbances of acid–base homeostasis. In: Weatherall D J, Ledingham J G G, Warrell D A (eds) Oxford textbook of medicine. Oxford University Press, Oxford, p 9.164–9.175

Don H 1987 Oxygen therapy. In Callam M L (ed) Current therapy in emergency medicine. B C Decker, Philadelphia p 345–348

Evans T R 1995 ABC of resuscitation. British Medical Association, London

Henry J, Volans G 1984 ABC of poisoning. British Medical Association, London

Jones R M 1989 Drug therapy in cardiopulmonary resuscitation. In: Baskett P J F (ed) Cardiopulmonary resuscitation, p 101

Roughton F J W 1964 Transport of oxygen and carbon dioxide. In: Fenn W O, Rahn H (eds) Handbook of physiology, American Physiological Society, Maryland vol 1, p 776

Royal College of Physicians of London 1991 Some aspects of the medical management of casualties of the Gulf War. February

Safar P, Bircher N G 1988 Cardiopulmonary cerebral resuscitation (3rd edn) Saunders, Philadelphia, p 212–219

Skinner D, Driscoll P, Earlam R 1996 ABC of major trauma. British Medical Journal, London

APPENDIX: Chemical Weapons

In the 1990–91 Gulf War it was considered possible that the chemical weapons of nerve gases and mustard gas would be used.

Nerve gases (e.g. Tabun)

These agents are organophosphorus compounds which act by inhibiting the enzyme acetylcholinesterase and therefore prevent the breakdown of acetylcholine at motor endplates. The symptoms and signs are the same as for organophosphorus insecticide poisoning, i.e. overactivity of the parasympathetic system and paralysis of the muscles of respiration. Early treatment involves the reversal of the effects of acetylcholine at muscurinic receptors by atropine, 2 mg being given intravenously every 10–15 minutes in severe poisoning. Management also involves the support of respiration, the reactivation of inhibited acetylcholinesterase by oximes (pralidoxime mesylate) and the suppression of convulsions by diazepam. Pretreatment with pyridostigmine (reversible inhibitor of acetylcholinesterase) protects a proportion of the total quantity of enzyme present against a subsequent attack by nerve gas.

Mustard gas (sulphur mustard)

Exposure to the liquid or vapour produces blistering of the skin and damage to the cornea and conjunctiva. Classically there is an asymptomatic latent period of up to 6 hours, before reddening of the skin, leading to blistering. Burns are initially superficial, and blister fluid does not contain free sulphur mustard.

Eye damage usually resolves over a number of weeks, but treat with saline irrigations, mydriatics, vaseline to prevent sticking of the eyelids, dark glasses and antibiotic drops.

Inhalation produces damage to the upper respiratory tract, with sloughing of the epithelium of the airways and nasal passages. The most severely affected patients need assisted ventilation with oxygen. Absorption leads to depression of the bone marrow and a fall in the white count, with a maximum effect at about 2 weeks' post-exposure.

In the First World War the death rate from mustard gas was 2% of those exposed, resulting from burns, respiratory damage and bone marrow depression.

3. Trauma

P. A. Driscoll   G. C. McMahon

INTRODUCTION

The objectives of this chapter are to:

- Discuss the mechanisms of injury commonly seen in clinical practice
- Revise those aspects of human anatomy important in trauma care
- Discuss the normal and pathophysiological response to trauma
- Describe the optimal organization for the management of the individual trauma victim and how this is altered in the multiple patient situation.

Size and extent of the problem

Trauma, as a major cause of death, is surpassed only by ischaemic heart disease and carcinoma. Indeed, it is the leading cause of death in either sex in people aged 1–35 years. In the UK, approximately 18 000 people die each year, but the USA can boast a figure approximately ten times greater. One-third of these victims are a result of road traffic accidents, and just under a third occur at home.

In addition to these fatalities, trauma also gives rise to a much larger group of people who have been permanently disabled. For every trauma death there are approximately 2–3 victims who are disabled, a proportion of whom will require continuing health-care facilities for life.

In the USA, there are 70 million non-fatal injuries per annum. These patients go on to occupy 12% of all hospital beds in that country. In the UK, 60 000 are annually admitted to hospital following road traffic accidents, and 26 000 from industrial incidents. Financially this costs the British tax payer £2.22 billion per annum, i.e. around 1% of the gross national product (World Health Organization estimation). In the USA, the figure is put at $75–100 billion – approximately equal to one and half times the whole military expenditure on the Gulf War.

Trimodal distribution of death following trauma

The first peak in mortality occurs at, or shortly after, the time of injury. These patients die of major neurological or vascular injury and most are unsalvageable with present-day technology, but 40% could be avoided by various prevention programmes.

The second peak occurs several hours after the injury. These patients commonly die from airway, breathing or circulatory problems and many are potentially treatable. This period is known as the 'golden hour', to emphasize the time following injury when resuscitation and stabilization are critical.

The final peak occurs days or weeks after the injury. These victims die from multiple organ failure (MOF), adult respiratory distress syndrome (ARDS) or overwhelming infection. It is now known that inadequate resuscitation in the immediate or early post-injury period leads to an increased mortality rate during this phase.

MECHANISM OF INJURY

Trauma can be divided into categories depending upon its causative mechanism:

- Blunt
- Penetrating
- Blast
- Burns.

In certain situations, for example following an explosion, a combination of mechanisms occurs. However, over 90% of trauma in the UK is a result of a blunt mechanism.

BLUNT TRAUMA

This mechanism of injury dissipates its force over a wide area, minimizing the energy transfer at any one spot and so reducing tissue damage. In low-energy impacts, the clinical consequences are dependent on the organs involved. In contrast, when high energies are involved, considerable tissue disruption can be produced, irrespective of the underlying organs.

Blunt trauma gives rise to three types of force:

1. *Shearing* results from two forces acting in opposite directions. Skin lacerations and abrasions following this tend to be irregular and have a higher risk of infection. They are also associated with more damage to the surrounding tissue and more excessive scarring than low energy penetrating trauma.

With regard to the abdominal viscera, shearing forces have a maximal effect at the points where the organs are tethered down. Common examples include the peritoneal attachments at the duodenojejunal flexure, the spleen and the ileocaecal junction as well as the vascular attachments of the liver.

2. *Tension* occurs when a force hits a tissue surface at an angle of less than 90°. It gives rise to avulsions and flap formation. Both are associated with more tissue damage and necrosis than that found after a shearing force.

3. *Compression* follows a force hitting a tissue surface at 90° and can result in significant damage and necrosis of the underlying structures. The site of the impact can usually be identified by the presence of contusion, haematoma (if a significant number of blood vessels are damaged), and possibly a breach in the surface tissue. In addition to this direct damage, compression forces may produce a sufficient rise in internal pressure to rupture the outer layer of closed gas or fluid-filled organs such as the bowel.

A combination of these forces frequently contribute to the pattern of injury seen in victims of blunt trauma. Typically multiple injuries occur, with usually one system being severely affected and one to two other areas damaged to a lesser degree. Overall, the UK incidence of life-threatening injuries in different systems is: head 50.2%, chest 21.8%, abdomen 23.9% and spine 8.55%. In excess of 69% of trauma victims also have orthopaedic injuries, but these are not usually life threatening.

Determining how these various forces result in patient injury is complicated. However, an important clue can be gained from members of the emergency services who have had the opportunity to inspect the scene. For example, a frontal impact with a 'bulls-eye' pattern on the windscreen, a collapsed steering column and indentations on the dashboard indicate that the driver of this vehicle may have sustained the following injuries:

- Facial fractures
- Obstructed airway
- Cervical injury
- Cardiac contusion
- Pneumothorax
- Flail chest/fractured ribs
- Liver and/or splenic injury
- Posterior dislocation of the hip
- Acetabular fracture
- Fractured femur
- Patella fracture
- Carpometacarpal injuries
- Tarsometatarsal injuries.

Following a frontal impact, the patient is at risk of sustaining a flexion–distraction type injury to the lumbar vertebrae if only a lap seat belt has been worn. This can produce a Chance fracture in addition to some or all of the injuries listed above. Motorcyclists, pedestrians and victims ejected from a car have a significant risk of multiple injuries, including head, spinal, wrist and lower limb damage.

A completely different pattern of injuries is produced in the patient who has sustained a rapid deceleration injury following a fall from a height onto a solid surface. If the victim lands on his feet, the following injuries could be expected:

- Tarsometatarsal injuries
- Calcaneal compression fractures
- Ankle fracture
- Tibial plateau fractures
- Pelvic vertical shear fracture
- Vertebral wedge fracture
- Cervical injury
- Dissecting thoracic aorta
- Ruptured main bronchi
- Avulsed liver.

Knowing the mechanism of injury will enable the trauma team to look for secondary injuries which may not be immediately apparent (see Ch. 2). It can also give a clue as to the degree of energy-transfer injury and, consequently, the level of tissue damage. Mechanisms that indicate a high energy transfer are:

- Road traffic accident
- Falls from a height
- Crushing.

PENETRATING TRAUMA

The clinical consequences of penetrating trauma are dependent on both energy transfer and local damage.

Energy transfer

Several factors affect the degree of energy transferred to tissues surrounding the track of the weapon or missile:

- The kinetic energy of the weapon or missile
- The mean presenting area of the weapon or missile
- The weapon or missile's tendency to deform and fragment
- Density of the tissues
- Mechanical characteristics of the tissues.

It follows that if the missile has a high velocity (e.g. a rifle bullet), then it will carry a considerable amount of kinetic energy, even though its mass may be small. It is important to realize that the crucial speed is the impact velocity, i.e. the speed of the missile when it hits the patient, not its initial velocity (i.e. the speed of the projectile when it leaves the barrel of the gun). Unlike the bullet, a knife has a much lower kinetic energy, because it is travelling at a much slower speed.

The neighbouring tissues may be injured when the kinetic energy of the missile is transferred to the surrounding structures. If the missile impacts in the tissue and fails to exit, all the kinetic energy will be transferred, and the maximum amount of damage will have been achieved for that particular missile. The chances of this occurring increase considerably if the missile tumbles or fragments once it enters the tissues.

With high energy transfer, neighbouring tissues are pushed away from the missile track and a temporary cavity is created. Although this lasts only a few milliseconds it can reach 30–40 times the diameter of the missile, depending on the amount of energy transferred to these tissues and their elastic properties. As the energy waves dissipate, the tissues rapidly retract to a permanent cavity formed by the immediate destruction of tissue in the direct path of the missile.

This has three consequences. Firstly, there is functional and mechanical disruption of the neighbouring tissues. The extent is related to energy transfer and the tissue characteristics. Solid organs, such as the liver and spleen, sustain more damage than the lungs and other low-density organs such as muscle, skin and blood vessels. These tissues have greater elastic properties, which minimizes the amount of damage they sustain.

Secondly, a core of any clothing that was originally over the skin surface is carried in front of the missile deep into the wound. The higher the velocity of the projectile, the finer the shearing of material and the wider it is spread. Further contamination can be caused by material being sucked into the wound from the negative pressure at the missile's exit site. These grossly contaminated wounds have a high chance of becoming infected.

Thirdly, as a general rule, if a missile traverses a narrow part of the body, then the exit wound is usually larger than the entry one. This is due to the temporary cavitation effect extending along the wound track. Conversely, the temporary cavitation effect would have finished if the missile had given up enough kinetic energy to behave as a low-energy missile before it left the body. Nevertheless, there are no absolute certainties, and variations in the relative sizes of exit and entry wounds are well recognized.

Local damage

An incision, produced by low-energy penetrating trauma (e.g. a stab wound), results in a wound with little oedema and inflammation, which heals quickly and with minimum scarring (see Ch. 32). However, low-energy transfer injuries can still be fatal, for example a stab wound to the heart. Consequently, the significance of a penetrating wound is also dependent upon the type and extent of the organs involved.

BLAST INJURIES

Following the detonation of a bomb, there is a sudden release of considerable energy. Initially, there is an almost instantaneous rise in pressure in the surrounding air known as the *shock front* (or blast wave). This moves through the surrounding air in all directions, faster than the speed of sound. As it spreads out it gets weaker as the distance from the edge of the band to the epicentre of the explosion increases.

Behind the shock front comes the *blast wind* which is movement of the air itself. As the blast wind rapidly spreads out from the epicentre, it carries fragments, either from the bomb or from surroundings debris. In view of the velocity at which they are travelling, many of these fragments can produce 'high energy transfer' wounds.

Bomb blasts can therefore injure people in a variety of ways.

Primary effect

This is a result of the shock front and mainly affects air-containing organs such as the lung, bowel and ears. Once the band of pressure hits the surface of the body it causes distortion, the magnitude and rate of onset of which has a direct effect on the extent of the tissue damage. In particular, the higher the rate, the bigger the pressure wave traversing the body. It is these waves which produce most of the damage associated with 'blast' lung, gut and tympanic membrane, with most of the pathology occurring at the air–tissue boundary. Pathological features of 'blast' lung, gut and tympanic membrane are:

- Haemorrhage into alveolar spaces
- Damage to alveolar septae
- Stripping of bronchial epithelium
- Emphysematous blebs produced on the pleural surface
- Contusion of the gut wall
- Leakage of blood into the gut lumen
- Perforation
- Rupture or congestion of the tympanic membrane.

If these pulmonary changes are extensive, a ventilation-perfusion (V/Q) mismatch will develop and hypoxia will result. High blast pressures may also lead to air emboli and, if they obstruct the cerebral or coronary arteries, sudden death can occur.

Secondary effects

These are the result of the direct impact of fragments carried in the blast wind. In most explosions, the lethal area for these fragments is much greater than that of the shock front. Furthermore, at distances outside this area, they can still produce considerable damage. The patient usually presents with multiple, extensive wounds of varying depth, which are grossly contaminated. As the distance from the epicentre increases, the wounds become more superficial.

Tertiary effects

These are a result of the dynamic force of the wind itself, which can be so great as to carry all or part of the patient along with it. This results in impact (deceleration) injuries and, in extreme cases, avulsive amputations.

In addition to these effects, the patient may also sustain injuries from falling masonry, as well as fires, toxic chemicals and flash burns. Acute and chronic psychological disturbance resulting from explosions are also well recognized.

BURNS

Thermal

These are the most common type of burns and are caused by heat from flames, scalds and contact with hot surfaces or flashes. Children and the elderly are the most frequent victims of scalds, but they are also the most prevalent type of industrial burn.

Chemical

Acids and alkalis release energy in the form of heat when they come into contact with biological tissue. Alkalis produce the most damage because they penetrate into deeper tissues. In contrast, acids react with the tissue surface to produce a barrier which inhibits further penetration.

Electrical

There are several factors that affect the severity of the injury:

- Type of current (AC or DC)
- The voltage of the shock
- Duration of the contact
- Resistance of the tissues
- The pathway in which the current travels.

Although the entrance and exit wounds are treated as thermal wounds, they do not give an accurate indication of the extent of the burn. This is because the electric current will have travelled through the body along the path of least resistance. For example, skin is highly resistant and consequently the current travels preferentially along arteries, veins, nerves, bones and tendons. It follows that the true extent of the tissue damage cannot be measured on superficial inspection.

RELEVANT ANATOMY

In addition to being aware of the mechanism of injury, the clinician should understand how the anatomical relationship of the body can have a profound effect on the type of injuries the patient sustains. Listed below are the more relevant aspects of each body system with regard to trauma. These are dealt with in the order they tend to be managed clinically (see Ch. 2):

- Airway
- Thorax
- Circulation
- Skull
- Face
- Abdomen and genitourinary system
- Bony pelvis
- Limbs
- Spinal column
- Skin.

AIRWAY

The important structures and surface landmarks of the upper airway are shown in Figure 3.1.

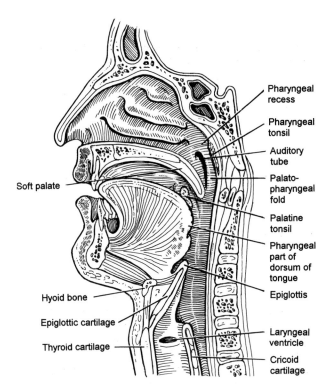

Soft palate

Hyoid bone

Epiglottic cartilage

Thyroid cartilage

Pharyngeal recess

Pharyngeal tonsil

Auditory tube

Palato-pharyngeal fold

Palatine tonsil

Pharyngeal part of dorsum of tongue

Epiglottis

Laryngeal ventricle

Cricoid cartilage

Fig. 3.1 Line diagram of the upper airway.

THORAX

Chest wall

The upper two ribs are extensively protected by the scapula and overlying muscle. Consequently, the patient has to be subjected to a considerable force for these structures to be broken. Therefore, when breaks do occur, there is a high chance of co-existing damage to vital structures such as the thoracic aorta, the main bronchi, the lungs and the spinal cord. It is therefore important that the clinician closely assesses these vital structures if fractures to the first two ribs are discovered during the resuscitation (see Ch. 2).

The lower six ribs overlie the abdominal cavity when the diaphragm is elevated during expiration. Therefore a penetrating wound in this area may perforate the diaphragm and enter the peritoneal cavity as well as causing pulmonary injury. Abdominal visceral involvement following penetrating to the lower chest is as follows:

- Stab wound   15%
- Gun shot wound   46%

Furthermore, fracture of these ribs can be associated with injury to the underlying liver and spleen. It follows

that trauma to this 'midzone' of the trunk may be associated with both abdominal and chest injuries.

A flail segment is when two or more ribs are fractured in two or more places. It also applies to the situation when the clavicle and first rib are similarly affected. In this case paradoxical movement of the chest may be visible on inspection. Nevertheless, in the early stages, the spasm of the chest wall musculature will splint these fractures, and so eliminate this sign. Later, however, the muscles fatigue and paradoxical movement becomes apparent. A flail segment can be a life-threatening condition, particularly if there is an underlying pulmonary contusion which adds to the hypoxia already produced as a result of the impaired ventilation.

As the neurovascular bundle lies underneath the ribs in the subcostal groove, these structure can be torn when ribs are fractured. When there are several fractures and/or significant disruption this can give rise to a massive haemothorax. Other sources for this degree of blood loss include the internal mammary artery and large lacerations of the lung surface which do not stop bleeding once the lung has been re-expanded following the insertion of a chest drain (see Ch. 2).

It is important for the clinician to remember that the pleural cavity and apex of the lung project above the clavicle. Consequently, a pneumothorax or lung injury can occur following penetrating injuries to the lower neck.

Trauma can lead to a one-way valve developing on the lung surface, allowing air into the pleural cavity during inspiration but blocking its escape during expiration. This will give rise to a tension pneumothorax unless the intrapleural pressure is relieved.

Mediastinum

The trachea, oesophagus and major blood vessels lie in close proximity to one another in the mediastinum. Consequently, penetrating injuries in this area may damage one or more of these structures. The surface landmarks of the mediastinum is medial to the nipple line anteriorly, or medial to the medial edges of the scapulae posteriorly.

CIRCULATION

The heart is covered with the tough, inelastic fibrous pericardium. In the healthy state, even a small collection of blood within the pericardium could create a pericardial tamponade, compromising ventricular filling and hence cardiac output. This condition usually follows penetrating trauma of the heart.

Blunt trauma to the heart can give rise to cardiac

contusion which, due to its anatomical location, may be associated with an overlying sternal fracture. This condition can lead to coronary artery occlusion due to a combination of vascular spasm, neighbouring tissue oedema and intimal tearing. As a result of the myocardial ischaemia the patient may develop dysrhythmias, infarction and impaired cardiac performance (see below). Significant blunt trauma can also rupture the chordae tendinae and, therefore, produce mitral or tricuspid incompetence.

The distal part of the arch of the aorta is anchored just inferior to the left subclavian artery. Patients who sustain deceleration injury of over 30 m.p.h. or falls over 30 feet have a significant risk of aortic disruption due to the mobile aortic arch shearing off the fixed descending aorta. In 10% of cases a dissecting thoracic aortic aneurysm results because the escaping blood is contained by the outer (adventitial) layer of the aorta. In the vast majority of cases, however, this outer layer is also breached, and the patient rapidly exsanguinates.

SKULL

The scalp is made up of five layers:

- **S**kin
- Sub**c**utaneous layer
- **A**poneurosis
- **L**oose (areolar) layer
- **P**eriosteum.

(A useful mnemonic to help remember these layers is SCALP.) The subcutaneous layer is very vascular and is divided into loculi by fibrous bands. The areolar layer is much looser and therefore has a greater capacity for expansion. This is the layer where scalp haematomas usually collect. Scalp wounds tend to pout open if the aponeurosis is breached.

The inside of the neurocranium is divided into two levels by a fibrous structure called the tentorium cerebelli (tent). The midbrain passes through the opening in the anterior aspect of this layer and is partially covered on its anterolateral aspects by the corticospinal tract. The oculomotor nerve leaves the anterior aspect of the midbrain and runs forward lying between the free and attached edges of the tent. In the intact state, there is free communication above and below the tentorium as well as between the intracranial and spinal subarachnoid spaces.

Following head trauma, the development of a mass lesion above the tent (e.g. from a haematoma or cerebral oedema) can cause a pressure gradient to develop. If this is unrelieved it can result in one or both medial surfaces of the temporal lobes herniating through the opening in the tent. In so doing, this brain tissue presses on, and damages, structures in this region, namely the oculomotor nerve and motor fibres in the corticospinal tract. This is called *tentorial herniation* and results in a fixed dilated pupil and weakness in the limbs. If the pressure increases further, the medulla and cerebellum are forced downwards into the foramen magnum – a process known as *coning*. This leads to compression of the vital centres, with disturbances of the cardiovascular and respiratory function.

The base of the neurocranium is irregular, with the sphenoid wings and the petrous processes projecting from its surface. Following acceleration and deceleration forces, the brain moves over the base of the skull. Consequently, its inferior surface can be damaged by colliding with these two large projections.

The internal surface of the neurocranium is lined with a thick, hard, fibrous cover called the *dura mater* (Fig. 3.2). Its blood supply is closely adherent to the bone surface and even groove it in places. Consequently these vessels can be torn when forces are applied to the overlying bone. The resulting haematoma collects between the bone and dura and is known as an *extradural haematoma*; 90% of these are associated with a fractured skull. The middle meningeal artery is the vessel most prone to this type of injury and the thin temperoparietal area is the commonest site.

The arachnoid mater is connected to the pia mater, across the cerebrospinal fluid (CSF) filled subarachnoid space, by thin fibrous strands. Running between these strands are bridging veins which carry blood from the brain to the venous sinuses. With age, the brain atrophies

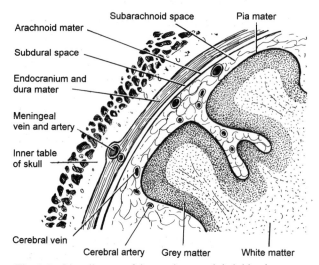

Fig. 3.2 Line diagram of the meninges and their blood supply.

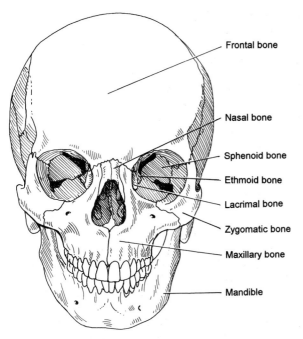

Fig. 3.3 Line diagram of the facial skeleton (individual bones labelled).

Frontal bone
Nasal bone
Sphenoid bone
Ethmoid bone
Lacrimal bone
Zygomatic bone
Maxillary bone
Mandible

and the subarachnoid space increases. This stretches the bridging veins and makes them more likely to tear following a head injury. The bleeding which results collects in the subdural and subarachnoid spaces.

MAXILLOFACIAL SKELETON

This consists of a complex series of mainly aerated bones which provide a firm but light foundation to the face (Fig. 3.3). The nasal, frontal and zygomatic–maxillary buttresses provide vertical support, with lateral stability coming from the zygomatic–temporal buttresses. Several of these bones, especially those making up the bony orbits, are closely associated with nerves and blood vessels which can consequently be damaged when these bones are broken or crushed following trauma. In addition, the associated bleeding and deformity can lead to obstruction of the patient's airway.

Nasoethmoidal–orbital fractures

These occur with trauma to the bridge of the nose or medial orbital wall. In view of their location they are associated with lacrimal injury, dural tears and traumatic telecanthus.

Blowout fractures

When a blunt object hits the globe it can cause the intraorbital pressure to rise such that the thin orbital floor breaks. It is commonly associated with a fracture of the medial orbital wall. The infraorbital nerve is usually damaged in the process, giving rise to infraorbital anaesthesia. Diplopia, especially to upward gaze, is also common and results from a combination of muscle haematoma, third-nerve damage, entrapment of periorbital fat and, in a minority of cases, true entrapment of extraocular muscles. Subcutaneous emphysema occurs if the fracture extends into a sinus or nasal antrum.

Zygomatic complex fractures

Blunt trauma can produce two types of zygomatic fracture. Zygomatic arch fractures are produced by a direct blow and can give rise to an open bite due to the fracture impinging on the temporomandibular joint. The more serious 'tripod' type of fracture involves the displacement of the whole zygoma. Consequently, there is a fractured intraorbital rim, diastasis of the zygomatic–frontal suture and disruption of the zygomatic–frontal junction. This is associated with lateral subconjunctival haemorrhage and infraorbital anaesthesia. In addition, the displacement leads to a downward angulation of the lateral canthus and either trismus or an open bite.

Fractures of the middle third of the facial skeleton

It takes approximately 100 times the force of gravity to break the middle third of the face. Consequently, patients with this condition have significant multisystem trauma in addition to the malocclusion, facial anaesthesia and visual symptoms described above.

Traditionally, the fractures are classified using the Le Fort system (Fig. 3.4). It should be remembered, however, that the grade of fracture is often asymmetrical, i.e. different on the right and left sides. The Le Fort I fracture runs in a transverse plane above the alveolar ridge to the ptergoid region. Le Fort II extends from the nasal bones into the medial orbital wall and crosses the infraorbital rim. Le Fort III detaches the middle third of the facial skeleton from the cranial base; it is therefore commonly associated with fractures of the base of the skull and bloody CSF rhinorrhoea and otorrhoea.

Mandibular fractures

These are the second most common facial fractures after nasal fractures. As with the pelvis, the mandible is a ring

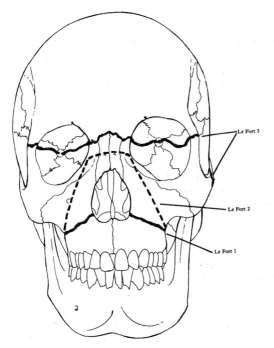

Fig. 3.4 Common sites of fracture of the midface.

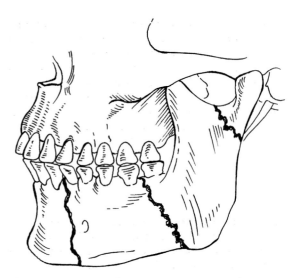

Fig. 3.5 Common sites of fracture of the mandible.

structure and is therefore rarely fractured in isolation. Usually there are multiple fractures or an injury to the temporomandibular joint. Common fracture sites are the condylar process, through the posterior alveolar margin, and through the alveolar margin anterior to the premolar teeth. In both of the latter cases the fracture extends to the lower border of the mandible (Fig. 3.5). Numbness of the lower lip on the affected side and malocclusion are common findings.

ABDOMEN AND GENITOURINARY SYSTEM

The contents of the abdomen occupy the following regions:

- The peritoneal cavity
- The retroperitoneum
- The pelvis.

Peritoneal cavity

This can be subdivided further into intrathoracic and abdominal regions. It is important to remember, however, that on expiration, the diaphragm rises to the level of the 4th intercostal space. As a result, several of the 'peritoneal' organs, such as the liver, spleen and stomach, actually lie within the bony thorax and are therefore at risk of injury if the patient suffers trauma to the lower chest.

Diaphragm

Injury to this structure is uncommon, and may occur as a result of both blunt and penetrating trauma. The former tends to occur with greater force than the latter, and usually leads to larger tears in the diaphragm through which abdominal contents may enter the thorax. Injuries to the diaphragm may be so slight that the patient is asymptomatic and the damage not discovered until weeks, months or even years later. In contrast when the tear in the diaphragm is large, the abdominal contents may herniate into the thoracic cavity, compromising the patient's respiration.

Liver and biliary tree

This is covered over a large part of its surface by the rib cage, which affords it some protection from injury. Although numerically less common than splenic injury, liver injuries account for more deaths as a result of unsuspected intra-abdominal haemorrhage. A high index of suspicion is essential when assessing trauma victims. Therefore, any injury to the right lower chest or upper abdomen should alert you to the possibility of underlying liver damage.

Due to their location, the gallbladder and extrahepatic biliary tract are usually damaged in association with other viscera. Liver trauma is the most common coexisting pathology (50% of cases), but there is a significant chance of the pancreas also being injured (17% of cases). As a consequence of this, the clinical presentation of trauma to the gallbladder and biliary tree is usually masked by symptoms resulting from damage to the surrounding viscera. This condition has an overall mortality of 16% due to coexisting organ injuries. Blunt trauma is the usual cause of gallbladder damage, and rupture is more likely when the gallbladder is distended, such as after a meal and during alcohol intoxication.

Spleen

As the spleen is the most commonly injured solid organ in the abdomen following blunt trauma, it is a frequent cause of shock in patients with abdominal injury. Any injury to the left lower chest or upper abdomen may lead to splenic injury, which can range from small tears to complete shattering of the organ.

Bowel

Injury to the stomach following blunt trauma is rare. However, the stomach is sometimes injured as a result of penetrating trauma, and usually presents as peritonitis. Damage to the small bowel may result from both blunt and penetrating trauma, as well as blast injuries.

Blunt trauma and blasts commonly cause bowel injury in one of three ways. Firstly, the force may squeeze the viscus between the anterior abdominal wall and the vertebral column. Secondly, the bowel may rupture as a result of a sudden increase in pressure within the lumen, such as may occur when the abdomen is compressed (the closed-loop phenomenon). Finally, the bowel may become ischaemic because of damage to the mesentery and its arteries. This usually arises when the abdomen is subjected to deceleration or shearing forces, and is particularly common at points where the bowel crosses the interface between the intra- and retroperitoneum. Examples of the latter include the duodenojejunal flexure and the ileocaecal junction. Blast injuries can also lead to multiple intestinal perforations and areas of infarction.

Penetrating injury to the bowel usually results in small tears in the bowel wall. Occasionally, the bowel may become completely transected.

Unlike injuries to the liver and spleen, trauma to the bowel is rarely immediately life-threatening. As with the stomach, the major problem is peritonitis, which develops over several hours as a result of leakage of bowel contents into the peritoneum.

Retroperitoneum

Injury to organs in this region are much more difficult to diagnose compared with those in the peritoneal cavity. The main reasons for this are that the viscera contained within this region are less accessible to physical examination and investigation.

Pancreas and duodenum

These may be injured as a result of both blunt and penetrating trauma, with the commonest mechanism being that of the unrestrained car driver impacting with the steering wheel.

Bowel

All of the caecum and ascending colon, as well as one- to two-thirds of the circumference of the descending colon lie within the retroperitoneal space. The remainder of the colon is located within the peritoneal cavity. Blunt or penetrating trauma can damage any part of the colon and cause leakage of the bowel contents. However, in cases of retroperitoneal perforation, the symptoms are usually ill-defined and slow to develop. This often leads to delays in diagnosis and increases the chances of abscess formation.

Vascular

The abdominal aorta is susceptible to damage as a result of penetrating injury. Severe trauma is almost invariably lethal, but lesser degrees of injury will manifest as hypotension and/or symptoms of ischaemia. If the haemorrhage is contained within the retroperitoneum then the hypotension may be mild and respond to fluid resuscitation. Later, a retroperitoneal haematoma may be visible as bruising in the flank or back (Grey Turner's sign).

The inferior vena cava (IVC) is susceptible to the same types of injury as the aorta. It can result in significant blood loss but this is usually less than that from an equivalent injury to the aorta because of the lower pressure within the vessel, and the relatively high pressure in the surrounding tissues. However, if this pressure is lost, as occurs in the presence of a large wound, haemorrhage from the IVC is severe and may be life-threatening.

Renal system

The kidneys are well protected by soft tissue in front and bone and muscle behind. As a result, isolated injury to the kidneys is uncommon barring sporting incidents. However, following major penetrating or blunt trauma, significant renal damage is associated with multiple organ injuries. Trauma to the ureters, as a result of either blunt or penetrating injury, is uncommon.

Pelvis

Injuries to the bladder and the posterior urethra are the most frequent types of urological trauma seen.

Urinary system

The bladder lies within the pelvis, but remember that, when full, it may extend as high as the umbilicus. This means that it is susceptible to injury following trauma to the lower abdomen. Injury to the bladder may follow compression of the abdomen, thus increasing intra-vesical pressure. More commonly, it is damaged as a result of penetrating injury from fragments of bone produced when the pelvis is fractured.

When the bladder is ruptured, the urine leaks into either the peritoneal cavity, causing peritonitis, or into the perineum and surrounding structures. The latter usually produces a less dramatic picture than intra-peritoneal leakage, but it is important to diagnose this condition early, as necrosis of the tissues will follow if it is missed.

The urethra is rarely injured in women, due to its short length. In men, injuries are divided into those above the urogenital diaphragm (posterior) and those below (anterior). This level is indicated by the sphincter urethrae. Posterior urethral injury usually arises as a result of pelvic fracture, and is therefore often associated with injuries to other body regions. Anterior urethral injury occurs as a result of blunt trauma to the perineum (e.g. falling astride a beam) and therefore is usually an isolated injury. If the rupture is complete, the patient will be unable to pass urine. In contrast, a lesser injury, such as a submucosal haematoma, will make micturition slow and painful, but possible.

Bowel and reproductive system

The pelvis also contains the rectum and the female reproductive organs. In addition to perforation from bony pelvic fragments following trauma, injuries to the rectum are similar to those described for the colon and bowel above. Injuries to the uterus are uncommon but can result from both blunt and penetrating trauma. Due to the increase in size, the chances of damage from either mechanism is increased during pregnancy.

Abdominal wall

In the fit, athletic individual this forms a firm muscular layer which can offer considerable protection from blunt trauma. The level of protection is much less in children and those with poor muscle development. Rupture of anterior abdominal muscles can occur spontaneously, for example following vigorous exercise or coughing. More commonly, however, these muscles are torn by compression from a seat belt in a deceleration injury. When this force is sufficient to produce an imprint of the overlying clothes and seat belt on the skin, there is a high probability of significant intra-abdominal injury.

Though penetrating trauma can breach the anterior abdominal wall, it may not necessarily cause intra-abdominal injury. The degree of damage sustained is dependent on the nature of the weapon used:

- Stab wound   35%
- Gunshot wound   90%.

Perineum

The penis can be subjected to both blunt and penetrating trauma. Fracture of the penis is rare but does occur following forceful bending of the erect organ. It leads to rupture of one or both corpora cavernosa, resulting in a large subcutaneous haematoma and detumescence.

The testes can be damaged by blunt or, rarely, penetrating trauma. Rupture of the testis following the former is uncommon because of the scrotal position, cremasteric retraction and the frictionless surface of the tunica vaginalis. All these features allow the testis to evade the direct effects of blunt trauma.

BONY PELVIS

The bones of the pelvis can only be separated if the ligaments joining them together are torn. When this occurs, structures which run close to the ligaments, i.e. vessels and nerves, can be damaged. The bleeding which results is usually venous, extraperitoneal and can be life-threatening. An open pelvic fracture is associated with a 50% mortality rate; however, some tamponading effect can be achieved if bones fracture whilst the ligaments remain intact. In these cases the degree of haemorrhage is less severe, and the mortality rate is reduced.

The bony pelvis is usually injured as a result of road traffic accidents or falls from a height. These mechanisms give rise to anteroposterior compression, lateral compression or vertical shear acting on the pelvis either singularly or in combination. They are all capable of producing pelvic instability and haemorrhage because of the vascular and bony damage.

The sciatic nerve lies close to the sacral wing. It is therefore not surprising that in 30% of fractures to this bone there is associated sciatic nerve damage. Similarly, the urethra and bladder are damaged in 20% of cases where there is disruption of the pubic symphysis.

LIMBS

Bone

The size, shape and consistency of bone varies with age. Old bones require less force to break them than young ones because they are more brittle and often osteoporotic. In children, fractures may involve the growth plate (physis), which if not accurately reduced can subsequently lead to deformity.

Bone is a living tissue with a generous blood supply and can bleed profusely after injury. Furthermore, blood loss from adjacent vessels and oedema in the surrounding tissues can be severe enough to cause hypovolaemic shock. The approximate blood loss with some closed fractures is:

- Pelvis   1.0–5.0 litres
- Femur   1.0–2.5 litres
- Tibia   0.5–1.5 litres
- Humerus 0.5–1.5 litres.

These volumes can be much higher if there is an open fracture (see below).

Nerves

In the limbs, nerves tend to lie close to the long bones in neurovascular fascial bundles. This close proximity is particularly noticeable around joints and makes them prone to nerve damage following fractures and dislocations.

Structure and function of a peripheral nerve

The neurons making up a nerve trunk are grouped into fascicles. In the more proximal segments there is considerable crossing over and rearrangement between fascicles, but more distally (below the elbow, for example) the fascicular arrangement is constant and predictable, and corresponds to the eventual motor and cutaneous branches. Some nerves, such as the ulnar nerve, have small numbers of well-defined fascicles; others, such as the median nerve, have large numbers of smaller ones.

Understanding the connective-tissue framework of the nerve is essential for thinking about nerve repair. The outermost layer is the epineurium, the chief charac-teristic of which is mechanical strength. It is usually in a state of longitudinal tension, which is why the ends of a cut nerve spring apart. Each fascicle is surrounded by perineurium; this functions as a blood–nerve barrier and determines the biochemical environment of the nerve tissue. The individual axons are invested in endoneurium, which forms conduits guiding each axon to the appropriate end organ.

The nerve is nourished by an internal longitudinal plexus of vessels, fed at intervals by perforators from the adventitia. This plexus becomes occluded if the nerve is subjected to undue tension, otherwise it can support the nerve trunk even when it has been lifted from its bed over quite a distance. The cell body and axonal parts of the neuron communicate with each other chemically by means of a highly efficient, two-way axoplasmic transport system. This carries transmitter substances centrifugally under normal conditions and structural proteins during regeneration after injury. It also carries, to the cell body, signalling molecules from the end organs or from axons which are damaged. In this way they can influence the nucleus in its control of the cell.

Vessels

Following trauma, the intimal layer may be the only part of a limb artery damaged. This can be very difficult to detect clinically, initially because distal pulses and capillary refill are maintained. Subsequently, the intimal tear can become a focus for both intravascular thrombosis formation and can give rise to distal embolization.

More overt acute signs are only seen if a significant area of the lumen is occluded. When all the layers of the artery are transected transversely, the vessel will go into spasm, due to constriction of the muscle fibres in the media, limiting the degree of blood loss. Conversely, if there is a partial or longitudinal laceration, the muscle spasm tends to keep the hole in the artery open, and blood loss continues.

Veins have little muscle fibre in their walls and therefore cannot contract when they are damaged. Consequently, blood continues to leak from the lumen until direct pressure is applied.

Limb compartments

These are regions in the limbs where skeletal muscle is enclosed by relatively non-compliant fascia. Running through these areas are blood vessels and nerves, the function of which can be affected if intracompartmental pressure rises above capillary pressure. This is most commonly seen in the four compartments around the tibia and fibula. Nevertheless, compartments also occur in the shoulder, forearm, hand, buttocks and thigh, and therefore these can also give rise to the compartment syndrome (see below).

SPINAL COLUMN

The stability of the vertebral column depends mainly on the integrity of a series of ligaments, including the intervertebral discs. Schematically, these can be divided into three vertical complexes. The anterior one consists of the anterior longitudinal ligaments and the anterior half of the intervertebral discs. The middle complex is made up of the posterior longitudinal ligaments and the posterior half of the intervertebral discs. The posterior complex is made up of the remaining intervertebral ligaments and joints, and is structurally the most important. If any two of these complexes are torn the vertebral column becomes unstable.

The spinal cord runs down the spinal canal to the level of the second (adult) or third (baby) lumbar vertebrae. The size of the space around the cord in the canal varies depending on the relative diameters of the spinal cord and spinal canal. In the region of the thorax it is very small because the spinal cord is relatively wide. In contrast, there is a large potential space at the level of C2. Consequently, injuries in this area are not automatically fatal because there is a potential space behind the dens. This has been described in *Steel's rule of three*:

One-third of the spinal canal area of C1 is occupied by the odontoid, one-third by the intervening space and one-third by the spinal canal.

The space in the spinal canal may be reduced in some patients due to spinal stenosis, or the presence of posterior osteophytes. An awareness of this space is therefore important because it controls the body's ability to adapt to injuries which further reduce the size of the spinal canal.

The incidents which commonly lead to spinal injury are:

- Road traffic accident   48%
- Falls   21%
- Violent acts   14%
- Sport   14%
- Other   3%.

Road traffic accidents account for approximately 50% of the spinal injuries in the UK and can result from side, rear or front collision. Ejection from a car increases the chance of a spinal injury to approximately 1 in 13. Rear-end collisions can produce hyperextension of the neck followed by hyperflexion (the 'whiplash phenomenon'). Unprotected victims, such as pedestrians hit by cars or motorcyclists, have a higher chance of sustaining a spinal injury compared to those who remain in the vehicle.

The sporting activities which are infamous for producing spinal trauma are rugby, especially after a collapse of the scrum, gymnastics, trampolining, horse riding, skiing and hang gliding. Diving is a common cause of neck injuries during the spring and summer months, particularly in young males who have recently drunk alcohol. The victim usually misjudges the depth of the water or dives from too steep an angle, hitting his head on a solid surface.

Due to the mechanism of injury, 50% of patients with spinal trauma have injuries elsewhere. In particular, 7–20% have head injuries, 15–20% have chest injuries and around 2.5% have abdominal injuries.

The common feature of all the mechanisms leading to spinal injury is that the vertebral column is subjected to a series of forces. These can act either singularly or in combination to produce flexion, extension, rotation, lateral flexion, compression and distraction. The vertebral column is usually injured at C5/C6/C7 and T12/L1. At these sites flexibility is reduced because the direction of the curve of the spine changes.

SKIN

The principal soft tissue in the body is the skin. With increasing age, there is a decrease in the amount of collagen in the skin and subcutaneous tissues as well as a weakening of the elastic fibres. These changes reduce the tensile strength of skin and thus allow extensive lacerations to develop with minor trauma. Similar effects are seen following long-term steroid use.

PATHOPHYSIOLOGICAL RESPONSE

Injury initiates many well-developed physiological responses. Consequently, clinicians dealing with trauma victims are presented with a combination of physiological changes, some of which are a direct result of the injury and others the body's response to the initial insult. The more important physiological changes are listed and described below:

- The metabolic response to injury
- Adult respiratory distress syndrome (ARDS)
- Shock and cardiovascular pathophysiology
- Coagulopathy
- Multiorgan dysfunction syndrome (MODS)
- Neuropathophysiology
- Spinal injuries
- Fractures
- Peripheral nerve injury

- Compartment syndrome
- Fat emboli
- Wound healing
- Burns.

THE METABOLIC RESPONSE TO INJURY

The response to injury can be usefully divided into three phases: the early, acute *ebb* phase, which is followed by either the *flow* phase if resuscitation and homoeostasis are able to overcome the initial insult, or by *necrobiosis* if treatment fails and death ensues (Fig. 3.6).

After very severe injuries the ebb phase may be short and necrobiosis may have already started by the time the patient reaches the Accident and Emergency (A&E) Department.

The ebb phase

This phase includes the pattern of physiological and metabolic changes associated with the preparation for fight or flight (the defence reaction). On this are the superimposed responses elicited by the hypoxia, tissue damage, nociceptive (from the Latin: *noceo* = to injure) afferent activity and fluid loss from the circulation associated with the injury. Broadly speaking, these changes are related to the severity of the injury.

The ebb phase is characterized by mobilization of energy reserves and changes in cardiovascular reflex activity. The latter corresponds to the clinical state commonly referred to as 'shock' (see below). A link between these factors is the increased activity of the sympathetic nervous system. This is initiated by the appreciation of danger, and is sustained by afferent neural impulses arising from the site of injury and cardiovascular reflexes triggered by reductions in blood pressure and volume. The increase in sympathetic activity is reflected by rises in plasma catecholamine concentrations which are directly related to the severity of injury. In addition, in the ebb phase there is a rapid secretion of hormones from the posterior and anterior pituitary as well as from the adrenal medulla.

Increased sympathetic activity stimulates the breakdown of liver and muscle glycogen leading, either directly or indirectly, to increases in plasma glucose levels. This hyperglycaemia is potentiated by the reduction in glucose utilization by skeletal muscle due to an inhibition (by the raised adrenaline levels) of insulin secretion and the development of intracellular insulin resistance. The mechanism of insulin resistance is unclear, although glucocorticoids may be involved.

The changes in carbohydrate metabolism in the ebb phase can be interpreted as defensive. In addition to providing a fuel for fight or flight, the hyperglycaemia

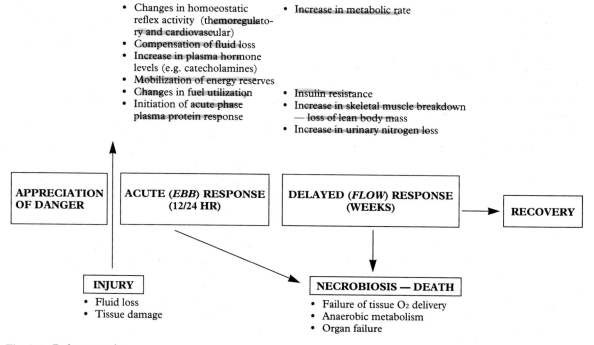

- Changes in homoeostatic reflex activity (themoregulatory and cardiovascular)
- Compensation of fluid loss
- Increase in plasma hormone levels (e.g. catecholamines)
- Mobilization of energy reserves
- Changes in fuel utilization
- Initiation of acute phase plasma protein response

- Increase in metabolic rate

- Insulin resistance
- Increase in skeletal muscle breakdown — loss of lean body mass
- Increase in urinary nitrogen loss

| APPRECIATION OF DANGER | ACUTE (*EBB*) RESPONSE (12/24 HR) | DELAYED (*FLOW*) RESPONSE (WEEKS) | RECOVERY |

INJURY
- Fluid loss
- Tissue damage

NECROBIOSIS — DEATH
- Failure of tissue O$_2$ delivery
- Anaerobic metabolism
- Organ failure

Fig. 3.6 Defence reaction.

may also play a role in the compensation for post-traumatic fluid loss, both through the mobilization of water associated with glycogen and through its osmotic effects. The decrease in glucose clearance associated with the development of insulin resistance can be considered as a mechanism for preventing the wasteful use of the mobilized carbohydrate, which is an essential fuel for the brain and the wound, at a time when the supply of nutrients may be limited.

The increases in sympathetic activity also cause mobilization of fat (triacylglycerol) in adipose tissue. Plasma concentrations of non-esterified fatty acids (NEFAs) and glycerol are raised after accidental injury in man, although the relationship with injury severity is complex. For example, plasma NEFA is lower after severe injuries than after moderate ones; this may be related to metabolic (e.g. stimulation of re-esterification within adipose tissue by the raised plasma lactate levels associated with severe injury) or circulatory (poor perfusion of adipose tissue) factors.

An increase in plasma cortisol, mediated by adrenocorticotrophic hormone (ACTH), occurs rapidly after all forms of injury, although the relationship with severity is, once again, complex. Unexpectedly low cortisol concentrations have been found after severe injuries which cannot be related to a failure of the ACTH response. It has been suggested that an impairment of adrenocortical blood flow in the severely injured is responsible.

The original description of the ebb phase characterized it as a period of depressed metabolism, and there is good evidence for this from experimental studies. The fall in metabolic rate following haemorrhage which is due to a reduction in tissue oxygen delivery can be reversed by transfusion; however, if hypovolaemia is accompanied by tissue damage, transfusion is less effective. It seems that neural impulses, associated with tissue injury ascending to the brain via the spinal cord, cause the release of noradrenaline in the hypothalamus which, in turn, leads to an inhibition of thermoregulatory heat production and, at ambient temperatures below thermoneutral, a fall in oxygen consumption and body temperature.

The evidence for such an inhibition of thermoregulatory heat production shortly after injury in man is, however, not nearly so clear. Indeed, what evidence there is suggests that oxygen consumption is maintained at or, more commonly, above normal levels shortly after injury in man. There is, however, clinical evidence for changes in the control of thermoregulation at this time; for example, severely injured patients do not shiver, despite having body temperatures below the normal threshold for its onset, and the selection of the ambient temperature for thermal comfort is modified.

In addition to modifying thermoregulation, nociceptive stimulation also modifies the cardiovascular response to fluid loss. For example, the heart rate response to simple haemorrhage is an initial tachycardia (mediated by the baroreflex) followed, as the severity of haemorrhage increases, by a bradycardia (mediated by the stimulation of neural afferents arising from the heart). This vagally induced bradycardia can be markedly attenuated, and blood pressure better maintained, if the blood loss is superimposed on a background of nociceptive stimulation. The sensitivity of the baroreflex is itself reduced by injury, although an increase is seen after haemorrhage. This impairment of the baroreflex, which can persist for several weeks after even quite modest injuries (e.g. fracture dislocation of the ankle), means that vasopressors such as vasopressin (ADH) released acutely after injury will be more effective in helping maintain blood pressure than normally, when the baroreflex buffers their pressor effects. This complex interaction between the cardiovascular responses to haemorrhage and injury may not be beneficial, as it has been demonstrated that the ability to tolerate haemorrhage is reduced by concomitant tissue damage. Thus it seems that the better maintenance of blood pressure after haemorrhage and injury is achieved at the expense of intense vasoconstriction in peripheral vascular beds. This may lead to further tissue damage and increase the likelihood of the development of multiple organ failure.

If the magnitude of tissue damage and fluid loss from the circulation is so severe that endogenous homoeostatic mechanisms are overwhelmed and resuscitation is inadequate, the phase of necrobiosis is initiated. This is characterized by a progressive imbalance between oxygen demand and supply in the tissues, leading to a downward spiral of anaerobic metabolism. As a result, irreversible tissue damage is initiated, leading to death. However, if treatment is successful and tissue oxygen delivery maintained, the ebb phase is followed by the flow phase.

The flow phase

The main features of the flow phase are increases in metabolic rate and in urinary nitrogen excretion. These are associated with weight loss and muscle wasting, which reach a maximum at 7–10 days after injury in uncomplicated cases. If sepsis and/or multiple organ failure supervene, this pattern of response may be prolonged for many weeks.

The increase in metabolic rate, which is directly related to the severity of injury, is due to a number of factors, probably the most important of which is an increased sympathetic drive secondary to an upward central resetting of metabolic activity. The wound, whether it is a fracture site or a burned surface, can be considered as an extra organ which is metabolically active and has a circulation which is not under neural control. The wound consumes large amounts of glucose which is converted to lactate; this in turn is carried to the liver, where it is reconverted to glucose. This is an energy-consuming process, which is reflected by an increase in hepatic oxygen consumption. Other factors that might contribute to the hypermetabolism are: increases in cardiac output (needed to sustain a hyperdynamic circulation); the energy cost of the latent heat of evaporation of water from, for example, the surface of the burn; and the energy costs of substrate cycling (metabolic processes which involve the expenditure of energy without any change in the amount of either substrate or product) and increased protein turnover.

Metabolic rates measured in the flow phase seldom exceed 3000–4000 kcal per day (twice normal resting metabolic expenditure), with the highest values noted after major burns. The levels of energy expenditure are often lower than expected and may be close to or even lower than values predicted from standard tables. The explanation for this is that the hypermetabolic stimulus of injury or sepsis is superimposed on a background of inadequate calorie intake, immobility and loss of muscle mass, all of which tend to reduce metabolic rate.

The hypermetabolism of the flow phase is fuelled by increases in the rates of turnover of both fat and glucose. Turnover of NEFAs is raised in relation to their plasma concentration, and the normal suppression of fat oxidation following the administration of exogenous glucose is not seen in these hypermetabolic patients. Both these changes have been attributed to increased sympathetic activity, although plasma catecholamine concentrations are not always increased at this time. The rate of hepatic gluconeogenesis is increased from a number of precursors (e.g. lactate and pyruvate from the wound and muscle, amino acids from muscle protein breakdown, and glycerol from fat mobilization). This increase in hepatic glucose production is not suppressed by the infusion of large quantities of glucose in patients with burns or sepsis. This apparent resistance to the effects of insulin is mirrored by the failure of peripheral glucose utilization to rise to the extent predicted from the raised plasma glucose and insulin concentrations. This insulin resistance in, for example, uninjured skeletal muscle seems to be an intracellular (postreceptor) change.

The balance between whole-body protein synthesis and breakdown is obviously disturbed in the flow phase.

It seems that the changes observed represent the interaction between the degree of injury and the nutritional state: increasing severities of injury cause increasing rates of both synthesis and breakdown, while undernutrition tends to depress synthesis. Thus, increasing nutritional intake ought to move a patient towards nitrogen balance; however, it seems that, despite advances in techniques for administering nutrients and modifications to the type and composition of feeding regimes, no amount of nitrogen is sufficient to produce a positive balance after severe injuries. Nevertheless, the use of anabolic agents, such as growth hormone, and manipulations of ambient temperature may be of advantage as the patient moves from the catabolic flow phase into the anabolic convalescent phase.

A major site of net protein loss is skeletal muscle, both in the injured area as well as distant from it. For example, after moderate injury the patient can lose 2 kg of lean body mass. The loss can be sufficient to compromise mobility, especially in the elderly, whose reserves of muscle mass and strength are already reduced. Although the changes in skeletal muscle are very obvious, the liver is another tissue in which changes in protein synthesis are of particular interest after injury. The liver is the source of the acute-phase reactants (e.g. C-reactive protein, fibrinogen and α_1-antitrypsin) the concentrations of which rise in response to infection, inflammation and trauma.

These metabolic changes, which cannot be attributed to starvation or immobility, can be mimicked to some extent by the infusion of the counterregulatory hormones glucagon, adrenaline and cortisol. However, the plasma concentrations required to elicit relatively modest increases in nitrogen excretion and metabolic rate and induce peripheral insulin resistance are much higher than those found in the flow phase, although they are similar to those noted in the ebb phase. It has been suggested that other factors must be involved, and the cytokines, most probably interleukin-6, released by activated macrophages may play an important role.

RESPIRATORY PATHOPHYSIOLOGY

The main functions of the lungs are oxygen (O_2) uptake and carbon dioxide (CO_2) elimination. To do this air has to get to the alveoli (*ventilation*, V), blood has to reach the pulmonary capillaries (*perfusion*, Q), and O_2 and CO_2 have to cross the gas–blood interface (*diffusion*). Finally, the balance between ventilation and perfusion (V/Q ratio) has to be correct. Impairment of any of these processes, can lead to hypoxaemia and hypercapnoea.

Adult respiratory distress syndrome (ARDS)

ARDS represents an example of a combined ventilatory, perfusion and diffusional pathology and is commonly associated with sepsis and multiple trauma. Although fairly rare in its fully developed state in general Intensive Care Units, the condition has a mortality rate of 50–60%.

The diagnosis is reserved for cases of acute lung injury where there is severe respiratory failure. It produces severe arterial hypoxaemia that is not corrected by conventional oxygen therapy. Pulmonary compliance and functional residual capacity are reduced. These changes result in tachypnoea, dyspnoea, hypoxaemia, cyanosis and increased work of breathing. The chest X-ray (initially normal) shows diffuse bilateral irregular infiltrates in the lung fields and ARDS may be mistaken for pulmonary oedema due to left ventricular failure. Evidence of other organ failure, such as hypotension and oliguria, is also usually present.

The diagnosis of ARDS depends on the presence of the above signs and symptoms along with the presence of an initiating factor (see below).

Aetiology

ARDS may be caused by, or is associated with, the following conditions:

- Direct lung injury due to lung trauma, i.e. blunt injury to the chest, resulting in pulmonary contusion, aspiration of gastric contents, near drowning, inhalation of toxic fumes and thermal injury to the respiratory tract, and bacterial, viral or drug-induced (e.g. bleomycin) pneumonia, radiation injury and oxygen toxicity
- Indirect causes (i.e. the primary insult is remote from the lungs) include sepsis, massive haemorrhage, multiple transfusions, shock from any cause, disseminated intravascular coagulation, massive burns, major and multiple trauma, pre-eclampsia, amniotic fluid embolism, pancreatitis, head injuries and cardio-pulmonary bypass.

The above list is not exhaustive and it has been suggested that any critical illness which leads to inadequate cellular oxygenation can precipitate the syndrome. The chances of developing ARDS increases with the number of risk factors: 25% for one risk factor; 42% for two and 85% for three.

The role of mediators in ARDS

The factors that trigger this syndrome are not fully understood. Clinical conditions associated with ARDS are thought to initiate abnormal behaviour and movement of neutrophils, platelets and monocytes (macrophages), causing the release of a wide variety of enzymes and factors. Neutrophils and platelets also attach themselves to capillary endothelium, damaging it and causing capillary leak. Abnormal macrophages release toxic oxygen radicals and add further to the existing capillary damage, thus causing widespread leakage of fluid into the tissues all over the body.

Despite diverse causative factors, the structural changes in the lungs follow a common pattern. Due to the capillary leak there is oedema of the lung tissue and movement of neutrophils and erythrocytes into the lung parenchyma. The lung lymph flow is increased and there is thickening of the alveolar capillary membrane. This results in impairment of oxygen diffusion and reduced lung compliance, because it is harder to distend an alveolus surrounded by fluid. Some of the fluid in the pulmonary parenchyma may leak into the alveoli, giving the characteristic appearance of a hyaline membrane. In the later stages of the disease, fibrosis may be seen.

Clinical and experimental evidence suggests that generalized capillary leak and defects in peripheral tissue oxygenation lead to other organ failure simultaneously with the lung failure. It is therefore worth remembering that ARDS is merely the pulmonary manifestation of a generalized disease causing failure of multiple organ systems (see below). Management must therefore be wide ranging and applied to the other organ systems as well (Fig. 3.7).

Clinical presentation

Not all patients presenting with sepsis and multiple trauma develop ARDS. The patients who develop ARDS have usually suffered hypoxia and/or hypotension at some stage in the management of their presenting problem. Untreated ARDS passes through four progressively worsening phases.

Phase I. This is the first stage in the development of ARDS and may start 16–24 hours after the onset of the presenting clinical condition. Apart from tachypnoea and tachycardia, no other abnormalities may be present. Chest X-ray at this stage is normal.

Phase II. This phase develops up to 48 hours after the initial insult and 12–24 hours after phase I. The patient appears clinically stable but shows increasing dyspnoea with cyanosis. The skin may appear moist. The effort of breathing is greatly increased and hypoxaemia is

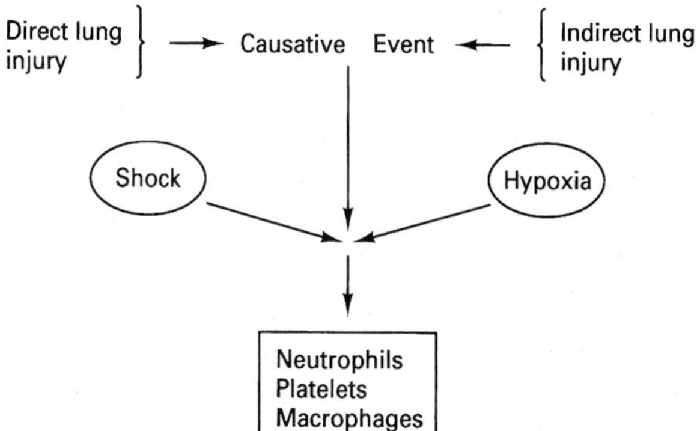

Direct lung injury } → Causative Event ← { Indirect lung injury

Shock   Hypoxia

Neutrophils
Platelets
Macrophages
(all activated)

Mediator release
toxic free radicals

Widespread endothelial damage

Cell destruction and
death

ARDS and multiple organ failure

Fig. 3.7 A simplified flow chart illustrating the development of ARDS.

present despite oxygen therapy. Clinically, only minor chest signs (such as inspiratory ronchi) may be present.

Phase III. This follows phase II and there is now marked tachypnoea and dyspnoea, with increasing involvement of the accessory muscles of respiration. Auscultation of the lung fields reveals high-pitched ronchi. Chest X-ray shows bilateral diffuse pulmonary infiltration. These are often most visible initially in the upper and middle lobes.

Phase IV. This is the terminal phase of ARDS if effective treatment has not been started. The patient shows increasing lethargy and restlessness and may lapse into a coma. There is respiratory and metabolic acidosis with severe hypoxaemia and hypotension. Urine output is usually low (<0.5 ml kg^{-1} h^{-1}). The prognosis at this stage is poor, even if effective treatment is started, as multiple organ failure has already set in.

Therapeutic intervention may alter many of these signs and phases, depending on when the treatment is started. Experience has shown that in phases I and II of ARDS the disease has a better prognosis if treated, as the lungs show only mild to moderate injury. Therefore it must be emphasized that the syndrome should be recognized and treatment started, preferably early in the disease process.

SHOCK AND CARDIOVASCULAR PATHOPHYSIOLOGY

Shock can be defined as inadequate organ perfusion and tissue oxygenation. It is therefore dependent upon pulmonary function (see above), oxygen delivery and release to the tissues and tissue oxygen consumption.

Oxygen delivery

This is governed by level of saturation of haemoglobin with oxygen, the haemoglobin concentration, the cardiac output, systemic vascular resistance and individual organ autoregulation.

The vast majority of oxygen carried in the blood is taken up by the haem molecule, with only a small amount dissolving in the plasma. The relationship between the Po_2 and oxygen uptake by haemoglobin is not linear, because each O_2 molecule added facilitates the uptake of the next O_2 molecule. This is known as the quaternary function of haemoglobin and it gives rise to a sigmoid oxygen association curve (Fig. 3.8). Furthermore, because haemoglobin is virtually fully saturated at a Po_2 of 100 mmHg (i.e. the level found in the normal healthy state), increasing the Po_2 further has little effect on oxygen transport.

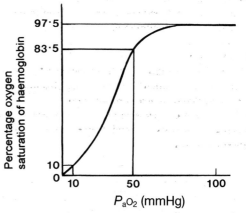

Fig. 3.8 Line diagram of the oxygen dissociation curve. (With permission from Driscoll, P, Gwinnutt, C, Jimmerson, C, Goodall, O, from Trauma Resuscitation: The Team Approach, Macmillan Press Ltd)

The affinity of haemoglobin for oxygen at a particular Po_2 (commonly known as the O_2–Hb association) is also affected by other factors. It is increased (i.e. shifting the curve to the left) by an alkali environment, low Pco_2, low concentrations of 2,3-diphosphoglycerate (2,3-DPG) in the red cells, carbon monoxide (CO) and a fall in temperature.

At first sight, it would seem logical that a greater haemoglobin concentration would allow more oxygen to be carried. However, increasing this leads to an increase in blood viscosity, which impedes blood flow, and so offsets this advantage. This normal haemoglobin concentration (as measured by haematocrit) is usually just above the point at which the oxygen transportation is optimal. Consequently, a slight fall in haemoglobin concentration actually increases oxygen transportation.

Oxygen release to tissue

At the tissue level, the capillary P_aO_2 is approximately 20 mmHg and the cellular Po_2 only 2–3 mmHg. This facilitates the release of oxygen by the haemoglobin molecule to the surrounding tissues. Local factors, such as an increase in P_aco_2, temperature, acidosis and an increase in 2,3-DPG have a similar effect.

Tissue oxygen consumption

In the normal subject, the total consumption of oxygen per minute (Vo_2) is constant throughout a wide range of oxygen delivery (Do_2). The normal Vo_2 for a resting male is 100–160 ml min^{-1} m^{-2} and the normal value of Do_2 in the same person is 500–720 ml min^{-1} m^{-2}. Therefore, tissues are taking up only 20–25% of the oxygen brought to it. This is known as the *oxygen extraction ratio* (OER) and demonstrates that normally there is great potential for the tissues of the body to extract more oxygen from the circulating blood.

Following trauma, both oxygen delivery and consumption can be affected. Tissue damage results in an early increase in consumption, despite the fact that the delivery of oxygen falls because of the reduced blood volume. The increase in consumption is achieved by increasing the extraction of oxygen from the blood. This compensatory response only works if the delivery of oxygen is greater than 300 ml min^{-1} m^{-2}. At levels below this the tissues cannot increase oxygen extraction any further. Oxygen consumption therefore progressively falls because it is now directly dependent on the rate of delivery to the tissues.

Compensatory mechanisms

When a sufficient cell mass has been damaged, the shocked state becomes irreversible and death of the patient is inevitable. Fortunately, the body has several compensatory mechanisms which attempt to maintain adequate oxygen delivery to the essential organs of the body and help prevent this stage being reached.

Circulatory control

Pressure receptors in the heart and baroreceptors in the carotid sinus and aortic arch trigger a reflex sympathetic response via control centres in the brain stem in response to hypovolaemia. The sympathetic discharge stimulates many tissues in the body, including the adrenal medulla, which leads to an increased release of systemic catecholamines, enhancing the effects of direct sympathetic discharge, particularly on the heart. This has the effect of preventing or limiting the fall in cardiac output by positive inotropic and chronotropic effects on the heart and by increasing venous return as a result of venoconstriction. Furthermore, selective arteriolar and precapillary sphincter constriction of non-essential organs (e.g. skin and gut) maintains perfusion of vital organs (e.g. brain and heart). Selective perfusion also leads to a lowering of the hydrostatic pressure in those capillaries serving non-essential organs. This also reduces the diffusion of fluid across the capillary membrane into the interstitial space, thereby decreasing any further loss of intravascular volume. Any reduction in renal blood flow is detected by the juxtaglomerular apparatus in the kidney, which releases renin. This leads to the formation of angiotensin II and aldosterone which, together with antidiuretic hormone released from the pituitary, increase the reabsorption of sodium and water by the kidney (reducing urine volume), which helps maintain the circulating volume. Renin, angiotensin II and ADH can also produce generalized vasoconstriction and so help increase the venous return. In addition, the body attempts to enhance the circulating volume by releasing osmotically active substances from the liver. These increase plasma osmotic pressure, and so cause interstitial fluid to be drawn into the intravascular space.

Oxygen delivery

Although sympathetically induced tachypnoea occurs, it does not produce any increase in oxygen uptake because the haemoglobin in blood passing ventilated alveoli is already fully saturated.

Causes of shock

Reduced venous return

The most common cause of shock in the trauma patient is haemorrhage. This may be occult, as the thorax, abdomen and pelvis have large potential spaces in which blood may collect. Significant haematomas can also develop in potential spaces in the body (e.g. the intrapleural and retroperitoneal spaces), as well as in muscles and tissues around the long-bone fractures. In addition, intravascular volume may be reduced by fractures as a result of leakage of plasma into the interstitial spaces. This can account for up to 25% of the volume of tissue swelling following blunt trauma.

The rate of blood returning to the heart is dependent on the pressure gradient created by the high hydrostatic pressure in the peripheral veins and low hydrostatic pressure in the right atrium of the heart. Any reduction in this gradient (e.g. tension pneumothorax or cardiac tamponade increasing right atrial pressure) will lead to a fall in the venous return to the heart. External compression on the thorax or abdomen can have a similar action in obstructing the venous return.

Cardiogenic

Both ischaemic heart disease and cardiac contusions have negative inotropic effects. Nevertheless, cardiogenic shock does not occur unless greater than 40% of the left ventricular myocardium has died or has been severely damaged. In cardiogenic shock the compensatory sympathetic and catecholamine response only serve to increase the myocardial oxygen demand and further increase the degree of ischaemia.

Certain dysrhythmias on their own significantly reduce cardiac performance. They are usually a result of pre-existing myocardial ischaemia, but can result *de novo* following cardiac contusion. It is also important to be aware all antiarrhythmic agents may have a significant negative inotropic effect and can therefore impede the patient's physiological response to the injury. Cardiac tamponade, in addition to its effect on venous return, also restricts ventricular filling.

Reduction of arterial tone

A spinal injury above T6 will impair the sympathetic nervous system outflow from the spinal cord below this level. As a consequence, both the reflex tachycardia and vasoconstriction responses to hypovolaemia are restricted to a degree proportional to the level of sympathetic block. With high level spinal injuries, generalized vasodilation, bradycardia and loss of temperature control can occur. This is known as *neurogenic shock*; it leads to a reduction in blood supply to the spinal column and so additional nervous tissue damage ensues. Any associated haemorrhage from the injury will aggravate this situation, further reducing spinal blood flow. In addition, these patients are very sensitive to any vagal stimulation. For example, pharyngeal suction can aggravate the bradycardia and lead to cardiac arrest.

In *septic shock*, circulating endotoxins commonly from Gram-negative organisms, produce vasodilation and impair energy utilization at a cellular level. In this type of shock tissue hypoxia can occur even with normal or high oxygen delivery rates because the tissue oxygen demand is extremely high and there is direct impairment of oxygen uptake by the cells. In addition, the capillary walls at the site of infection become leaky due to the endotoxin. Later on this becomes more generalized, allowing sodium and water to move from the interstitial to the intracellular space. With time, this leads to hypovolaemia, and the condition becomes indistinguishable from hypovolaemic shock.

Further cellular damage by endotoxins causes the release of proteolytic enzymes. These paralyse precapillary sphincters, enhance capillary leakage and increase hypovolaemia. The situation is aggravated by the endotoxin acting as a negative inotrope on the myocardium. It follows that in the late stage of sepsis there are several causes of the shock state.

COAGULOPATHY

This is defined as inappropriate intravascular activation of the coagulation and fibrinolytic systems, causing depletion of platelets, coagulation and fibrinolytic factors. It is associated with the formation of platelet-fibrin thrombi in the microvasculature and raised fibrin degradation products in the plasma.

Massive blood transfusion, with resulting dilution of platelets and coagulation factors, and hypothermia are the usual causes of coagulopathy in trauma victims. However, injury and damage to the microvascular endothelium are also common initiating factors. This can be in the presence of either low tissue blood flow (e.g. hypoxia, thromboxanes and leukotrienes) or high tissue blood flow (e.g. endotoxins, cytokines such as tumour necrosis factor, interleukins and free radicals).

By vascular occlusion, coagulopathy can give rise to end-organ ischaemia, infarction and failure. At the same time it can lead to haemorrhage and uncontrolled bleeding at many sites, such as surgical wounds, the pulmonary system, the gastrointestinal tract, and retroperitoneal and intracranial spaces.

MULTIORGAN DYSFUNCTION SYNDROME (MODS)

This is a deadly condition which still carries a mortality rate of around 60%. As its name implies many organs of the body are effected. ARDS (see above) may represent just one part of this syndrome. It is the final common pathway of many disease processes, but with regard to trauma it usually results from prolonged hypoperfusion. Conditions that lead to MODS are:

- Prolonged inadequate perfusion
- Persistent infection
- Persistent inflammatory source (e.g. pancreatitis and dead tissue).

It is suspected that an essential process which occurs in the development of MODS is the adhesion of leukocytes to endothelial cells lining blood vessels. This occurs in virtually all organs of the body, but particularly the lungs, liver and intestine. Three separate families of molecules are involved in this process: selectins, the immunoglobulin superfamily and the integrins. The process leads to the migration of white cells into the interstitial space and the release of proteases and reactive oxygen species. This, in turn, gives rise to a disseminated inflammatory response which presents clinically as MODS.

In managing these patients it is important to realize that the normal relationship between oxygen delivery to tissue (Do_2) and oxygen consumption (Vo_2) is altered. In MODS, partly due to the marked increase in Vo_2, tissues become flow dependent (i.e. reliant upon Do_2). Consequently, any hypovolaemia, pulmonary disease or myocardial dysfunction will jeopardize the delivery of oxygen even further, and so increase the degree of tissue hypoxia and organ dysfunction.

NEUROLOGICAL PATHOPHYSIOLOGY

Head injuries are common. Over 10 million people per year present to A&E departments in the USA after sustaining a head injury. In the UK the figure is approximately 1.4 million, or 11% of all A&E attendances. Of all trauma deaths 50–70% are associated with this type of injury, with 4000 children dying each year in the USA alone, due to the resulting brain damage.

Intracranial pressure (ICP)

As the neurocranium is a rigid box in the adult, the pressure generated inside it, i.e. the ICP, is dependent on the relationship between its volume and its contents. In the normal state the latter consists of the brain, CSF,

blood and blood vessels. Together, these produce an ICP of 5.8–13 mmHg in the horizontal position.

If the ICP is to be kept at normal levels, any increase in the volume of one component must be accompanied by a decrease in either or both of the other components. CSF can be displaced into the spinal system and its absorption increased. The volume of cerebral venous blood within the dural sinuses can also decrease. Furthermore, the brain is a compliant organ, so it can mould to accommodate changes. Once the limit of these compensatory mechanisms is reached, the ICP rises.

Head trauma results not only in mass lesions but also in an increase in the permeability of the intracerebral microvasculature. This leads to interstitial oedema and cerebral swelling, making the brain relatively 'stiff'. Consequently, the brain has less ability to adapt to changes in the intracranial contents. This situation is worsened if ventilation is impaired, as hypoxia produces additional cerebral swelling. Hypercarbia results in vasodilatation of the blood vessels in the uninjured parts of the brain (see below), thereby increasing intracranial pressure.

Alterations in the intracranial contents, including haematoma, not only produce an elevation in the ICP, but also make the brain, CSF and blood less adaptable to any further additions. In this situation, even a small rise in volume of the intracranial contents causes a steep rise in the ICP. Eventually, tentorial herniation occurs, causing pupillary dilatation (III N compression) and motor weakness (corticospinal tract compression). With a further rise in ICP coning occurs and the vital centres are compressed. *Cushing's response* includes:

- Decrease in the respiratory rate
- Decrease in the heart rate
- Increase in the systolic blood pressure
- Increase in the pulse pressure.

Without treatment, pontine compression gives rise to a further deterioration in motor function and bilateral pupillary constriction. In the preterminal situation, pupillary dilatation returns, the heart rate increases, the respiratory rate becomes very slow and irregular and the blood pressure falls. Finally, there is a respiratory arrest from haemorrhage or infarction of the brain stem.

Cerebral perfusion

To supply the brain with oxygenated blood there needs to be adequate ventilation and cerebral perfusion. The ability to carry out the latter is dependent on the mean arterial pressure (MAP), the resistance to blood flow due to the ICP and, to a lesser extent, the central venous pressure (CVP).

In the multiply injured patient, not only is the ICP rising due to the head injury, but also the MAP may be falling because of blood loss from an extracranial trauma. In these situations, therefore, the cerebral perfusion pressure (CPP) is markedly reduced. If the CPP is 50 mmHg or less, cerebral ischaemia will develop. As described above, this leads to additional brain swelling and further rises in ICP as the cycle perpetuates itself. A CPP less than 30 mmHg causes death.

Consciousness

This is dependent on two features: a network of neurons in the midbrain and brain stem, known as the reticular activating system; and both cerebral cortices. If either or both of these features are damaged, then consciousness is lost. Hypercapnia, from any cause, can lead to a reduction in the level of consciousness. Mild hypoxia tends to make the patient restless, and only when it is profound does a fall in consciousness result.

Other important causes of an alteration in the conscious level can be remembered from the mnemonic 'TIPPS on the vowels':

Trauma	Alcohol
Infection	Epilepsy
Poisons	Increase in ICP
Psychiatric	Opiates
Shock	Uraemia/metabolic

Clinically, the level of consciousness is measured from the best eye opening, verbal and motor responses using the Glasgow Coma Scale (G koma = a deep sleep):

Eye opening	Score	Verbal response	Score	Motor response	Score
Spontaneous	4	Orientated	5	Obeys commands	6
To speech	3	Confused	4	Localizes to pain	5
To pain	2	Inappropriate words	3	Withdraws	4
None	1	Inappropriate sounds	2	Flexion to pain	3
		None	1	Extension to pain	2
				None	1

The Scale is an objective measure of the condition and can be used to monitor the patient's progress. The three scores are added; the minimum score is 3 and any score below 8 carries a poor prognosis.

Fractures

Skull fractures usually result from direct trauma and are classified as being linear, depressed or open. The term 'open' is used when there is a direct communication between the brain surface and either the scalp or mucous membrane laceration.

Primary and secondary brain injury

Primary brain injury is the neurological damage produced by the causative event, e.g. the blow to the head. It is now also suspected that progressive primary brain damage may occur subsequently due to endogenous neurochemical changes leading to further cellular injury. Secondary brain injury is the neurological damage produced by subsequent insults such as hypoxia, ischaemia, hypovolaemia, metabolic imbalance, infection and elevations in the ICP.

A purely focal injury can follow a contact force. However, there is usually sufficient associated diffuse brain injury to produce an altered level of consciousness from a temporary disruption of the reticular formation. Furthermore, a space-occupying lesion is often accompanied by a swollen brain due to primary and secondary brain damage. This accelerates the rise in intracranial pressure and the development of additional brain damage. Consequently, the trauma patient invariably has diffuse and specific neurological injuries.

The presenting signs and symptoms from a focal injury depend on the site injured, as different parts of the brain carry out different functions. A focal lesion above the tentorium can produce ipsilateral unilateral herniation of the medial part of the temporal lobes (diffuse brain injuries tend to be bilateral). This produces an ipsilateral fixed dilated pupil in 90% of cases, and contralateral hemiplegia. With further rises in the ICP the brain stem begins to be compressed and the patient develops the signs described previously.

Selective herniation of the cerebellum through the foramen magnum can be produced by an expanding posterior fossa intracranial haematoma. This can lead to a whole collection of presenting signs, the most common being pupil dilatation, respiratory abnormalities, bradycardia, head tilt and cranial nerve palsies. Most alarming is the sudden respiratory arrest due to distal brain stem compression. This is the only cerebral haematoma to do this without a preceding deterioration in conscious level. It is a rare condition but must be considered early on, especially in patients who are found to have an occipital fracture.

Concussion

Concussion occurs when the head has been subjected to minor inertial forces. The patient is always amnesic of the event and there may also be post- and antegrade amnesia. A transient loss of consciousness (usually less than 5 minutes) may occur. On examination, these patients do not have any localizing signs, but there can be nausea, vomiting and headache. Originally it was thought that no organic brain damage occurred in this condition. This has been found not to be the case – microscopic changes occur and, while the net effect of one episode is minor, the effect of more than one episode can be cumulative.

Diffuse axonal injury (DAI)

This is a result of widespread, mainly microscopic, disruption of the brain consisting of axonal damage, microscopic haemorrhages, tears in the brain tissue and interstitial oedema. As a consequence, it can cause prolonged periods of coma (days or weeks) and has an overall mortality rate of 33–50%. Autonomic dysfunction giving rise to high fever, hypertension and sweating are also common in this condition.

The brain, lying under the impact point of a contact force, is subjected to a series of strains resulting from the inward deformation of bone and the shock waves spreading out from the site of impact. Strain can also occur as the base of the brain impinges on projections on the base of the skull. These strains produce gross neurological damage, with haemorrhages, neuronal death and brain swelling. The patient therefore invariably loses consciousness at the time of the incident and has usually developed neurological signs by the time he is examined by a doctor. The most common signs are an altered consciousness level, hemiparesis, ataxia and seizures.

The brain is not fixed inside the neurocranium but floats in a bath of CSF tethered by the arachnoid fibres and blood vessels. If the head moves due to an accelerating or decelerating force, the skull, and then the brain, will move in the direction of the force. As a consequence, strains develop in the brain tissue and small blood vessels opposite the impact point. This gives rise to the contusional changes described previously. Another factor giving rise to injury is that the brain will continue to move until it collides with the opposite side of the skull or its base. The result is a brain which can be injured in two places, with the site furthest from the impact being the most severely injured. This is known as a *contra coup injury*.

Acute intracranial haematoma

In the majority of cases, extradural haematomas (EDHs) develop in the temporoparietal area following a tear in the middle meningeal artery. However a small number are due to tears in one of the venous sinuses inside the neurocranium. As the source of the haematoma is usually arterial, the EDH develops quickly and produces a rapid rise in the intracranial pressure.

The 'classic' presentation of an EDH (Fig. 3.9) only occurs in approximately one-third of patients. The rest are either unconscious from the time of the impact or do not lose consciousness at the scene of the injury but go on to develop neurological signs. The most common clinical signs are a deterioration in the consciousness level and pupil-size changes.

Acute intradural haematoma (IDH)

This is a collective term used for both subdural (SDH) and intracerebral (ICH) haematomas. They frequently co-exist, and are 3–4 times more common than EDHs. SDHs usually develop in the temporal lobe and can be bilateral. Following an inertial force, some of the bridging veins tear and blood collects in the subdural space.

- Transient loss of consciousness at the time of the injury from a momentary disruption of the reticular formation.

- Patient then regains consciousness for several hours, the lucid period.

- Localising signs develop with neurological deficits, headache and eventually unconsciousness from the developing EDH, which causes the ICP to rise.

Fig. 3.9 Classic history of an extradural haematoma (EDH).

Occasionally, a SDH develops with no accompanying ICH. Rarer still is the solitary presence of an ICH. When this occurs it is often found in the frontal lobes.

Small ICHs can also be produced by inertial forces, and their volume can increase over time. Depending on their location, ICHs may cause localizing signs or a rise in the intracranial pressure and a deterioration in the clinical state of the patient.

The forces needed to produce an IDH are greater than those needed to produce an EDH and an IDH is usually associated with cerebral contusion and cortical lacerations. Consequently, the patient commonly loses consciousness at the time of the injury. Fits (which are commonly focal), a deteriorating conscious level, contralateral hemiparesis and unilateral pupil dilatation are the usual signs. If a solitary SDH occurs, the patient may have a lucid period followed by a gradual deterioration in the neurological state. This takes longer to develop than in the case of an EDH, because the source of bleeding is venous rather than arterial. If only a few bridging veins are torn and there is plenty of intracranial space due to brain atrophy, then it can take several days for symptoms to develop.

Subarachnoid haemorrhage (SAH)

This can occasionally follow a head injury. The patient often develops severe headaches and photophobia, but other signs of meningism can occur. Any test for neck stiffness should not be done until injury to the cervical spine has been ruled out both radiologically and clinically (see Ch. 2).

PATHOPHYSIOLOGY OF SPINAL INJURIES

In the UK, 10–15 people per million of the population suffer spinal injuries each year (Table 3.1). The commonest site is the cervical spine, mainly because most people are injured following a road traffic accident.

Primary neurological damage

This is a neurological injury resulting directly from the initial insult. It is usually due to blunt trauma which produces abnormal movement in the vertebral column. In severe cases this leads to ligamental rupture and fractures of the vertebrae. These movements reduce the space around the spinal canal and also allow bone and soft tissue to impinge directly on the cord. The potential space around the spinal cord may already be small, so the chance of neurological damage is increased.

Less commonly, the primary spinal damage is caused by penetrating trauma. A localized area of injury is the usual result of stabbings. Much more extensive areas of destruction and oedema occur when the spinal cord is subjected to a large force such as a gunshot.

Secondary neurological damage

This is deterioration of the spinal cord after the initial insult. The three common causes are mechanical disturbance of the back, hypoxia and poor spinal perfusion. These effects are additive.

Hypoxia can result from any of the causes mentioned above, but significant spinal injury on its own can also produce hypoxia. The reasons for this are listed in Table 3.2. The common underlying problem is usually a lack of respiratory muscle power following a high spinal lesion. Lesions above T12 will involve the intercostal muscles. Injuries above the level of C5 will also block the phrenic nerve and consequently paralyse the diaphragm.

Inadequate spinal perfusion results from either general hypovolaemia or a failure of the spinal cord to regulate its own blood supply. This failure in autoregulation can occur after cord injury. A fall in mean arterial pressure will therefore produce a reduction in spinal perfusion. Conversely, if the pressure is increased too much, then a spinal haemorrhagic infarct could develop.

Secondary damage leads to interstitial and intracellular oedema, which further aggravates the deficient spinal perfusion. As this oedema spreads, neurons are squeezed and an ascending level of clinical deterioration is produced. With high spinal injuries, this process can lead to secondary respiratory deterioration.

Table 3.1 Sites of spinal injuries

Site	Blunt trauma	Penetrating trauma
Cervical	55%	24%
Thoracic	35%	56%
Lumbar	10%	20%
Multiple	10%	

Table 3.2 Respiratory failure in spinal injury

Tetraplegic	Paraplegic
Intercostal paralysis	Intercostal paralysis
Phrenic nerve palsy	
Inability to expectorate	
V/Q mismatch	

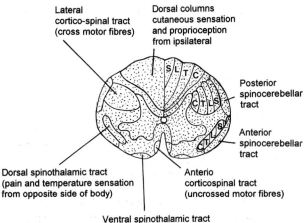

Lateral cortico-spinal tract (cross motor fibres)

Dorsal columns cutaneous sensation and proprioception from ipsilateral

Posterior spinocerebellar tract

Anterior spinocerebellar tract

Dorsal spinothalamic tract (pain and temperature sensation from opposite side of body)

Anterio corticospinal tract (uncrossed motor fibres)

Ventral spinothalamic tract (crude touch and pressure from opposite side of body)

S : sacral area
L : lumbar area
T : thoracic area
C : cervical area

Fig. 3.10 Cross-section of the spinal cord demonstrating the longitudinal tracts. (With permission from Driscoll, P, Gwinnutt, C, Jimmerson, C, Goodall, O, from Trauma Resuscitation: The Team Approach, Macmillan Press Ltd)

Partial spinal cord injury

Anterior spinal cord injury

This is due to direct compression or obstruction of the anterior spinal artery. It affects the spinothalamic and corticospinal tracts (Fig. 3.10), resulting in a loss of coarse touch, pain and temperature sensation and flaccid weakness. This type of injury is associated with fractures or dislocations in the vertebral column.

Central spinal cord injury

This is usually found in elderly patients with cervical spondylosis. Following a vascular event the corticospinal tracts are damaged, with flaccid weakness resulting. In view of the anatomical arrangement in the centre of the cord, the upper limbs are affected more than the legs and hands.

Sacral fibres in the spinothalamic tract are positioned laterally to corresponding fibres from other regions of the body (Fig. 3.10). It follows that anterior and central injuries, which are primarily affecting the midline of the spinal cord, may not affect the sacral fibres. This leads to the phenomenon of 'sacral sparing' in which sensation is lost below a certain level on the trunk but pinprick appreciation is retained over the sacral and perineal area.

Lateral (Brown–Sequard syndrome)

This results from penetrating trauma. On the side of the wound, at the level of the lesion, all sensory and motor modalities are disrupted. However, below this level there is a contralateral loss of pain and temperature sensation and an ipsilateral loss of muscle power and tone.

Posterior spinal cord injury

This is a rare condition. It results in a loss of vibration sensation and proprioception.

Spinal shock

This term refers to the totally functionless condition occasionally seen after spinal injury. The patient has generalized flaccid paralysis, diaphragmatic breathing, priapism, gastric dilatation and the autonomic dysfunction associated with neurogenic shock. Beevor's sign, i.e. movement of the umbilicus when the abdomen is stroked, may be present.

This state can last for days or weeks, but areas of the cord are still capable of a full recovery. Parts which are permanently damaged give rise to spasticity once the flaccid state resolves. Upper motor neuron reflexes will return, below the level of the lesion, if there has been a complete transection of the cord. This is seen as exaggerated responses to stimuli; however, there will be no sensation.

During this stage these patients are at risk of developing pressure sores, deep venous thrombosis, pulmonary emboli and acute peptic ulceration with either haematemesis or, occasionally, perforation.

FRACTURES

Following trauma. The fracture occurs in normal bone as a result of trauma. The type of fracture depends on the direction of the violence. For example, a twisting injury will cause a spiral or oblique fracture, whereas a direct blow usually causes a transverse fracture. Axial compression frequently results in a comminuted or burst fracture.

Stress fracture. The underlying bone is normal and the abnormal load placed on the bone would not be sufficient to cause a fracture on its own. However, the load is repetitive. This type of fracture is most frequently seen in individuals undertaking increased amounts of unaccustomed exercise, such as the 'march' metatarsal fracture in army recruits.

Pathological fracture. In this case the underlying bone is weak, perhaps as a result of metastatic cancer or metabolic bone disease, and gives way under minimal trauma.

Fracture repair

When a fracture occurs, not only is the bone broken, but the surrounding tissues are also damaged. Initially, the bone ends are surrounded by a haematoma which includes the surrounding injured tissues. Within hours, however, an aseptic inflammatory response develops, comprising polymorphonuclear leukocytes, lymphocytes, macrophages and blood vessels. Later, fibroblasts infiltrate the area.

Within this organized fracture haematoma, bone develops either directly or following the development of cartilage with endochondral ossification. At the same time osteoclasts develop and resorb the necrotic bone ends. The initial bone that is laid down (callus) consists of immature woven bone. This is gradually converted to stable lamellar bone with consolidation of the fracture. Resorption takes place within the bone trabeculae as recanalizing Haversian systems bridge the bone ends.

There are basically two types of callus. The first is the primary callus response, which is due to the proliferation of committed osteoprogenitor cells in periosteum and bone marrow. These cells produce directly membranous bone, and this response is a once-only phenomenon limited in duration. The second callus is inductive or external callus, which is derived from the surrounding tissues. This callus is formed by pluripotential cells. A variety of factors, including mechanical and humoral factors, may induce these mesenchymal cells to differentiate to cartilage or bone.

The mediators for callus formation are not fully understood, but it is likely that the fracture ends emit osteogenic substances such as bone morphogenetic protein into the surrounding haematoma. This is in addition to mediators such as interleukin-1 and growth factors which are released from the fracture haematoma. Angiogenic factors probably play an important role in the vascularization of the fracture haematoma. Movement of the fragments increases the fracture exudate. Consequently, rigid fixation minimizes the granulation tissue and external callus. It may also retard the release of morphogens and growth factors from the bone end. Reaming of the intramedullary canal may cause additional bone damage. Weight bearing stimulates growth factors and prostaglandins, which act as biochemical mediators.

PERIPHERAL NERVE INJURY

Blunt trauma to a nerve may produce a temporary block in the conduction of impulses, but leave intact the axonal transport system. The axon distal to the injury does not die, and complete functional recovery can be expected; this is called *neuropraxia*. More severe trauma will interrupt axonal transport and cause Wallerian degeneration: the distal axon dies, the myelin sheath disintegrates and the Schwann cells turn into scavenging macrophages which remove the debris. The cell body then embarks on a preprogrammed regenerative response which is usually known as *chromatolysis*, since it involves the disappearance of the Nissl granules which are the rough endoplasmic reticulum of the normal cell. An entire new set of ribosomes appear, dedicated to the task of reconstruction. By their efforts, axon sprouts emerge from the axon proximal to the lesion and grow distally. Injury of this severity is known as *axonotmesis*. It eventually produces a good functional result because the endoneurial tubes are intact and the regenerating axons are therefore guaranteed to reach the correct end organs.

Laceration or extreme traction produces neurotmesis, which also leads to Wallerian degeneration distally and chromatolysis proximally, followed by either cell death or axonal regeneration. In this case, however, the final functional result is bound to be much worse than in any injury which leaves the endoneurial tubes intact. Not only do the axon sprouts have to transverse a gap filled with organizing repair tissue, but they also need to grow down its original conduit at a rate of approximately 1 mm per day. Axons which fail to enter the distal stump may form a tender neuroma; the symptoms arising from this may be exceedingly troublesome. Progress may be monitored clinically by the Tinel sign (electric feelings in the territory of the nerve produced by light percussion over regenerating axon tips) whether in the distal portion of the nerve or in a neuroma.

Motor axons have the capacity to produce collateral sprouts once they enter muscle, leading to abnormally large motor units with relatively good return of strength. Sensory axons often fail to reinnervate the specialized receptors which form the basis for the sense of touch and this, together with the mismatching of axons with conduits, means that sensory recovery is invariably poor, except in the very young. In the hand this means a poor functional result.

COMPARTMENT SYNDROME

Following injury, muscle swelling is contained within these compartments and there is a rise in tissue pressure. Necrosis of nerves and muscles, resulting from tissue ischaemia, will ensue once the compartment pressure exceeds capillary pressure. This is known as a compartment syndrome and the pressure required to produce these effects is estimated to be about 40 mmHg below the mean arterial pressure. If left untreated, fibrotic contractures may develop. Alternatively, areas of muscle may infarct giving rise to rhabdomyolysis, hypovolaemia, hyperkalaemia, hyperphosphataemia, high levels of uric acid and metabolic acidosis.

A compartment syndrome can result from a variety of causes:

- Crushing injury
- Open or closed fracture
- Prolonged compression of a limb in an unconscious patient
- Restoration of blood flow to a previously ischaemic limb.

Crush injuries occur in a variety of ways:

- Trapped under fallen masonry
- Trapped in a car following a road traffic accident
- Prolonged use of the pneumatic antishock garment
- Prolonged compression of an extremity by the patient's own body.

Such injuries may result in rhabdomyolysis secondary to ischaemia. In addition, there is often associated bone damage and the abnormal biochemical levels found with muscle infarction.

Until the limb is released, there is little systemic effect. However, once reperfusion starts, plasma and blood leaks into the surrounding soft tissues. In severe cases this can cause hypovolaemia. The combination of hypovolaemia and myoglobinaemia can lead to acute renal failure, and hyperkalaemia may precipitate a cardiac arrest. Ultimately, the devitalized tissue has a high chance of becoming infected, resulting in the release of further toxins systemically.

FAT EMBOLISM

In this condition, lipid globules are formed mainly from circulating plasma triglycerides, which are normally carried by very-low-density lipoproteins (VLDLs). In trauma, this is commonly a result of the release of lipid globules from damaged bone marrow adipocytes into the circulation. However, it can also occur with increased peripheral mobilization of fatty acids and increased hepatic synthesis of triglycerides or reduced peripheral uptake and clearance of plasma VLDLs (Fig. 3.11).

It gives rise to thromboembolism of the microvasculature, with lipid globules and fibrin-platelet thrombi. As several organs can be effected, there is a wide range of possible clinical presentations. Pulmonary changes include ventilation-perfusion (V/Q) mismatch, impaired alveolar surfactant activity and segmental hypoperfusion. Cerebral effects include ischaemia, infarction and oedema. The heart can also be affected such that there is a fall in mechanical performance and arrhythmias. Renal affects can lead to lipiduria with tubular damage, and ischaemic glomerular-tubular dysfunction. Skin can manifest its involvement by capillary endothelial disruption and petechial haemorrhage.

To diagnose thromboembolism there has to be either: fat globules in body fluids (e.g. sputum, urine, or lipid emboli in retinal vessels on fundoscopy); histological demonstration of intracellular and intravascular aggregation of lipid globules with Sudan black stain; or evidence of pulmonary and at least one other organ-system dysfunction.

PATHOPHYSIOLOGY OF WOUND HEALING

Soft-tissue injuries heal by a complex series of cellular events leading to connective-tissue formation and repair by scar formation. The process is continuous, but it is convenient to consider it in three phases.

Phase 1: inflammation

Tissue injury, with disruption of vessels, activates platelets and initiates the coagulation cascade, producing a clot in the wound and generating biologically active substances which cause vasodilatation, increased capillary permeability and oedema. These substances are also chemotactic to polymorphonucleocytes (PMNs) and monocytes, and act as potent growth factors for fibroblasts and endothelial cells.

PMNs are present in the wound within a few hours and their numbers increase during the first 24–48 hours. Macrophages, arising by local proliferation and from circulating blood monocytes, are present within 24 hours and both cell types act to remove cellular debris, foreign material and bacteria by phagocytosis. PMNs prevent infection and remove necrotic tissue, but their role is not essential to tissue repair as clean wounds will heal in the absence of PMNs. In contrast, macrophages are critical to wound healing and a reduction in their numbers will slow or stop wound healing. Part of this central role is due to the secretion by macrophages of growth factors which stimulate proliferation of fibro-

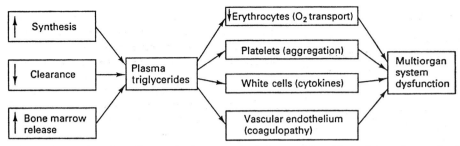

Fig. 3.11   The mechanism of interaction between raised plasma triglycerides and the pathogenesis of multiorgan system dysfunction in fat embolism.

blasts, endothelial cells and smooth muscle cells and extracellular matrix deposition by fibroblasts. These processes start after 3–4 days and are characteristic of phase 2 of wound healing.

Phase 2: cell proliferation and matrix formation

As tissue debris and clot are removed, fibroblasts migrate into the wound. Endothelial migration and proliferation produce new capillaries, and matrix synthesis of collagen, proteoglycans and glycoproteins occurs. Production of this granulation tissue occurs in all adult wound healing and is prominent in open wounds left to heal by secondary intention, but less obvious is incised, primarily repaired wounds. Epithelial migration and proliferation re-establishes epidermal continuity and the clot covering the surface of the wound is lost. As matrix production, and particularly collagen synthesis, continues, the mechanical strength of the wound increases, with approximately 50% of the normal strength of skin regained by 6 weeks after injury.

Phase 3: matrix remodelling

For practical purposes a wound is healed by the end of phase 2, but significant changes occur during phase 3. The latter is prolonged and in children may last 2 years or more. The scar becomes less vascular and less cellular, while collagen synthesis and degradation continue. Reorientation of collagen fibrils occurs and the tensile strength of the scar increases (although not to the level of undamaged tissue). However, the normal tissue structure is not restored and, because of its inelastic nature, the scar may cause long-term problems by restricting function and growth.

Wound contracture

In wounds where tissue loss has occurred, which are left to heal by secondary intention, contraction of granu-lation tissue reduces the size of the tissue defect. There is some evidence that the cell responsible for this process is the myofibroblast, although the exact role of this cell is unresolved. Even though reducing the size of the tissue deficit is of benefit in wound healing, the distortion and scar formation produced by the process inhibit function in certain areas of the body (particularly on the face and around joints).

PATHOPHYSIOLOGY OF BURNS

For the first 24–48 hours after a major burn there are fluid shifts. Leakage of intravascular water, salt and protein occurs through the porous capillary bed into the interstitial space. This, in turn, results in loss of circulating plasma volume, haemoconcentration and hypovolaemia, the severity of which increases with the severity of the burn. In a burn over 15% of the total body surface area (TBSA), the capillary leak may be systemic, causing generalized oedema and a significant fall in blood volume.

Shock associated with burn injuries

The effect on the circulation is directly related to the size and severity of the burn wound. The body compensates for this loss of plasma with an increase in peripheral vascular resistance, and the patient will appear cool, pale and clammy (see Circulatory control, p. 38). However, this compensation will only be effective in maintaining circulation for a period of time, depending on the severity of the burn and the presence of other injuries. Ultimately, the patient will demonstrate signs of hypovolaemic shock as the cardiac output falls. During this time it is rarely possible to keep the circulating volume within normal limits. The end of the shock phase in the adequately resuscitated burn is usually marked by a diuresis. This occurs approximately 48 hours after the burn and is usually associated with fluid balance which is more like that of a normal patient.

A burn of greater than 25% TBSA almost always requires intravenous fluid administration to expand the depleted vascular volume. However, shock can occur with a burn involving as little as 15% TBSA, as a result of complicating factors such as age, pre-existing disease and other major injuries. In these circumstances, a burn of 25–40% becomes a potentially lethal injury.

Depth of burn and cause of burn

The diagnosis of the depth of burn is not always easy. If doubtful, it should be reassessed at 24 hours using only non-stick dressings between examinations.

Superficial burns

These are typically wet, pink and blister but there can also be white areas among the pink. They are always sensitive to pin prick. Superficial burns epithelialize in 14 days from the epithelial-producing elements (hair follicles and sweat glands) and from the edges of the wound. They heal with normal-quality skin, although there can be some pigmentation changes. Superficial burns include: scalds by non-boiling liquids; some chemical burns; and the edges of areas of flame burns and flash burns.

Deep dermal burns

This is an important depth of burn to diagnose. They are pink but do not blanch on pressure (called the *zone of stasis*), there are more areas of whiteness and they can blister. They are dull to pin prick, prone to contracture and struggle to heal in 3–4 weeks. Healing is by epithelialization from the reduced number of epithelial-producing elements and from the edge of the wound. The final result of healing is either poor-quality skin or hypertrophic scar. There is some degree of wound contraction and marked pigmentation change (either hyper- or hypopigmentation). Deep dermal burns include: scalds; contact burns; chemical burns; and flame burns in areas of thick skin, e.g. the back and in concave areas.

Full-thickness burns

These are usually obvious and have no sensation to pin prick. The diagnosis between deep dermal and full thickness burns can be difficult and sometimes is only made at surgery. They can only heal naturally by epithelialization from the wound edge and by wound contraction, leaving contracted poor-quality scars. In the acute situation, circumferential full-thickness burns around limbs and the chest can act as tourniquets, impeding the distal circulation and respiration, respectively. Urgent escharotomy is required in these situations (see Ch. 21).

Full-thickness burns are caused by many scald injuries with near-boiling water, especially in the thin skin of the elderly or young patient. Even tea or coffee with milk can produce burns in the deep dermal and full-thickness range. Chemical burns such as those due to hydrofluoric acid, most flame burns, and virtually all electrical burns with a voltage of 220–240 V or above can also give rise to full-thickness burns. Most contact burns are full thickness in unconscious patients, e.g. postepilepsy or due to alcohol or drug intake. Similarly, they occur in denervated skin, e.g. diabetes and neuropathies. Burns below the deep fascia do occur, e.g. some contact burns, scalds in non-accidental injury in children and high-voltage electrical burns. The latter are particularly prone to destroy muscle groups.

Staphylococcal toxic shock syndrome

This can occur in children even with relatively small superficial burns. If a child with even a 1% burn becomes unwell, toxic shock syndrome must be considered and the specific treatment with fresh frozen plasma and anti-staphylococcal antibiotics started immediately.

Response of the respiratory system to inhalation injury

The lungs themselves are rarely injured from 'burning', even with blast injuries that cause air to be inspired under pressure. Usually laryngeal spasm occurs from the heat of the inspired gases, thereby protecting the lower airway and lungs from exposure.

The upper airway may receive thermal burns and tissue swelling can develop very rapidly in these vascular tissues. The mouth and oropharynx in particular can cause acute respiratory obstruction. Oedema from these injuries may also involve the vocal cords. Dramatic changes in the patient's ability to maintain his airway have been observed over a short period of time following this type of injury. Documentation from the prehospital-care providers concerning the mechanism of injury and the changes in respiratory status en route to hospital allows the team to anticipate airway problems.

The lung parenchyma is frequently damaged by inhaled gases or chemicals that are released by the fire or explosive event in which the patient is involved. Common sources of these are building and home decorating materials, particularly polyvinyl chloride (PVC), polyurethane, urea formaldehyde as well as acrylic fibres, orlon and nylon. Symptoms may be absent initially, but develop with time and rehydration during the resuscitation period. The lung responds initially with irritation, inflammation and progressing oedema. The reaction frequently includes a decrease in surfactant levels and a decrease in pulmonary macrophages, and may result in haemorrhagic tracheobronchitis. This leads to a decrease in lung compliance which is seen as an increase in the work of breathing and an impairment of diffusion through the alveolar membrane.

In view of the very large surface area of the lung, fluid requirements for resuscitation may increase by as much as 50% of the calculated values if a severe inhalation injury has been sustained. The severity of the injury will not be related to the TBSA burn size, but rather to the length of time and intensity of exposure to the inhalation. Accurate information from the prehospital-care providers relative to these conditions is vital in planning the patient's care and anticipating respiratory complications.

Carbon monoxide intoxication

> Carbon monoxide intoxication is the biggest cause of death in people caught in house fires, or other types of closed-space fires.

Carbon monoxide (CO) affects the body in two ways. Firstly, it inhibits the cellular cytochrome oxydase system, causing inhibition of cellular metabolism. Secondly, it has over 200 times the affinity for binding to haemoglobin compared with oxygen. It therefore blocks the ability to transport oxygen to active tissues, causing cellular hypoxia. This is usually demonstrated firstly in alterations in the patient's mental state, ranging from mild anxiety or nervous behaviour to drowsiness and eventual unconsciousness. The inhibition of the cytochrome oxidase system in the brain is another cause for extended periods of unconsciousness. Carbon monoxide also combines with myoglobin in the patient's muscle cells, causing weakness.

The duration of the patient's exposure to carbon monoxide is significant, as short exposures to a high concentration may cause high carboxyhaemoglobin levels but not cause significant metabolic effects (usually acidosis with bicarbonate deficit). These are usually more severe in patients with low-level exposures of a longer duration. Carboxyhaemoglobin levels greater than 10% are significant and levels greater than 50% are generally lethal.

20% hyperbaric O₂

Cyanide poisoning

When the polyurethane foam in modern furniture burns a thick black smoke is produced. This not only contains carbon monoxide and the corrosive substances mentioned above but also cyanide gas. The latter is another metabolic poison which has a similar effect to carbon monoxide in preventing the tissues from utilizing oxygen. Cyanide gas is difficult to measure but should be assumed to be present if the carbon monoxide level is greater than 10%.

ORGANIZATION

THE ROLE OF THE TRAUMA TEAM IN THE CARE OF THE INDIVIDUAL PATIENT

A fully integrated team of trained nurses and doctors needs to be present to deal with a trauma victim when they arrive at the hospital. It has been shown that the most efficient team organization is achieved by simultaneously having each team member carry out individual tasks. This process is known as *horizontal organization*. However, if tasks are to be performed simultaneously, precise allocation of tasks to team members is essential. Each procedure needs to be divided into manageable units and allocated to individual team members by a designated nursing and medical team leader. These tasks must be divided evenly among the team to prevent overloading of any particular member.

When these organizational changes are introduced significant reductions in resuscitation times can be achieved (Fig. 3.12). In particular, the time required to carry out the life-saving procedures is shortened and this is known to correlate with the short- and long-term survival of the patient.

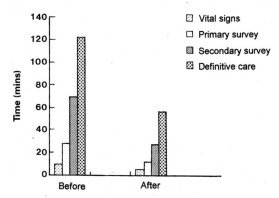

Fig. 3.12 Changes in time for stages of resuscitation following the introduction of horizontal organization and task allocation.

ORGANIZATION DURING A MAJOR INCIDENT

For the health services a major incident exists when the number and severity of live casualties, or its location, requires special arrangements. With regard to a hospital, these special arrangements should deal with the personnel and organizational changes required in the hospital as well as the provision of a Medical Incident Officer (MIO) and a mobile medical team. The latter two should only be provided if they are fully equipped and adequately trained.

Hospitals are usually notified of a major incident by ambulance control using a specified form of words such as 'Major incident declared'. They will also relay as much relevant information as possible, which will include:

- The nature of the incident
- The site of the incident
- The number of casualties
- Special considerations
- Requirements for a MIO or mobile medical team.

As this information will change frequently, it is essential that communication with ambulance control and, later on, with the scene, is maintained throughout the incident.

Once the incident has been declared, the hospital switchboard will call in key personnel who will take up predetermined roles. Part of these responsibilities consists in delegating to specific personnel the further summoning of staff.

One of the problems encountered during a major incident is that personnel have to carry out tasks which are not part of their daily routine. Furthermore, they will not be familiar with the command structure. It is therefore important that the plan has clear guidelines regarding responsibilities and that the tasks allocated diverge as little as possible from the normal daily routine. Action cards should also be available to instruct each member of staff on their immediate duties, responsibilities and priorities.

Additional equipment will be required both for the hospital and at the scene. As there is no time to organize this once the incident has started, it is essential that this extra stock is already in place and immediately accessible.

At each receiving hospital there should be a single entry point through which all patients pass. This point should be manned by the Chief Triage Officer who is usually the duty A&E consultant whose job is rapidly to reassess and recategorize patients triaged at the scene of the incident and allocate them to the most appropriate part of the A&E department (see below). These areas must be appropriately staffed and equipped. Resuscitation and definitive care of the individual patient can then follow the principles described in Chapter 2.

TRIAGE

Triage principles should be employed whenever the number of casualties exceeds the capacity to provide optimum care. Thus appropriate situations for the use of triage range from the road accident with two casualties and only one helper, to major disasters where there may be many victims. Whatever the situation modern triage is dynamic rather than static; continual reassessment allows priorities to be changed according to the changing state of the patient, and depending on the stage of care.

Categories

The categories into which casualties are sorted are generally referred to as 'priorities'. The five-category system shown in Figure 3.13 is widely used. The first priority group consists of patients who require immediate life-saving treatment, for example airway clearing or thoracostomy for tension pneumothorax. The second group comprises those patients requiring urgent treatment (generally surgery) whose lives are not in immediate danger. The aim is to deliver definitive care to these patients within 6 hours. The third group is made up of patients who can withstand a delay to definitive care of more than 6 hours.

The fourth group includes patients who have injuries which are either so severe as to be non-survivable, or are such that the time taken to treat them would seriously compromise the treatment of other casualties. Circumstances will dictate whether such a group has to be defined. Casualties in this category are treated expectantly until all first-priority patients have been treated. Their evacuation and treatment, should they survive long enough, therefore begins after category 1 cases and before category 2. The final category consists of the dead.

Category	Priority	Name	Colour
1	First	Immediate	Red
2	Second	Urgent	Yellow
3	Third	Delayed	Green
4	Fourth	Expectant	Blue
5		Dead	White

Fig. 3.13 The five-category system.

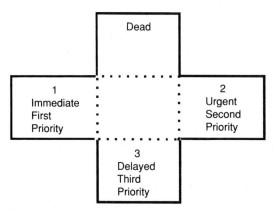

Fig. 3.14 Single card and cruciform triage labels.

Triage methods

Initial triage decisions are made on the basis of a primary survey of the airway, breathing and circulation. Priority cases are identified at this stage. Later a physiological score is obtained using the revised trauma score (respiratory rate, systolic blood pressure and Glasgow Coma Scale). If enough time is available and conditions are satisfactory a secondary survey can be undertaken. This approach has the advantage that it is quick and allows more to be done if time allows.

Triage documentation

Once triage decisions have been made using the categories and methods described above, it is important that the casualties are clearly marked by priority. This is usually achieved by using triage labels. Labels should be visible, clearly marked by priority (both by colour and text), easily attached, and allow for easy changes in priority as the casualty's condition changes. Space should be available for notes on diagnosis and treatment. Two types of label are in widespread use: the single card system (such as the Thames label) and the cruciform system (such as the Cambridge label). These types are depicted in Figure 3.14. The cruciform label is suitable for use during dynamic triage, and can be used from point of injury to point of definitive care. The single label appears simpler to use, but is much more limited in application.

TRAUMA SEVERITY SCORING

This allows the severity to be assessed, the prognosis to be estimated and comparisons to be made between treatment methods within a centre or between trauma centres. Such scores must be interpreted sensibly, especially in individual cases.

Injury Severity Score (ISS) describes the anatomical severity of an injury. The body is divided into 6 regions and the severity of injury is graded from 1 (minor) to 6 (unsurvivable). The highest grading scores, from three separate regions, are squared and added together to make the final score.

Revised Trauma Score (RTS) measures the physiological derangement. It combines the Glasgow Coma Scale score, the Respiratory function score 0 (nil)–4, and Systolic blood pressure 0 (nil)–4 (BP>89). The final score is calculated after weighting the individual scores, using a simple computer programme.

TRISS is a number derived from the ISS, RTS, the age of the patient and the mechanism of injury (i.e. blunt or penetrating). It enables the likely outcome to be predicted for an individual against a large database.

SUMMARY

Trauma is an important clinical problem. In order to be effective in trauma care, the clinician needs a good understanding of the biomechanics of injury and how they relate to specific anatomical regions of the body. In addition, one needs to be aware of both the physiological and pathophysiological response to trauma, as this has direct implications for optimum patient resuscitation.

Those responsible for managing trauma patients should also work in an effective team. This requires tasks to be allocated prior to the patient arriving and the carrying out of these tasks simultaneously. This will reduce the time taken for the team to complete the life-saving procedures.

Preparation for the occurrence of a major incident, which for the health service is defined as a situation in which the number and severity of live victims, or its location, requires special arrangements, is paramount in trauma management. The success of this is directly dependent on the level of preplanning, communication and team work.

ACKNOWLEDGEMENTS

Thanks are also due to Richard A. Cowie, Charles S. Galasko, Roop Kishen, Roderick Little, Kevin Mackaway-Jones, David Marsh, Mohamed Y. Rady, Stewart Watson, David J. Whitby and D. Yates.

FURTHER READING

Advanced Life Support Group 1995 Major incident medical management and support. BMJ Publications, London

Barton R (ed) 1985 Trauma and its metabolic problems. British Medical Bulletin 41 (3)

Barton R 1987 The neuroendocrinology of physical injury. Baillière's Clinical Endocrinology and Metabolism 13 (2): 355–374

Barton R, Frayn K, Little R 1990 Trauma, burns and surgery. In: Cohen R, Lewis B, Alberti K, Denman A (eds) The metabolic and molecular basis of acquired disease. Baillière Tindall, London, p 684–717.

Beale R, Grover E, Smithies M, Bihari D 1993 Acute respiratory distress syndrome (ARDS): no more than a severe acute lung injury? British Medical Journal 307: 1335–1339

Bessey P, Wilmore D 1988 The burned patient. In: Kinney J, Jeejeebhoy K, Hill G, Owen O (eds) Nutrition and metabolism in patient care. W B Saunders, Philadelphia, p 672–700

Colucciello S 1995 The treacherous and complex spectrum of maxillofacial trauma: etiologies, evaluation and emergency stabilisation. Emergency Medicine Reports 16: 59–70

Cole R, Shakespeare P 1990 Toxic shock syndrome in scalded children. Burns 16: 221–224

Cuthbertson D 1980 Alterations in metabolism following injury: part 1. Injury 11: 175–189

Driscoll P, Vincent C 1992 Organising an efficient trauma team. Injury 23: 107–110

Driscoll P, Vincent C 1992 Variation in trauma resuscitation and its effects on patient outcome. Injury 23: 111–115

Driscoll P, Gwinnutt C, LeDuc Jimmerson C, Goodall O 1994 Trauma resuscitation: the team approach. Macmillan, London

Fong Y, Moldawer L, Shiners G, Lowry S 1990 The biologic characteristics of cytokines and their implication in surgical injury. Surgery, Gynecology and Obstetrics 170: 363–378

Frayn K 1986 Hormonal control of metabolism in trauma and sepsis. Clinical Endocrinology 24: 577–599

Gann D, Amaral J 1989 Endocrine and metabolic responses to injury. In: Schwartz S, Shires G, Spence F (eds) Principles of surgery, 5th edn. McGraw-Hill, New York, p 1–68

Greenberg C, Sane D 1990 Coagulation problems in critical care medicine. Critical Care: State of the Art 11: 187–194

Grundy D, Swain A 1994 ABC of spinal cord injury, 2nd edn. British Medical Association, London

Irving M, Stoner H 1987 Metabolism and nutrition in trauma. In: Carter D, Polk H (eds) Butterworths international medical reviews: trauma surgery 1. Butterworths, Oxford, p 302–314.

Matthay M A 1990 The adult respiratory distress syndrome: definition and prognosis. Clinics in Chest Medicine 11 (4): 575–580

Moore J, Moore E, Thompson J 1980 Abdominal injuries associated with penetrating trauma in the lower chest. American Journal of Survery 140: 724–730

Murphy P G, Jones J G 1991 Acute lung injury. British Journal of Intensive Care 1 (3): 110–117

Mubarak S, Hargens A 1983 Acute compartment syndromes. Surgical Clinics of North America 63: 539–565

Proctor J, Wright S 1995 Abdominal trauma: keys to rapid treatment. In: Bosker G (ed) Catastrophic emergencies. Diagnosis and management. American Health Consultants, Atlanta, GA, p 65–74

Repine J 1992 Scientific perspective on adult respiratory distress syndrome. Lancet 339: 466–469

Stoner H 1986 Metabolism after trauma and in sepsis. Circulatory Shock 19: 75–87

Stoner H 1995 The metabolic and nutritional aspects of trauma – an historical introduction. International Journal of Orthopaedic Trauma 5: 60–68

Taylor R, Norwood S 1988 The adult respiratory distress syndrome. In Civetta J, Taylor R, Kirby R (eds) Critical care. Lippincott, Philadelphia, p 1057–1068

Wilmore D 1977 The metabolic management of the critically ill. Plenum, New York

4. Investigations

M. C. Pietroni

GENERAL

A useful investigation is one that alters management. Occasionally, it is easier, quicker and cheaper to ask for a specialist opinion. Sometimes patients in the outpatient department are investigated by trying to answer one question at a time. This results in repeated outpatient visits, and is not only wasteful of resources, but may lead to harmful clinical delays. Reassurance and certainty, on the other hand, are purchased at a price. Moving from a position of 95% certainty to 100% certainty is often very expensive. When using investigations it is vital to understand that the need to manage risk, while at the same time remaining accountable to the patient and to society for the way in which money is spent, requires a delicate balance.

All doctors need to understand the need for this balance to be struck between open access to investigations and the intelligent use of resources. One radiological investigation a week less per Senior House Officer or Registrar in a unit of four to six trainees would produce the salary of another doctor for the unit.

Investigations guide the management of problems. Successful investigations provide data. There is still a need to interpret this in the clinical context. Whenever investigations produce unexpected information, go back to your clinical findings, review and reflect. Your original working hypothesis may have been wrong. It is the intelligent management of problems that matters. In the course of good management the diagnosis emerges.

Ask yourself: Why am I doing this investigation? Does it discriminate, is it reliable, is it safe and is it cost-effective? Should I do an endoscopy or a barium contrast study? What will I lose and what will I do if this investigation does not provide the information I seek?

If you first state the question you want answered, you may find you use certain investigations less often. You may find you reject certain investigations as being incapable of answering your question definitively. Bear in mind the problems of false-positive and false-negative results, especially in radiological contrast studies and biopsies.

Following 'What is the question I want answered?' comes 'what do I need to know?' Do not collect data indiscriminately. When investigating a problem organize your knowledge, examine your problem, explore your attitude, assess your skills and acknowledge your constraints. You will usually work by pattern recognition and hypothesis testing rather than on a blank slate to which you gradually add data. The two most important questions are: What is the likely cause here? and What must I not miss? Ask yourself, in addition: What is the urgency here? Failure to ask these three questions leads to inappropriate investigations in all the surgical specialties, especially when pursuing ill-defined abdominal pain (in general surgery), vague back pain (in orthopaedic surgery), 'cystitis' in young women (in urology), chronic catarrhal pharyngitis (in ear, nose and throat (ENT) surgery), ill-defined and long-standing headaches (in neurosurgery), and all the other chronic problems that overload the outpatient departments of all the surgical specialties.

The experienced surgeon has a working hypothesis within a few minutes of taking a history. The anatomical area of the problem, the physical process at play and the pathology are generally identified in that order. The purpose of investigations is to reduce the management options and to seek to obtain crucial information once, not repeatedly. Sometimes an impasse is reached. Pause, reflect, reconsider, and perhaps postpone for a while a decision, using time as a diagnostic tool. If you rush to make a decision where there is no indication for urgency you will make mistakes. A high negative laparotomy rate in a surgeon usually indicates an unwillingness to use time in this way, perhaps because of organizational constraints. Avoid the temptation to do a laparotomy in the middle of the night just because of the difficulties you might encounter if the need for surgery emerges the next day.

Having asked the right question, and chosen the

correct investigation, do make an effort to see the report and apply the correct interpretation. Then go on to make the correct management decision.

This is especially important if the investigation yields unexpected findings. Do not blindly accept the situation. A negative biopsy may need to be repeated, a blood sample may have been incorrectly obtained or, worse still, labelled with another patient's name. Almost all investigations are operator dependent and as such they express opinions. Opinions depend on experience and expertise. All doctors are fallible. Go back to the radiologist or histopathologist and ask their opinion in the light of your clinical hypothesis. They may enlighten you with their insight into the fallibility of their methods of investigation. Sometimes these investigations may need to be repeated by a more experienced operator.

Establish the diagnosis

Investigations are commonly used to establish a diagnosis. Ask yourself: Is the problem likely to be structural or functional? Structural problems are best investigated by displaying altered anatomy. Select the appropriate radiology or endoscopy. Functional problems are best investigated by studying function using biochemical, radioisotope or organ excretion studies. In the gut, pressure and motility studies come into this category. For example, the history and examination will guide you in patients with dysphagia. If the pattern points to carcinoma of the oesophagus the patient needs an endoscopy. If the diagnosis suggested is a motility problem then a barium meal followed, if necessary, by pressure studies is more appropriate.

In orthopaedic surgery you may need to decide between tumours and infection in bone. Choose the investigation most likely to give you the answer to the question you pose. Is an X-ray, a bone scan or a biopsy the best way? This will not only depend on the local circumstances (e.g. tibia or spine) but also on the expertise available in your hospital.

Exclude alternative diagnoses

It may happen that you are reasonably certain of your diagnosis but that an important alternative must be excluded because of its consequences. Do not be wasteful of resources. You cannot do a barium enema on all patients with irritable bowel syndrome whenever they present, an intravenous urogram (IVU) on all patients with urinary infection, or magnetic resonance imaging (MRI) scan on all patients with backache, just because you wish to exclude cancer. Try and establish in your mind the degree of certainty that is appropriate to the clinical situation you face.

Evaluate the extent and severity of disease

Once the diagnosis is firm you may wish to assess the extent and severity of the disease. This usually applies to cancer. You want to know something about the extent of local and systemic spread, because this will influence clinical decisions about the indications for surgery, and operative decisions about the extent of the resection required. Bear in mind the limitations of the techniques available to you. Metastatic spread can only be demonstrated once the lesion is beyond a certain size. Local infiltration and nodal involvement is difficult to demonstrate in its early phases. Weight loss may abolish fat planes that allow computed tomography (CT) scans in oesophageal and pancreatic cancer to show these boundaries. Bone scans and chest X-rays may not show up small lesions.

Evaluate the whole system

If one part of a system is affected should you assess the whole system? Should you be screening certain patients for unrelated disease? These questions may arise in patients with vascular disease, diabetes, joint disease, tuberculosis, cancer and, in recent times, increasingly with human immunodeficiency virus (HIV) infection.

Exclude incidental disease

Patients requiring surgery need to be fit for anaesthesia. Investigate the cardiovascular system in those at risk and especially in those with a recent history of myocardial ischaemia or those with rhythm disorders. It is here that a cardiological opinion may be better that indiscriminate investigations. Establish the adequacy of lung function, especially in patients with a history of asthma and obstructive airways disease. You want to know about respiratory reserve and ventilatory function. Use blood gases and expiration volume flow rates here. Patients with significant weight loss suffer malnutrition and have reduced albumin levels. In all surgical specialties this reduces healing rates. This may affect the timing of surgery, especially if an anastomosis is contemplated. Diabetics need careful investigation, not only to ensure satisfactory control but also to assess whether other systems are involved. Exclude sickle cell disease (see below).

Satisfy medicolegal requirements

Lastly, investigations are often used for medicolegal purposes. Probably more money is wasted on skull X-ray in patients with mild head injuries than in any other situation. How will the management of the patient change? Would it not be better to X-ray the cervical spine? Medicolegal considerations may well sometimes override common sense. Nevertheless, in the field of penetrating foreign bodies it would be wrong not to X-ray the part since it is well known that foreign bodies can frequently be present with minimal signs. Do not discard moles without histology. A patient may at a subsequent date develop a melanoma and the absence of a histology report will be difficult to justify.

HAEMATOLOGY

Most laboratories now use analysers that give all the common haematological indices when only a haemoglobin (Hb) estimation is required. Be careful to interpret these values in the light of the patient's general condition. For example, dehydrated patients have a high Hb and packed cell volume (PCV, haematocrit) because of haemoconcentration. Patients who are heavy smokers or who have chronic obstructive airways disease also have raised Hb levels. Remember that patients with rheumatoid arthritis often have a low Hb. Allow for this if such a patient is to have an operation on their joints. Do not be misled into overtransfusing patients. There are serious risks attached, especially in paediatric and neurosurgery.

The Hb level by itself is insufficient to establish the transfusion requirements in acute blood loss. In the first few hours after blood loss it cannot answer the question: 'How much blood has been lost?' The body's physiological responses to shock produce a reduction in the capacity of the circulation. It is only after many hours that haemodilution produces a representative cellular/plasma ratio, when the PCV is a better guide.

The level of the white blood cell (WBC) count is a valuable indicator but not an accurate diagnostic tool. When raised it gives useful corroborative evidence of infection. When normal it does not exclude infection. By itself it cannot answer the questions: Has this patient got appendicitis? and Is there postoperative sepsis somewhere? Remember that the WBC count is also raised in the presence of tissue necrosis (e.g. burns in plastic surgery) and need not necessarily imply infection.

In the presence of overwhelming sepsis a low or normal WBC level indicates an inability of the patient's immune system to react to infection. Levels of 15–18 × 10^9 WBC per litre generally indicate intermediate degrees of infection, while levels over 20 × 10^9 WBC per litre suggest life-threatening sepsis. Trends are more useful than absolute levels. A falling WBC count in a clinically improving patient suggests response to treatment.

It is possible to label granulocytes with radioactive phosphorus, technetium or indium. The cells aggregate in septic foci and can be localized using a γ-camera if the site of infection cannot be detected clinically. CT scanning has generally superseded this test.

Always seek the haematologist's help when analysing bleeding disorders and coagulopathies. In the presence of massive blood loss and whenever six or more units of blood have been transfused, check the platelet count, the prothrombin time (PT) and the kaolin cephalin clotting time (KCCT) to identify any prolonged bleeding tendency. The result may indicate the need to infuse platelets or fresh frozen plasma. In cases of suspected disseminated intravascular coagulopathy (DIC) the haematologist's help is essential. Measure fibrinogen degradation products and fibrinogen titres and measure the thrombin time. These results will assist in assessing the need for platelets, cryoprecipitate and fresh frozen plasma.

Patients with deep venous thrombosis (DVT) or pulmonary embolism (PE) require anticoagulation. Use the activated partial thromboplastin time (APTT) for heparin therapy and the PT for patients on warfarin. The laboratory results will usually be expressed as international normalized ratios (INR), to aid therapeutic adjustments. Measure heparin levels in the circulating blood or factor-10 levels in cases of massive thrombosis, where heparin consumption can be unpredictable. Once the patient has been stabilized the frequency of testing can be gradually reduced to once weekly and eventually to once monthly. Sometimes there is a background predisposition to DVT and PE which may be congenital. It may be wise to check on protein C, protein S, antithrombin 3, lupus anticoagulant and anticardiolipin antibody, if you suspect this may be the case (recurrent DVT and PE, or if there is a family history).

Perform a sickle cell test on all patients from the Middle East, the Indian subcontinent and on those of African and Mediterranean extraction. Hypoxia and dehydration are especially dangerous in these patients as a sickle cell crisis may be so induced.

When ordering blood for cross-matching do not overestimate the need. Order blood grouping, saving the serum for operations of medium severity such as nephrectomy, cholecystectomy and thyroidectomy. The transfusion of blood postoperatively is rarely required here.

Discuss cases of suspected lymphoma with the

haematologist. It may be that if the peripheral blood picture shows involvement (as in chronic lymphatic leukaemia), peripheral blood marker studies will lessen the need for lymph-node biopsy. This will avoid the need for a general anaesthetic, and a bone marrow sample can be taken under local anaesthetic instead. If you do need a lymph-node biopsy (see below) then do not forget that the haematologist can help as well as the histopathologist. Immunocytochemistry can give valuable prognostic information and can distinguish between T-cell and B-cell lymphomas. Formalin fixation destroys this information. Collect the dry lymph node in liquid nitrogen or, if this is not available, cut the node sharply in half and do an imprint on a slide, which is then air dried.

HISTOPATHOLOGY

A biopsy is a sample of tissue. Ensure that it is a representative sample. Ensure that the histopathologist receives the correct specimen, in the correct container in the best possible condition, labelled correctly and with full information. The pathologist can comment only on the tissue presented by the surgeon. The more information you give the more useful and detailed is the pathologist's report. The best results follow personal contact between surgeon and histopathologist, both of whom understand the other's difficulties. Cytology refers to the examination of cells and is inherently not as reliable as histology, which looks at architectural detail too.

Cytological examination of the spun-down deposit of fluids can often diagnose cancer. This is the simplest way to diagnose malignancy in pleural effusions and in ascites. Urine cytology is also useful, especially as a monitoring test in patients with known urothelial tumours. Avoid painful, expensive procedures when simple ones will do. Sputum cytology, when positive, may avoid the need for bronchoscopy and biopsy.

Fine-needle aspiration (FNA) cytology is a valuable diagnostic tool in lesions of the breast and thyroid. In recent years it has been used for most solid masses that are accessible to a needle. This applies in ENT surgery (head and neck cancers), in urology (prostatic cancer) and in lung surgery (lung neoplasms). Radiologically guided aspirates can also be obtained from organs within the abdominal cavity.

Take FNA of palpable breast lesions when you wish to establish the diagnosis preoperatively or when you think you can avoid surgery. The finding of malignant cells establishes the diagnosis, but a negative result does not exclude malignancy. Positive and negative results are operator dependent, so interpret them with care. Look closely at the wording of the report: 'malignant cells not seen' is not a useful report. You need to know whether the sample collected was adequate and whether normal cells were seen; only then is the absence of malignant cells a useful conclusion. FNA reports as well as being positive and negative can be expressed along a spectrum of indeterminacy.

FNA is particularly useful with impalpable breast lesions. These are usually shown on mammography as clusters of microcalcification. Ensure your FNA sample is taken with radiological guidance. Seek your histopathologist's attitude to a positive FNA result. If you wish to proceed to definitive breast surgery it may be preferable first to obtain histological proof of cancer. Centres with great expertise will accept a cytological result alone.

The cytologist can say that a thyroid lesion is a neoplasm or a papillary cancer, but the distinction between a follicular adenoma and a follicular carcinoma is not easily made by this method. Invasion of the capsule is the key factor and FNAs and even needle biopsies do not supply this tissue.

In neurosurgery, needle biopsy under X-ray control often avoids the need for open biopsy and hence avoids craniotomy. Similarly, in orthopaedics, needle biopsy may sometimes avoid the need for open biopsy (e.g. in the spine). However, the presence of calcium makes the collection of suitable specimens difficult. TruCut® needle biopsy may produce an adequate core from many tissues.

The best biopsy is the whole lesion. You only need a biopsy if you have different management options in mind. Most skin lesions are best removed in toto. If you must sample the lesion, take a representative portion. In the rectum and colon orientate your specimen on a piece of filter paper before immersing it in formalin. This preserves the normal architectural relationships of the layers. Avoid taking biopsies of polyps. Take the whole lesion. If this is not possible, ensure you sample the base (not the tip) of the lesion. With bladder tumours you want to know about the stalk and the base of papilliferous lesions. Take biopsies appropriately. You need to know about invasion. At gastroscopy do not biopsy the centre of the ulcer; this just yields necrotic tissue. Take several samples at the periphery. At oesophagoscopy you may want to establish a diagnosis of oesophagitis, but you also need to know the nature of the mucosa proximally. Take labelled biopsies at intervals of 2 cm.

Try not to take biopsies of lymph nodes. Wherever possible take at least one whole node and do not crush or alter its anatomy. When this is not possible, take a wedge, preserving if possible the capsule. The pathologist is not just giving a report on cellular detail but also on altered anatomy. Remember to send a sample to the microbiologist if you suspect tuberculosis. Immunocytochemistry will be required with lymphomas. Either send an unfixed sample in liquid nitrogen or carry out an imprint as mentioned before.

The smaller the sample the greater is the degree of expertise required of the pathologist. This can be a problem with deep-seated organs (abdominal masses, liver and pancreas) where only a needle biopsy is available. Sample carefully. A false-negative result may be due to a sampling error.

Remember that the pathologist is able not only to make the diagnosis but also to give you useful information about prognosis. You want to know about clearance margins, depth of invasion, cellular differentiation, number of nodes and presence or absence of metastases. Evidence of vascular invasion in the tumour may predict future haematogenous deposits. Make it easy for him by giving as much information as possible. Label and orientate your specimen and identify specific portions you want examined when sending very large specimens.

MICROBIOLOGY

A pus swab only briefly contains a representative sample of organisms from an infected source. Some organisms die because they are anaerobic (e.g. *Streptococcus faecalis*) because they are delicate (e.g. *Neisseria*), or because the other organisms in the sample proliferate faster and overwhelm them. Therefore lose no time between taking the swab and transferring it to an appropriate medium for culture. If pus is available then collect a quantity and send that, rather than a swab, to the microbiologist. Pus swabs (in Stewart's transport medium) should be stored at 4°C when taken at night. Do ensure they are sent to the laboratory the next day.

Taking swabs for culture without careful thought may cause you to miss the diagnosis. Make sure you ask the correct question in order to select the best method of answering it. For example, the detection of amoebic dysentery is not accomplished by taking a swab for culture but by examining a fresh specimen immediately under the microscope. If you can see blood-stained mucus through the sigmoidoscope then take a sample of that rather than sending a stool specimen. When investigating diarrhoea send three fresh stool specimens taken on three separate days.

Tell the microbiologist whether the urine specimen you send is a midstream specimen or a catheter specimen. Always interpret the culture report in the light of the microscopy report. More than 15 pus cells per microlitre of urine is generally taken as a significant result. Remember that tuberculosis may present as a sterile acid pyuria. Occasionally, pus cells are seen in great numbers in the absence of any growth on culture. This usually implies a recent operation (e.g. a transurethral resection of the prostate) or the presence of an antibiotic. Do let the microbiologist know about antibiotic therapy.

This is especially important when taking blood cultures. Whenever possible, take blood before starting antibiotic therapy. If this is not possible then let the microbiologist know. He will add β-lactamase to the culture medium in order to neutralize the effect of penicillin or cephalosporin.

When investigating urethral discharges remember that non-specific urethritis and chlamydial infections are difficult to diagnose. Special transport media are required. The gonococcus is a delicate organism and fresh samples swiftly examined are vital to establishing a bacteriological diagnosis.

Always seek the help of the microbiologist whenever you deal with superadded infection, especially in transplant patients and in the immunocompromised (as in HIV infections or in patients on chemotherapy). *Pneumocystis carinii* is the commonest opportunistic infection here. The picture can, however, become quite complicated, partly because several infective agents can become involved (bacterial, viral or fungal) and partly because the picture may change from day to day.

It is a wise precaution to test all jaundiced patients or those with a history of jaundice for the hepatitis antigen. A positive result for hepatitis B alerts medical, nursing and laboratory staff of the risks of needle-stick injury. Testing for HIV seropositivity is a controversial subject. It is well known that the incidence is highest in homosexuals, their partners and offspring, and in drug addicts. Confining HIV testing to this group may well miss many others who may be carriers. At present there is no consensus on who should be tested, when the test should be done or how often it should be repeated. There are complicated and unresolved questions over the rules of consent. Naturally the implications of a positive result are enormous. It seems wise therefore to obtain informed consent and to perform the test whenever the clinical need seems appropriate. You will need to counsel patients carefully both before doing the test and afterwards if the result is positive.

BIOCHEMISTRY

Modern laboratories use the autoanalyser. All the common biochemical indices are measured even if only one has been requested. The results are expressed as concentrations per unit volume of blood. Blood loss, dehydration, infusion and transfusion will therefore affect the result. This is especially important when dextrose or lipids are being infused. Avoid a tourniquet if you want calcium levels. Potassium leaches out of cells, so avoid delay in delivering the sample for analysis.

Remember you are sampling plasma. You are only indirectly discovering what is going on inside cells. Potassium levels, for instance, reflect poorly the intracellular potassium. The plasma amylase is only transiently raised in the plasma during pancreatitis. Hormone, enzyme and drug levels are affected by the levels of the plasma proteins, so allow for this when interpreting results.

You need information about electrolyte balance in patients with dehydration and intestinal obstruction. Sodium, potassium and bicarbonate levels will assist you in judging fluid and acid–base balance. The rate at which laboratory values change will dictate how often these tests should be performed. There is no need to repeat these tests on a daily basis if the changes are not clinically significant. The body's homoeostatic mechanisms are usually very good, but if the physiology of the lungs or kidneys is impaired then you will need information more often.

Be careful with dehydrated patients who have diabetes as well as intestinal obstruction. Use glucose and potassium levels as well as the electrolytes in gauging transfusion requirements. Keep an eye on the levels of urea and creatinine. Any element of renal failure in addition will make therapeutic judgements difficult.

In surgery the investigation of the jaundiced patient is now a radiological rather than a biochemical exercise. However, the balance between the levels of bilirubin, alkaline phosphatase and the transaminases will give valuable additional information. Obstruction is always characterized by high bilirubin and alkaline phosphatase levels. The latter often lag behind the bilirubin when the obstruction has been relieved. Hepatocellular damage is usually reflected more in the transaminases, which are then disproportionately raised.

Use hormone assays intelligently when investigating thyroid disease. There is scarcely ever a need for all the thyroid function tests to be performed. What do you want to know? Hypothyroidism is reflected in a low total thyroxine (T4) and high levels of thyroid-stimulating hormone (TSH), while hyperthyroidism will produce high levels of total T4 and triiodothyronine (T3). Measuring the levels of free T3 and T4 is not necessarily helpful unless the total levels are misleading in patients with protein abnormalities, the pregnant and the elderly. If your patient is on maintenance therapy, judge his control clinically. Do not be swayed by the biochemical levels. Thyrotoxic patients controlled with propranolol will still have abnormal biochemical levels even though they are well controlled clinically.

IMAGING

Radiology

Once again phrase the question you want answered and then choose the right investigation. Too many indiscriminate radiological examinations are carried out. Discuss difficult cases with the radiologist. Remember that X-rays are shadows. An X-ray report is an expression of an opinion on the interpretation of shadows on a particular occasion. It is not infallible. Plain X-rays are used for the demonstration of differences between penetration characteristics of different tissues in a particular locality. They are of course unsurpassed in the demonstration of fractures and tumours of bone. However, secondary deposits in an osteoporotic spine may be difficult to outline. Choose a bone scan.

X-ray the skull and whole cervical spine in recent severe head and neck trauma, after immobilizing the spine. The presence or absence of a skull fracture does not often alter the management of the patient, but it is most important not to miss cervical spine fractures. You will need to immobilize the head and neck as a matter of urgency if such a fracture exists.

The chest X-ray is excellent for outlining lung tumours since they are outlined by relatively normal air-containing lung. It is easy to miss masses near and behind the mediastinum, however, and the straight line of a left lower lobe collapse can be missed behind the left heart border if the X-ray penetration is not exactly right. In the presence of past surgery or radiotherapy to the lung the chest X-ray does not easily discriminate between past events and a new tumour. Choose CT or MRI (see below).

Use plain X-rays in the renal tract when looking for renal calculi but remember that uric-acid stones are not opaque. Be careful how you interpret calcified lesions and learn to distinguish the difference between phleboliths and calculi.

Plain X-rays are invaluable in outlining hollow organs in the abdomen because of the contrast between air-containing bowel and surrounding tissues. Classically, in perforated peptic ulcer, free air is seen beneath the diaphragm. Because of this they are helpful in intestinal obstruction. The position, but not the nature, of the obstruction can usually be inferred. Small bowel can usually be distinguished from large bowel by the disposition of the loops and the presence of the ladder pattern of the valvulae conniventes.

Contrast studies

The investigation of disease in hollow organs is traditionally accomplished by using contrast media. The organ is then outlined. Double-contrast studies with air enable fine mucosal details to be identified in the gastrointestinal tract. Use this examination when you wish to outline polyps of the small bowel or mucosal abnormalities in small bowel malabsorption states, in Crohn's disease and in ulcerative colitis. Cancers of the stomach, colon and rectum can also be usefully outlined this way. Endoscopy, however, is usually a quicker and more certain way of establishing the diagnosis, especially since there is simultaneous access to biopsy. A negative endoscopy is more reliable than a negative barium study. Use barium studies when you wish to outline gross disease, or for the small bowel where the organ is not generally accessible to endoscopy. Local factors in your hospital will determine whether upper gastrointestinal endoscopy and colonoscopy are easily obtained. If they are then use this facility in preference to barium studies. Of course, barium studies can be used in addition, especially by surgeons who do not do their own endo-scopies.

Barium studies are better than endoscopy for the assessment of functional disease of a hollow organ. Better still, for motility disorders use oesophageal or rectal manometry. Barium, and especially cine barium, studies of swallowing and defaecation give good pictures of the functioning organ. Manometry will quantify the problem.

The bladder is, of course, normally investigated by cystoscopy, but contrast radiology has a place, especially in the demonstration of reflux (especially in children). The bladder is filled with contrast and pictures are taken during micturition (micturating cystogram).

Mammography

Plain X-rays of the breast (mammograms) use high-resolution X-ray films and rays with special penetration characteristics. The dosage is low and mammograms may be repeated on several occasions for screening pur-poses. Be reluctant to use them in women under the age of 45 years since the younger breast is denser than the postmenopausal breast. The fine spiculate calcification of breast cancer is difficult to recognize against the dense stroma in younger women.

Tomography

Differences in penetration characteristics can be enhanced by using tomography, and an extension of this process is CT scanning. CT scanning gives superb cross-sectional views of any region of the body. Pictures can be enhanced either by adding contrast media to hollow organs or by simultaneous arteriography.

CT scanning has revolutionized the investigation of disease. It is now the investigation of choice in urology, ENT surgery, and pulmonary and general surgery, for outlining problems in the neck, chest and abdomen whenever the questions posed are:

- How extensive is this lesion?
- Has it spread into adjacent structures?
- Is it resectable?

In appropriate cases a CT-guided needle biopsy will also give a histological diagnosis.

MRI

MRI is the latest advance in this field. External magnets cause realignment of the protons of hydrogen nuclei. They then resonate and emit signals which can be picked up. This allows a three-dimensional image to be con-structed and pictures may be taken from any angle. MRI is particularly useful in the central nervous system as lipids have a high content of hydrogen atoms. It is the investigation of choice in neurosurgery for the accurate delineation of tumours in the central nervous system. In orthopaedic surgery it has virtually replaced myelo-graphy; in spinal surgery MRI gives valuable information about cartilage, and hence can help cut down on the need for diagnostic (as opposed to therapeutic) arthro-scopy, especially in the knee. The distinction between vessels, tumour, inflammatory lesions and surgical scars is more easily demonstrated using MRI than CT scan-ning in all surgical specialties.

Ultrasound examination

Ultrasound examination of the abdomen is, of course, quicker and cheaper than and may give the answer just as reliably as CT or MRI in many cases, but you are more likely to move from ultrasound to CT or MRI than vice versa when the first investigation has failed. An exception is with carcinoma of the pancreas. Weight loss has caused the fat to disappear and the outlines may appear blurred or indistinct on CT, whereas the ultra-sound scan may readily outline a pancreatic mass.

Ultrasound is particularly useful in the biliary and urogenital systems. The contrast between fluid-filled organs, normal tissue and stones leads to variations in echogenicity. Portable systems now make this a valuable diagnostic tool in the outpatient department. Be careful in your interpretation of negative results. Small uncalci-fied stones may be missed. If there is any clinical doubt about the common bile duct use endoscopic chol-angiography rather than ultrasound. Ultrasound is of primary importance in establishing whether a lesion is solid or cystic. For this reason it is particularly useful in the breast, in the thyroid and in testicular lesions. It may also answer this question in the chest, abdomen or pelvis. It is especially useful in the pelvis because the urine-filled bladder provides a better contrasting background than does air-filled bowel. Intracavity and intraluminal ultrasound are more recent advances. Tumour extent can be gauged in the oesophagus, vagina and rectum. Rectal endosonography can, in addition, help in outlining complex sphincter defects.

Cannulation of ducts and tubes

Tubal anatomy can be displayed by cannulation and the injection of dye. It is a useful investigation in salivary gland surgery for showing ectasia of ducts, in urology for showing urethral abnormalities and in pancreatobiliary surgery for showing abnormalities of biliary and pancreatic ductular anatomy. It is particularly useful in the investigation of sinuses and fistulae, especially if a communication with other organs is suspected, either because of infection, or because of congenital anomalies in children. In orthopaedics such investigations may be used to demonstrate communication with artificial prostheses. However, this method of investigation has particular value in the vascular system.

The vascular system

The standard imaging technique for the vascular system is the retrograde (Seldinger) transfemoral arteriogram. The catheter is passed up the aorta and films are taken of the arterial tree. The procedure, although invasive, is safe and produces reliable pictures. There is a risk of initiating intimal dissection or dislodgement of a thrombus in the presence of severe aortic disease or in the presence of aneurysms. Some surgeons feel that the presence of an aortic aneurysm is a contraindication to the retrograde transfemoral route. Always look carefully at the aortic bifurcation. If there is any doubt about disease at this level the radiologist should take lateral views. In the presence of a proximal lesion the distal arterial tree is sometimes difficult to demonstrate. Beware of attributing this to distal occlusion when the cause is really one of underfilling. Look carefully at the region of the origin of the profunda artery and the popliteal trifurcation. The vessels in the leg are often overlain by bony outlines and a good peroneal artery can easily be missed behind the fibular shadow. Look carefully for patency of the dorsal pedal arch.

If the femoral artery is impalpable or occluded then choose a translumbar or axillary (or brachial) route. In most specialized centres a more popular alternative would be digital subtraction angiography (DSA). Indeed, this has supplanted femoral arteriography in many vascular units. The translumbar route gives excellent pictures, but there are dangers of haematoma, haemorrhage and intimal dissection. It should be avoided in the presence of aneurysmal disease. If the puncture site is above the renal arteries there are risks associated with too much contrast entering the renal circulation too suddenly.

The axillary or brachial route requires more expertise and should be performed only by radiologists who do this on a regular basis. Once again there is a problem with local vessel damage and with haematoma. Occasional damage to the brachial plexus has been reported.

Venography and lymphangiography may be important investigations in venous disease and lymphatic and lymph-node disease.

DSA should now be available to most vascular centres. The dye is injected via a peripheral vein. Large quantities are required, and this occasionally gives rise to problems of hypotension. The pictures obtained are often almost as good as with conventional arteriograms, but dilutional problems result in inferior pictures of the distal vascular tree.

Doppler ultrasound

Learn to use Doppler ultrasound scans on all your vascular patients. Do it yourself and get used to the problems of siting the probe accurately and using the correct angulation. Do not press too hard, as you will occlude the vessel. Accustom yourself to the sharp-peaked biphasic waveform of normal vessels. Obstructed vessels show a low-frequency long-duration waveform with very little delay before the next waveform. The portable Doppler ultrasound is an invaluable tool in the outpatient department, the ward and the operating theatre, and you should learn to diagnose problems by ear. Sophisticated machinery in the vascular laboratory gives you a paper readout with an analysis of waveform characteristics. Use this together with vascular imaging to establish the site of the lesion, its severity and whether it can be relieved or not. Use Doppler ultrasound in conjunction with a proximally placed sphygmomanometer cuff to find the occluding pressure. The two lower-limb pressures can be compared with each other and with the pressure in the arm (Pressure index = Ankle pressure/Arm pressure). This gives you an idea of the severity of the problem. You can use this as a simple non-invasive monitoring tool in the outpatient department.

Duplex scanning is the most recent development in this field. A combination of ultrasound scanning and measurements of the velocity of the flowing blood allows a computer-generated image of the vessel to be displayed. It is not invasive and is therefore repeatable. It is a useful screening test, especially in the surveillance of infrageniculate anastomoses.

Radioimaging

Radioimaging is a method of outlining a problem within an organ by using radioisotopes. The radioisotope chosen is one that has a particular affinity for the organ under investigation. The resulting pictures are called 'radioactive scans'. They do not have the anatomical clarity of other methods, but they highlight changes in physiology in the organ. When used in the investigation of thyroid disease, they demonstrate increased, reduced or absent function in a palpable lump. You might be able to show other impalpable lesions or a retrosternal thyroid enlargement. Subtraction scans may demonstrate a parathyroid adenoma by taking two types of scan (one demonstrating vascularized organs and the other the thyroid) and subtracting one from the other. Use liver scans or pancreatic scans to help you distinguish between tumours and benign lesions already shown in the liver, spleen and pancreas on CT scanning. Gallium scanning helps in distinguishing between hepatomas and secondary deposits in the liver.

Use bone scans when looking for lesions in the spine which may be too small to show with conventional radiography. It is the increased vascularity of the lesion (inflammatory or malignant) which reveals its presence. You will still need to seek confirmation of its nature by other means (e.g. biopsy). Absent vascularity, as for example in avascular necrosis of the head of the femur, can help in distinguishing between fractures and secondary deposits.

Radioactive scans in the genitourinary tract are used in showing dynamic as opposed to anatomical differences. Conventional iodine-based contrast radiology gives poor pictures in the presence of obstruction. Use DTPA (diethylene tetramine pentaacetic acid) to show the pelvis and ureter, or DMSA (dimercaptosuccinic acid) to show the cortex or when you suspect the presence of differences in function between the two kidneys (e.g. renal artery stenosis or after long-standing obstruction on one side has been relieved). In some units there has been a move recently to using MAG 3 in these instances because this gives structural as well as functional information in one session. Its use is limited by its expense.

ENDOSCOPY

Tubes and cavities are accessible to endoscopy. This is the most direct way in which to recognize anatomical and pathological alterations of normality. All forms of endoscopy share common features. There must be easy access to the organ or tube, which generally requires to be cleaned and emptied of its contents. Fibre optics has made accessibility and illumination much easier, but there are still hazards and traps for the unwary. Large tumours in the stomach are easy to recognize, but mucosal infiltration and lack of distensibility can be missed. In the colon, small polyps can be missed, as can the subtle changes of inflammatory disease. Faecal loading can interfere with adequate sigmoidoscopy in the outpatient department.

In the bronchial tree, systematic examination of all the bronchial orifices is required to ensure a comprehensive report. In the bladder, debris from infection can hide underlying pathology. All forms of endoscopy are operator dependent, therefore interpret reports with care.

Laparoscopy has been used for diagnostic purposes in gynaecology for many years but has only recently been recognized for this purpose in general surgery. Thoracoscopy and mediastinoscopy have their place in thoracic surgery. In orthopaedic surgery, arthroscopy has contributed to preoperative evaluation and can determine the presence of lesions in the knee that are undetected by physical examination of the patient.

5. Decision-making

R. M. Kirk

Surgical practice varies remarkably. A patient with a particular condition may be treated expectantly by one surgeon and operated on by another. In theory, once the diagnosis of a common condition is made, it should be possible to determine the best action from previous trials. However, many important surgical and other decisions cannot be made with mathematical precision. There is no unanimity of opinion about the correct treatment of many conditions. Reliable trials have been carried out on relatively few human illnesses. There are innumerable papers containing much conflicting evidence. From those we read, each of us interprets selectively, depending upon our character, philosophy and previous experience. We often cannot logically justify why we made a particular decision, any more than we can give the real reasons why we studied medicine, chose a surgical career, or chose a particular life partner.

Attempts to apply reason may be thwarted because the problem is complex, with too many imponderables. Very often the aspects that can be tested objectively are unimportant, while the crucial aspects are not amenable to objective testing in our present state of knowledge. This should not deter us from attempting to deduce the implications of different courses of action. Some surgeons appear to get better results than others; perhaps they have exceptional inborn technical skills, but often they make a higher percentage of decisions that prove to be correct. Those of us who are less 'lucky' need to study how they make their decisions, and copy them. The great golfer Gary Player is reputed to have said, 'The more I practise and the harder I try, the luckier I get'.

Incomplete information

Decision-making is facilitated if all the required information is available. However, in surgical practice we never have a complete knowledge of the physical and psychological state of the patient and of the extent and severity of the pathological condition. Moreover, it is often necessary to take some action even before all the available information reaches us. Do not make this an excuse for failing to obtain all possible information.

Discriminating features

A frequent cause of failure, especially among inexperienced clinicians, is indiscriminate overcollection of information, resulting in confusion. Long lists can be composed of the presenting features of recognized conditions, but if all the features are given equal 'weight' the possible interpretations are multiplied. Identify the cardinal features (Latin: *cardinis* = a hinge, i.e. on which the diagnosis hinges), and base decisions on them.

Distracting pressures

It is rare to have just a single patient on whom to concentrate. Other patients and other activities need attention. Rank these demands in order of priority, remembering that this order is not static. In the extreme circumstances of battles and major disasters the calls may be overwhelming. Select those patients whose lives can be saved by quick action, setting aside for the moment those requiring too much time and those whose lives are not endangered. This often agonizing series of decisions is called 'triage' (Old French: *trier* = to pick, select).

Insight

The solution to a puzzle often appears apparently spontaneously as the result of a shift in the way that the problem is viewed. For this reason, when time permits, put aside the subject when an impasse is reached and reconsider it later. Remarkably, your conclusions may have altered. Discuss it with someone else if possible, since laying out the problem often clarifies your views.

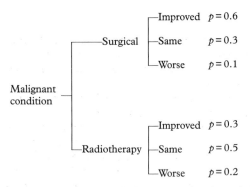

Fig. 5.1   A simple decision tree comparing the probability
(*p*) of outcomes for two methods of treating a malignant
condition.

Decision tree

In limited areas reliable information exists on outcomes
in well-defined circumstances, allowing comparisons of
differing treatments. For example, suppose a malignant
condition might be amenable to operation or radiotherapy. If reliable reports are available on outcome, a
decision tree can be constructed with the probability of
the patient being better, the same or worse after a defined
interval. All the probable outcomes for a particular
course of action should add up to 1 (Fig. 5.1). However,
each outcome has a subjective value, called a 'utility'. A
high utility value indicates a desirable result, a low value
indicates an undesirable result. The utility is multiplied
by the probability to produce an 'expected utility'. The
sums of the expected utilities for each or all the possible
courses of action can be compared. The course of action
gaining the highest expected utility should be the preferred one (Fig. 5.2).

Objective evidence that can be constructed in this way

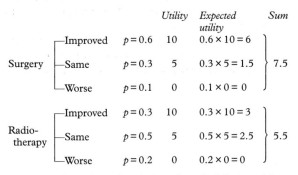

Fig. 5.2   The utility (subjective benefit or disability) resulting
from the outcome is graded from 10 (good) to 0 (bad). The
product of probability (*p*) and utility is the 'expected utility'.
Finally, the sum of the expected utilities for each decision can
be compared. The course scoring the highest mark is the
preferred one, in this case, surgery.

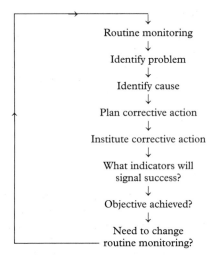

Fig. 5.3   The essential part played by planned monitoring
after taking a decision and acting on it. There is no point at
which this can be relaxed until the patient is fully recovered.
As the circumstances change and effective action is taken, the
response must be checked and, when correction is achieved,
routine monitoring must be continued.

may be difficult to accumulate. However, the considerations that go into the construction of a decision
tree make a worthwhile exercise when trying to decide
between courses of action. The patient's view of 'utility'
may differ from yours, and must be included in the
equation.

Provisional decisions

All decisions must be provisional. They rest on incomplete knowledge and on the interpretation of events at
the time they are made. The situation may alter rapidly
due to progression of the presenting condition and to
the effects of your management. The initial plan may be
called the 'strategy'. By monitoring and responding to
the situation you alter the tactics. Too often, initially
good management fails because it is not reviewed and
revised in the light of subsequent changes. Decide what
needs to be monitored as an indicator of deterioration
and recovery (Fig. 5.3). Be willing to accept early that
your actions are incorrect, and change tactics. Most
people find the admission of error to be painful and few
will not, for this reason, accept that they have made a
mistake. Such people should not take up a surgical
career.

Anticipation

Actively look for predictable features that will affect your decisions. After selecting a course of action, do not totally reject the ones you have passed over. Consider the ill-effects your action may produce if you have misjudged the condition, and be ready to change it if necessary. Your management may, of itself, produce predictable effects that should be anticipated, recognized, and corrected if necessary.

Preparation

Standard reactions are appropriate in certain conditions. When they have gained general approval they are often produced as 'protocols', or sets of rules. Examples are the management of respiratory obstruction, cardiac arrest and external haemorrhage. Of course, standard management will not save everyone and indeed may rarely be inappropriate. Nevertheless, such routines are likely to save the greatest number of lives. Whenever you can identify a routine reaction that is safe and acceptable, learn it and practise using it. Regrettably, many medical practitioners prove to be inexpert when tested in procedures such as administering cardiac resuscitation.

Personal and acquired experience

In the distant past clinicians based their decisions on their own experience, supplemented by advice from those colleagues with whom they came into contact. Their reaction to a condition was determined by what they had seen or heard previously. With the availability of written treatises they were given access to wider experience. We are fortunate in being able to survey the accumulated experience of our colleagues throughout the world. However, it remains our own responsibility to view what we read critically. The validity of a report must be judged on the clarity and logic of the investigation and the soundness of the interpretation. It is not always necessary to be a competent statistician to detect flaws in the construction of an experiment or the conclusions drawn from the findings (see Ch. 36).

Personal audit

Whether or not others review your results, make sure that you look back on your successes and failures. A successful outcome does not necessarily signify that you have acted wisely, nor does failure necessarily denote that your actions were at fault. Sometimes you conclude that the patient has recovered in spite of errors in your management. At other times you may console yourself that your decisions were correct but the problems were overwhelming or there were factors which you could not be aware of. Identify, admit and learn from your mistakes. Some people, claiming to be experienced, have merely repeated the same mistakes over a long period. Remember the statement of the novelist, Thomas Hardy: 'Experience is as to intensity, not as to duration'.

Essentials for good decisions

1. Identify the discriminating features which override less reliable, perhaps contradictory, features.

2. Do not be obsessed with your personal, perhaps limited, experience, which may not be typical.

3. Critically read the surgical literature to determine the best action to take in standard circumstances. Keep up to date, since evidence gathered at one time is not necessarily of permanent value, as fresh assessments are made.

4. If you make a decision to act, do not continue doggedly with it. The decision only applies at the time that it was made.

5. Constantly monitor the condition of the patient to note the effect of the action and be ready to change course if necessary.

6. Whenever you have a difficult decision to make ask yourself: 'If my selected course of management fails, can I justify it to the patient, to my peers and, most importantly, to myself?'

7. Do not be too proud to ask advice. Outlining the problem to a colleague often clarifies your own thoughts.

8. Learn from your mistakes – and your successes.

6. Influence of coexisting disease

R. M. Jones

About half of adult patients presenting to the surgeon will have a coexisting disease unrelated to the pathological process necessitating surgery. The proportion is increased in the elderly and patients presenting for emergency surgery. The morbidity and mortality associated with surgery and anaesthesia are increased in patients with coexisting disease and the more significant the coexisting disease the greater the risk (Buck et al 1987, Campling et al 1993). The medical diagnoses most commonly associated with an increase in surgical morbidity and mortality are:

- Ischaemic heart disease
- Congestive cardiac failure
- Arterial hypertension
- Chronic respiratory disease
- Diabetes mellitus
- Cardiac arrhythmias
- Anaemia.

It can be seen that pre-existing cardiac-related problems account for the most significant increase in operative risk. The aims of management of patients presenting for surgery with pre-existing medical disease(s) are three-fold:

- To diagnose the presence of pre-existing medical disease and make an accurate assessment of the degree of the problem
- To ensure that the patient's medical condition is optimized before surgery
- To consider the potential for drug interactions arising from the use of anaesthetic and other drugs administered in the operative and perioperative period with those that the patient is taking long term.

The National Confidential Enquiry into Perioperative Deaths for 1990 (Campling et al 1992) emphasized the importance of discussion between surgeon and anaesthetist before a decision to proceed in a particular patient. All patients presenting for surgery should have a full clinical history and examination performed, including details of concurrent drug therapy, previous medical history and history of allergy. Depending on the nature of the coexisting medical disease and that of the planned surgery, additional specialized investigations may subsequently be needed. Young (<45 years), fit patients undergoing minor elective surgery do not need routine blood haematology or chemistry, a chest X-ray or an electrocardiogram (ECG).

CARDIOVASCULAR DISEASE

Coronary artery disease

Coronary atherosclerosis is the commonest type of cardiovascular disease; it is probably the single most common underlying factor in the production of operative morbidity and mortality (Aitkenhead et al 1989). The preoperative evaluation must include an assessment of diseases associated with the development of coronary atherosclerosis, e.g. systemic arterial hypertension, diabetes mellitus and smoking. The degree of activity that precipitates symptoms of myocardial ischaemia must be assessed and the presence or absence of congestive heart failure should be noted (does the patient also become breathless on exertion?). Patients with a degree of heart failure in addition to ischaemia have often had a previous myocardial infarction and may be taking digoxin. Concurrent drug therapy should be noted and, almost without exception, this should be continued until the time of surgery (see Concurrent drug therapy, p. 80). The drugs most frequently encountered are:

- Nitrates (e.g. glyceryl trinitrate)
- β-Adrenergic antagonists
- Calcium antagonists
- Angiotensin enzyme converting inhibitors
- Digoxin.

It is important to remember that the preoperative ECG is normal in 20–50% of patients with proven ischaemia. Smokers should be encouraged to stop smoking at least

4-6 weeks

12 hours before surgery in order to decrease the percentage of carboxyhaemoglobin present in the blood and to minimize the cardiovascular side-effects of nicotine. It is also important to differentiate chest pain of gastro-intestinal origin (e.g. hiatus hernia) from ischaemic cardiac pain. This may necessitate a specialist opinion and subsequent investigations such as a thallium scan.

The basis of management depends on the fact that myocardial ischaemia will occur whenever the balance between myocardial oxygen supply and demand is disturbed such that demand exceeds supply. The major determinants of myocardial oxygen supply are:

- The coronary perfusion pressure (the aortic diastolic pressure minus the left ventricular end-diastolic pressure)
- Diastolic time.

The major determinants of myocardial oxygen demand are:

- Increasing heart rate
- Increasing inotropic state
- Afterload, which is the impedance to left ventricular ejection (the systemic arterial pressure is an approximate determinant of afterload)
- Preload, which is the left ventricular end-diastolic pressure.

In the perioperative period factors that decrease supply and/or increase demand must be avoided. It can be seen that an increase in heart rate and an increase in preload will be especially deleterious as they will increase myocardial oxygen demand and decrease myocardial oxygen supply. During the perioperative period a decrease in systemic arterial pressure to a significant degree (a decrease in diastolic pressure greater than 20% of the patient's normal resting diastolic pressure is a useful guide) must not be allowed to occur because this decreases coronary perfusion pressure, which is very poorly tolerated in patients with multiple sites of coronary artery narrowing. Good pain management post-operatively is essential, as the presence of pain will lead to hypertension and tachycardia. This may mean referring the patient to the hospital's acute-pain team. In addition, after major surgery especially intra-abdominal or intrathoracic, supplemental oxygen should be administered for 24 hours and consideration given to providing supplemental oxygen overnight for the first 4 post-operative days.

Arterial hypertension

Moderate or marked, long-standing, untreated hypertension increases perioperative morbidity and mortality, and is a significant risk factor for the production of coronary atherosclerosis. Patients with sustained systemic arterial hypertension (systolic >160 mmHg, diastolic >110 mmHg) should be satisfactorily stabilized on antihypertensive therapy before elective surgery of any type or duration. The untreated or inadequately treated hypertensive responds in an exaggerated manner to the stress of surgery, with a resultant increase in operative morbidity and mortality. Patients with long-standing moderate to marked hypertension should be assumed to have coronary atherosclerosis, even in the absence of overt signs and/or symptoms of ischaemic heart disease, and managed appropriately. Antihypertensive therapy is associated with its own unique considerations for anaesthetic and surgical management, the specific issues depending upon the medication the patient is taking (see Concurrent drug therapy, p. 80).

Heart failure

This implies an inadequacy of heart muscle secondary to intrinsic disease or overloading. The latter may be due to an increase in volume (an increase in intravascular volume or valve incompetence) or pressure (systemic arterial hypertension or aortic stenosis). It is usual for one ventricle to fail before the other, but disorders that damage or overload the left ventricle are more common (e.g. ischaemic heart disease and systemic arterial hypertension), and hence symptoms attributable to pulmonary congestion are usually the presenting ones. Left ventricular failure is the most common cause of right ventricular failure and if this supervenes dyspnoea may actually decrease as right ventricular output decreases, leading to a reduction in pulmonary congestion. Conventionally, congestive heart failure refers to the combination of left and right ventricular failure with evidence of (and symptoms relating to) systemic and pulmonary venous hypertension. Physiologically, heart failure may be thought of as the failure of the heart to match its output in order to meet the body's metabolic needs. Treatment is aimed at normalizing this imbalance. Thus, cardiac output can be improved or metabolic needs decreased. Traditionally, digitalis glycosides have been thought of as mediating their beneficial effects by improving cardiac output. Vasodilators can also be used to decrease peripheral demand.

In the preparation of the patient before surgery, digitilization remains the basis of treatment for the patient in heart failure (although its value in failure that is predominantly right sided is open to question). Digitilization is particularly indicated in patients with atrial fibrillation or flutter, and when congestive heart failure is marked or of recent onset. Diuretics still have a role, but with the increase in use of vasodilators this is a diminishing one. The operative mortality and morbidity of patients with well-compensated heart failure is small; however, surgery in the presence of decompensated heart failure is associated with a particularly high mortality and, if the operation cannot be delayed, peri- and intraoperative haemodynamic monitoring should be comprehensive. For major surgery this would indicate the use of a balloon-tipped pulmonary artery catheter; measurement of cardiac output and pulmonary capillary wedge pressure (a determinant of left ventricular preload) will allow the construction of ventricular function curves to guide in the selection of appropriate cardiovascular therapy. Postoperative admission to a high-dependency unit or an intensive-care facility (with the ability to measure and adjust preload, afterload and cardiac output) is indicated.

Congenital heart disease

Eisenmenger's syndrome is the commonest form of symptomatic congenital heart disease seen in adult patients. This consists of pulmonary hypertension with a reversed or bidirectional shunt usually through a large atrial or ventricular septal defect. Patients have a very high pulmonary vascular resistance and this renders the underlying defect inoperable (short of heart/lung transplantation), although they may live for many years and patients up to the age of 50 or 60 years may be encountered who present for incidental non-cardiac surgery. Systemic arterial hypotension in the perioperative period will increase right-to-left shunting and worsen hypoxia. Other problems include air embolus during surgery as well as postoperative thrombo-embolism and infective endocarditis. Because of the danger of life-threatening haemoptysis, patients are usually not taking prophylactic anticoagulants. However, preoperative subcutaneous heparin is usually safe, and early ambulation should be encouraged to minimize the risks of thromboembolism. All patients should receive prophylactic antibiotics. During the siting of intravenous lines it is important to avoid getting air in the tubing.

Acquired valvular heart disease

Mitral stenosis

This is nearly always of rheumatic origin, but symptoms do not appear until the valve area is reduced to less than 2.5 cm^2, i.e. half the normal valve area. This may take 20 years following the episode of rheumatic fever. As valve area decreases below 2 cm^2, an increase in left atrial pressure is required at rest to maintain cardiac output. A valve area below 1 cm^2 is classified as severe mitral stenosis and is associated with a left atrial pressure in excess of 20 mmHg, and even at rest cardiac output may be barely adequate; there is pulmonary hypertension. Eventually right ventricular failure supervenes and atrial fibrillation is common. Patients with mild to moderate mitral stenosis and sinus rhythm tolerate surgery well. All patients should receive antibiotic prophylaxis. Fluid balance should be carefully monitored, as overtransfusion may precipitate pulmonary oedema whereas undertransfusion will compromise left ventricular filling. Similarly, changes in heart rate are poorly tolerated, and during surgery the anaesthetist will use a technique which minimizes changes in cardiac parameters. If major surgery is to be undertaken, with the possibility of large blood loss, consideration should be given to monitoring pulmonary capillary wedge pressure by means of a balloon-tipped flow-directed catheter. Unless the patient is taking oral anticoagulants a local anaesthetic technique may be used for surgery, but a high spinal or epidural block may be associated with adverse cardiovascular effects (systemic arterial hypotension) and should be employed with caution.

Patients who are dyspnoeic at rest and have a fixed and reduced cardiac output present a significant risk during surgery. Digoxin should be continued up until the time of operation and plasma electrolytes checked, as hypokalaemia will increase the incidence of cardiac rhythm disturbances. These patients may have to be ventilated electively postoperatively.

Aortic stenosis

Valvular aortic stenosis is commonest in elderly males, although it may occur at any time of life. The aetiology is diverse and includes congenital, rheumatic, senile and mixed forms. It must be remembered that it is most common in patients in whom the incidence of ischaemic heart disease is also high. As in mitral stenosis, moderate degrees of stenosis of the aortic valve do not appreciably increase the risks of surgery. However, severe aortic stenosis is associated with an increased perioperative morbidity and mortality. Systemic arterial hypotension must be avoided at all times, because it will compromise coronary perfusion. Thus, peripheral vasodilatation, hypovolaemia and myocardial depression are all poorly tolerated. A change in cardiac rhythm is also poorly tolerated, as the atrial component to ventricular filling is essential to maintain normal cardiac output. For major procedures it is advisable to monitor left ventricular filling pressure, as higher than normal filling pressures are needed to maintain cardiac output.

Table 6.1 Cardiomyopathies: diagnosis and treatment

	Congestive (dilated)	Hypertrophic (obstructive)	Restrictive
Presenting signs/symptoms	Heart failure	Syncope	Heart failure
	Rhythm disturbance	Dyspnoea	Eosinophilia
	Systemic emboli	Angina Rhythm disturbance Systolic murmur appearing during long-standing hypertension	
Treatment	Diuretics Vasodilators Antiarrhythmics Anticoagulants	Antiarrhythmics β-Adrenergic antagonists Anticoagulants	Steroids Cytotoxic agents

Cardiomyopathies

Using echocardiography, three principal forms of cardiomyopathy are described:

1. Congestive or dilated cardiomyopathy: this may be associated with toxic, metabolic, neurological and inflammatory diseases. There is decrease in contractile force of the left or right ventricle, resulting in heart failure.

2. Hypertrophic or obstructive cardiomyopathy: this is an autosomal dominantly inherited condition, in which there is hypertrophy and fibrosis which mainly affects the interventricular septum, but may involve the whole of the left ventricle.

3. Restrictive cardiomyopathy: this is a rare form of cardiomyopathy and the main feature is the loss of ventricular distensibility due to endocardial or myocardial disease. Restrictive cardiomyopathy in many ways resembles constrictive pericarditis, and the endocardial disease may produce thromboembolic problems.

Table 6.1 summarizes the treatment and management of these patients.

Disturbances of cardiac rhythm

Atrial fibrillation

This is the most commonly encountered disturbance of cardiac rhythm and it is important to define the disease process causing the fibrillation. These are:

- Ischaemic heart disease
- Rheumatic heart disease, especially mitral stenosis
- Pulmonary embolism
- Bronchial carcinoma
- Thyrotoxicosis
- Thoracotomy.

If there appears to be no underlying cause, the rhythm disturbance is usually termed 'lone atrial fibrillation'. The atrial discharge rate is usually between 400 and 600 impulses per minute, but the atrioventricular (AV) node cannot conduct all these impulses, so that some fail to reach the ventricle or only partially penetrate the node, and this results in a block or delay to succeeding impulses. Ventricular response is therefore irregular, but seldom more than 200 impulses per minute; the use of drugs or the presence of disease of the AV node often causes the response rate to be lower than this. The medical management of patients with atrial fibrillation must include the management of the underlying cause of the rhythm disturbance. It is important to ensure that the fibrillation is well controlled, i.e. that the response rate of the ventricle is not too rapid. Digitalis alkaloids remain the primary method of slowing AV nodal conduction, but if these fail to control the response rate, verapamil or β-adrenergic antagonists are usually effective. If surgery is urgent the latter may be given by slow intravenous injection (e.g. using propranolol, administering 1-mg aliquots every 2–3 minutes to a maximum of 10 mg with the aim of decreasing the ventricular response rate to less than 100 beats per minute).

Intravenously administered verapamil should not be used in conjunction with β-adrenergic antagonists as this may precipitate complete heart block. Occasionally, cardioversion will restore sinus rhythm, although this is unusual if the atrial fibrillation is of long standing.

Atrial flutter

The causes of this disturbance of cardiac rhythm are similar to those of atrial fibrillation, and the perioperative considerations are principally those of the underlying disease process. Atrial flutter is less commonly seen than atrial fibrillation. Although control of ventricular rate is more difficult in flutter, unlike fibrillation cardioversion is often successful. In patients with a very rapid ventricular rate, verapamil administered intravenously will often reduce the rate and may be used in an emergency; occasionally it will restore sinus rhythm.

Heart block

There are two basic types of heart block:

- Atrioventricular heart block
- Intraventricular conduction defects.

Atrioventricular heart block. This may be incomplete (first- or second-degree AV block) or complete (third-degree AV block). In first-degree heart block the PR interval of the ECG exceeds 0.21 seconds, but there are no dropped beats and the QRS complex is normal. It does not always imply significant underlying heart disease, but is seen in patients on digitalis therapy. It is important not to expose the patient to any drug in the perioperative period which will further decrease AV nodal conduction (e.g. halothane anaesthesia, β-adrenergic antagonists or verapamil).

There are two types of second-degree heart block: Mobitz types 1 and 2. Mobitz type 1 block is also known as the 'Wenckebach phenomenon' and this is usually associated with ischaemia of the AV node or the effects of digitalis. There is a progressive increase in the length of the PR interval until the impulse fails to excite the ventricle and a beat is dropped. As a generalization, patients with this type of heart block do not require a pacemaker prior to surgery, and should it be necessary the administration of atropine will often establish normal AV conduction. Mobitz type 2 block is less common than type 1; it is a more serious form of conduction defect and may be a forerunner to complete AV block. The atrial rate is normal and the ventricular rate depends on the number of dropped beats, but it is commonly 35–50 beats per minute. The net result is that of an irregular pulse. The ECG indicates that there are more P waves then QRS complexes, but the PR interval, if present, is normal. It is probably acceptable to undertake minor surgery in patients with Mobitz type 2 block without the need for the insertion of a prophylactic pacemaker. However, in these circumstances drugs such as atropine and isoprenaline should be immediately at hand, and the means for temporary pacing should be available. Prophylactic pacemaker insertion is indicated for major surgery, especially if this is likely to result in significant blood loss and associated haemodynamic instability.

Third-degree heart block is also termed 'complete heart block'. It may result from conduction defects located within the AV node, bundle of His, or the bundle branch and Purkinje fibres. An escape pacemaker emerges at a site distal to the block (e.g. if the impulses are blocked within the AV node, the bundle of His usually emerges as the subsidiary pacemaker). In general, the more distal the site of the escape pacemaker, the more likely is the patient to suffer symptoms such as dyspnoea, syncope or congestive heart failure and to need permanent ventricular pacemaker therapy. Pacemaker therapy is always indicated before surgery, although in emergency situations (such as complete heart block appearing intraoperatively) various drugs may be tried to increase the heart rate. Atropine may be of value if the escape pacemaker is junctional. Isoprenaline may be of value if the escape pacemaker is more distal.

Intraventricular conduction defects. Left bundle branch block is always associated with heart disease. The QRS complex is wide (>0.12 seconds). A hemiblock occurs if only one of the two major subdivisions (anterior and posterior) of the left bundle is blocked. The QRS complex is not prolonged in left hemiblocks. Left anterior or posterior hemiblock may occur with right bundle branch block and it is generally considered that left anterior plus right bundle branch block is not an indication for temporary pacemaker therapy before surgery, but that left posterior plus right bundle branch block is an indication for a pacemaker. The latter patients are at risk of developing complete heart block. Right bundle branch block is not invariably associated with underlying heart disease. The principal significance lies in its association with a left posterior hemiblock, as there is then a risk of complete heart block; in these patients a temporary pacemaker is indicated before surgery and anaesthesia.

Pacemakers

The patient with a pacemaker can safely undergo surgery and anaesthesia, but it is important to review the medical condition that gave rise to the need for pacemaker therapy. The usual indications for a pacemaker are:

- Congenital or acquired complete heart block
- Sick sinus syndrome
- Bradycardia, associated with syncope and/or hypotension.

Acquired complete heart block is probably the commonest indication, the underlying cause for this usually being ischaemic heart disease. The patient should be specifically asked about the return of symptoms such as syncope, which may indicate that the pacemaker is failing to capture the ventricle (or atria if an atrial pace-maker is present). The heart rate should be within a couple of beats per minute of the pacemaker's original setting. It is important to determine the type of pacemaker that has been implanted and the time when it was put in.

All patients with pacemakers are normally reviewed regularly in a pacemaker clinic. Whenever a pacemaker is in situ, atropine, adrenaline and isoprenaline should be available for use in the event of pacemaker failure. During surgery, diathermy is usually safe, but some precautions are needed (Simon 1977):

- The indifferent electrode of the diathermy should be placed on the same side as the operating site and as far away from the pacemaker as possible
- The use of diathermy should be limited to short bursts of 1–2 seconds at intervals not greater than every 10 seconds
- The anaesthetist should check the patient's pulse when the diathermy is used for inhibition of pacemaker function (Simon 1977, Aitkenhead & Barnett 1989).

RESPIRATORY DISEASE

Asthma

Patients with asthma have bronchospasm, mucus plugging of airways and air trapping. These result in a mismatch of ventilation and perfusion and total effective ventilation may be severely impaired. A number of exogenous and endogenous stimuli may produce reversible airway obstruction. The most active chemical mediators are histamine and the leukotrienes. Expiration is prolonged, functional residual capacity and residual volumes are increased and vital capacity is decreased. Bronchospasm may be aggravated by anxiety, by instrumentation of the upper airway, by foreign material or irritants in the upper airway, by pain, and by drugs. The latter include morphine, papaveretum, unselective β-adrenergic antagonists, and various anaesthetic drugs including tubocurarine and antocholinesterases. In taking the clinical history, special attention should be paid to factors which precipitate an attack, and the patient's normal drug therapy should be reviewed. If possible, the timing of surgery should be arranged to coincide with a period of remission of symptoms. The patient's normal bronchodilator therapy should be continued up until the time of surgery, and consideration should be given to the provision of preoperative chest physiotherapy. It is important to allay preoperative anxiety, and suitable premedication should be prescribed. Diazepam, pethidine, promethazine and atro-

pine are free from bronchospastic activity. If the patient is taking steroid therapy, additional doses may be needed during the perioperative period (see Concurrent drug therapy, p. 80). In the postoperative period, careful attention should be paid to pain management, together with the use of nebulized or intravenous bronchodilators if this is necessary. Local anaesthetic techniques are often suitable in the severe asthmatic undergoing suitable surgery and appropriate techniques can be used to provide postoperative analgesia (e.g. epidural blocks). In the perioperative period, the following are indications for the use of intermittent positive pressure ventilation in asthmatics:

- Distress and exhaustion
- Systemic arterial hypotension or significant disturbance of cardiac rhythm
- An arterial oxygen tension of less than 6.7 kPa or an arterial carbon dioxide tension of greater than 6.7 kPa, associated with an increasing metabolic acidosis in the face of maximum medical therapy.

Chronic bronchitis and emphysema

A patient with chronic bronchitis will have had a cough with sputum production on most days for 3 months of the year for at least 2 years. The patient with emphysema will have destruction of alveoli distal to the terminal bronchioles and loss of pulmonary elastic tissue. Patients with chronic bronchitis are often smokers (see below), and have irritable airways leading to coughing and some degree of reversible airways obstruction in response to minimal stimulation. Patients with emphysema experience airway closure with air trapping and, therefore, inefficient gaseous exchange. Chronic bronchitis and emphysema commonly coexist in the same patient. Many of the considerations in the perioperative period that apply to the asthmatic patient also apply to patients with chronic bronchitis and emphysema; there are, however, some additional points to note. These diseases are usually slowly progressive and may eventually result in a respiratory reserve which is so low that the patient is immobile and dyspnoeic at rest, and even speaking and eating may be difficult. It is important that elective surgery should take place during the months in which symptoms are least noticeable; this is usually during the summer. Every effort should be made to persuade smokers to quit their habit. If the patient requires major surgery, and if the disease is severe, elective tracheostomy and postoperative ventilation may be called for. These will facilitate the clearing of secretions, and thus gaseous exchange, during the postoperative period when diaphragmatic splinting and pain or respiratory depression may cause acute respiratory insufficiency.

Smoking

Cigarette smoking has wide-ranging effects on the cardio-respiratory and immune systems and on haemostasis (Jones 1985). It is a common cause of perioperative morbidity, and smokers have about six times the incidence of postoperative respiratory complications compared with non-smokers. Smokers may have arterial carbon monoxide concentrations in excess of 5%; the resultant carboxyhaemoglobin decreases the amount of haemoglobin available for combination with oxygen, and inhibits the ability of haemoglobin to give up oxygen (i.e. the oxygen dissociation curve is shifted to the left). Carbon monoxide also has a negative inotropic effect. Nicotine increases heart rate and systemic arterial blood pressure. Thus, carbon monoxide decreases oxygen supply, while nicotine increases oxygen demand and this is of particular significance in patients with ischaemic heart disease. In these patients, it is especially important that patients stop smoking for 12–24 hours before surgery; this will result in a significant improvement in cardiovascular function (the elimination half-lives of carbon monoxide and nicotine are a few hours).

However, the respiratory effect of smoking, especially mucus hypersecretion, impairment of tracheobronchial clearance, and small airway narrowing take at least 6 weeks before there is any improvement in function after smoking cessation. Similarly, the effects of smoking on immune function (smokers are more susceptible to postoperative infections) require at least 6 weeks before improvement occurs. Many smokers will complain that they find it difficult to clear their mucus if they stop smoking, and will use this as an excuse not to stop smoking before surgery; there may be some substance to this claim, but it does not outweigh the benefits of stopping. It is important that the risks of smoking are emphasized to smokers, and they should be encouraged to stop smoking for as long as possible before elective surgery.

ENDOCRINE DYSFUNCTION

Thyroid gland

Excluding diabetes, disorders involving the thyroid gland account for about 80% of endocrine disease. There are two practical issues for the surgeon and anaesthetist. Firstly, there are problems related to the local effects of a mass in the neck. These include airway problems and the potential for difficult tracheal intubation. Secondly, there are problems associated with the generalized effects of an excess or deficiency of hormone. Patients with hyperthyroidism must be made euthyroid and properly prepared before surgery. Propylthiouracil (average daily dose 300 mg) inhibits hormone synthesis and blocks the peripheral conversion of thyroxine to triiodothyronine. As a generalization, the larger the gland the longer it takes to achieve the euthyroid state. The vascularity of the gland can be considerably decreased by 7 days' treatment with potassium iodide solution. Propranolol is an alternative treatment to thiouracil, and 60–120 mg daily for 2 weeks may be the only treatment required, and is now routinely used at many centres.

The management of the properly prepared patient should cause few problems. An emergency operation in a poorly or non-prepared patient is associated with significant risk and should be avoided if possible. Cardiovascular complications are potentially life-threatening and intravenous propranolol should be considered before induction of anaesthesia (using 0.5–1.0 mg increments every 5 minutes to decrease the resting heart rate by 10 beats per minute). Disturbances of cardiac rhythm, hypoxia and hyperthermia may all occur. If appropriate, a local anaesthetic technique may be the method of choice. Hypothyroidism is not uncommon, especially in elderly patients. Cardiac output is low and blood loss is poorly tolerated. However, blood transfusion must be given with caution in order to avoid overloading the circulation. It has been said that in hypothyroidism the respiratory centre is less responsive to hypoxia and hypercarbia, so that it may be necessary to ventilate patients electively in the postoperative period. These patients are especially sensitive to opioid analgesics and these should be used with caution in the perioperative period. The patient's temperature should be monitored and measures take to prevent hypothermia; hypothermia will aggravate the circulatory and respiratory depression.

Pituitary gland

In hypopituitarism, the varying involvement of the several hormones which the anterior pituitary produces leads to a variety of clinical presentations; amenorrhoea in females and impotence in males are common presenting features. If hypopituitarism is unrecognized, there is a greatly increased perioperative risk of hypoglycaemia, hypothermia, water intoxication and respiratory failure. If the diagnosis is known, planned substitution therapy is indicated before surgery. Oral hydrocortisone (15 mg twice daily) is administered. This is increased during the operative period; thyroxine is also given and the dose slowly increased to about

0.15 mg daily and the plasma thyroxine level is measured.

Acromegaly is caused by excessive production of pituitary growth hormone. This results in overgrowth of bone, leading to an enlarged jaw and kyphoscoliosis, as well as connective tissue and viscera. There is cardiomegaly, early atherosclerosis and systemic arterial hypertension, and diabetes mellitus is common. Management should include consideration of all associated conditions and the anaesthetist will carefully assess the patient, as tracheal intubation may be difficult.

Deficiency of antidiuretic hormone results in diabetes insipidus. A water deprivation test is used to differentiate diabetes insipidus from compulsive water drinking, and measurements are made of urine and plasma osmolarity. When the plasma osmolality reaches about 295 mOsmol kg normal patients will concentrate their urine, but patients with diabetes insipidus cannot do so. If the syndrome is differentiated from compulsive water drinking, the operative management of these patients is usually uncomplicated. The patient should receive a bolus of 100 milliunits of vasopressin intravenously before surgery and during the operation 100 milli units h^{-1} are administered by continuous infusion. Isotonic solutions, such as 0.9% sodium chloride, may then be administered with minimal risk of water depletion or hypernatraemia. Plasma osmolality should be monitored perioperatively (the normal range is 283–285 mOsmol kg).

Adrenal gland

Adrenocorticol insufficiency is known as Addison's disease. It may present in acute and chronic forms and may be due to disease of the gland itself or to disorders of the anterior pituitary or hypothalamus. A patient with adrenocortical insufficiency undergoing surgery presents a major problem. The cardiovascular status of the patient and the blood glucose and electrolytes must be measured. The patient is prepared by infusing isotonic sodium chloride and glucose solutions, in order to correct hypernatraemia and hypoglycaemia. The day before surgery, an intramuscular injection of 40 mg methylprednisolone is administered. Before induction of anaesthesia a further 100 mg hydrocortisone is administered, and for major surgery an infusion of hydrocortisone should be given during the operation. Hydrocortisone has approximately equal glucocorticoid and mineralocorticoid effects. Postoperatively, the dose of hydrocortisone is decreased from 100 mg twice daily to a replacement dose of about 50 mg daily.

Adrenocorticol hyperfunction is commonly iatrogenic. Whatever the aetiology, these patients will have glucose intolerance manifest as hyperglycaemia or frank diabetes mellitus, systemic arterial hypertension (possibly associated with heart failure) and electrolyte disturbances, especially hypokalkaemia and hypernatraemia. Protein breakdown leads to muscle weakness and osteoporosis. Muscle weakness will be aggravated by obesity, and respiratory function should be carefully assessed before surgery, as well as postoperatively. Osteoporosis may lead to vertebral compression fractures and patients should be positioned during surgery with great care. Prolonged immobilization after surgery will lead to further demineralization of bone, and hypercalcaemia may lead to the formation of renal calculi. Vitamin D therapy may therefore be needed in the postoperative period.

Aldosteronism may be primary (an adrenocortical adenoma – Conn's syndrome), or secondary, in which the condition is associated with an increase of plasma renin secretion (e.g. the nephrotic syndrome and cardiac failure). Patients will have hypokalaemia and hypernatraemia, which may be associated with systemic arterial hypertension. If the diagnosis is made before surgery, the administration of spironolactone (up to 300 mg daily) will reverse hypertension and hypokalaemia.

Phaeochromocytoma

These catecholamine-secreting tumours may produce sustained or intermittent arterial hypertension. During surgery, arterial hypertension and disturbances of cardiac rhythm are common, due to the release of adrenaline and noradrenaline into the circulation. Prolonged secretion of these produces not only arterial hypertension but also a contracted blood volume; α- and β-adrenergic blockade will help to reverse both these effects. It is important that preoperative α-adrenergic blockade is not complete, for the following reasons:

- It may cause preoperative postural syncope
- It may cause difficulties in controlling the profound hypotension that sometimes occurs after tumour removal
- A rise in systemic blood pressure on tumour palpation is a useful sign in searching for small tumours or metastases.

Phenoxybenzamine is the agent usually used to induce partial α-adrenergic blockade. Careful preoperative preparation using α- and β-adrenergic blockade, as well as the introduction of anaesthetic techniques that promote cardiovascular stability, have greatly decreased the mortality of patients undergoing surgery for removal of a phaeochromocytoma, from 30–45% in the early 1950s to less than 5% recently.

Pancreas

Diabetes mellitus

Even minor surgery is associated with an increase in basal metabolic rate and protein breakdown with nitrogen loss and some degree of glucose intolerance. Thus, surgery in a patient with pre-existing glucose intolerance, whether this is known or not, will further exacerbate metabolic derangement. Diabetes is also a potent risk factor in the development of coronary artery disease and patients may have diabetic neuropathy which may cause autonomic nervous system dysfunction, leading to a lability in arterial blood pressure. Before surgery, the cardiovascular status of the patient should be carefully reviewed and the blood pressure taken both supine and erect to test for the possibility of autonomic neuropathy; the preoperative control of blood glucose is assessed and should be adequate. In the perioperative period it is important to monitor the patient by estimating blood glucose concentrations, rather than urinary glucose measurements, which are too insensitive for appropriate surgical patient management. It is important to treat ketoacidosis before surgery, including urgent surgery, if at all possible. Sepsis markedly increases insulin requirements. Patients undergoing cardiac bypass surgery may also have increased insulin requirements.

Table 6.2 summarizes the regimes suitable for minor and more major surgery in diabetics that are either controlled by diet alone, by oral hypoglycaemic agents, or with insulin.

Chlorpropamide is a sulphonylurea with a very long duration of action, and hypoglycaemia is a particular concern in patients taking this agent; it should be stopped 48 hours before planned surgery and the blood sugar measured regularly after the patient becomes nil by mouth.

Patients taking long-acting insulin preparations should be converted to Actrapid insulin (8 hourly, using the same total insulin dose), and surgery should be scheduled for the early morning if possible. A number of regimes for the infusion of dextrose–insulin have been described, but the common aim is to maintain the blood glucose at $6-12$ mmol l^{-1}. One method is to add 10 mmol of KCl and 6–12 units Actrapid insulin (the precise dose depending upon the blood sugar measured 1 hour before surgery) to 500 ml of 5% dextrose and to give 100 ml h^{-1} starting half an hour before surgery,. The blood sugar is measured at least 2 hourly during surgery and the amount of insulin adjusted to maintain the blood sugar between 6 and 12 mmol l^{-1}. Following surgery blood sugar and plasma potassium are measured at least 4 hourly.

Postoperatively, as soon as the patient starts eating, those who are normally treated with oral hypoglycaemics may need subcutaneous insulin for a few days before oral therapy is recommended. Patients normally treated with insulin can be converted to 8-hourly Actrapid insulin to a total equal to the normal preoperative dose. After 3 days the original regime can usually be restarted (i.e. using long-acting insulins). In the perioperative period lactate-containing fluids (e.g. Hartmann's solution) should be avoided in diabetics. If oral feeding has not started within 72 hours of surgery, consideration should be given to the institution of parenteral nutrition.

Obesity

Life expectancy is decreased by obesity, and operative morbidity and mortality increase with increasing weight. In moderate obesity, the patient presenting for surgery should be instructed to decrease weight and given dietary advice appropriate to the patient's social and

Table 6.2 Severity of diabetes

	Type of surgery	
	Minor	Intermediate/major
Controlled by diet	No specific precautions	Measure blood glucose 4-hourly: if >12 mmol l^{-1} start dextrose–insulin infusion. Avoid i.v. dextrose
Controlled by oral agents	Omit medication on morning of operation and start when eating normally postoperatively	Omit medication and monitor blood glucose 1–2 hourly; if >12 mmol l^{-1} start dextrose–insulin infusion
Controlled by insulin	Unless very minor procedure (omit insulin when nil by mouth) give dextrose–insulin infusion during surgery and until eating normally postoperatively	

economic circumstances. They should also be examined carefully for the presence of conditions with which obesity is commonly associated; these include diabetes mellitus and systemic arterial hypertension. Patients who are double or more their ideal weight are usually termed 'morbidly obese'. These patients present a number of problems to both surgeon and anaesthetist. Their preoperative cardiorespiratory status should be assessed carefully and, as these patients are at an increased risk of inhalation of gastric contents, all should receive appropriate antacid therapy before surgery. Obesity is one of a number of conditions that will lead to an increase in postoperative deep vein thrombosis and associated thromboembolic phenomena; obese patients should receive appropriate preoperative prophylaxis for this. Transport and positioning of morbidly obese patients may cause difficulties, and occasionally two standard operating tables used side by side may be needed. Intravenous access may be difficult, and non-invasive methods of monitoring arterial blood pressure may be inaccurate. Therefore, an intra-arterial line is indicated for all but the most minor procedures. This will also enable arterial blood gases to be monitored in the intra- and postoperative periods. Patients may need continued ventilatory support after surgery.

BLOOD DISORDERS

Primary blood disorders produce a wide range of clinical manifestations, which may affect any organ in the body. Conversely, there are nearly always some changes in the blood accompanying general medical and surgical disorders. Thus, haematological investigations form an important part of the assessment and subsequent monitoring of most disease processes.

Anaemia

This is defined clinically as a reduction in haemoglobin level below the normal range for the individual's age and sex. It becomes clinically apparent when the oxygen demand of the tissues cannot be met without the use of compensatory mechanisms. Although the level of haemoglobin at which elective surgery should be postponed will vary according to the precise medical status of the patient and the type of surgery planned, as a generalization a level of 10 g dl^{-1} is commonly accepted as one below which preoperative anaemia should be treated before surgery. It is important to realize that blood transfusion to raise the haematocrit should be carried out at least 48 hours before the preoperative procedure, as this period of time will allow full recovery of the stored erythrocytes' oxygen-carrying capacity. In order to min-

imize the risk of transmitting the human immuno-deficiency virus (HIV), blood transfusion should be undertaken only if the urgency of surgery necessitates this. Tissue oxygenation appears to be maximal at around a haemoglobin concentration of 11 g dl^{-1} (tissue oxygenation depends upon cardiac output, peripheral vascular resistance, blood viscosity and blood oxygen-carrying capacity). Patients with ischaemic heart disease are likely to suffer more from the consequences of decreased oxygen-carrying capacity from untreated anaemia, and it is especially important to treat preoperative anaemia in these patients.

Haemoglobinopathies

These are characterized by the presence of abnormal haemoglobins in the blood. Haemoglobin S is an abnormality in the amino acid sequence of the haemoglobin. When a deoxygenated haemoglobin molecule becomes distorted, this may lead to capillary occlusion and tissue hypoxia. The disease is inherited and it may be in the heterozygous or homozygous form. The former (HbAS) does not usually cause problems during surgery as the molecular distortion, known as 'sickling', only occurs at very low oxygen saturations. However, in the homozygous state (HbSS), there is a real risk of sickling during surgery and this may cause tissue infarction. Screening tests are available for the presence of haemoglobin S and electrophoresis is used to determine the exact nature of the abnormality. During surgery it is important to avoid low oxygen tensions and thus an elevated inspired oxygen concentration is used, and the patient is kept warm and well hydrated in order to maintain cardiac output and avoid circulatory stasis. If very major surgery is planned, where there is the possibility of perioperative hypoxia, for example pulmonary surgery, an exchange transfusion should be considered in an attempt to raise the levels of haemoglobin A to 40–50%. Patients with haemoglobin C and haemoglobin SC should be managed in a similar way to those with haemoglobin SS.

Bleeding and coagulation disorders

As a generalization, purpura, epistaxis and prolonged bleeding from superficial cuts are suggestive of a platelet abnormality and bleeding into joints or muscle is suggestive of a coagulation defect. Both forms may be congenital or acquired and it may be possible to differentiate these from the patient's history, a recent onset being indicative of an acquired disorder. A family history should be sought but it must be remembered that the absence of other relatives with a positive history does not exclude an hereditary bleeding diathesis (one-third of haemophilia patients show no family history). Many systemic diseases may be complicated by bleeding, as may treatment with a number of drugs which can cause bone marrow depression leading to thrombocytopenia.

Platelet disorders

Thrombocytopenia arises from a number of causes:

- Failure of megakaryocyte maturation
- Excessive platelet consumption
- Hypersplenism.

Bone marrow disorders leading to failure of maturation may be due to hypoplasia or infiltration. Increased consumption occurs in disseminated intravascular coagulation, idiopathic thrombocytopenic purpura and certain viral infections. Sequestration in an enlarged spleen occurs in lymphomas and liver disease. Spontaneous bleeding does not usually occur until the platelet count has decreased to $30 \times 10^9 \, l^{-1}$. Treatment has to be directed at the underlying disease, but thrombocytopenia resulting in clinically important bleeding necessitates a platelet transfusion. Ideally, the count should be increased to $100 \times 10^9 \, l^{-1}$, but transfusing platelets until a clinically acceptable effect is attained is often performed. Routine major surgery should not be undertaken in the presence of an abnormal platelet count until the result is confirmed and the cause identified.

Haemophilia

Before surgery in patients with haemophilia A or B the concentration of the coagulation factors should be increased to a level that will minimize bleeding, and this concentration should be maintained until healing has occurred. It is important to seek specialist advice in determining the dosage of factors required. Cryoprecipitate and fresh frozen plasma or factor IX fraction are used to manage bleeding episodes, but the patients should be tested for antibodies to the products. If these are present, only life-saving operations should be contemplated. If cryoprecipitate or freeze-dried factor IX concentrate are administered, complications include viral hepatitis and allergy, and adrenaline and hydrocortisone should always be immediately at hand during their administration.

RENAL DISEASE

Chronic renal failure

This is said to be present when chronic renal impairment, from whatever cause, results in abnormalities of plasma biochemistry. Usually, this happens when the glomerular filtration rate (GFR) has fallen to less than $30 \, ml \, min^{-1}$. Management before surgery depends on the severity of the renal failure. Patients in late and terminal degrees of chronic renal failure (GFR < $10 \, ml \, min^{-1}$) may already have commenced on dialysis. If not, dialysis should be performed before surgery if at all possible. Dialysis does not reverse all the adverse effects of chronic renal failure; for example, systemic arterial hypertension and pericarditis may still be present. In addition, patients who are dialysed very soon before surgery may have cardiovascular lability during anaesthesia and surgery because they may have a relatively contracted blood volume. These patients are also vulnerable to infection, anaemia, blood coagulation defects, electrolyte disturbances and psychological problems. It is important to define the degree of renal failure present before surgery, and review the dialysis regime. Blood biochemistry, coagulation and haemoglobin must be checked. There should be a careful assessment of cardiorespiratory function and the patient's normal medication should be reviewed. The latter may well include antihypertensive drugs (see Concurrent drug therapy, p. 80). A careful search should be made for the presence of occult infection and all patients should have a preoperative chest X-ray. The susceptibility to infection is compounded in transplant patients by the administration of immunosuppressive drugs, and prophylactic antibiotics may be necessary preoperatively and postoperatively. Chest physiotherapy may also be needed. Procedures such as arterial or central venous cannulation must be carried out under strict aseptic conditions. Before, during and after surgery, fluid and electrolyte balance must be very carefully monitored.

The nephrotic syndrome

The clinical association of heavy proteinuria, hypoalbuminaemia and generalized oedema is usually referred to as the 'nephrotic syndrome'. The hypoalbuminaemia is the result of urinary albumin loss and the syndrome becomes apparent if more than 5 g of protein are lost per day, and the plasma albumin concentration falls to less than $30 \, g \, l^{-1}$. It is important to define the underlying cause of the nephrotic syndrome. Before surgery, the plasma protein and electrolyte levels must be estimated and corrected as indicated. An albumin infusion (up to 50 g) will restore circulating blood volume and may in itself initiate a diuresis. An alteration in plasma proteins will cause changes in drug effect due to an alteration in drug binding. The anaesthetist may use more conservative doses of some drugs. Central venous cannulation is advisable for all but the most minor surgery.

HEPATOCELLULAR DISEASE

The patient with pre-existing liver disease is at an increased risk during surgery, especially if the pressure gradient across the liver is greater than 12 mmHg, suggesting a significant degree of portal hypertension. Perioperative mortality is probably in excess of 50% in the presence of marked ascites, raised bilirubin, reduced albumin (<25 g l^{-1}) and prolonged prothrombin time. In contrast to obstructive jaundice, if hepatocellular disease is responsible for decreased prothrombin synthesis, parenteral administration of vitamin K will not correct the situation. In patients with hepatocellular disease, the safety of hospital personnel must be borne in mind and all patients should be screened routinely for hepatitis B. Infection-control precautions should be instituted if this is positive. In the presence of excess bleeding, especially if clotting factors are known to be reduced preoperatively, fresh blood and plasma should be transfused. Blood should be given slowly in the presence of moderate to severe liver disease, because citrate clearance will be reduced. The presence of jaundice from whatever cause brings with it some specific problems in the operative period.

Obstructive jaundice

The haemoglobin of red cells is the major source of bilirubin. Jaundice due to biliary tract obstruction which decreases the gastrointestinal uptake of vitamin K will often cause a prolonged prothrombin time. This usually responds to intramuscular vitamin K, 10 mg daily for 2 days preoperatively. There is an increased incidence of postoperative renal failure in patients with preoperative jaundice. The precise cause is unclear; it may be due to endotoxin produced from the patient's own bowel flora, or to obstruction of renal tubules by pigment. It is especially important to maintain good hydration and urine output intraoperatively as well as postoperatively. It is therefore essential to monitor urine output closely, and if this falls below 30 ml h^{-1} mannitol should be used. Mannitol is an osmotic diuretic and 250 ml of 10% solution should be infused over 30 minutes. During surgery, close monitoring of cardiac status should be undertaken; jaundice itself tends to cause a bradycardia, although other rhythm disturbances may occur. As in all situations, if the prothrombin time is prolonged,

regional anaesthetic techniques are contraindicated.

NEUROLOGICAL DISEASE

Multiple sclerosis

The aetiology of this disease of temperate climates has become clearer in recent years. It appears that in genetically susceptible individuals activated T cells and macrophages responding to environmental triggers interact with type-1 astrocytes, causing a disruption of the blood–brain barrier and a leak of immune mediators into the nervous system. This causes demyelination. Patients may present for incidental surgery or surgery associated with alleviation of the complications, e.g. implantation of extradural stimulating electrodes. In order to decrease perioperative morbidity, careful preoperative examination is needed. Patients may have a labile autonomic nervous system associated with postural hypotension. Muscle atrophy may lead to significant kyphoscoliosis and this may result in a restrictive form of pulmonary disease. Urinary tract infections commonly occur, but the patient must be carefully examined to identify other infective foci. An elevation in temperature is the one definite factor known to precipitate an exacerbation of the disease, so that all but the most urgent surgery should be postponed until the patient is free from infection. Epilepsy is not uncommon in patients with multiple sclerosis.

Epilepsy

This term refers to a variety of types of recurrent seizure produced by paroxysmal neuronal discharge from various parts of the brain. Seizures may have a cerebral cause (e.g. tumour) or be due to a systemic disorder (e.g. uraemia or hypercalcaemia). The symptomatology is variable and seizures may cause total loss of consciousness or only a minimal alteration in awareness. The disease occurs in all age groups, with an incidence of about 1%. About 75% of patients have no recognizable underlying cause. If there is an underlying cause, the surgical management should take this into account. Otherwise management is usually uncomplicated; it is important that the patient's usual anticonvulsant medication be continued until the time of surgery and restarted as soon as possible postoperatively, if necessary using parenteral drug administration (see Concurrent drug therapy, p. 80). Anticonvulsant drugs such as phenytoin lead to induction of liver microsomal enzymes, and thus the patient's response to a variety of drugs that may be given during the perioperative period may be altered.

Myasthenia gravis

This is an autoimmune disease of the neuromuscular junction, involving the postjunctional acetylcholine receptors. Specific autoantibodies have been identified and microscopic changes in the membrane demonstrated. The disease is characterized by muscle weakness of fluctuating severity, most commonly affecting the ocular muscles. Facial and pharyngeal muscle weakness also occurs, leading to dysarthria and dysphagia. It can occur at any age in life, but is most frequently seen in the fourth decade. There is an association with thymic enlargement and thymomas, both benign and malignant. About two-thirds of patients without a thymic tumour will improve after thymectomy, although the outlook is less good for patients with tumour, whether this is excised or not. Inhibitors of the enzyme cholinesterase (e.g. edrophonium, neostigmine and pyridostigmine) are used in the treatment of myasthenia gravis, as are drugs which suppress the immunological response and eliminate circulating antibodies. The latter has now become the first line of treatment, and 90% of patients will benefit from the use of azathioprine or steroids.

Patients may present for thymectomy or incidental surgery, and the surgical management depends upon the nature of the operation and severity of the disease. As usual, the patient's normal medication must be continued up until the time of surgery. If the disease is severe, or major thoracic or upper abdominal surgery is planned, elective postoperative ventilation is advisable and, occasionally, a tracheostomy will be required, but this should only be needed if ventilation is prolonged and excess secretions are a problem. Respiratory failure in myasthenic patients may be secondary to either a myasthenic or a cholinergic crisis. Assisted ventilation should be instituted and anticholinesterase drug therapy stopped, and then cautiously reintroduced after testing with small doses of intravenous endrophonium (2–5 mg). Elective postoperative ventilation may also be advisable for lesser forms of surgery, including thymectomy, if the patient's preoperative vital capacity is less than 2 litres or there is a history of intercurrent respiratory problems. Following surgery, the requirements for anticholinesterase and other drug therapy may be changed and it is important to titrate drug dosage against clinical response. It should be remembered that overtreatment can cause weakness just as can undertreatment. Postoperatively, the adequacy of ventilation can best be assessed by repeated blood gas measurement and, therefore, before surgery there are advantages to the placement of an intra-arterial line. This will also facilitate accurate cardiovascular monitoring during surgery.

ALCOHOLISM AND DRUG ABUSE

Addiction is characterized by psychological dependence, change in tolerance and a specific withdrawal syndrome. Drugs including alcohol are used by susceptible individuals in order to obtain oblivion or excitement. Aetiological factors include psychiatric illness, personality disorders and social pressures. It should be remembered that many addicts abuse more than one drug. In general, it is advisable to maintain normal doses of the addict's usual drug in the immediate pre- and postoperative periods. The perioperative period is not the best time to attempt to wean a patient from an addiction and it may only serve to precipitate an acute withdrawal reaction. Addicts may not admit to their addiction and the first sign that there is a problem may be the appearance of a withdrawal syndrome.

Specific organ damage may result from drug addiction. Alcohol gives rise to liver damage and can progress to cirrhosis, and thus a change in protein synthesis, altered glycogen storage and susceptibility to hypoglycaemia. In addition, alcoholics are prone to bleeding, especially from the gastrointestinal tract, and there may be hypomagnesaemia. They may also have cardiomyopathy, and careful assessment of cardiovascular status is necessary in the alcoholic patient. Solvent or glue sniffers may have hepatic or renal damage and bone marrow suppression. Addicts to opioids will often have used contaminated needles and syringes, and there is a high incidence of hepatitis and liver damage and also of infection with the HIV virus (see below). If sudden hypotension occurs in the operative or postoperative period in a narcotic addict, and if other obvious causes are excluded, this may respond to the administration of intravenous morphine.

PSYCHIATRIC DISEASE

Anxiety and concern are a normal reaction of patients to forthcoming surgery and anaesthesia. A significant proportion of the population will suffer from an affective disorder at some time in their lives. A depressive illness is the commonest affective disorder and treatment may involve psychotherapy, antidepressant drug therapy or, if the disorder is severe, electroconvulsive therapy. It is important that the patient's preoperative drug therapy is continued, although both tricyclic antidepressants and monoaminoxidase inhibitors significantly interact with the drugs used during anaesthesia (see Concurrent drug therapy, p. 80). Before surgery both a psychiatrist and an anaesthetist should be consulted. Many anaesthetists would prefer that the drugs be continued up until the time of surgery, and their anaesthetic technique modified to take account of the potential for drug interactions.

It should not be forgotten that severe affective disorders are accompanied by a very significant mortality rate in terms of suicide, and supportive drug therapy should not automatically be withdrawn before planned surgery unless there is a very good reason to do so. The post-operative course in patients with a depressive illness may be more prolonged and these patients should be treated with appropriate forbearance.

ACQUIRED IMMUNE DEFICIENCY SYNDROME (AIDS)

This is caused by infection with a retrovirus, the human immunodeficiency virus (HIV). Infection is most common in homosexual men and in users of drugs that are injected by needles which can be infected. However, it may also be seen in patients who have received infected blood products (e.g. haemophiliacs). The disease is not very infectious and is transmitted primarily in blood, and there is little evidence to support transmission via saliva or airborne transmission. It is thought that the risk of infection in medical and allied professions is low, unless accidental inoculation has occurred. The issue of routine preoperative screening is controversial.

SURGERY IN THE ELDERLY

Although patients over the age of 65 years comprise only 22% of the surgical caseload, they are reported to account for 79% of perioperative deaths (Buck et al 1987). The mortality of surgery in elderly patients is significantly higher in those suffering from serious coexisting medical conditions. In a study of 100 000 surgical operations, the relative risk of dying within 7 days, comparing patients over 80 with those under 60

years, was 3, but the risk factor comparing patients having symptomatic medical disease with those having none was over 10 (Cohen et al 1988). Not only do elderly patients have an increased likelihood of coexisting disease, but physiological function in general decreases with age. As a generalization, many physiological functions (e.g. cardiac output, glomerular filtration rate and renal blood flow) decrease by about 1% per annum after the age of 30 years. Respiratory function also declines with age (maximum breathing capacity decreases from about $100 \ 1 \ min^{-1}$ at 20 years to $30 \ 1 \ min^{-1}$ at 80 years). The elderly are also more sensitive to the majority of drugs that might be used in the perioperative period (e.g. diazepam has a half-life measured in hours that is approximately equal to subject age in years). As in all other situations where a patient presents for surgery with a significant coexisting disease, the morbidity and mortality associated with surgery can be reduced to a minimum after careful preoperative evaluation and by optimizing the patient's condition.

CONCURRENT DRUG THERAPY

It is a general rule that any patients stabilized on long-term drug therapy should continue to take their normal medication until the time of surgery, and that this should be recommenced as soon as possible following surgery. If the patient is unable to take drugs by mouth, then appropriate parenteral administration is required. This is especially important for patients taking drugs such as antiepileptics, antiarrhythmics or antihypertensives. A thorough knowledge of the pharmacokenetic and pharmacodynamic profile of the individual drugs is needed, in order that the appropriate doses and interval between doses is arrived at for parenteral administration. A number of drugs (e.g. propranolol) undergo extensive

Table 6.3   Some important drugs the administration or dosage of which needs to be modified before surgery

Oral contraceptives	Maintain for minor or peripheral procedures and institute prophylaxis against deep vein thrombosis, before surgery. Stop one complete monthly cycle before abdominal (especially pelvic) surgery
Anticoagulants	Stop oral agents several days before surgery and substitute heparin if continued anticoagulant is necessary. The action of heparin can be rapidly reversed with protamine
Agents used in diabetes	See section on diabetic management
Levodopa	Omit dose before surgery
Monamine oxidase inhibitors	Significant potential for drug interactions, causing severe physiological disturbance. Discuss with psychiatrist and anaesthetist and treat each case on its merits
Steroids	Supplement with hydrocortisone 100 mg i.v. 30 minutes before surgery, repeated 3-hourly during surgery, reducing slowly postoperatively to the patient's preoperative dose. Treat similarly if taking large dose regularly, any time during 3 months before surgery

first-pass liver metabolism after oral administration, and drugs such as this need much lower doses administered parenterally than they do orally. Admission to hospital for surgery gives the opportunity to review the appropriateness of long-term drug therapy and dosage; this may be especially important in elderly patients as they are more likely to suffer from toxic symptoms. The nature of some operations may mean that the need for continued drug therapy has to be reviewed post-operatively, or the dosage of the drugs may need to be altered. An example of this would be a myasthenic patient undergoing thymectomy. Although the majority of patients stabilized on long-term therapy should continue their normal drugs up until the time of surgery, there are a number of drugs whose administration or dosage will need to be modified before surgery (see Table 6.3 for the more important examples of these).

REFERENCES

Aitkenhead A R, Barnett D B 1989 Heart disease. In: Vickers M D, Jones R M (eds) Medicine for anaesthetists. Blackwell, London

Buck N, Devlin H B, Lunn J N 1987 The report of a confidential enquiry into perioperative deaths. Nuffield Provincial Hospitals Trust, London

Campling E A, Devlin H B, Hoile R W, Lunn J N 1992 The report of the national confidential enquiry into perioperative deaths, 1990. London

Campling E A, Devlin H B, Hoile R W, Lunn J N 1993 The report of the national confidential enquiry into perioperative deaths 1991/1992. London

Cohen M M, Duncan P G, Tate R B 1988 Does anesthesia contribute to operative mortality? Journal of the American Medical Association 260: 2859–2863

Jones R M 1985 Smoking before surgery: the case for stopping. British Medical Journal 290: 1763–1764

Simon A 1977 Perioperative management of the pacemaker patient. Anesthesiology 46: 127–131

7. Haematological assessment and blood component therapy

A. B. Mehta

This chapter outlines the management of surgical patients who have a haematological cytopenia (anaemia, thrombocytopenia and, to a lesser extent, leucopenia) or an abnormality of blood plasma constituents, and focuses on replacement therapy. Anaemia and excessive bleeding are symptoms and not diagnoses. An accurate diagnosis is an essential initial step in the formulation of a management plan. In the majority of hospitals, a clinical haematologist will be available to advise you on optimum use of laboratory diagnostic facilities and interpretation of results. Make sure you discuss problems early, and take advice on the appropriate specimens to send and tests to order. If a result is puzzling, go and discuss it with the haematologist.

PREOPERATIVE ASSESSMENT

Growing pressure on hospital beds and increasing use of day surgery means that the preoperative assessment should, wherever possible, be performed prior to admission. The key aims are to assess a patient's fitness to undergo surgery and anaesthesia, anticipate complications, arrange for supportive therapy to be available perioperatively and to liaise with the appropriate specialist physician regarding non-surgical management. A full history and physical examination are mandatory. Laboratory evaluation begins by an assessment of the full blood count (FBC) (which is performed by automated analysers and gives the haemoglobin concentration, red cell indices, white cell count, white cell differential and platelet count). If the FBC shows changes in more than one cell line (e.g. anaemia plus thrombocytopenia and/or leucopenia) or is in any other way indicative of intrinsic bone marrow disease (e.g. blood film showing leukaemic infiltration) surgery must be deferred pending a full haematological assessment.

Anaemia

Anaemia is defined as a reduction in haemoglobin concentration below the normal range after correction for age and sex (approximately $13-16$ g dl^{-1} in males, $11.5-15$ g dl^{-1} in females). A classification of anaemia is given below:

- *Decreased red cell production*
- Haematinic deficiency:
    Iron, vitamin B_{12}, folic acid, other
- Marrow failure:
    Aplastic anaemia
    Leukaemia
    Pure red cell aplasia
- *Abnormal red cell maturation*
- Myelodysplasia
- Sideroblastic anaemia
- *Increased red cell destruction*
- Inherited haemolytic anaemia (e.g. sickle cell anaemia, thalassaemia)
- Acquired haemolytic anaemia:
    immune (e.g. autoimmune)
    non-immune (e.g. microangiopathic haemolytic anaemia, disseminated intravascular coagulation)
- *Effects of disease in other organs*
    Anaemia of chronic disorder
    Renal, endocrine, liver disease.

Important clues regarding the cause of anaemia are gained from examination of red cell indices. The following alterations in red cell indices offer a clue to the cause of anaemia:

- *Lowered Mean Cell Volume (MCV)/Mean Cell Haemoglobin (MCH)*
- Iron deficiency
- Thalassaemia trait
- Homozygous thalassaemia
- Hyperthyroidism
- *Raised MCV*
- Megaloblastic anaemia

– Hypothyroidism
– Liver disease
– Reticulocytosis
– Myelodysplasia
– Aplastic anaemia
– Paraproteinaemia
– Alcohol abuse
● *Normochromic normocytic*
– Anaemia of chronic disease
– Renal failure
– Bone marrow infiltration
– Haemorrhage.

A reduction in MCV and MCH (microcytic hypochromic picture) is highly suggestive of iron deficiency, which in turn is most frequently due to haemorrhage. Nutritional deficiency leads to a well-compensated anaemia of gradual onset. Malabsorption (due to pernicious anaemia, coeliac disease, or after gastrectomy) or poor dietary intake are the commonest causes. Blood component therapy should be avoided wherever possible and the underlying cause of the anaemia should be specifically treated.

Haemoglobinopathies. These are inherited disorders of haemoglobin synthesis which lead to a life-long haemolytic anaemia. Patients with sickle cell disease (HbSS, HbSC or HBS/thalassaemia) in general require exchange transfusion before major surgery, whereas intermediate and minor surgical procedures can be carried out safely without transfusion in the majority of patients. Particular attention should be paid to the hydration of the patient and to oxygenation during anaesthesia. Patients with sickle cell disease may develop painful crisis due to infarcts in tissues and organs, before, during or after an operation; this is best managed by symptomatic treatment, but occasionally may require blood transfusion.

Excessive bleeding

Significant numbers of patients with an inherited or acquired defect of coagulation (Table 7.1) which leads to peri- and postoperative complications cannot be detected preoperatively. However, a full history may reveal features such as excessive bleeding at times of previous surgery, bleeding while brushing teeth, nose bleeds, a family history of bleeding disorders, spontaneous bruising, a history of renal or liver disease and a relevant drug history. A coagulation screen (prothrombin time (PT), activated partial thromboplastin time (APTT) and thrombin time (TT)) and platelet count should be done in any patient with a suspected bleeding disorder, but disordered platelet

Table 7.1 Bleeding disorders associated with excessive bleeding which may cause peri- or postoperative complications

Disorder type	Cause
Congenital	
Clotting factors	Haemophilia A, B
	von Willebrand's syndrome
Platelets	Congenital platelet disorders
Vessel wall	Hereditary haemorrhagic
	telangectasia
Acquired	
Clotting factors	Drugs (anticoagulants, antibiotics)
	Liver disease
	DIC (in sepsis)
Platelets – function	Drugs (aspirin, NSAIDs)
	Liver disease, renal disease,
	myeloproliferative disorders,
	paraproteinaemic disorders
Platelets – number	Autoimmune thrombocytopenia
	Hypersplenism
	Aplastic anaemia, myelodysplasia
Vessel wall	Drugs (steroids)
	Vasculitis
	Malnutrition

DIC, disseminated intravascular coagulation; NSAIDS, nonsteroidal anti-inflammatory drugs.

function can be difficult to detect. A bleeding time is the time taken for firm clot formation following a standard skin incision (normal range 3–10 minutes) and is the best in vivo test of platelet function.

Anticoagulant therapy

The dose of oral anticoagulants (e.g. warfarin) is adjusted to maintain the international normalized ratio (INR, which is a measure of the ratio of the patient's PT to that of a control plasma) within a therapeutic range. The dose of heparin, which is a parenteral anticoagulant, is monitored by measurement of the ratio of the patient's PTT to that of control plasma. For elective surgery in patients on oral anticoagulants, the challenge is to balance the risk of haemorrhage if the INR is not reduced against the risk of thrombosis if the INR is reduced for too long or by too great an amount. For minor surgery (e.g. dental extraction) it is normally sufficient to stop the oral anticoagulant for 2 days prior to the procedure and restart with the usual maintenance dose immediately afterwards. For high-risk patients (e.g. those with prosthetic heart valves) or for patients undergoing more extensive procedures, it is necessary to stop warfarin and give heparin (either subcutaneously or by continuous intravenous infusion) under close haematological supervision to provide thrombosis prophylaxis. Patients on anticoagulants who present for emergency surgery or who have bled as a result of anticoagulant therapy may need reversal of the anticoagulant. This can be done with vitamin K in association with either fresh frozen plasma (FFP) or a concentrate of factors II, IX, X and VII.

ARRANGING INTRAOPERATIVE BLOOD COMPONENT SUPPORT

Elective surgery

For most surgical patients, *red cells* are best ordered as plasma reduced cells. Place your request at least 24 hours in advance; this allows the laboratory to establish the recipient's blood group and also to screen serum for the presence of atypical antibodies ('group and save' procedure). If no atypical antibodies are found, the subsequent cross-match can be simplified substantially. Many hospitals now operate a 'maximum blood order schedule' (MBOS) which indicates the recommended number of units to be cross-matched for the more common surgical procedures. For many procedures (e.g. appendicectomy and uncomplicated or laparoscopic cholecystectomy) analysis of blood usage indicates that blood does not have to be cross-matched if a 'group and save' has been electively performed, as compatible blood can be issued, if required, within 10–15 minutes. The operation of a MBOS schedule improves efficiency within the blood bank and can also simplify ordering by junior doctors.

Other blood components should be discussed pre-operatively with a clinical haematologist. Elective surgery in patients with thrombocytopenia or congenital and acquired disorders of coagulation should only be undertaken after careful preoperative assessment and transfusion therapy.

Preoperative autologous transfusion

Preoperative donation of 2–4 units of red cells (typically 1 unit per week) for autologous transfusion at or after operation is increasingly practised. Longer term storage of cryopreserved autologous units is reserved for patients with multiple red cell antibodies who are unable to receive standard donor blood. Directed donations from family or friends are not recommended in the UK, primarily because of confidence in the general safety of donor blood and concern that coercion may inhibit voluntary withdrawal of unsuitable donors. Autologous donations may not be given by patients with active infection, unstable angina, aortic stenosis and severe hypertension. A haemoglobin level of >10 g dl^{-1} is maintained with oral iron supplements, and trials have failed to show

a consistent advantage in using recombinant human erythropoietin (rhEPO) to accelerate haemopoiesis. Elective orthopaedic and gynaecological surgery are two areas where up to 20% of patients may be suitable for autologus donation.

A number of issues mitigate against the wider applicability of this procedure.

- late cancellation of surgery can lead to waste
- criteria for transfusion of donated units should be identical to those for ordinary units (they should not be used simply because they are available)
- current UK guidelines stipulate that autologous units be tested for the same range of markers of transmissible disease as homologous donations, which increases costs and leads to ethical dilemmas if positive results are obtained
- hospitals must operate secure laboratory and clinical protocols to ensure proper identification of autologous units and separation from homologous donation
- the practice is likely to be associated with increased cost, and benefits are difficult to quantify.

Emergency surgery

Patients who are in clinical shock (e.g. due to sepsis or haemorrhage) or actively bleeding require preoperative clinical and laboratory assessment and should be stabilized if possible prior to surgery. The aims in treating acute haemorrhage resulting in acute blood volume depletion are initially to maintain blood pressure, circulating volume and colloid osmotic pressure, and later to restore the haemoglobin level. Appropriate initial therapy is with a synthetic plasma substitute.

Whole blood is an appropriate form of replacement in acute haemorrhage as it will restore plasma volume as well as haemoglobin. It will not correct disordered coagulation or elevate the platelet count, and FFP and/or platelet transfusions may be indicated. Fully compatible blood is unlikely to be available in less than 1 hour. If blood is required sooner you may request group-compatible units (approximately 10 min). Non-cross-matched blood (group O, rhesus negative) can be made available in approximately 5 minutes, but always take a pretransfusion sample so that a retrospective cross-match can be performed.

BLOOD COMPONENTS

The supply of whole blood and plasma in the UK is based on volunteer, healthy donors. Over 90% of donated blood is separated into its various constituents to allow prescription of individual components and preparation of pooled plasma from which specific blood products are manufactured (Table 7.2). The collection and processing of blood products is organized within the UK by the National Blood Authority (NBA). The hospital laboratory is primarily concerned with issuing appropriate components, compatibility testing and ensuring accurate documentation. These functions of a hospital transfusion laboratory require regulation and monitoring. Most hospitals have standard protocols which are issued to all medical staff and detail the range of components available, together with procedures and indications for their use. The Hospital Transfusion Committee provides a forum whereby clinical laboratory users meet with local transfusion specialists. The responsibilities of such a committee are to organize audit so that activity can be assessed against protocols, and to provide information on use of resources, the appropriateness of such use, and to provide a mechanism whereby the audit loop can be completed (i.e. to amend practice where it can be shown to deviate from protocol, or vice versa). Accurate documentation is of paramount importance, so that the ultimate fate of each component can be traced from donor to recipient.

BLOOD GROUPING AND COMPATIBILITY TESTING

Red cells carry antigens which are typically glycoproteins or glycolipids attached to the red cell membrane. Antibodies to the ABO antigens are naturally occurring, whereas antibodies to other red-cell antigens appear only after sensitization by transfusion or pregnancy to cause haemolytic transfusion reactions and haemolytic disease of the fetus and newborn.

Table 7.2 Blood constituents available for clinical use

Whole blood*	
Blood components*	Red cells – plasma reduced
	– leukocyte poor
	– frozen
	– phenotyped
	Platelets
	White cells (buffy coat)
	Fresh frozen plasma
	Cryoprecipitate
Plasma products	Human albumin solution
	Coagulation factor concentrate
	Immunoglobulin – specific
	– standard human

*These products are not heat treated, and all may transmit microbial infection.

Naturally occurring antibodies are principally of the immunoglobulin M (IgM) type and are detectable by suspension of cells with diluted antibody at room temperature. They are therefore termed 'complete' antibodies. Immunoglobulin G (IgG) antibodies are termed 'incomplete' as their reactions can only be demonstrated using special techniques (e.g. enzyme treatment of red cells, addition of albumin to reaction mixture, use of antihuman globulin, and microscopical examination for agglutination). Compatibility testing entails suspension of group-compatible red cells from a donor pack with recipient serum, incubation (at room temperature, 37°C) to allow reactions to occur, and examination for agglutination to ensure that no reaction has occurred. Atypical 'incomplete' (IgG) antibodies in recipient serum will coat incubated donor red cells and their presence is demonstrated by adding antihuman globulin, which leads to agglutination (antihuman globulin or Coomb's test). Many hospitals now use less labour-intensive solid-phase techniques in which reagents are provided already suspended in plastic tubes; donor red cells are added, followed by incubation, centrifugation and non-microscopic examination for reactions.

RED CELL TRANSFUSION

Major indications are haemorrhage, anaemia (once the cause has been established) and bone marrow failure.

Whole blood (1 unit usually contains 450 ml) is available for the treatment of acute haemorrhage with hypovolaemia. Fresh whole blood (<5 days after collection) is preferable for neonates and may have value in patients with haemostatic defects, though accurate diagnosis of the defect with appropriate correction by drugs or blood components (e.g. FFP or platelets), if indicated, is preferred. Granulocytes and platelets lose function, many coagulation factors lose activity and aggregates of aged platelets, leukocytes, fibrin strands and cellular debris are formed.

Plasma-reduced red cells are whole blood from which plasma has been removed to allow the use of plasma for the preparation of other blood components. The red cells are usually suspended in optimum additive solution (OAS), e.g. SAG-M (sodium chloride, adenine, glucose and mannitol), to give a total volume of 350 ml. These preparations have a shelf-life of 35 days when stored at 4°C. During storage the concentration of the red cell 2,3-diphosphoglycerate (2,3-DPG) gradually falls, which increases their oxygen affinity and reduces the amount of oxygen they can deliver to tissues. Red cells in OAS are generally considered unsuitable for neonates.

Leukocyte depleted red cells have been passed through a bedside leukocyte filter to remove contaminating white cells. They are given to patients who are sensitized to HLA, granulocyte and platelet antigens (e.g. multiply transfused patients) who experience febrile reactions during transfusion.

Phenotyped red cells correspond as closely as possible to the red cells of the recipient. *Frozen red cells* are only available from NBA Transfusion Centres, and may be useful in rare patients with multiple antibodies.

PLASMA SUBSTITUTES

These include products based on hydroxyethyl starch (HES), dextran (a branch-chained polysaccharide composed of glucose units) and modified gelatin. Such components remain in the circulation longer than crystalloid solutions (up to 6 hours for modified gelatin and up to 24 hours for some high molecular weight starch-based products). Other advantages are that they are relatively non-toxic, inexpensive, can be stored at room temperature, do not require compatibility testing and do not transmit infection. Adverse effects include anaphylaxis, fever and rash, such effects being more frequent with starch-based products. Dextran can also impair coagulation and platelet function and can interfere with compatibility testing, so that samples for this must be taken prior to therapy. The maximum dose of synthetic plasma expanders is approximately 20–30 ml/kg. Patients receiving larger volumes or with significant evidence of other organ failure (e.g. pulmonary or renal disease, or a bleeding diathesis) may be given albumin.

PLATELET TRANSFUSIONS

Platelet concentrates are available as single units (prepared from 1 unit of whole blood within a few hours of collection), pooled platelets (usually equivalent to 5 single units) or as platelets collected using a cell separator. A single unit contains approximately 5×10^{10} platelets in 50–60 ml of fresh plasma and, when stored in a platelet agitator, has a shelf-life of 4–6 days. The standard adult dose is 5 units; group compatible (but not cross-matched) units are given.

Indications

Indications for platelet transfusion are:

1. Thrombocytopenia ($<50 \times 10^9 \, l^{-1}$) in the presence of significant bleeding or prior to an invasive procedure. Such transfusions are only rarely required if platelet destruction is antibody mediated.
2. Prophylactic transfusions in patients after chemotherapy or with failure of marrow production. In clini-

cally stable patients with no fever or coagulopathy the count can safely be allowed to fall to $5 \times 10^9 \, l^{-1}$.

3. Others, including platelet function defects (in the presence of bleeding or prior to surgery), DIC, dilutional thrombocytopenia following massive transfusion and following cardiopulmonary bypass (CPB) surgery (see below).

White cell transfusions are now rarely used as there are few data demonstrating clinical efficacy.

FRESH FROZEN PLASMA (FFP)

FFP is prepared by centrifugation of donor whole blood within 6 hours of collection and frozen at $-30°C$. It may be stored for up to 12 months and is thawed prior to administration. It has a volume of approximately 200 ml. It is a source of all coagulation and other plasma proteins. Compatibility testing is not required, but group-compatible units are used. FFP from group AB donors may be used if the recipient blood group is unknown. Although 2–4 units are usually administered, the volume and frequency of administration should be assessed separately for each patient. FFP is not heat sterilized and the possibility of viral transmission must be borne in mind.

Indications

Indications for FFP transfusion are:

1. Coagulation factor replacement: coagulation tests and a platelet count must be performed prior to use. Patients with disseminated intravascular coagulation (DIC), who have undergone massive transfusion or CPB, who are at risk of bleeding or have coagulation abnormalities may benefit.
2. Liver disease: in the presence of bleeding or prior to invasive procedures, in conjunction with vitamin K.
3. Haemolytic uraemic syndrome (HUS) or thrombotic thrombocytopenia purpura (TTP): FFP replacement, often in conjunction with plasma exchange, is indicated. Cryoprecipitate-poor FFP is also available and is useful in this setting.
4. Reversal of oral anticoagulation or thrombolytic therapy.

Cryoprecipitate is prepared from FFP, is rich in fibrinogen, fibronectin and factor VIII, is stored at $-30°C$ for up to 12 months and thawed prior to infusion. Its low volume makes it useful in patients with DIC following massive transfusion, and occasionally in liver or renal disease.

PLASMA PRODUCTS

The following products are derived from pooled human plasma, but have undergone a manufacturing process designed to concentrate the component and to sterilize it, thus markedly reducing the risk of viral infection.

Albumin solution

This is available as 5%, 20% and 20% salt-poor formulations in a variety of dose units. It does not contain coagulation factors. Indications for 5% albumin are replacement of plasma proteins and expansion of plasma volume, as in hypoproteinaemia following burns (after the first 24 hours) and as a part of the replacement fluid in large-volume plasma exchange. Albumin solutions may play a role in restoration of circulatory volume in haemorrhage, shock and multiple organ failure, but the view that administration of colloid and crystalloid solutions is preferable (it is certainly cheaper) is gaining popularity. The indications for 20% albumin are replacement of plasma proteins in severe hypoproteinaemia in renal or liver disease, after large-volume paracentesis, following massive liver resection and in some cases of Gram-negative septicaemia.

Coagulation factor concentrates

These are manufactured from pooled fractionated human plasma and are available as freeze-dried powder which is reconstituted prior to use. Factor VIII concentrate is used for treatment of haemophilia A and von Willebrand's disease.

Factor IX concentrate contains factors IX, X and II and is used for treatment of bleeding complications in inherited deficiencies of these factors. Given with vitamin K, it is also used in treatment of oral anticoagulant overdose, and in severe liver failure. Its use carries a risk of provoking thrombosis and DIC. Other concentrates include the naturally occurring anticoagulant factors protein C and antithrombin III (see below), and factors VII, XI and XIII; they are used in the corresponding congenital deficiencies.

Immunoglobulins

These are prepared from pooled donor plasma by fractionation and sterile filtration. Specific immunoglobulins include hepatitis B and herpes zoster and can provide passive immune protection. Standard human immunoglobulin for intramuscular injection is used for prophylaxis against hepatitis A, rubella and measles, whereas hyperimmune globulin is prepared from donors with high titres of the relevant antibodies for prophylaxis of tetanus, hepatitis A, diphtheria, rabies, mumps, measles, rubella, cytomegalovirus and *Pseudomonas* infections. Intravenous immunoglobulin is used as replacement therapy in patients with congenital or acquired immune deficiency and in autoimmune disorders (e.g. idiopathic thrombocytopenic purpura).

ADVERSE CONSEQUENCES OF BLOOD TRANSFUSION

In general, transfusion of blood and blood products is a safe and effective mode of treatment. Avoid administrative and clerical errors by rigorous adherence to procedures for checking, and rigorous documentation when ordering, prescribing, issuing and administering blood and blood components.

IMMUNE COMPLICATIONS

ABO-incompatible red cell transfusions will lead to life-threatening intravascular haemolysis of transfused cells, manifesting as fever, rigors, haemoglobinuria, hypotension and renal failure (immediate haemolytic transfusion reaction (HTR)). In the anaesthetized patient, persistent hypotension and unexplained oozing from the wound may be the only signs.

Atypical antibodies arising from previous transfusions or pregnancy may cause intravascular haemolysis, but more commonly lead to extravascular haemolysis in liver and spleen and may be delayed for 1–3 weeks (delayed HTR). Typical manifestations are jaundice, progressive anaemia, fever, arthralgia and myalgia. Diagnosis is easily established by a positive direct antiglobulin test (DAT) and a positive antibody screen. Non-haemolytic febrile transfusion reaction (NHFTR) usually occurs within hours of transfusion in multitransfused patients with antibodies against HLA antigens or granulocyte-specific antibodies. The reaction is due to pyrogens, released from granulocytes damaged by complement in an antigen–antibody reaction. It presents as a rise in temperature with flushing, palpitations and tachycardia, followed by headache and rigors. Hypersensitivity reactions to plasma components may cause urticaria, wheezing, facial oedema and pyrexia, but can cause anaphylactic shock (e.g. in patients with congenital IgA deficiency who have anti-IgA antibodies following previous sensitization).

Treatment

Stop the transfusion immediately in all cases except for the appearance of a mild pyrexia in a multiply transfused

∠385

patient. Check clerical details and send samples from the donor unit and recipient for analysis for compatibility and haemolysis. Recipient serum is analysed for the presence of atypical red cell leucocyte HLA and plasma protein antibodies. Treat severe haemolytic transfusion reactions with support care to maintain blood pressure and renal function, to promote diuresis and treat shock. Intravenous steroids and antihistamines may be needed, with the use of adrenaline in severe cases. Management of NHFTR consists of administration of antipyretics (e.g. paracetamol) and, for severe symptoms, 100 mg of hydrocortisone intravenously can also be given. Prevent NHFTR by administering blood filtered through one of the specific leukocyte depletion filters (e.g. Sepacell R-500 and Pall RC-100).

TRANSMISSION OF INFECTION

Blood transfusion is an important mode of transmission of a range of protozoal, bacterial and viral infections. Bacterial infections can occur through failure of sterile technique at the time of collection or due to bacteraemia in the donor (especially if organisms such as *Yersinia* which can survive at 4°C are incriminated). Donors at risk of malaria are not eligible to donate. Transmission of syphilis is now very rare.

Viral infection

Transmission of viruses may occur in spite of mandatory screening because: serological tests may not have had time to become positive in a potentially infectious individual; the virus may not have been identified; or the most sensitive serological tests may not be routinely performed (e.g. antihepatitis B core antibodies). The risk of transmission is much lower, although still present, for those blood products which have undergone a manufacturing and sterilization process.

Viruses that are transmissible by blood transfusion are:

- *Plasma-borne viruses*
  - Hepatitis B and its variants
  - Hepatitis A (rarely)
  - Hepatitis C
  - Other unidentified hepatitis viruses
  - HIV-1 and HIV-2 (also cellular)
  - Parvovirus
- *Cell-associated viruses*
  - Cytomegalovirus
  - Epstein–Barr virus
  - HTLV-1 and HTLV-II.

Hepatitis B vaccine should be given to hepatitis B virus negative recipients of pooled plasma products or repeated red cell transfusion.

OTHER COMPLICATIONS

There is increasing evidence that transfusion of blood components can cause immunosuppression in the recipient. This may lead to earlier relapse or recurrence of malignant disease after surgical removal of malignant tumours (shortened disease-free interval) as well as an increased incidence of postoperative infection. These effects are probably due to defective cell-mediated immunity and are reduced by the use of leukocyte-depletion filters. Circulatory overload may result from the infusion of large volumes in patients with incipient heart failure. Iron overload occurs in patients who have received repeated red cell transfusions and these patients require iron chelation therapy. Graft-versus-host disease may be caused by transfusion of T-lymphocytes into severely immunosuppressed hosts, and cellular components should be irradiated prior to transfusion to severely immunodeficient patients.

INTRAOPERATIVE ASSESSMENT

Rapid bleeding confined to one site is usually due to a surgical problem. Suspect haemostatic failure in a high-risk patient with multiple sites of bleeding or an unusual bleeding pattern and confirm it by appropriate laboratory tests. The following tests are useful in assessing the degree of blood loss and should serve as a guide for determining need for replacement therapy:

- *Oxygen-carrying capacity of blood*
  - Haemoglobin concentration
  - Pulse oximetry
- *Haemostatic function*
  - Coagulation screen:
    prothrombin time (PT)
    activated partial thromboplastin time (APTT)
    thrombin time (TT)
    platelet count
  - Thromboelastography.

Quantification of intraoperative blood loss is imprecise. Clinical evaluation must be accompanied by laboratory tests (Table 7.3) and many of the latter cannot be performed outside the main laboratory. Thromboelastography is a useful and rapid test whereby a graphical recording is produced of in vitro blood clot formation and dissolution, and provides a global test of coagulation and fibrinolysis which can be performed rapidly within the operating suite in high-risk patients.

Table 7.3 Results of laboratory tests as an aid in differential diagnosis of excessive bleeding

Cause of bleeding	Laboratory test				
	PT	APTT	TT without protamine	TT with protamine	Platelet count
Loss of platelets	N	N	N	N	↓↓
Lack of coagulation factors	↑↑	↑↑	N	N	N or ↓
Excess of heparin	↑	↑↑	↑	N	N or ↓
Hyperfibrinolysis	↑	↑	↑↑	↑↑	N or ↓
DIC	↑↑	↑↑	↑↑	↑↑	↓↓
Massive blood transfusion	↑	↑	N	N	↓
Vitamin K deficiency	↑↑	↑	N	N	N

Key: N, normal; ↑↑, markedly raised; ↑, mildly raised; ↓↓, markedly decreased; ↓, mildly decreased.

Intraoperative autologous transfusion

Normovolaemic haemodilution involves removal of 1–2 units of whole blood during induction of anaesthesia, with replacement by crystalloid, reducing the haematocrit to 25–30%. Surgery is usually well tolerated, the collected blood can be returned later during the operation, and there is no need to undertake virological testing of the unit.

Salvage of blood lost during an operation is accomplished using a simple device (e.g. Solcotrans) or a cell saver (e.g. Haemonetics Cell Saver IV). Blood shed into the thoracic or abdominal cavity is aspirated and mixed with anticoagulant. It can then be returned to the patient (Solcotrans) or the red cells can be washed, suspended in saline and transfused to the patient (Haemonetics Cell Saver IV). The use of a cell saver may considerably reduce the number of units required for transfusion. Contraindications for the use of the blood-salvage procedure is exposure of blood to a site of infection or the possibility of contamination with malignant cells.

Methods of reducing intraoperative blood loss

Meticulous surgical technique clearly plays a major role, but there is increasing interest in the use of pharmacological agents to improve haemostasis. Desmopressin (DDAVP) improves platelet function by increasing plasma concentrations of von Willebrand factor, but has not been convincingly shown to reduce blood loss in cardiac surgery. Aprotinin is a serine protease inhibitor which inhibits fibrinolysis and has been shown to reduce blood loss and operative morbidity in cardiac surgery (particularly in repeat procedures) and major hepatic surgery (e.g. liver transplantation).

SPECIAL SITUATIONS

Massive blood transfusion

This is defined as transfusion of a volume of blood greater than the recipient's blood volume in less than 24 hours. Blood-group-specific, compatible whole blood or red cell preparations can be transfused, usually using an in-line microaggregate filter. A pressure infusor or a pump and blood warmer will provide more rapid administration. FFP and platelet concentrates (from the same blood group as the red cells) may also be required.

Complications include:

1. Cardiac abnormalities (ventricular extrasystoles, ventricular fibrillation (rarely) and cardiac arrest) due to the combined effect of low temperature, high potassium concentration and excess citrate with low calcium concentration. They can be prevented by using a blood warmer and a slower rate of transfusion, particularly in patients with hepatic or renal failure. Routine administration of calcium gluconate is unnecessary and may even be dangerous unless the ionized calcium concentration in the plasma can be monitored.

2. Acidosis in the patient with severe renal or liver disease may be aggravated by the low pH of stored blood.

3. Failure of haemostasis manifests as local oozing and, infrequently, as a generalized bleeding tendency due to the lack of coagulation factors and platelets in stored blood. Laboratory assessment is essential (see above). FFP (1–2 units) corrects the abnormalities of coagulation and should be given prophylactically after every 10 units of blood. Platelet transfusion may be required when the platelet count is lower than $50 \times 10^9 \, 1^{-1}$, particularly if the patient is bleeding.

4. Adult respiratory distress syndrome (ARDS), also

called non-cardiogenic pulmonary oedema, occurs in severely ill patients after major trauma and/or surgery. Clinical features include progressive respiratory distress, decreased lung compliance, acute hypoxaemia and diffuse radiographic opacification of the lungs. The mortality is high; post-mortem studies show widespread macroscopic and microscopic thrombosis in the pulmonary arteries. Local disseminated intravascular coagulation, microvascular fluid leakage and embolization of leukocyte aggregates and microaggregates from stored blood all contribute to pathogenesis. Management consists of stopping the transfusion, administering corticosteroids and providing supportive treatment to combat pulmonary oedema and hypoxia by using oxygen and positive-pressure ventilation.

Transfusion in open heart surgery

This requires cardiopulmonary bypass (CPB) for maintaining the circulation with oxygenated blood. In adults blood is not required for priming of the heart–lung machine, but it is needed in neonates and small children. Usually 4 units of blood (ideally less than 5 days old) are initially cross-matched (6–8 units for repeat procedures). The use of albumin solutions either for priming the heart–lung machine or postoperatively is unnecessary.

Bleeding associated with CPB is due to activation and loss of platelets and coagulation factors in the extracorporeal circulation, failure of heparin neutralization by the first dose of protamine, activation of fibrinolysis in the oxygenator and pump, and/or disseminated intravascular coagulation in patients with poor cardiac output and long perfusion times. Management requires: administration of 4–8 units of platelet concentrates when the platelet count is less than $30 \times 10^9 l^{-1}$; transfusion of 2–4 units of fresh frozen plasma to correct the loss of coagulation factors; neutralization of excess heparin by protamine (1 mg of protamine neutralizes approximately 100 IU of heparin); administration of tranexamic acid (or a similar antifibrinolytic agent) when hyperfibrinolysis is confirmed by laboratory testing; treatment of disseminated intravascular coagulation, in the first instance by correcting the underlying cause (e.g. poor perfusion, oligaemic shock, acidosis or infection) and then by transfusion of FFP and platelet concentrates, as required.

Prostatic surgery

This may be followed by excessive urinary bleeding due to local fibrinolysis related to the release of high concentrations of urokinase. Antifibrinolytic agents, which include ϵ-aminocaproic acid (EACA) and tranexamic acid are often helpful in reducing clot dissolution, but should be used cautiously as fibrinolytic inhibition can lead to ureteric obstruction in patients with upper urinary tract bleeding.

Liver disease

This warrants special mention as the liver is an important site of manufacture of the components as well as the regulatory factors of the coagulation and fibrinolytic pathways. Vitamin K is required for hepatic synthesis of the coagulation factors II, VII, IX and X as well as the coagulation inhibitors proteins C and S. Impaired vitamin K absorption can occur in biliary obstruction and patients should receive 10 mg vitamin K by intramuscular injection preoperatively. The liver is also the site of manufacture of factor V and fibrinogen (factor 1), the regulatory factors antithrombin III and α_2-antiplasmin, and defects of both platelet function and number (e.g. thrombocytopenia due to complicating hypersplenism) can occur. These patients are at increased risk of DIC and renal failure, and require assessment by a gastroenterologist as well as a haematologist.

POSTOPERATIVE ASSESSMENT

Anaemia, coagulopathy and excessive bleeding in the immediate postoperative period are often due to the operation or its complications. Blood component therapy commenced intraoperatively for the management of special situations (see above) must be continued postoperatively.

Patients with excessive bleeding and clinical evidence of haemostatic failure require laboratory assessment (Table 7.3). The trauma of surgery triggers both the coagulation and fibrinolytic pathways and places patients at increased risk of DIC. Do not routinely use red cell transfusions to correct postoperative anaemia (e.g. to maintain the haemoglobin concentration arbitrarily greater than 10 g dl^{-1}) as this practice has not been shown to improve wound healing or aid surgical recovery. Thromboprophylaxis is an important aspect of postoperative care (see Ch. 31).

FUTURE DIRECTIONS

The field of transfusion medicine is rapidly developing and there is increasing awareness of the risks of homologous blood. The advent of recombinant DNA technology has already led to use of recombinant erythropoietin, but granulocyte and granulocyte–

monocyte colony stimulating factors are in routine use to elevate the white cell count in leukopenic patients. Recombinant thrombopoietin is likely to be available in 1996 and will revolutionize platelet transfusion therapy. Synthetic oxygen carriers ('artificial blood') have been under development for many years. Perfluorocarbons dissolve oxygen but function only in high concentrations of ambient oxygen and are only useful for short-term perfusion in the Intensive Care Unit setting (e.g. following coronary angioplasty). Recombinant haemoglobin solutions and liposomal haemoglobin are under active development.

FURTHER READING

American Association of Blood Banks 1993 Blood transfusion therapy: a physician's handbook, AABB, Virginia 4th edn

British Committee for Standards in Haematology 1990 Guidelines for implementation of a maximum surgical blood order schedule. Clinical and Laboratory Haematology 12: 321–327

British Committee for Standards in Haematology, Blood Transfusion Task Force 1993 Guidelines for autologous transfusion. 1. Pre-operative autologous donation. Transfusion Medicine 3: 307–316

Contreras M (ed) 1990 ABC of transfusion. British Medical Journal, London

Hunt B J 1991 Modifying perioperative blood loss. Blood Reviews 5: 168–176

McClelland D B L (ed) 1989 Handbook of transfusion medicine. HMSO, London

Williamson L 1994 Homologous blood transfusion: the risks and alternatives. British Journal of Haematology 88: 451–458

8. Fluid, electrolyte and acid–base balance

W. Aveling   C. Hamilton-Davies   6/47

FLUID COMPARTMENTS

Every medical student knows that man is mostly water. For the surgeon the key to fluid and electrolyte balance is a knowledge of the various fluid compartments. An adult male is 60% water; a female, having more fat, is 55% water; newborn infants are 75% water. The most important compartments are the intracellular fluid (ICF) – 55% of body water – and the extracellular fluid (ECF) – 45%. ECF is further subdivided into the plasma (part of the intravascular space), the interstitial fluid, the transcellular water (e.g. fluid in the gastrointestinal tract, the cerebrospinal fluid (CSF) and aqueous humour) and water associated with bone and dense connective tissue which is less readily exchangeable and of much less importance. The partitioning of the total body water (TBW) with average values for a 70-kg male, who would contain 42 litres of water, is shown in Figure 8.1 (Edelman & Leibman 1959).

To understand fluid balance one needs to know from which compartment or compartments fluid is being lost in various situations, and in which compartments fluids will end up when administered to the patient. For practical purposes we need only consider the plasma, the interstitial space, the intracellular space and the barriers between them.

The capillary membrane

The barrier between the plasma and interstitium is the capillary endothelium, which allows the free passage of water and electrolytes (small particles) but restricts the passage of larger molecules such as proteins (the colloids). Although no one has demonstrated holes in the membrane, capillaries behave as if they had pores of 4–5 nm in most tissues. Kidney and liver have larger pores, and brain capillaries are relatively impermeable. The osmotic pressure generated by the presence of colloids on one side of a membrane which is impermeable to them is known as the colloid osmotic pressure (COP).

Only a small quantity of albumin (mol. wt. 69 000) crosses the membrane and it is mainly responsible for the difference in COP between the plasma and the interstitium. The COP is normally about 25 mmHg and tends to draw fluid into the capillary, while the hydrostatic pressure difference between capillary and interstitium tends to push fluid out. This balance was first described by Starling (1896).

Staverman (1952) introduced the concept that different molecules will be 'reflected' to a different extent by the membrane. This term, the reflection coefficient, varies between zero (all molecules passing through the membrane) and + 1 (all molecules reflected). In disease states when the capillary membrane becomes leaky the reflection coefficient will fall. Flow across the membrane is represented by the equation:

$$V = K_f S[(P_c - P_{IF}) - \sigma(\pi p - \pi_{IF})]$$

where V is the rate of movement of water, K_f is the capillary filtration coefficient, S is the surface area; P_c and P_{IF} are the capillary and interstitial hydrostatic pressures, πp and π_{IF} are the plasma and interstitial oncotic pressures, and σ is the reflection coefficient.

The cell membrane

The barrier between the extracellular and intracellular space is the cell membrane. This is freely permeable to water but not to sodium ions, which are actively pumped out of cells. Sodium is therefore mainly an extracellular cation, while potassium is the main intracellular cation. Water will move across the cell membrane in either direction if there is any difference in osmolality between the two sides. Osmolality expresses the osmotic pressure across a selectively permeable membrane and depends on the number of particles in the solution, not their size. Normal osmolality of ECF is 280–295 mOsm kg^{-1}. Since each cation is balanced by an anion, an estimate

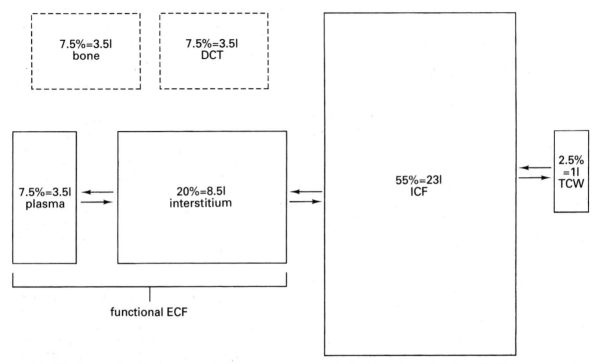

Fig. 8.1   Distribution of total body water in a 70 kg man. ECF, extracellular fluid; ICF, intracellular fluid; DCT, dense connective tissue; TCW, transcellular water.

of plasma or ECF osmolality can be obtained from the formula:★

Osmolality (mOsm kg^{-1})
= 2(Na$^+$ + K$^+$) + Glucose + Urea (mmol l^{-1})

Note that the colloids contribute very little to total osmolality as the number of particles is small, although as we saw above they play an important role in fluid movement across the capillaries.

Movement of water between compartments

Consider what happens when a patient takes in water, either by drinking or in the form of a 5% glucose infusion, the glucose in which is soon metabolized. It will rapidly distribute throughout the ECF with a result-ant fall in ECF osmolality. Since osmolality must be the same inside and outside cells, water will move from ECF to ICF until the osmolalities are the same. Thus 1 litre of water or 5% glucose given to a patient will distribute

★ Osmolality is expressed per kilogram of solvent (usually water), whereas osmolarity is expressed per litre of solution. The presence of significant amounts of protein in the solution, as in plasma, means that the osmolality and osmolarity will not be the same.

itself throughout the body water. In spite of being infused into the intravascular compartment (3.5 litres) it will be distributed throughout the body water space (42 litres) of which only 3.5/42, approximately 7.5%, is intravascular. For this reason approximately 13 litres of 5% glucose will need to be infused to increase the plasma volume by 1 litre. By a converse argument we can see that someone marooned on a life raft with no water will lose water from all compartments.

Normal saline (0.9%) contains Na$^+$ and Cl$^-$ at con-centrations of 150 mmol l^{-1}. If this is infused into a patient it will stay in the ECF because the water tends to follow the sodium ion and osmolality matches that inside the cells thus there is no net movement of water into the cells. Thus a volume of normal saline given intravascularly will tend to distribute throughout the extracellular space. The extracellular fluid makes up approximately 45% of the body water with the plasma volume being approximately 7.5%, and therefore 1/6 will remain intravascular and 6 litres will need to be given to increase the plasma volume by 1 litre. Equally, a patient losing electrolytes and water together, as in severe diarrhoea, loses the fluid from the ECF and not the ICF.

Finally, consider the infusion of colloid solutions (e.g.

albumin, starch solutions and gelatins). The capillary membrane is impermeable to colloid and thus the solution stays in the plasma compartment (there are, of course, circumstances in which it can leak out). A burned patient losing plasma loses it from the vascular compartment and initially there is no shift of fluid from the interstitial space. As blood pressure falls, hydrostatic pressure in the capillary falls, and if colloid osmotic pressure is maintained the Starling forces will draw water and electrolytes into the vascular compartment from the interstitium. Because there are only 3.5 litres of plasma, losses from this compartment lead to hypoperfusion and reduced oxygen transport to tissues and are potentially life-threatening. The use of hypertonic saline as a resuscitation fluid has become topical lately with reports of improved survival (Mattox et al 1991), the mechanism being the transfer of water into the intravascular space in the short term, leading to better tissue perfusion.

Since the plasma is part of the ECF, any loss of ECF results in a corresponding decrease in circulating volume and is potentially much more serious than loss of an equivalent volume from the total body water. For example, compare a man losing 1 litre a day of water, because he is marooned on a life raft, with a man losing 1 litre a day of water and electrolytes, due to a bowel obstruction. The man on the life raft will lose 7 litres in a week from his total of 42 litres body water, i.e. a 17% loss. The plasma volume will fall by 17%, which is survivable. The man with a bowel obstruction, on the other hand, loses his 7 litres from the functional ECF of 12 litres, i.e. a 58% loss. Losing more than half of the plasma volume is not compatible with life.

NORMAL WATER AND ELECTROLYTE BALANCE

We take in water as food and drink and also make about 350 ml per day as a result of the oxidization of carbohydrates to water and carbon dioxide, known as the metabolic water. This has to balance the output. Water is lost through the skin and from the lungs; these insensible losses amount to about 1 litre a day. Urine and faeces account for the rest. A typical balance is shown in Table 8.1.

Table 8.1 Average daily water balance for a sedentary adult in temperate conditions

Input (ml)		Output (ml)	
Drink	1500	Urine	1500
Food	750	Faeces	100
Metabolic	350	Lungs	400
		Skin	600
Total	2600	Total	2600

Table 8.2 Daily water requirements by body weight

Weight (kg)	Water requirements
0–10	$4 \text{ ml kg}^{-1} \text{ h}^{-1}$
10–20	$40 \text{ ml h}^{-1} + 2 \text{ ml kg}^{-1} \text{ h}^{-1}$ for each kg > 10 kg
>20	$60 \text{ ml h}^{-1} + 1 \text{ ml kg}^{-1} \text{ h}^{-1}$ for each kg > 20 kg

The precise water requirements of a particular patient depend on their size, age and temperature. Surface area ($1.5 \text{ l H}_2\text{O/m}^2$ daily) is the most accurate guide, but it is more practical to use weight, giving adults 30–40 ml kg^{-1}. Children require relatively more water than adults, as set out in Table 8.2. Requirements for the first 10 kg should be added to the requirements for the next 10 kg and likewise added to subsequent weight. Therefore, for a 25 kg child the basal requirements per hour should be $(10 \times 4) + (10 \times 2) + (5 \times 1) = 65$ ml h^{-1}.

The average requirements of sodium and potassium are 1 mmol kg^{-1} day^{-1} of each. Humans are very efficient at conserving sodium and can tolerate much lower sodium intakes, but they are less good at conserving potassium. There is an obligatory loss of potassium in urine and faeces and patients who are not given potassium will become hypokalaemic. As potassium is mainly an intracellular cation there may be a considerable fall in total body potassium before the plasma potassium falls.

PRESCRIBING FLUID REGIMES

In prescribing fluid regimes for patients, we need to consider three things:

- Basal requirements
- Continuing abnormal losses over and above basal requirements
- Pre-existing dehydration and electrolyte loss.

Intraoperative fluid balance needs special consideration, as all three of the above apply. Normally nourished patients who are nil by mouth for a few days during surgery do not in general need feeding intravenously, although some work has shown early feeding to lead to better postoperative recovery. Only in special circumstances is intravenous feeding required; this topic is outside the scope of this chapter.

Basal requirements

We have seen above the daily requirements of water and electrolytes. If we look now at the various crystalloid solutions that are available (Table 8.3), we can design

Table 8.3 Content of crystalloid solutions

Name	Known as	Na$^+$	Cl$^-$	K$^+$ (mmol l^{-1})	HCO$_3^-$	Ca^{2+}	Calculated (mOsm l^{-1})
Sodium chloride 0.9%	Normal saline	150	150				300
Sodium chloride 0.9%, potassium chloride 0.3%	Normal saline + KCl	150	190	40			380
Sodium chloride 0.9%, potassium chloride 0.15%	Normal saline + KCl	150	170	20			340
Ringer's lactate	Hartmann's	131	111	5	29 (as 12 lactate)		280
Glucose 5%	5% dextrose						280
Glucose 5%, potassium chloride 0.3%	5% dextrose + KCl		40	40			360
Glucose 5%, potassium chloride 0.15%	5% dextrose + KCl		20	20			320
Glucose 4%, sodium chloride 0.18%	Dextrose saline	30	30				286
Glucose 4%, sodium chloride 0.18%, potassium chloride 0.3%	Dextrose saline + KCl	30	70	40			366
Glucose 4%, sodium chloride 0.18%, potassium chloride 0.15%	Dextrose saline + KCl	30	50	20			326
Sodium chloride 0.45%	Half normal saline	75	75				150
Sodium chloride 1.8%	Twice normal saline	300	300				600
Sodium bicarbonate 8.4%	–	1000			1000		2000
Sodium bicarbonate 1.4%	–	167			167		334

fluid regimes for basal requirements. Normal saline, Hartmanns, 5% dextrose and dextrose saline are the most commonly used. Note that their osmolalities are similar to that of ECF, i.e. they are isotonic with plasma. The purpose of the glucose is to make the solution isotonic, not to provide calories, although a small amount of glucose does have a protein sparing effect during the catabolism that follows major surgery and trauma. Our standard 70-kg patient can be provided with the 24-hour basal requirements of 30–40 ml kg^{-1} of water and 1 mmol kg^{-1} of sodium in any of the ways shown in Table 8.4.

Potassium

None of these regimes supply significant amounts of potassium. Potassium chloride can be added to the bags and is supplied as ampoules of 20 mmol in 10 ml or 1 g (= 13.5 mmol) in 5 ml. Bags of crystalloid are available with potassium already added and this is safer than adding ampoules. It cannot be stressed enough that potassium can be very dangerous because hyperkalaemia causes cardiac arrhythmias and asystole. It should never be injected as a bolus. There have been a number of tragedies reported to the medical defence societies in which potassium chloride ampoules were mistaken for sodium chloride and used as 'flush', with fatal conse-

quences. Hyperkalaemia may also occur if potassium supplements are given to anuric patients. For this reason, you should usually wait until you are certain of reasonable urine output before adding potassium to the regime postoperatively. Safe rules for giving potassium are:

- Urine output at least 40 ml h^{-1}
- Not more than 40 mmol added to 1 litre
- No faster than 40 mmol h^{-1}.

Table 8.4 Basal water and sodium regimes for a 70-kg patient on intravenous fluids

Solution	Volume (ml)	Na$^+$ (mmol)	K$^+$ (mmol)
5% glucose	2000	–	
0.9% saline	500	75	
5% glucose	2000	–	–
Hartmann's	500	65.5	2.5
4% glucose	2500	75	–
0.18% saline			

Continuing loss

Patients with continuing losses above the basal requirements need extra fluid. The commonest example in anaesthetic and surgical practice is the patient with bowel obstruction. Fluid can be aspirated by a nasogastric tube to assess both volume and electrolyte content. Saline with added potassium should be given to replace it. Dextrose saline is not an appropriate fluid for this purpose because it only contains Na 30 mmol l^{-1}, and 5% glucose is even worse. Hyponatraemia will result if these solutions are used to replace bowel loss.

To keep track of the fluids, a fluid balance chart should be kept. This records all fluid in (oral and intravenous) and all fluid out (urine, drainage, vomit, etc.). Every 24 hours these are totalled, an allowance is made for insensible losses and the balance, positive or negative, is recorded. Any patient on intravenous fluids should have a daily balance, daily electrolyte measurements and a new regime prescribed every day. The instruction 'and repeat' should never be used in fluid management and has led to disasters in the past.

Correction of pre-existing dehydration

Patients who arrive in a dehydrated state clearly need to be resuscitated with fluid over and above their basal requirements. Usually this will be done intravenously. The problems are:

- To identify which compartment or compartments the fluid has been lost from
- To assess the extent of the dehydration.

The fluid used to resuscitate the patient should be similar in composition and volume to that which has been lost. From what we know about the movement of fluid between compartments (see above) and the patient's history, one can usually decide where the losses are coming from. As we have seen, bowel losses come from the ECF, while pure water losses are from the total body water. Protein-containing fluid is lost from the plasma and there may sometimes be a combination of all three types of loss.

Assessment of deficit

In estimating the extent of the losses, the patient's history, clinical examination, measurement and laboratory tests all play a part. A dehydrated patient may be thirsty, have dry mucous membranes, sunken eyes (and in infants fontanelles) and cheeks, loss of skin elasticity and weight loss. They will feel weak and, in severe cases, will be mentally confused. The cardiovascular system responds with tachycardia and peripheral vasoconstriction, so that the patient feels cold. Eventually, blood pressure and cardiac output fall, at which point the vital organs (brain, liver and kidneys), which up to now have been protected, are affected. Clouding of consciousness and oliguria are signs of severe dehydration. Weight, pulse, blood pressure and urine output are essential and simple measurements in the assessment and treatment of fluid loss, although these may be misleading as sympathetic drive from the nervous system may maintain blood pressure until very late.

Venous pressure. Equally important is the measurement of central venous pressure (CVP). An intravenous catheter is inserted into a central vein. The tip should lie within the thorax, usually in the superior vena cava or right atrium. In this position, blood can be aspirated freely and there is a swing in pressure with respiration. The pressure is usually measured by an electronic transducer but can be done quite simply by connecting the patient to an open-ended column of fluid and measuring the height above zero with a ruler.

The zero point for measuring CVP is the fifth rib in the midaxillary line with the patient supine (this corresponds to the position of the left atrium). The normal range for CVP is 3–8 cmH$_2$O (1 mmHg = 1.36 cmH$_2$O). A low reading, particularly a negative value, confirms dehydration, but CVP measurements are of more use as a guide to the adequacy of treatment. The response of the CVP to a fluid challenge of 200 ml colloid tells you more about the state of the circulation than a single reading. A dehydrated patient's CVP will rise in response to the challenge but then fall to the original value as the circulation vasodilates to accommodate the fluid. If the response to the challenge is a sustained rise (5 minutes after the challenge) of 2–4 cmH$_2$O this indicates a well-filled patient. If the CVP rises by greater than 4 cmH$_2$O and does not fall again this indicates overfilling or a failing myocardium.

The CVP reflects the function of the right ventricle which usually parallels left ventricular function. In cardiac disease, either primary or secondary to systemic illness, there may be disparity between the function of the two ventricles. The left ventricular function can be assessed by the use of a balloon-tipped catheter (Swan–Ganz) in a branch of the pulmonary artery. When the balloon is blown up to occlude the vessel the pressure measured distally gives a good guide to the left atrial pressure. This is called the pulmonary capillary wedge pressure (PCWP) and is normally 5–12 mmHg. In certain circumstances the CVP may be high when the PCWP is low, which then indicates that although the right atrium may be well filled the filling state of the systemic circulation is low. Here, as with the fluid challenge of the CVP, management of the filling status of the patient should be by means of fluid challenging the PCWP. Similar changes in level apply.

Work performed by Shoemaker et al (1988) demonstrated that the Swan–Ganz catheter could be used to treat patients to oxygen delivery/consumption goals when undergoing high-risk surgery. They found that those who achieved goals of:

- Oxygen delivery[*] > 600 ml min^{-1} m^{-2}
- Oxygen consumption[†] > 170 ml min^{-1} m^{-2}
- Cardiac index > 4.5 l min^{-1} m^{-2}

demonstrated an improved outcome. However, one argument is that these patients are self-selecting and that they would have had a good outcome anyway as they are able to achieve these goals thus, demonstrating better cardiovascular function.

Boyd et al (1993) also demonstrated an improvement in outcome in patients treated with dopexamine to achieve these goals, but again the same arguments apply. It has been shown that if critically ill patients are subjected to a similar style of management by driving their cardiovascular systems to achieve these goals with inotropes, then this group fare worse than a control group (Hayes et al 1994).

In summary, it would seem to be a reasonable form of management to attempt to achieve delivery/consumption goals in the cardiovascularly fit subjects undergoing high-risk surgery. However, in patients with cardiovascular disease these goals should probably be sought only with the use of fluid and agents that offload the left ventricle such as glyceryl trinitrate, thus reducing myocardial work. This should be performed under Swan–Ganz monitoring of cardiac function or the more recent non-invasive Doppler cardiac output monitor.

For those patients in whom these goals are non-attainable, attention should be turned to ensuring an otherwise meticulous perioperative course.

One other recent measure of occult hypovolaemia has been the measurement of gut intramucosal pH (pHi). This has been demonstrated to be the area that first suffers during haemorrhagic blood loss (Price et al 1966) and thus possibly the first to develop an acidosis due to anaerobic metabolism. Assessment can be made of this by means of a saline-filled balloon passed into the gut lumen which equilibrates with the CO_2 generated in the gut mucosa. From this, intramucosal pH can be derived. This value again has been related to outcome following high-risk surgery (Mythen et al 1993) and studies are currently being devised to investigate the effects of resuscitating patients to a pHi end-point.

[*] Oxygen delivery = Cardiac output × Hb × Arterial saturations × 1.34.
[†] Oxygen consumption = Cardiac output × Hb × (Arterial – Mixed venous saturations) × 1.34.

Quantification of plasma and ECF loss

If plasma is lost from the circulation, the plasma remaining still has the same albumin concentration, although the volume is diminished. Since no red cells are lost they become concentrated, resulting in a rise in haematocrit. Plasma is of course part of the ECF, so that losses of fluid and electrolytes without protein loss will cause a rise in haematocrit but also a rise in plasma protein concentration (Fig. 8.2). Changes in plasma albumin and haematocrit thus provide a good guide to ECF losses, while only haematocrit is of use in monitoring plasma loss (Robarts et al 1979).

In ECF depletion, the total amount of albumin stays the same although its concentration goes up. If Pr_1 is the initial albumin concentration and Pr_2 is the concentration after dehydration it can be shown that:

$$\% \text{ Fall in ECF volume} = \left(1 - \frac{Pr_1}{Pr_2}\right) \times 100$$

For example, if the albumin rises from 35 to 45 g l$^-$

$$\% \text{ Fall in ECF volume} = \left(1 - \frac{35}{45}\right) \times 100 = 22\%$$

By a similar argument one can calculate the fall in plasma volume as follows:

% Fall in plasma volume

$$= 100 \left[1 - \left(\frac{Hct_1}{100 - Hct_1} \times \frac{100 - Hct_2}{Hct_2}\right)\right]$$

For example, if the haematocrit (Hct) rises from 40% to 50%:

% Fall in plasma volume

$$= 100 \left[1 - \left(\frac{40}{60} \times \frac{50}{50}\right)\right] = 33\%$$

Haematocrit and plasma albumin are thus very useful in the assessment of ECF and plasma losses; much more so than the sodium which, though being lost, does not change in concentration.

A practical application of this from the paper by Robarts et al (1979) is shown in Figures 8.3 and 8.4. Figure 8.3 shows the results in a patient with acute pancreatitis. The plasma volume has fallen 30% (as determined by a rise in haematocrit), but the rest of the ECF volume is unchanged as there was no change in plasma protein concentration. After giving 1.5 litres of plasma, the plasma volume has been restored. By contrast, Figure 8.4 illustrates a patient who had lost ECF through the bowel; both the haematocrit and the plasma protein estimations show a 25% fall in plasma, and hence ECF, volume. As saline is administered, the values

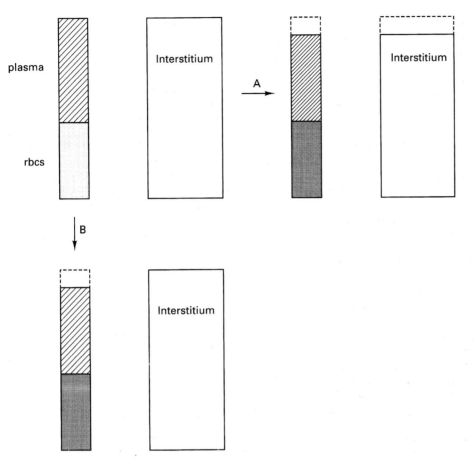

Fig. 8.2 **A** Loss of ECF leading to a rise in albumin concentration and haematocrit. **B** Loss of plasma leading to a rise in haematocrit but no change in albumin concentration.

return to normal. Table 8.5 summarizes the changes in volume and composition of various compartments in (1) isotonic fluid loss, (2) loss of water in excess of electrolytes, and (3) loss of sodium in excess of water. The corresponding expansion of compartments is also shown. It is a useful exercise to work through the various boxes predicting what change, if any, will occur. In the case of water loss (from both ECF and ICF) remember that the red cells are part of the ICF, so when water is lost from both compartments the haematocrit may not change. Similarly, when there is hypotonic expansion, red cells increase in volume as part of the ICF and with the simultaneous expansion of ECF there may again be no change in haematocrit.

Water and electrolyte replacement

Having assessed the amount of deficit, as discussed above, we come to the question of what to give to restore the situation. A look at the composition of various body fluids (Table 8.6) shows us that ECF losses of water and electrolytes should be replaced with either normal saline or Ringer's lactate with added potassium (see Basal requirements, p. 95). The only hypotonic secretions are saliva and sweat. The sodium content of sweat varies and responds to aldosterone. Gastric secretion, though having a sodium content of only 50 mmol l^{-1}, is isotonic with ECF because of the hydrogen it contains. Where the losses are primarily of gastric secretion, e.g. pyloric stenosis, one might think it necessary to supply hydrogen ions. In fact, the kidney compensates by retaining hydrogen and excreting sodium and bicarbonate, so that the net effect is a loss of sodium and chloride. Normal saline with potassium should therefore be used in rehydration.

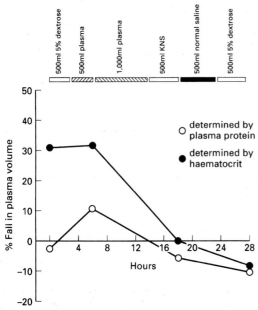

Fig. 8.3 Changes in plasma volume as determined by changes in plasma protein and haematocrit, during treatment of acute pancreatitis (see text).

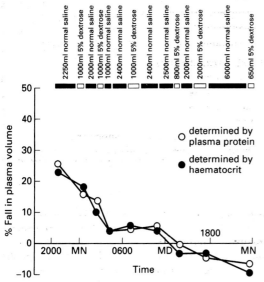

Fig. 8.4 Changes in plasma volume as determined by changes in plasma protein and haematocrit, during treatment of bowel obstruction (see text).

Plasma replacement and plasma substitutes

When we need to replace lost plasma there is a choice between giving plasma prepared from donated blood or one of the synthetic plasma substitutes. Human plasma protein fraction (HPPF) or human albumin solution (HAS) is prepared by separating red cells from donated blood. A bottle contains plasma from several donors and has been pasteurized to prevent the transmission of disease (e.g. hepatitis or human immunodeficiency virus (HIV)). It contains 4.5% albumin, has no clotting factors and is stable at room temperature. The main disadvantage is its cost (£40 in the UK, 1991), which reflects its limited availability. A number of solutions containing molecules large enough to stay within the capillaries and generate colloid osmotic pressure are available as plasma substitutes (Table 8.7).

Dextrans. The dextrans are glucose polymers available in preparations of different molecular weights. There is a large range of molecular weights in the solution. Dextran 70 is so called because the average molecular weight is supposed to be 70 000. In fact, the number-average molecular weight which is much more relevant to the colloid osmotic pressure, is 38 000 (see footnote to Table 8.7) (Webb et al 1989). Dextran 40 has smaller molecules and can be nephrotoxic. Dextran 110 has larger molecules. Neither of these will be considered further. Dextran 70 is quite a good plasma substitute, but its use has declined in popularity because of its adverse effects on coagulation and cross-matching and the relatively high incidence of allergic reactions.

Gelatins. Gelatin solutions are prepared by the hydrolysis of bovine collagen. They have the advantage over dextrans of not affecting coagulation and having a low incidence of allergic reactions. Being of smaller average particle size they stay in the intravascular space for a shorter time. Haemaccel contains potassium and calcium ions, which can cause coagulation if mixed with citrated blood in a giving set. Haemaccel stays a shorter time in the circulation, 30% of the molecules being dispersed to the interstitial tissues in 30 minutes. Gelofusin is probably preferable from this point of view.

Hetastarch. Six per cent hetastarch in saline has become available in the last few years. It has the largest average molecular weight of any of the plasma substitutes and therefore stays in the circulation longer. The dose should be limited to 1500 ml/70 kg; more can cause coagulation problems. About 30% of a dose is taken up by the reticuloendothelial system without apparent detriment to its function. Smaller molecules (mol. wt. <50 000 Da) are filtered by the kidneys. Larger ones are broken down by plasma amylase until small enough for real excretion.

Choice of solution for plasma expansion. The intravascular space can be expanded by the use of crystalloid solutions, e.g. saline, but because the fluid spreads throughout the ECF, 6 litres of crystalloid are needed to expand the plasma by 1 litre. In an emergency

Table 8.5   Changes resulting from three kinds of expansion and contraction of body fluids

Acute change	Example	Change in ECF vol	Change in ICF vol	Change in [Na]	Change in [Hct]	Change in [protein]
Loss H$_2$O + NaCl	Cholera	↓	→	→	↑	↑
Loss H$_2$O > Na	Excess sweating	↓	↓	↑	→	↑
Loss Na > H$_2$O	Addison's	↓	↑	↓	↑	↑
Isotonic expansion	Saline infusion	↑	→	→	↓	↓
Hypertonic expansion	2 × normal saline	↑	↓	↑	↓	↓
Hypotonic expansion	5% glucose infusion	↑	↑	↓	→	↓

Table 8.6   Electrolyte content and daily volume of body secretions

	Na	K (mmol l^{-1})	Cl	Volume (litres daily)
Saliva	15	19	40	1.5
Stomach	50	15	140	2.5
Bile, pancreas, small bowel	130–145	5–12	70–100	4.2
Insensible sweat	12	10	12	0.6
Sensible sweat	50	10	50	Variable

crystalloid is useful. All the battle casualties in the Falklands War were resuscitated in the field with Hartmann's solution.

5% glucose should not be used from choice as it is distributed throughout both ECF and ICF compartments; thus 13 litres are needed to increase the intravascular space by 1 litre. For most patients with acute hypovolaemia the best combination of advantages at low cost is offered by succinylated gelatin (Gelofusin). Being relatively short acting it is particularly useful as a holding measure until blood becomes available.

In continuing hypovolaemia hetastarch gives more prolonged expansion and its larger molecules are better retained in the circulation when the capillaries are leaky, e.g. in septicaemic shock.

Blood loss and blood transfusion

So far we have talked about plasma loss and plasma expansion. Most of what has been said about the assessment and replacement of plasma volume applies to blood loss. Transfusion of donated blood is possible in most circumstances, but has several disadvantages to be weighed against the fact that only haemoglobin carries oxygen. With a haemoglobin of 14 g dl^{-1}, evolution has equipped us with spare capacity as far as oxygen-carrying capacity is concerned. Indeed, as haematocrit falls, the decrease in oxygen carrying is compensated by better tissue perfusion due to reduced blood viscosity. It has been shown that the best balance between oxygen carrying and viscosity occurs around a haematocrit of 30%. It is also suspected that blood transfusion at the time of surgery for certain cancers leads to immuno-

---

Box 8.1   The hazards of blood transfusion

Any transfusion
- Transmission of disease, e.g. AIDS, malaria (donor blood screened for HIV, hepatitis, syphilis)
- Bacterial contamination
- Pyrogenic reactions (antibodies to white cells)
- Incompatibility reactions
- ± Haemolysis (clerical error commonest cause)

Massive transfusion
- Hypothermia
- Hyperkalaemia
- Citrate toxicity
- Acidosis
- Microaggregate embolism, 'shock lung'
- Dilution and consumption of clotting factors

---

logical suppression and poorer long-term survival. On the other hand, blood transfusion prior to transplant procedures improves graft survival. Since the AIDS scare there is greater reluctance on the part of the public to accept blood transfusion. For all these reasons, as well as the hazards of blood transfusion listed in Box 8.1, the expense of blood and rarity of some blood groups, one is reluctant to transfuse blood. In practical terms, operative blood loss up to 500 ml can be replaced with saline, remembering that six times as much will be needed (see above), or plasma substitutes. Only if more than 1 litre of blood has been lost in a healthy adult should one consider giving blood.

Rather than supply whole blood, it is more efficient

Table 8.7   Characteristics of colloid solutions

Name	Brand name	No. average* mol. wt.	Mol. wt. range	Na$^+$/K$^+$/Ca^{2+} (mmol l^{-1})	$t_{\frac{1}{2}}$ in plasma	Adverse reactions (%) Mild	Severe	Effect on coagulation	Cost (UK 1991)
Human plasma protein fraction	HPPF	69 000	69 000	150 5 2	20 days	0.02	0.004	None	£40
Dextran 70 in saline 0.9% or glucose 5%	Macrodex Lomodex 70 Gentran 70	38 000	<10 000–>250 000	150 – –	12 h	0.7	0.02	Inhibit platelet aggregation Factor VIII↓ Interfere with cross-match	£3.66 £4.11
Polygeline (degraded gelatin)	Haemaccel	24 500	<5 000–>50 000	145 5 6.25	2.5 h	0.12	0.04	None	£3.81
Succinylated gelatin	Gelofusin	22 600	<10 000–>140 000	154 0.4 0.4	4 h	0.12	0.04	None	£3.16
Hydroxyethyl starch 6% in saline (Hetastarch)	Hespan	70 000	<10 000–>10^6	154 – –	25 h	0.09	0.006	> 1.5 g kg^{-1} day^{-1} can cause coagulopathy	£15.39

*Number-average molecular weight should not be confused with weight-average molecular weight, which is usually quoted by the manufacturers. No average molecular weight is more appropriate.

Box 8.2   Blood products

- Plasma-reduced blood (packed cells)
- Washed red cells: if transfusion reaction a problem
- Plasma protein fraction (HPPF)
- Fresh frozen plasma (FFP): contains clotting factors more dilute than the concentrates below
- Cryoprecipitate: rich in factor VIII
- Factor VIII concentrate: even richer in VIII
- Factors II, VII, IX and X concentrate
- Factor XI concentrate
- Fibrinogen
- Platelet concentrate

---

for the transfusion service to separate it into components as listed in Box 8.2. Blood cross-matched for patients undergoing surgery usually comes as plasma-reduced blood ('packed cells'). This is more viscous than whole blood and needs to be given with appropriate amounts of crystalloid or colloid solution to restore the volume.

The quantity of blood lost is assessed clinically as outlined above, and at operation by watching the suction bottle and weighing swabs, but this generally underestimates the loss. In operations such as transurethral resection of prostate, measurement of haemoglobin in the irrigating fluid gives an accurate measure of blood loss. In acute blood loss, haematocrit and haemoglobin concentrations do not change until the blood remaining in the patient has been diluted by shift of fluid from the interstitial space or intravenous infusion. Plasma-reduced blood and whole blood more than 1 day old (which it almost always is) contain no viable platelets and a few clotting factors. The same applies to plasma

protein fraction. In massive transfusion both dilution and consumption of clotting factors make it necessary to send blood for a clotting screen and give platelets and fresh frozen plasma (FFP) according to the results. As a rule, one gives a unit of FFP for every 4–6 units of stored blood transfused.

Intraoperative fluid balance

During an operation everything we have discussed so far may be going on at the same time. The patient is starved for 6–12 hours, there may be blood loss, plasma loss, ECF loss and evaporation of water from exposed bowel. As part of the stress response to surgery the patient retains water and sodium. The importance of careful monitoring in major surgery will be obvious; this includes accurate assessment of blood loss, haemodynamic variables and urine output.

As a rule of thumb, in intra-abdominal surgery Hartmann's solution 5 ml kg^{-1} h^{-1} may be given up to 2 litres. This will compensate for starvation, ECF loss, evaporation and some blood loss. Blood or colloids may have to be given in addition. If the patient is being treated in an attempt to achieve oxygen delivery/consumption goals then continually fluid challenging the CVP in cardiovascularly healthy patients, or the PCWP in those with cardiac dysfunction, should be performed to maintain an optimal haemodynamic state.

For the first 36 hours postoperatively there is water retention and there is sodium retention lasting 3–5 days. Obligatory potassium loss of 50–100 mmol per day continues. If additional sodium is given it is simply retained, although the urine may show an increase in sodium output. Provided that intraoperative losses have been replaced by the end of the operation one should give the basal requirements (30–40 ml kg^{-1} day^{-1} H_2O + 1 mmol kg^{-1} day^{-1} Na^+ and K^+) plus additional blood or colloid if there is significant wound drainage. Remember, not to start potassium until urine output is established; the operation of inadvertent bilateral ureteric ligation is not unknown.

ACID–BASE BALANCE

Claude Bernard was the first to recognize that to function effectively the body needs a stable *milieu interieur*. The hydrogen ion concentration is the most important contribution to this. An acid is a hydrogen ion (proton) donor and a base accepts hydrogen ions. Throughout life the body produces hydrogen ions and they must be excreted or buffered to keep the internal environment constant.

Terminology and definitions

Hydrogen ion activity

Hydrogen ion activity is traditionally expressed in pH units, pH being the negative log_{10} of the hydrogen ion concentration:

$$pH = -\log[H^+] = \log \frac{1}{[H^+]}$$

Hydrogen ion concentration can also be expressed directly in nanomoles per litre (Table 8.8). Note that the pH is a log scale, so that each 0.3 unit fall in pH represents a doubling of hydrogen ion concentration.

Acidosis and alkalosis

The normal ECF pH is 7.36–7.44 (44–36 nmol l^{-1}). Acidaemia is a blood pH below this range and alkalaemia a pH above it. Acidosis is a condition that leads to acidaemia or would do if no compensation occurred, but the terms 'acidosis' and 'acidaemia' are often used loosely to mean the same thing, which is not strictly correct. Alkalosis and alkalaemia are defined in a similar way.

Respiratory acidosis. A fall in pH resulting from a rise in the P_{CO_2} is a respiratory acidosis, e.g. opiate overdose leading to hypoventilation causes a rise in P_{CO_2}.

Respiratory alkalosis. This is a rise in pH due to a lowering of the P_{CO_2}, such as occurs in hyperventilation.

Metabolic acidosis. This is a fall in pH due to anything other than carbon dioxide (sometimes referred to as non-respiratory acidosis). There is a primary gain of acid or loss of bicarbonate from ECF.

Metabolic alkalosis. This is a rise in pH from non-respiratory causes. There is either a gain in bicarbonate or a loss of acid from the ECF.

Compensatory changes. If the initial problem is respiratory, the result is called a *primary respiratory acidosis* or alkalosis. If the respiratory problem persists for more than a few hours the kidney will excrete or retain bicarbonate to try and compensate for the respiratory disturbance. This is referred to as *secondary or compensatory metabolic acidosis* or alkalosis.

Thus a primary respiratory acidosis may be accompanied by a secondary metabolic alkalosis. For example, chronic obstructive airways disease leads to a rise in the P_{CO_2}: primary respiratory acidosis. To compensate for this the kidney retains bicarbonate, leading to a rise in ECF bicarbonate: secondary or compensatory metabolic alkalosis.

In the same way primary respiratory alkalosis (e.g. the hyperventilation that occurs at high altitude) will be compensated by a secondary metabolic acidosis. Where the first disturbance is metabolic, e.g. the build-up of acid in diabetic ketoacidosis, the primary metabolic acidosis will cause hyperventilation (secondary respiratory alkalosis), which will tend to restore the pH to normal. This respiratory compensation for a metabolic change happens much more rapidly than the metabolic compensation for a respiratory problem.

The fourth possible combination of changes is to have a metabolic alkalosis (e.g. loss of H^+ in pyloric stenosis) compensated by a respiratory acidosis. However, hypoventilation (respiratory acidosis) leads to a fall in P_{O_2}, which stimulates ventilation so that in practice compensatory respiratory acidosis is not usually seen.

In deciding which is the primary and which is the secondary change it is important to realize that the compensatory changes do not bring the pH back to normal; they bring it back *towards* the normal range. In other words, even after compensation the measured pH is altered in the direction of the primary problem (acidosis or alkalosis). Compensatory mechanisms merely make the disturbance in pH less than it otherwise would have been. It is also important to consider the history. Examiners may give candidates blood gas results to interpret, but in real life blood gases come from patients. Knowing that a patient is an unconscious diabetic breathing spontaneously, rather than an anaesthetized patient on a ventilator, certainly helps one's interpretation.

Buffers

Buffers are substances which by their presence in solution minimize the change in pH for a given addition of acid or alkali. Three-quarters of the buffering power of

Table 8.8 Conversion table for pH units and hydrogen ion concentration

pH unit	H^+ (nmol l^{-1})
8.00	10
7.70	20
7.44	36
7.40	40
7.36	44
7.10	80
7.00	100

the body is within the cells; the rest is in the ECF. Proteins, haemoglobin, phosphates and the bicarbonate system are all important buffers. The particular importance of the bicarbonate system is that carbon dioxide is excreted in the lungs and can be regulated by changes in ventilation. Bicarbonate excretion in the kidney can also be regulated. The lungs are responsible for the excretion of 16 000 mmol per day of acid and the kidneys for only 40–80 mmol per day. The formation of carbonic acid from carbon dioxide and water is catalysed by carbonic anhydrase (present in red cells). The reaction may go in either direction:

$$H^+ + HCO_3^- \rightleftharpoons H_2CO_3 \rightleftharpoons H_2O + CO_2$$

The Henderson–Hasselbalch equation is derived from this and expresses the relationship between the bicarbonate concentration, the carbon dioxide and the pH:

$$pH = pK + \log \frac{[HCO_3^-]}{[H_2CO_3]}$$

The carbonic acid can be expressed in terms of carbon dioxide, so that a more useful form of the equation is:

$$pH = pK + \log \frac{[HCO_3^-]}{0.03 \, P\text{CO}_2}$$

As this is a buffer system which minimizes changes in pH, we can see that if the carbon dioxide rises so will the bicarbonate, to keep $[HCO_3^-]/P\text{CO}_2$ constant. Similarly a fall in bicarbonate will be accompanied by a fall in $P\text{CO}_2$ to prevent a change in pH.

Interpretation of acid–base changes

As the patient's acid–base status varies, three things are changing at once: pH, $[HCO_3^-]$ and $P\text{CO}_2$. Blood gas machines measure $P\text{O}_2$, pH and $P\text{CO}_2$ directly. The actual bicarbonate $[HCO_3^-]$ is calculated from the Henderson–Hasselbalch equation. Blood gas machines also derive other variables which help in the interpretation of the acid–base status. These are as follows.

Standard bicarbonate (SBC)

This is the concentration of bicarbonate in the plasma of fully oxygenated blood at 37°C at a $P\text{CO}_2$ of 5.3 kPa (40 mmHg). In other words, it tells you what the bicarbonate would be if there was no respiratory disturbance. Looking at the standard bicarbonate therefore tells you what is going on on the metabolic side. Normal standard bicarbonate is 22–26 mmol l^{-1}. Values above this indicate metabolic alkalosis and those below, metabolic acidosis.

Base excess (BE)

This is the amount of strong base or acid that would need to be added to whole blood to titrate the pH back to 7.4 at a $P\text{CO}_2$ of 5.3 kPa and 37°C. It tells you the same thing as standard bicarbonate, namely the metabolic status of the patient. Normal base excess is obviously zero (± 2 mmol l^{-1}). Positive base excess occurs in metabolic alkalosis, and negative base excess (sometimes called base deficit) indicates metabolic acidosis. The base excess is an in vitro determination in whole blood. It is also known as the actual base excess (ABE) or the base excess (blood) (BE b).

Standard base excess (SBE)

This is an estimate of the in vivo base excess and takes into account the difference in buffering capacity between the patient's ECF and the blood that was put in the blood gas machine. Interstitial fluid, having less protein and no haemoglobin, has a lower buffering capacity than blood. SBE is therefore 1–2 mmol l^{-1} greater than BE, but this makes very little difference in practice. SBE is sometimes called base excess (e.c.f.).

Total carbon dioxide (TCO_2)

This is the total concentration of carbon dioxide in the plasma as bicarbonate and dissolved carbon dioxide.

$$T\text{CO}_2 = [HCO_3^-] + (P\text{CO}_2 \times \text{Solubility})$$

Oxygen saturation (O$_2$ sat.)

The percentage saturation of haemoglobin by oxygen is derived from the haemoglobin oxygen dissociation curve and the measured $P\text{O}_2$. The normal value is >95%. This value should not be relied upon to be accurate, as other forms of haemoglobin such as carboxyhaemoglobin will be included as oxyhaemoglobin. If this is suspected (e.g. in burns patients) then a co-oximeter should be used to determine the level of oxyhaemoglobin.

Table 8.9 Printout from a blood gas machine with normal values

Temp	37°C
pH	7.36–7.44 (44–36 nmol l^{-1})
PCO_2	4.6–5.6 kPa (35–42 mmHg)
PO_2	10.0–13.3 kPa (75–100 mmHg)
HCO_3^-	22–26 mmol l^{-1}
TCO_2	24–28 mmol l^{-1}
SBC	22–26 mmol l^{-1}
BE	−2 to +2 mmol l^{-1}
SBE	−3 to +3 mmol l^{-1}
O_2 sat.	>95%
Hb	11.5–16.5 g dl^{-1}

PO_2 and inspired oxygen (F_IO_2)

To interpret the PO_2 one needs to know the age of the patient and the F_IO_2. Normal arterial PO_2 declines with age. Roughly speaking $PO_2 = 100 -$ age in years/3 mmHg or $13.3 - 0.044 \times$ Age kPa.

The expected alveolar PO_2 (P_AO_2) can be predicted from the inspired oxygen by the simplified alveolar gas equation: $P_AO_2 = P_IO_2 - P_ACO_2/R$, where R is the respiratory exchange ratio (normally 0.8). In dry gas P_IO_2 (in kPa) = Fractional inspired oxygen (F_IO_2)%. Alveolar gas is saturated with water vapour (6.3 kPa), for which allowance must be made. If the $F_IO_2 = 40\%$ and the $PCO_2 = 5.3$:

$$P_AO_2 = \frac{(40 - 40 \times 6.3)}{100} - \frac{5.3}{0.8} = 30.85 \text{ kPa}$$

As an approximate rule of thumb one can deduct 10 from the $F_IO_2\%$ to give the expected P_AO_2 in kPa (e.g. if $F_IO_2 = 50\%$ then P_AO_2 is approximately 40 kPa). The difference between the estimated P_AO_2 and the measured arterial PO_2 is called the (A–a) PO_2 gradient. It is normally 0.5–3 kPa.

Without considering the inspired oxygen it is not possible to comment sensibly on the observed P_AO_2. A rough calculation of the (A–a) PO_2 gradient should be made when commenting on blood gas results. Some machines even calculate this for you as well!

A blood gas machine usually prints out the variables shown in Table 8.9. There is often a haemoglobin measurement and the temperature of measurement (37°C) is quoted.

Temperature correction

The blood gas machine operates at 37°C. Because gases are more soluble in liquid at lower temperatures (as drinkers of cold lager will know) the blood gases would be different if measured at another temperature. Blood gas machines are programmed to correct the gases if you tell the machine the patient's actual temperature. However, there has been much debate as to whether it is appropriate to correct for temperature. Suffice it to say that the protagonists of not correcting for temperature (the alpha stat theory) hold sway and one should probably act on the blood gases as measured at 37°C and not the temperature-corrected values.

The anion gap

For electrochemical neutrality of the ECF the number of anions must equal the number of cations. The main cations are sodium and potassium and the main anions are chloride, bicarbonate, proteins, phosphates, sulphates and organic acids.

Normally, only Na^+, K^+, HCO_3^- and Cl^- are measured in the laboratory. Thus, when we add the normal values for these they do not balance:

Cations		Anions	
Na^+	140	Cl^-	105
K^+	5	HCO_3^-	25
Total	145	Total	130

The difference is known as the *anion gap* and represents the other anions not usually measured. Anion gap $= (Na^+ + K^+) - (HCO_3^- + Cl^-) = 11\text{–}19$ mmol l^{-1}. Its significance is that in certain metabolic acidoses (e.g. ketoacidosis or lactic acidosis) the anion gap will be increased by the presence of organic anions. However, in metabolic acidosis in which chloride replaces bicarbonate (e.g. bicarbonate loss due to diarrhoea), the anion gap will be normal.

Plan for interpreting blood gases

1. Check for internal consistency. Remember that the machine only measures pH, PCO_2 and PO_2. If it measures any of these wrongly, which is not infrequent, the derived variables will be wildly abnormal too. If the results do not fit with the clinical picture, suspect the machine. Example: a patient on a ventilator in theatre with an end-tidal carbon dioxide of 5% has the following gases:

PO_2	13.0
pH	7.64
PCO_2	5.1
HCO_3^-	37.5
TCO_2	38.5
SBC	39.0
BE	+15
SBE	+16
O_2 sat.	99%

It is much more likely that the pH has been measured wrongly than that the patient has a gross metabolic alkalosis.

2. Look at the pH. Remember the pH change is always in the direction of the primary problem acidosis or alkalosis.

3. Look at the P_{CO_2}. Abnormality of the P_{CO_2} indicates the respiratory component.

4. Look at the base excess or standard bicarbonate. Both give the same information, i.e. the metabolic acid–base status after correcting for the P_{CO_2}.

5. Calculate the anion gap.

6. Look at the P_{O_2} and calculate the A–a gradient.

Examples of abnormal blood gases

pH	7.51	The alkalaemia is due to primary
P_{CO_2}	3.7	respiratory alkalosis (low P_{CO_2}).
P_{O_2}	29	There is no metabolic
HCO_3^-	22.1	compensation (normal base
T_{CO_2}	23.6	excess). The P_{O_2} would be
SBC	25	expected if breathing 40%
BE	+ 1.1	oxygen $P_{I}O_2 - 10 = (40 - 10) =$
SBE	+ 2	30. The patient is
O_2 sat.	100%	hyperventilating.
(F_IO_2 40%)		

pH	7.28	A respiratory acidosis with high
P_{CO_2}	7.33	P_{CO_2} due to hypoventilation.
P_{O_2}	9.21	Again no metabolic
HCO_3^-	25.2	compensation (normal SBC and
T_{CO_2}	28.4	BE). Low P_{O_2} due to
SBC	22.3	hypoventilation.
BE	- 1.9	
SBE	- 2.5	
O_2 sat.	91%	
(F_IO_2 air)		

pH	7.35	Again a respiratory acidosis
P_{CO_2}	9.33	(high P_{CO_2}) but this time
P_{O_2}	7.11	compensated by metabolic
HCO_3^-	39.1	alkalosis (high SBC and positive
T_{CO_2}	41.2	base excess). This is typical of
SBC	32.4	chronic obstructive airways
BE	+ 8.2	disease with renal
SBE	+ 9.1	compensation.
O_2 sat.	85%	
(F_IO_2 air)		

pH	7.21	The acidaemia (low pH) is
P_{CO_2}	4.0	primarily due to a metabolic
P_{O_2}	13.3	acidosis (low SBC, base excess
HCO_3^-	11.5	- 15). Compensatory
T_{CO_2}	12.8	respiratory alkalosis (low P_{CO_2}),

SBC	9.3	does not return the pH to
BE	- 15.2	normal. P_{O_2} normal.
SBE	- 16.4	
O_2 sat.	99%	
(F_IO_2 air)		

pH	7.36	The pH is in the normal range
P_{CO_2}	4.21	despite low P_{CO_2} (respiratory
P_{O_2}	10.49	alkalosis) and low standard
HCO_3^-	17.6	bicarbonate (metabolic
T_{CO_2}	18.5	acidosis). The important thing
SBC	17.8	here is the P_{O_2}. It is apparently
BE	- 6.2	in the normal range but not
SBE	- 6.9	when breathing 60% oxygen.
O_2 sat.	96%	The (A–a) P_{O_2} gradient is
(F_IO_2 60%)		roughly 40 kPa. These gases are
		typical of a patient with adult
		respiratory distress syndrome.

Treatment of acid–base disturbances

As in any other field of medicine, treatment should be directed at the underlying cause. Correcting the P_{CO_2} is usually possible by taking over the patient's ventilation and adjusting the minute volume to give the desired P_{CO_2}.

Treatment of a metabolic acidosis is more controversial. It was traditional to treat a metabolic acidosis by giving sodium bicarbonate according to the formula (Base excess × Body weight in kg/3) mmol starting by giving half the dose; 8.4% sodium bicarbonate contains 1 mmol ml^{-1}.

It is now argued that, particularly in a hypoxic state such as exists at cardiac arrests, bicarbonate administration may do more harm than good (Graf & Arieff 1986). The bicarbonate generates carbon dioxide which crosses easily into cells, making the intracellular acidosis worse. If ventilation is impaired the carbon dioxide generated is unable to escape via the lungs. The traditional practice of giving 50–100 mmol bicarbonate at a cardiac arrest is probably unjustified. In metabolic acidosis due to poor perfusion of tissues the best way to manage this is to correct the perfusion defect which may be achieved, in some instances, by improving oxygen delivery using fluids, vasodilators or inotropes. This may involve the use of invasive monitoring such as Swan–Ganz catheterization in order to guide therapy. Treatment of the metabolic acidosis due to sepsis is controversial and, even though goal-directed therapy may not be universally accepted, most will still try to achieve reasonably high oxygen delivery targets. In sepsis, however, this does not give the anticipated rise in oxygen consumption after allowing for the rise in oxygen consumption due to increased myocardial work required to achieve the delivery. Sepsis appears to involve a defect in tissue oxygen uptake/utilization.

There is still a place for bicarbonate therapy in acidosis due to diarrhoea, renal tubular acidosis and uraemic acidosis. As outlined above, the base excess is used to calculate the dose; 8.4% sodium bicarbonate is hyperosmolar and must be given into a large central vein. Accidental subcutaneous administration can cause tissue necrosis. One must also bear in mind that each millimole of HCO_3^- is accompanied by Na^+ and it is easy to overload the patient with sodium. Frequent blood gas and electrolyte analyses must be made during treatment with bicarbonate.

REFERENCES

Boyd O, Grounds R M, Bennett E D 1993 A randomised clinical trial of the effect of deliberate peri-operative increase of oxygen delivery on mortality in high-risk surgical patients. Journal of the American Medical Association 270: 2699–2707

Edelman I S, Leibman J 1959 Anatomy of body water and electrolytes. American Journal of Medicine 27: 256, 277

Graf H, Arieff A I 1986 Use of sodium bicarbonate in the therapy of organic acidosis. Intensive Care Medicine 12: 285–288

Haes M A, Timmins A C, Yau E H 1994 Elevation of systemic oxygen delivery in the treatment of critically ill patients. New England Journal of Medicine 330: 1717–1722

Mattox K L, Maningas P A, Moore E E 1991 Prehospital hypertonic saline/dextran infusion for post-traumatic hypotension. Annals of Surgery 213: 482–491

Mythen M G, Purdy G, Mackie I J 1993 Post-operative multiple organ dysfunction syndrome associated with gut mucosal hypoperfusion, increased neutrophil degranulation and C-1-esterase inhibitor depletion. British Journal of Anaesthesia 71: 858–863

Price H L, Deutsch S, Marshall B E 1966 Haemodynamic and metabolic effects of haemorrhage in man with particular reference to the splanchnic circulation. Circulation Research 18: 469–474

Robarts W M, Parkin J V, Hobsley M 1979 A simple clinical approach to quantifying losses from the extracellular and plasma compartments. Annals of the Royal College of Surgeons of England 61: 142–145

Shoemaker W C, Appel P L, Kram H B 1988 Prospective trial of supranormal values of survivors as therapeutic goals in high-risk surgical patients. Chest 94: 1176–1186

Starling E H 1896 On the absorption of fluids from the connective spaces. Journal of Physiology 19: 312–326

Staverman A 1952 Apparent osmotic pressure of solutions of heterodisperse polymers. Rec Trav Chim 71: 623–633

Webb A R, Barclay S A, Bennett E D 1989 In vitro colloid pressure of commonly used plasma expanders and substitutes. Intensive Care Medicine 15: 116–120

9. Nutritional support

J. J. Payne-James

The metabolic response to injury – such as multiple trauma, major surgery and sepsis – is synonymous with increased demands for nitrogen and energy. Oral feeding is the optimum method of administering additional nutrients to a nutritionally compromised patient with increased needs. Sip feeds and oral diet supplementation are important ways of increasing nutrient intake and are therefore widely used in hospitals and community practice.

Many hospitalized patients, however, will not be appropriate for oral feeding. For these patients other routes of administration must be sought. Artificial nutrition support (provision of nutrient substrates by other than the oral route) is therefore indicated for many critically ill patients such as those in the postoperative period.

It is often considered surprising that malnutrition can be considered a problem in hospitals. Hill et al (1977) and Bistrian et al (1976) showed almost two decades ago incidences of malnutrition of up to 60% of hospital patients. Despite advances in the practice of clinical nutrition, McWhirter & Pennington (1994) recently established that 40% of patients were undernourished at the time of admission to hospital, and over half of those patients had no nutritional data documented in their case notes. Malnutrition is still a significant problem in hospitals. The aim of nutritional support should therefore be to identify the malnourished (or potentially malnourished) patient, and to correct or improve the nutritional status such that morbidity and mortality are minimized. Patients require nutritional support because studies have demonstrated poorer outcomes of treatment in patients who are malnourished. Worse outcome caused by impairment and eventual failure of physiological protein-dependent functions may be manifested as increased infection rates (e.g. chest, urinary or wound), slower healing, wound breakdown and dehiscence, and death. Identification of the patients suffering from protein energy malnutrition (PEM) is not always straightforward. Some assessment

of the nutritionally compromised patient is possible by measuring a variety of parameters, including biochemical (e.g. serum albumin, transferrin and retinol-binding protein), anthropometric (e.g. triceps skin-fold thickness (TSF) and midarm muscle circumference (MAMC)), immunological (e.g. lymphocyte count and delayed hypersensitivity skin-testing) and dynamometric (e.g. hand-grip strength). However these markers may have poor sensitivity or specificity when used alone.

INDICATIONS FOR NUTRITIONAL SUPPORT

In the absence of a single specific measure of nutritional state it is necessary for the practising clinician to define groups of patients who should receive nutritional support. All patients admitted to hospital, even for elective procedures, should have a nutritional assessment, the results of which should be recorded clearly in the notes, with the decision made about whether nutritional support is required. The routine history and clinical examination of a patient should enable patients to be placed in one of the following four groups:

1. Obvious severe malnutrition (recent or long term) (>10% recent weight loss; serum albumin <30 g l^{-1}; gross muscle wasting and peripheral oedema).

2. Moderate malnutrition (some nutritional parameters suggestive of depletion; dietary history shows impaired nutrient intake in preceding 2–4 weeks or more; there may be no obvious physical evidence of malnutrition).

3. Normal or near-normal nutritional status (but underlying pathology is likely to result in malnutrition if nutritional support withheld, e.g. trauma patients, ventilated patients).

4. Normal nutritional status which is unlikely to be affected by illness.

There are specific aspects of bedside clinical assessment which assist with this nutritional classification (Payne-James & Wicks 1994). Height and weight must

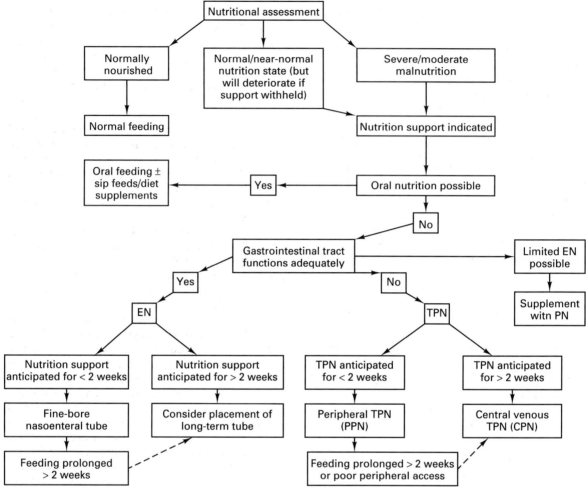

Fig. 9.1   Flow chart of options when nutritional support is required. CPN, central venous parenteral nutrition EN, enteral nutrition; PN, parenteral nutrition; PPN, peripheral parenteral nutrition; TPN, total parenteral nutrition.

be recorded and compared with standardized charts. Protein and energy balance may be estimated from the dietary history, and from the assumption that the maximum requirements of protein and energy for hospitalized patients are 1.5 g kg^{-1} per 24 h and 40 kcal kg^{-1} per 24 h, respectively. Body composition can be assessed clinically. Hill (1992) has described the 'positive finger–thumb test' when the dermis can be felt between finger and thumb when pinching triceps and biceps skinfolds. Body composition studies suggest that, when positive, the body mass is composed of <10% fat. Hill has also described the 'positive tendon–bone test' when tendons are prominent to palpation and bony prominences of the scapula are apparent – at which point patients have lost >30% of body protein stores. Additionally,

look for and record loss of muscle power, peripheral oedema, skin rashes, angular stomatitis, gingivitis, nail abnormalities, glossitis, paraesthesia and neuropathy.

Once the patient has been classified into one of the four groups above, a decision can be made as to whether nutritional support is indicated. If it is considered that nutritional support is required, the best route of administration must be chosen. Figure 9.1 illustrates the decision-making process. These routes are explored in more detail below. The key rule to be observed when choosing the optimal route of access is that: *the enteral route should be used as the technique of choice in all patients with a normal or near-normal functioning, accessible gastrointestinal tract.*

ENTERAL AND PARENTERAL NUTRITION FOR SURGICAL PATIENTS

Until recently, the gut has been considered to be an unimportant organ during critical illness caused by injury or infection. In the last few years the metabolic role of the gastrointestinal (GI) tract in both fasting and stressed states has been elucidated. It is now accepted that the GI tract is frequently a reservoir for bacteria that may cause systemic infections, by allowing bacterial translocation across the gut wall. Gut-derived endotoxin may therefore be the link between GI failure and multiple organ failure in patients without overt clinical evidence of infection. The relationship between GI bacteria, systemic host defences and injury in the development of bacterial translocation is represented in simplified form in Figure 9.2. In summary, enteral nutrition can improve antibacterial host defences, blunt the hypermetabolic response to trauma, maintain gut mucosal mass, maintain gut barrier function and prevent disruption of gut flora.

The potential role of early enteral alimentation in preserving intestinal barrier function cannot be overstated (Deitch et al 1990). Work continues to determine whether dietary manipulation (e.g. provision of glutamine or fibre) can prevent bowel atrophy and maintain intestinal mass. However, for the majority of critically ill patients (including those after surgery) the GI tract is an appropriate and desirable route for nutritional support, as long as there is no evidence of bowel dysfunction – such as abdominal distension, vomiting and large volume nasoenteral aspirates. Small intestinal function is maintained postoperatively (as the main sites of 'ileus' are the stomach and colon), and enteral nutrition (EN) may be delivered safely into the small bowel immediately after intra-abdominal surgery (including major aortic reconstruction). It is often suggested that bowel anastomosis is a contraindication to EN in the early postoperative period, but studies have confirmed its safety. EN should be considered the first choice for feeding patients with severe head injuries, and should be commenced early as aggressive nutritional support confers benefit on outcome.

Studies have been undertaken to investigate the effects of EN in patient groups which previously would have been given total parenteral nutrition (TPN). Kudsk et al (1992) undertook a prospective study investigating 98 trauma patients with an Abdominal Trauma Index (ATI) of >15 who were randomized to receive either EN or TPN feeding within 24 hours of injury. The aim of the study was to examine the effects of the two regimens on outcome in the first 15 days of hospitalization. All patients had laparotomy for management of intra-abdominal injuries and had a needle catheter jejunostomy placed at that time. The EN group had significantly fewer episodes of pneumonia, intra-abdominal abscess and line sepsis. EN patients with penetrating injuries had significantly fewer infections, and this was also observed in those needing >20 units of blood, those with an ATI >40 and in those requiring reoperation within 72 hours. Thus there was a significantly lower incidence of septic morbidity in EN-fed patients (compared with TPN-fed patients) after blunt and penetrating trauma, and this difference was enhanced with the most severely injured patients. Moore et al (1992) undertook a meta-analysis which included data from eight previously published randomized trials comparing the outcome of high-risk surgical patients fed either by early EN or TPN. Only 18% of EN patients compared with 35% of TPN patients developed postoperative septic complications.

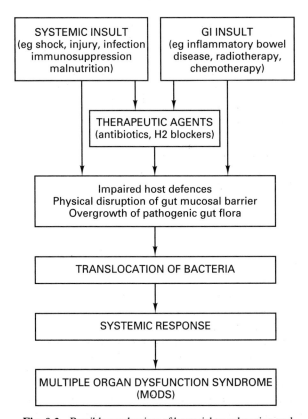

Fig. 9.2 Possible mechanism of bacterial translocation and multiple organ failure.

PERIOPERATIVE NUTRITION

The way in which nutritional support (including supplementation and EN) should be used in the preoperative period is summarized in Box 9.1. The length of preoperative nutritional support should not be such that the patient's condition can deteriorate as a result of progression of the disease. Postoperative nutrition should be considered for any patient who fails to have an adequate oral intake (as assessed by a dietitian) 5 days after surgery. Postoperative TPN should be considered when oral or enteral nutrition is not anticipated within 7–10 days in previously well-nourished patients or within 5–7 days in previously malnourished or critically ill patients. For some patients it may be clear at the time of operation that adequate oral intake will not be possible (because of major oropharyngeal/maxillofacial surgery) for some time postoperatively, or that normal gut function will take more than a few days to recover (major upper GI resection). In cases such as these it may be advisable to insert routes of access (e.g. gastrostomy, jejunostomy or central lines) while the patient is still in the operating theatre and still anaesthetized. If unexpectedly rapid recovery ensues, these may be removed; but, if they are required, the patient is not then subject to, and the surgeon does not have to arrange, placement at a later date.

These are all general principles and each case must be assessed individually. The reason for operation, the degree of malnutrition and expected postoperative course are all important in making this decision. A severely malnourished elderly patient who is a smoker, requiring oesophagectomy, would be a candidate for preoperative nutritional support. A patient with a pro-

longed exacerbation of inflammatory bowel disease unresponsive to medical management who presents with a perforated viscus requires surgery first and nutritional support later.

ENERGY AND NITROGEN REQUIREMENTS

Most surgical patients in need of nutritional support are metabolically stressed, septic or have been subject to trauma (accident or operation). These patients (particularly those with burns or head injuries) are likely to be hypermetabolic as a result of the normal neuro-endocrinological response to injury. Specific energy requirements may be determined from indirect calorimetry, but this is not practical for most clinicians. In general, energy requirements are rarely more that 2200–2400 kcal per 24 hours for surgical patients to achieve positive energy balance. Thus 35–40 kcal kg^{-1} per 24 hours will be appropriate for most patients, and this will be supplied as a mixture of carbohydrate and fat. Nitrogen requirements are often considerably greater than normal, and in hypermetabolic, stressed and injured patients nitrogen balance may be impossible to achieve until the primary pathology has been treated. The amount of nitrogen administered should ideally: minimize net losses without wasting administered nitrogen; permit maintenance of the patient's lean body mass, allowing an adequate supply of nitrogen for repair; and allow active repletion of lean body mass in the previously compromised patient. For most adult patients, 14–16 g nitrogen will be appropriate. Those patients with increased energy needs will require increased nitrogen and amounts of up to 0.4 g kg^{-1} per 24 hours have been suggested.

Monitoring

The main parameters that should be considered when monitoring a patient receiving nutrition support are:

- Diet charts
- Weight
- Haematology
- Biochemistry
- Anthropometry
- Dynamometry.

Diet charts (for patients on enteral nutrition) enable an accurate record of the patient's actual versus prescribed intake to be kept, and the charts will allow correction of intake problems to be undertaken. These charts are also of importance during the changeover from enteral feeding to oral nutrition. Weighing is the simplest but most valuable way to ensure that the nutrition regimen prescribed for a particular patient is satisfactory. A steady increase in weight of 1–2 kg per week suggests adequate nutrition in those requiring body mass repletion. Remember, however, that weight gain may result from water retention. Basic haematological and biochemical parameters should be measured at the commencement of nutrition. Initially, close monitoring of the plasma potassium, phosphate and glucose are important, particularly in the severely malnourished patient. In patients on long-term feeding, vitamin levels or trace-element levels may be required if clinically indicated. The plasma proteins albumin, transferrin and thyroid binding pre-albumin can all be useful markers for indicating a response to nutritional support over a period of time. Anthropometric and dynamometric measurements are often considered as research tools, but they can offer sensitive and effective measurement of the efficacy of nutritional support over a period of time.

Nitrogen balance

Nitrogen balance is frequently used as an assessment technique for monitoring day-to-day progress of nutritional support. One of the aims of nutritional support should be to place the patient in positive nitrogen balance. This is often difficult or impossible to achieve in the very stressed or catabolic patient. The components of nitrogen balance are those of whole-body protein turnover, which represents the difference between whole-body protein synthesis and breakdown. It is a measure of metabolic state rather than nutritional status. In most patients nitrogen balance can be calculated from urinary and faecal nitrogen losses and, whenever possible, 24-hour collections of urine should be undertaken on all patients receiving nutritional support. Faecal output is often negligible. There is a reasonable correlation between urinary urea excretion and total urinary nitrogen, with urea accounting for about 80%. Adjustments must be made for plasma urea levels and a figure of 2–3 g allowed for other routes of loss, including faeces. These figures are not appropriate for the severely ill patient, where the urinary urea may represent considerably less than 80% of the total nitrogen because of excessive excretion of ammonium and other non-urea nitrogenous compounds. In many centres total urinary nitrogen is measured routinely by chemiluminescence, obviating the need to estimate output from urea values.

ENTERAL NUTRITION (EN)

Types of enteral diet

There are three main types of nutritionally complete enteral diet appropriate for the surgical patient: polymeric, predigested (or elemental), and disease specific.

Polymeric diets are indicated for the vast majority of patients with normal or near-normal GI function. They contain whole protein as a nitrogen source, energy is derived from triglycerides and glucose polymers, while electrolytes, trace elements and vitamins are included in standardized amounts. Generally, one of two polymeric diets, a standard or an energy (nitrogen dense) diet, is prescribed. The standard polymeric diets contain approximately 6 g nitrogen per litre with an energy density of 1 kcal ml^{-1}. The energy (nitrogen dense) diets contain between 8 and 10 g nitrogen per litre and an energy density of 1–1.5 kcal ml^{-1}. Polymeric diets are suitable for over 90% of patients with normal or near-normal GI function. In a few patients with very severe exocrine pancreatic insufficiency or with intestinal failure because of short bowel syndrome, intraluminal hydrolysis may be severely impaired, thereby limiting diet assimilation. In such cases a *predigested or elemental diet* may be indicated. These diets have a nitrogen source derived from free amino acids or oligopeptides. Energy is derived from glucose polymer mixture predominating with polymers of chain length >10 glucose molecules. The fat source consists of a combination of long and medium-chain triglycerides. Specially formulated *disease-specific diets* have been developed for patients with disorders such as encephalopathy associated with chronic liver disease, and respiratory failure. Malnourished patients with cirrhosis who present with encephalopathy, or who have a previous history of episodes of encephalopathy, present a difficult problem of nutritional management. Branched-chain amino acid enriched diets have been advocated to normalize plasma amino acid profiles with the aim of improving nutritional state and preventing worsening of encephalopathy. Patients with respiratory failure on ventilators are adversely affected by diets with high carbohydrate loads which increase carbon dioxide production. Diets with higher fat energy component allow earlier weaning from a ventilator as a result of decreased carbon dioxide production and reduced respiratory quotient.

Much research is being undertaken on the use of nutrition substrates or supplements designed to modify or modulate the metabolic response to stress and the immune response. Such substrates include fish oils, arginine, glutamine and nucleotides. Although experimental work is promising, no clinical recommendations can yet be given (Heyland et al 1994).

Route of administration

Most patients will require nutritional support for less than a month. For these patients the best method of enteral delivery is via a fine-bore nasogastric feeding tube. The most frequent complication (less than 5% of patients) is tube malposition at insertion, generally into the trachea and bronchi. If the presence within the bronchus has not been recognised then accidental intrapulmonary aspiration of feed may occur. This complication occurs most commonly in patients with altered swallowing, diminished gag reflex or those who have had upper airway or pharyngeal surgery. In patients who are alert and orientated, tube positioning may be confirmed by aspiration of gastric contents and auscultation of the epigastrium. If aspiration or auscultation is unsuccessful, X-ray confirmation of the position of the tube is essential, and must be undertaken routinely in all patients with altered consciousness, altered cough or gag reflex, who are mechanically ventilated or who have had upper airway surgery. In some patents nasogastric delivery of nutrients may not be appropriate because of an increased risk of regurgitation and/or pulmonary aspiration of feed (Box 9.2).

All patients in the groups indicated in Box 9.2 and those with gastric atony or paresis for any reason should at least be considered for postpyloric nasoduodenal or nasojejunal feeding to reduce the risk of regurgitation or aspiration. Placement of fine-bore tubes beyond the pylorus remains a problem. Techniques using metoclopramide, manipulation of the tube at the bedside or under fluoroscopic control have all been tried, with varying success. For the surgical patient in whom postoperative feeding is anticipated, placement at laparotomy is advised. In other cases a fine-bore tube of appropriate length may be introduced pernasally, and if spontaneous passage has not occurred after 12–24 hours endoscopic or fluoroscopic positioning is undertaken.

Box 9.2
Patient groups/diseases with risk of gastric atony or paresis:

- Critically ill
- Diabetes with neuropathy
- Head injury
- Hypothyroidism
- Neuromotor deglutition disorders
- Postabdominal surgery
- Recumbent patients
- Intensive Care Unit/ventilated patients

For some patients other routes of administration may be more appropriate than or preferable to the nasoenteral route.

Pharyngostomy and oesophagostomy are used by a few surgical enthusiasts. Surgically placed gastrostomies are still used for long-term administration of feed for patients with progressive deglutition disorders (motor neurone disease or multiple sclerosis), but the percutaneous endoscopically placed gastrostomy (PEG) is now the technique of choice for long-term administration of enteral nutrition. This technique has a lower morbidity and mortality compared with the conventional surgical placement. The technique of needle catheter jejunostomy (NCJ), whereby a fine catheter is inserted either as a separate surgical procedure or concurrently at the time of abdominal surgery, is increasingly used. It has been suggested that an NCJ could be recommended for: (a) patients who are malnourished at the time of surgery; (b) patients undergoing major upper GI surgery; (c) patents who may receive adjuvant radiotherapy or chemotherapy after surgery; and (d) patients undergoing laparotomy after major trauma. The availability of this route means that TPN with its attendant risks may be avoided.

Reservoirs and giving sets

Enteral diets may be dispensed from different-sized containers ranging from 500 ml to 2 litres in volume. The policy of using larger reservoirs improves the ratio of administered diet/prescribed diet and reduces the amount of handling time needed. Giving sets should be changed every 24 hours as there is a risk of contamination of the diet container with bacteria spreading retrogradely up the giving set from the patient.

Infusion versus bolus administration

Bolus feeding of enteral diets, where typically 200–400 ml of feed is instilled into the stomach via a nasogastric tube over a period ranging from 15 minutes to 1 hour, was the standard method of administration for many years. This is a poor method of administering an enteral diet, because it has greater incidence of side-effects such as bloating and diarrhoea, in addition to which a considerable amount of nursing time is required and feeds may often be accidentally omitted. A continuous infusion either by gravity feed or by using a peristaltic pump is therefore the method of choice. A continuous overnight infusion followed by disconnection during the day may be the optimal technique, as nutritional parameters may also be improved in this way.

> **Box 9.3**
> Complications of enteral nutrition:
>
> **Feeding tube related**
> - Malposition
> - Unwanted removal
> - Blockage
>
> **Diet and diet-administration related**
> - Diarrhoea
> - Bloating
> - Nausea
> - Cramps
> - Regurgitation
> - Pulmonary aspiration
> - Vitamin, mineral, trace element deficiencies
> - Drug interactions
>
> **Metabolic/biochemical**
>
> **Infective**
> - Diets
> - Reservoirs
> - Giving sets

Starter regimens

Starter regimens (diluting the feed or reducing the volume) only results in limiting the intake of diet in the first few days of feeding, thereby prolonging the length of negative nitrogen balance. The incidence of GI side-effects is unchanged in patients with normal bowel, or those with inflammatory bowel disease, when a full-strength, full-volume diet is used to commence enteral nutrition. Therefore, in general, starter regimens should not be used.

Commencing enteral feeding

For those patients who are immobile or confined to bed, or with altered consciousness, the head of the bed should be elevated by 20° or 30° to help reduce the risk of regurgitation and pulmonary aspiration. In most adult patients with no other metabolic or fluid balance problems, 2–2.5 litres of diet are prescribed on a daily basis. This volume is infused from day one.

Complications

The potential complications of enteral nutrition are summarized in Box 9.3.

Tube blockage most commonly occurs after disconnection of the giving set from the feeding tube, and the residual diet solidifies. This complication may be prevented by flushing the tube with water after disconnection. An obstructed tube may occasionally be unblocked by instilling pancreatic enzyme or cola.

Diarrhoea occurs in about 10% of patients. The definition of diarrhoea as 'passage of too loose or too frequent stools, or both, sufficient to have been observed by patient and nursing staff' is useful in clinical practice. Its aetiology is multifactorial with a strong association with concomitant antibiotic therapy. Hypoalbuminaemia may play a role. Symptomatic treatment (with antidiarrhoeals such as codeine phosphate or loperamide) is appropriate, and only rarely does enteral feeding have to be discontinued. Antibiotics that are no longer clinically indicated should be stopped.

Nausea and vomiting rarely occur and may result from slowed gastric emptying. Antiemetics may be of benefit. The symptoms of bloating, abdominal distension and cramps most commonly occur following inadvertent too rapid administration of feed, and are very similar to the symptoms described in association with bolus-type feeding.

Enteral diets will interact with enterally administered drugs (e.g. theophylline, warfarin, methyldopa and digoxin). Failure of drug therapy in previously stable patients receiving EN support must be assumed to be feed related until proved otherwise.

TOTAL PARENTERAL NUTRITION (TPN)

The successful use of intravenous nutrition (total parenteral nutrition) in maintaining body weight and allowing growth to progress normally was first demonstrated by Dudrick et al (1968) over 20 years ago. TPN plays an essential role in the management of some acutely ill patents. Up to 25% of patients in hospital requiring nutrition support need it administered via the parenteral route. TPN can be considered for all malnourished or potentially malnourished patients with non-functioning and/or non-accessible GI tract. Four main areas need to be considered when providing TPN for a patient (see Box 9.4).

Access

TPN solutions have high osmolalities. As a result, administration of TPN solutions into peripheral veins can result in rapid development of thrombophlebitis and line failure. This problem has been overcome by using central venous catheters to deliver TPN solutions into large veins such as the superior vena cava (SVC), most commonly via the subclavian or internal jugular veins. Getting access to, and the presence of central venous

Box 9.4

Considerations for TPN:

- Access route (peripheral or central)
  - techniques
  - complications
  - delivery
- Nutrients
- Monitoring
- Complications
  - metabolic
  - catheter-related

Box 9.5

Central venous catheter complications:

Insertion-related
- Air embolism
- Arterial puncture
- Cardiac arrhythmias
- Catheter embolus
- Chylothorax
- Haemopericardium
- Haematoma
- Haemothorax
- Hydro/TPN-thorax
- Malposition
- Neurological injury
- Pneumothorax

Late complications
- Catheter infection, or sepsis
- Catheter displacement
- Central venous thrombosis
- Luminal occlusion

---

catheters within these veins, give rise to certain complications, the most well recognised of which are listed in Box 9.5. These catheter-insertion complications represent most of the serious complications associated with TPN.

A variety of routes, catheters and techniques of insertion are available. The two main methods of insertion are: blind percutaneous puncture of a vein; and open surgical exposure. The advantages of the percutaneous technique in experienced hands are that insertion is quick and may be done under local anaesthesia at the patient's bedside, as long as sterile procedure is observed. A catheter should be used that is inserted by

the Seldinger technique so that guidewire exchange of catheters is possible. Complications should occur in less than 5% of patients and are dependent on operator experience. Open surgical exposure generally requires an operating theatre and, occasionally, general anaesthesia. However, there are three groups of patients where catheter insertion should always be undertaken by using the open surgical technique if possible, because the risks associated with development of complications are more likely to be serious. These are patients with chronic respiratory disease, those on a ventilator, and those with severe clotting disorders.

The majority of catheters used for TPN in the UK are single-lumen central venous catheters. Most of these are inserted with a short subcutaneous tunnel fashioned to allow the catheter to exit away from the point of vein penetration. Strict catheter-care protocols should be followed and monitored by an infection-control or nutrition nurse to minimize the incidence of catheter-related sepsis. If a patient on TPN develops a pyrexia and leucocytosis in the absence of any other focus of infection, then the central venous catheter should be considered the source of infection. However, all other possible sources of infection should be considered and culture of sputum, urine, wound and other sites is mandatory.

Renewed interest in the feasibility of administering TPN by the peripheral route (peripheral parenteral nutrition (PPN)) has identified a number of methods which have been investigated to reduce the incidence of peripheral vein thrombophlebitis, including the use of heparin, in-line filtration, cortisol, buffering, locally applied glyceryl trinitrate patches and using fine-bore cannulas. Reducing the osmolality by altering the formulation of carbohydrate energy components and nitrogen source may also have a role, and specially formulated commercial mixtures have been shown in clinical studies to be suitable for PPN. Thrombophlebitis cannot be totally abolished, however, but it should be borne in mind that most courses of TPN rarely last more than 10–14 days. For many patients now, TPN should be administered peripherally if it is anticipated that support will be needed for less than 2 weeks. In this manner the risks associated with placement of central venous catheters are avoided. PPN is now widely used in many centres in the UK.

TPN nutrients

Macronutrients consist of energy sources, nowadays consisting of carbohydrate (glucose) and lipid emulsions. Most regimens consist of a combination in proportions up to 50% : 50%. Nitrogen sources are most commonly L-amino acids.

Box 9.6
Metabolic complications of TPN in order of frequency:

- Hyperglycaemia
- Hypoglycaemia
- Hypophosphataemia
- Hypercalcaemia
- Hyperkalaemia
- Hypokalaemia
- Hypernatraemia
- Hyponatraemia
- Other (particularly after long-term feeding): deficiencies of folate, zinc, magnesium, other trace elements, vitamins and essential fatty acids

Micronutrients are electrolytes, trace elements and vitamins, deficiencies of which may present interesting clinical problems. Commercial sterile solutions of the parenteral nutrition requirements may be mixed together safely in a single container (generally made of ethylvinyl acetate), an all-in-one bag (AIO), the contents of which can be infused safely over a given period. Mixing of these solutions is undertaken in a sterile laminar flow room. AIO bags can be used effectively in clinical practice, and solutions can be compounded and stored for several weeks without deleterious effect. Compatibilities of solutions vary, and if in doubt manufacturers should be consulted for advice.

Monitoring

It is important that an accurate record of the administration of TPN is maintained. TPN should be administered using infusion pumps or flow-control devices. In the first week of TPN administration, blood glucose should be measured 6-hourly, as many patients will develop some degree of insulin resistance because of their underlying pathology and may require exogenous insulin administered by injection/infusion, or occasionally incorporated in the TPN regimen. Electrolytes should be measured daily to allow correction of initial electrolyte imbalance and fluctuations, and to detect changes before severe metabolic/biochemical changes can affect the patient's clinical status. Liver function tests should be monitored to observe changes in serum albumin, and to detect TPN-related hepatobiliary dysfunction (see below).

Metabolic complications

A wide variety of metabolic complications can occur with TPN, and the results of a study documenting complications in order of frequency are listed in Box 9.6.

Although wide ranging, these complications only occurred in under 5% of patients, the majority of whom were in intensive care. A specific complication of TPN of multifactorial aetiology is the development of hepatic dysfunction. This is characterized by elevated hepatic enzymes, intrahepatic cholestasis and fatty infiltration of the liver. This is generally self-limiting and hepatic function returns to normal after cessation of TPN. Certain methods of reducing the incidence and degree of hepatobiliary dysfunction have been proposed (Box 9.7).

NUTRITION SUPPORT TEAM

A multidisciplinary nutrition support team is the best way of optimizing the nutritional care of hospitalized patients. The different members of the team can provide expert advice within their own specialty. Input to the team should come from clinicians, dietitians, pharmacists, nurses, chemical pathologists and microbiologists. The multidisciplinary approach ensures the most appropriate administration of nutrition support, and minimizes complications.

FURTHER READING

Payne-James J J, Silk D B A 1991 Hepatobiliary dysfunction

Box 9.7
Practical and theoretical methods by which the incidence and degree of hepatobiliary dysfunction with TPN may be reduced:

- Oral feeding, where possible (even if small volume)
- Stopping TPN
- Cyclic administration of TPN
- Avoid sepsis
- Avoid unnecessary surgical procedures
- Reduce non-protein calories
- Reduce glucose calories
- Review amino acid profile of TPN solution
- Use of lipid (as calories and supplier of essential fatty acids)
- Carnitine supplementation
- Taurine supplementation

associated with total parenteral nutrition. Digestive
Diseases 9: 106–124

Payne-James J J, Grimble G K, Silk D B A (eds) 1995 Artificial
nutrition support in clinical practice. Edward Arnold,
London

REFERENCES

Bistrian B R, Blackburn G L, Vitale J, Cochran D, Naylor J
1976 Prevalence of malnutrition in general medical patients.
Journal of the American Medical Association 235: 1567–
1570

Deitch E A et al 1990. The role of intestinal barrier and
bacterial transleration in the failure development of systemic
infection and Multiple Organ failure. Arch Surg 125: 403–
404

Dudrick S J, Wilmore D W, Vars H M, Rhoads J E 1968 Long-
term total parenteral nutrition with growth, development
and positive nitrogen balance. Surgery 64: 134–142

Heyland D K, Cook D J, Guyatt G H 1994 Does the
formulation of enteral feeding products influence infectious
morbidity and mortality rates in the critically ill patient? A
critical review of the evidence. Critical Care Medicine 22:
1192–1202

Hill G L 1992 Body composition research: implications for
the practice of clinical nutrition. Journal of Parental and
Enteral Nutrition 16: 197–218

Hill G L, Blackett R L, Pickford I et al 1977 Malnutrition in
surgical patients. Lancet i: 689–692

Kudsk K A, Croce M A, Fabian T C et al 1992 Enteral versus
parenteral feeding. Effects on septic morbidity after blunt
and penetrating abdominal trauma. Annals of Surgery 215:
503–513

McWhirter J P, Pennington C R 1994 Incidence and
recognition of malnutrition in hospital. British Medical
Journal 308: 945–948

Moore F A, Feliciano D V, Andrassy R J et al 1992 Early
enteral feeding, compared with parenteral, reduces
postoperative septic complications. The results of a meta-
analysis. Annals of Surgery 216: 172–183

Payne-James J J, Wicks C 1994 Key facts in clinical nutrition.
Churchill Livingstone, London

10. Clinical pharmacology

M. Schachter

INTRODUCTION AND DEFINITIONS

A decade ago an eminent professor of clinical pharmacology could foresee a time when every district general hospital would have its own clinical pharmacologist. This has not happened and does not seem imminent. Indeed, many clinicians have reservations about the role of clinical pharmacology as a specialty, except perhaps within the pharmaceutical industry. In fact, clinical pharmacologists themselves have very divergent views on their role. They have their own subspecialties and no one person can pretend to have comprehensive knowledge of all medicines. But clinical pharmacology does provide a framework of principles for evaluating the uses and dangers of new drugs, for comparing them with established agents, for detecting and even predicting both wanted and unwanted interactions, and for defining the ways in which drugs are handled in man. It is also involved in monitoring the effect of age, pregnancy and intercurrent disease on the use of drugs. This role is increasingly reinforced by the drug information services within hospital pharmacies, with access to extensive literature from many sources and to vast computerized databases. The readers of this chapter will already be aware, with more or less enthusiasm, that surgeons are major prescribers of drugs of all kinds from analgesics to antibiotics. Some reminders of clinical pharmacological principles may therefore be helpful, starting with a few definitions, particularly relating to pharmacokinetics. These terms will be used frequently in other parts of the chapter. This will obviously not be an overview of all the drugs that might be used in surgical practice, but will rather consider the principles of drug usage in some of the circumstances outlined above.

Half-life (or half-time)

This is almost always a measure of the rate of decline of drug plasma concentration, though occasionally it may have other meanings. The half-life (often written as $t_{\frac{1}{2}}$) is often easy to calculate, since the rate of decline of the drug concentration is usually exponential: if plotted as the logarithm of the concentration against time one therefore obtains a straight line (Fig. 10.1). However, in other instances the relationship is much more complex.

A knowledge of $t_{\frac{1}{2}}$ is clearly essential for the rational use of any drug (though prescribing practice does not always reflect this!). It allows the prescriber to calculate how rapidly a drug is eliminated from the body, under both normal and under pathological conditions. Equally important, it is an indication of the rate of accumulation of a drug during regular, fixed-interval dosing. For all practical purposes the $t_{\frac{1}{2}}$ is the only variable which determines the rate at which a drug accumulates under these circumstances, as well as the time taken for plasma levels to reach a steady state (that is, where input and output of the drug are in approximate balance). This takes about five half-lives (Fig. 10.2). There is, of course, one special case of 'multiple' dosing of particular importance in surgical practice, namely intravenous infusion. This can be considered as the administration of an infinitely large number of separate doses separated by infinitesimally small time intervals. It still needs the same number of half-lives to reach steady state, but with a much smoother increase in plasma levels. Finally, another issue arises from the inflexible interaction of half-life and steady-state plasma drug concentrations. For drugs with a long $t_{\frac{1}{2}}$ the time required to reach steady state may be unacceptably long. Therefore a loading dose may be given to achieve a therapeutic level which can then be maintained as the steady-state concentration. Digoxin is much the best known example of this, with a $t_{\frac{1}{2}}$ of about 40 hours even in the presence of normal renal function. Of course, a loading dose may also be given for a drug with a short $t_{\frac{1}{2}}$ if a very rapid effect is essential (for instance, gentamicin, with $t_{\frac{1}{2}}$ of 2–3 hours).

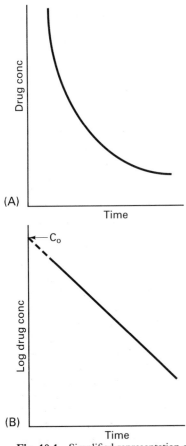

(A)

(B)

Fig. 10.1   Simplified representation of change in drug concentration with time: (A) linear concentration scale; (B) logarithmic scale. C_0 is the theoretical concentration at time zero used in calculating the volume of distribution.

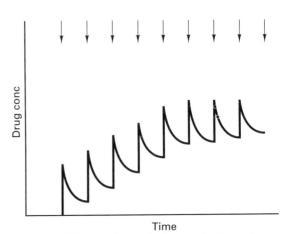

Fig. 10.2   Diagram of step-wise increase in plasma drug concentration when a drug is administered (arrows) at intervals of approximately one half-life. Steady-state concentration is reached in about 5.5 half-lives: note that this is not necessarily a *therapeutic* level.

Volume of distribution

Many find this the most confusing term in pharmacokinetics. The volume of distribution (or, more correctly, the apparent volume of distribution, abbreviated V_d), has units of litres per kilogram. This leads in some instances to absurd figures totalling several thousand litres. This is obviously not physically real, but does nevertheless have practical relevance. The V_d is calculated on the assumption that a drug distributes itself instantaneously throughout the body, with a concentration designated as C_0 (see Fig 10.1). It is therefore most appropriate to think of V_d as an indicator of the extent to which a drug is distributed in the tissues. Therefore:

$$V_d = \text{Dose}/C_0$$

Plasma and extracellular fluid may make only a modest

contribution to the total volume. In this context plasma protein is *not* a tissue and, as a result, highly protein-bound drugs (such as warfarin and the sulphonylureas) have V_d values approximating to plasma volume. On the other hand, very lipid-soluble drugs (tricyclic antidepressants and neuroleptics, for instance) may have enormous volumes of distribution.

Knowledge of the V_d of a particular drug may be useful in designing dosage regimes, though in practice it is not often used. V_d is related to $t_{\frac{1}{2}}$ and clearance (see below) by a simple equation:

$$\text{Clearance} = (V_d \times 0.7)/t_{\frac{1}{2}}$$

In other words, $t_{\frac{1}{2}}$ may be altered either by changes in clearance or in V_d. The clinical relevance of this is discussed in other sections of this chapter. Knowledge of V_d can also help in the evaluation of potential drug interactions: drugs with very large V_d values are, as already noted, likely to have low levels of plasma protein binding. They are therefore very unlikely to displace highly protein-bound drugs such as warfarin; of course, the converse is also true.

Clearance

This is a widely used term the exact meaning of which is not always appreciated. It is defined as that fraction

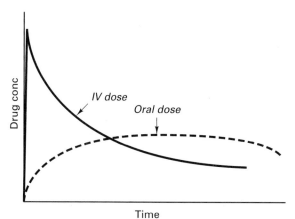

Fig. 10.3 Diagram to illustrate the calculation of bioavailability: the ratio of the area under the oral administration curve to that under the intravenous curve over a specified period.

of V_d from which the drug is removed per unit time. It is usually expressed as millilitres per minute or millilitres per minute per kilogram. Total clearance is the sum of clearances by all routes of elimination, both renal and non-renal. The most familiar example of clearance is not of a drug, but of endogenous creatinine which is used as an index of renal function. Much the most important of the non-renal routes is, of course, hepatic metabolism (e.g. corticosteroids and pethidine, among many others). Some drugs are metabolized elsewhere, in the plasma (suxamethonium) or in the gut wall (salbutamol). The latter is often described as 'first-pass' metabolism, though this term is also used for extensive metabolism of a drug in the liver.

Bioavailability

This term describes the proportion of the oral dose of a drug which reaches the systemic circulation, compared to intravenous dosing. It can easily be calculated from the areas under the time–concentration curves after intravenous and oral doses, respectively (Fig. 10.3). The main determinants of bioavailability are absorption and first-pass metabolism. Bioavailability may differ after chronic dosing, as compared to a single dose: metabolic enzymes may be induced or saturated during prolonged treatment. *It must be appreciated that different brands and* *formulations of a particular drug may have widely differing bioavailability.*

DRUGS IN THE YOUNG AND OLD

Neonates, infants and children

There is no lower age limit either for surgical intervention or drug therapy, but it must be appreciated that babies cannot be regarded simply as small adults. Every aspect of drug handling is drastically different in neonates and infants, as compared to adults. Firstly, the adult body has a lower water content than the neonate's (about 60% compared to 75%). Changes in fat content are less dramatic, but fat represents 12–15% of body weight in the neonate and 18–20% in most adults (much more in some, of course!). Renal function is initially poor in neonates, with a glomerular filtration rate only 5–10% of that in the adult. However, adult values are reached in 3–6 months. Tubular function is also immature in the very young. Hepatic function presents a more complex picture. Some enzyme systems are grossly underdeveloped in neonates (chloramphenicol glucuronidation is a notorious example), but other processes are fully active (most sulphation for instance). In general, however, oxidative systems are not fully mature and this can be of clinical importance, as with anticonvulsants and theophylline. The single most important alteration in gastrointestinal function is the increase in gastric acidity with age. Higher pH leads to increased absorption of some drugs, such as amoxycillin and flucloxacillin. Gastric emptying is also impaired in the neonate. Finally, the blood–brain barrier is relatively permeable in the very young. This can have serious consequences both in disease (kernicterus) and after drug administration, as in the case of the antidiarrhoeal opiates diphenoxylate and loperamide. These can cause significant, even fatal, central nervous system (CNS) depression in infants. All these considerations emphasize the importance of using the minimum number of drugs at the lowest possible doses: no different from any other patient, in fact! The principal difficulty lies in the calculation of the appropriate dose. Several approaches are possible, and none is universally applicable. Adjusting dose to surface area is considered the most appropriate method for neonates, but may not be accurate enough in premature babies. In these, weight may be a more reliable guide, and this is sometimes also used in older children. Another system matches the age to a fixed percentage of the adult dose: for example, 12.5% at 1 month, 25% at 1 year, 50% at 7 years, 75% at 12 years. This is safe with relatively non-toxic drugs with a high therapeutic index, but is too approximate for more hazardous agents.

Drugs and the elderly

The clinical pharmacology of the elderly has become a subspecialty in its own right. This is very welcome, and hardly surprising. The number of patients over the age of 65 years is rising rapidly in all developed countries, as is the number of those over 80 or even 90 years. In parallel, the number of available drugs is also increasing, though at a rate constrained by the escalating costs of drug development and the growing anxiety of most governments at the budgetary implications of drug prescribing. This section summarizes some of the most important considerations in prescribing for the elderly.

It is sensible to assume that old patients will show increased sensitivity to the therapeutic and adverse effects of most drugs. Much of this can be explained by pharmacokinetic changes which are relatively easy to quantify. However, there are also examples where there seem to be alterations in pharmacodynamic responsiveness. These are usually poorly understood, but may be of considerable clinical relevance. For instance, it is well known that many CNS depressants, such as benzodiazepines, have an enhanced effect in the elderly: there is more prolonged sedation, often accompanied by confusion, disorientation or even hallucinations. For many benzodiazepines, including lorazepam and nitrazepam, conventional pharmacokinetic parameters differ little in the elderly and in young adults. The exaggerated response is often attributed to 'hypoxia', but the evidence for this is rarely convincing. This is in fact part of a broader area of ignorance: we know little about the determinants of individual response to psychoactive drugs, at any age. Similarly, warfarin often produces a disproportionate fall in clotting factor synthesis in the old, in the absence of impaired drug clearance or of significant interactions with other drugs. Another poorly understood phenomenon is the increased likelihood of diuretic-induced hypokalaemia. In some other instances there is a better understanding of the mechanisms of change. In the elderly there is a generalized reduction in adrenoceptor, particularly cardiovascular β_1-adrenoceptor, density. Consequently, the therapeutic efficacy of both β-agonists and β-antagonists (in angina and hypertension) is likely to be impaired. It should be noted that response to β_2-agonists in asthma seems to be undiminished. A final example is the increased frequency and severity of drug-induced hypotension in aged patients, possibly due to impaired baroreceptor reflexes.

Much more is known about the altered pharmaco-kinetics characteristic of the elderly. Drug absorption is not greatly affected, in the absence of specific gastrointestinal disease. Body composition is significantly different, with reduced muscle mass and total body weight, and a relative reduction in body water. There is thus a compensatory increase in the percentage of bodily fat, though this may be drastically reversed in the very old. Plasma albumin concentration is often reduced, but this is rarely of practical importance. Changes in V_d are complex and not always easy to predict. As examples, V_d is higher for some benzodiazepines, including diazepam and chlordiazepoxide, and for gentamicin. By contrast, it is lower for digoxin and ethanol.

Renal function declines with age. This is true both of glomerular filtration rate and of tubular function, though the former is usually of greater clinical relevance: this will be considered in greater detail below. Many important drugs are affected, including digoxin, the aminoglycoside antibiotics, tetracycline and lithium. Of these, the tetracyclines (except doxycycline and minocycline) should be avoided if there is significant renal impairment. Plasma levels of the other drugs can be monitored. Some other drugs (methyldopa and methotrexate are examples) are cleared by both renal and non-renal routes, and therapeutic monitoring is not usually available. If these drugs cannot be avoided doses can be reduced on an empirical basis, based on plasma creatinine levels or, preferably, on creatinine clearance. Changes in hepatic metabolism are more complex and more difficult to summarize. They are less often of therapeutic importance. There is usually a reduction in hepatic blood flow, reflecting diminished cardiac output, and this leads to reduced clearance of some highly metabolized drugs, such as propranolol and (probably) lignocaine. On the other hand, the clearance of other extensively metabolized drugs, including warfarin and ethanol, hardly changes with ageing.

From the clinician's point of view these are not necessarily the most challenging problems in prescribing for the aged. The real difficulties can be summarized as follows:

1. The elderly often have multiple illnesses, and tend to be prescribed numerous drugs – often far too many. This inevitably leads to additive side-effects and great potential for drug interactions.

2. There is a high incidence of non-compliance amongst the elderly, for a variety of reasons, notably failure to understand the prescriber's instructions and unwillingness (sometimes justified!) to take medication.

3. As an extension of the first two points, patients may be taking non-prescribed medication, often of unknown composition.

Box 10.1

Drugs to be avoided in pregnancy

In early pregnancy – potentially teratogenic
- Cytotoxic drugs
- Sex steroids
- Warfarin
- Retinoids
- Anticonvulsants (most) (risks of drug withdrawal may outweigh possible teratogenic effect)
- Tetracyclines

In later pregnancy – fetal and perinatal effects
- Sex steroids
- Warfarin
- Tetracyclines
- Sulphonamides
- Chloramphenicol
- Alcohol
- Tobacco
- Non-steroidal anti-inflammatory drugs
- Sulphonylureas

May be used if essential but *caution*
- Any CNS depressant
- Lithium (probable teratogen, only use in first trimester if withdrawal considered dangerous)
- Antithyroid drugs
- Corticosteroids (probably teratogenic, but may be essential, e.g. in severe asthma)

These points are, of course, relevant for any patient, of any age.

DRUGS IN PREGNANCY

Unfortunately, prescribing is often unavoidable in pregnancy as, sometimes, is surgical intervention. Although there are considerable alterations in drug handling (increased plasma volume and glomerular filtration rate, decreased plasma albumin) this rarely necessitates alterations in drug usage. The overriding anxiety is the possibility of toxic effects on the fetus. Some of the most important teratogens and other drugs with potentially adverse actions are listed in Box 10.1.

DRUG USAGE IN DISEASE

Drugs in renal disease

It has already been pointed out that renal impairment almost inevitably accompanies ageing. Although this is significant it is rarely very severe. However, in many cases much more abnormal renal function has to be taken into account when using drugs. The consequences of diminished renal function are more complex than is often appreciated. Naturally, renal elimination of many drugs and their metabolites is impaired, but there are also changes in drug distribution. The plasma protein binding of many drugs, particularly acidic drugs such as phenytoin, warfarin and salicylates, is reduced. The reduction is proportional to the severity of renal failure, and may have several causes. Firstly, there may be low plasma albumin due to proteinuria. Secondly, many endogenous acidic metabolites accumulate during renal failure, and these can compete for binding sites with the acidic drugs. The importance of these changes should not be overemphasized, as they often have been. Nonetheless, for drugs that are affected it will mean a higher free, unbound, fraction in plasma: since this is the pharmacologically active component of the drug it will effectively lower the therapeutic range of the drug. It must be remembered, though, that the increased free fraction will also increase the clearance.

Many drugs will require dosage adjustment in the presence of renal failure: a few, discussed below, should be avoided altogether. In cases where a drug is used in reduced dosage the target steady-state blood level (if there is one) is the same as in healthy individuals. This can be achieved in two ways: by reducing the unit dose, or by increasing the dosage interval. Both approaches are used in practice. Digoxin is produced in a low-dose formulation (0.0625 mg against the standard dose of 0.25 mg) specifically for use in the elderly or in other patients with renal impairment. Occasionally, the standard dose unit is used at 2- or 3-day intervals, but this is generally done in hospital since prolonged dosage intervals tend to have an unfavourable effect on patient compliance. By contrast, the aminoglycosides tend to be administered at prolonged intervals, but at standard unit doses. These drugs are classical examples of the usefulness of therapeutic plasma drug level monitoring to minimize toxicity in circumstances where drug clearance may be abnormal. In fact, nomograms have been constructed which allow reasonable estimates of desirable dosages even if drug assays are not available. The nomograms are based on creatinine clearance or, if this is not known, on plasma creatinine. However, measurement of plasma drug levels is always preferable. For most other drugs this degree of monitoring is not available and dosage adjustment must be empirical. Important examples of such drugs are:

- Atenolol, sotalol
- Cephalosporins (most)
- Lithium – *always monitor*
- Cimetidine, ranitidine (less significant).

Box 10.2 lists some drugs that should be avoided in renal failure.

Drugs in liver disease

Given the central role of the liver in drug handling, and so many other metabolic processes, it is to be expected that liver disease would have a dramatic impact on drug usage. This is the case, but in fact most of the problems arise from abnormal responses to drugs rather than from pharmacokinetic anomalies. These can be very complex, for several reasons. Firstly, severe liver disease is often accompanied by some degree of renal failure. Secondly, as in renal disease, but often to a greater extent, plasma albumin levels may be depressed because of diminished synthesis. Thirdly, cirrhosis is often associated with an increase in total liver blood flow, but with a variable degree of shunting of blood within the liver. This can lead to increased flow to metabolically inactive areas. It will be seen that the ultimate effect can be very difficult to predict, but can lead to increased bioavailability and possible toxicity of several important drugs such as metoprolol, propranolol, labetalol and chlormethiazole. Predictably, the clearance of many extensively metabolized drugs is reduced. These include theophylline, phenytoin, verapamil, chloramphenicol and most benzodiazepines.

This leads to consideration of drugs to avoid in severe liver disease. The following are among the more important:

1. *All CNS depressants*, including benzodiazepines and opiate analgesics. These may precipitate or aggravate hepatic encephalopathy.

2. *Diuretics*, which may cause hyponatraemia and hypokalaemia and hence increase the likelihood of encephalopathy. However, the aldosterone antagonist spironolactone is widely used in cirrhosis-associated ascites.

3. *Warfarin and other oral anticoagulants*, since there is already decreased synthesis of clotting factors.

4. *Potentially hepatotoxic drugs*, such as rifampicin and tetracyclines.

Drugs in heart failure

Severe heart failure can have far-reaching effects on drug disposition. Reduced cardiac blood flow will lead to diminished perfusion of gut, liver and kidneys. The absorption of some drugs (for example, hydrochlorothiazide and frusemide) is therefore impaired. Hypoperfusion of the liver will diminish clearance of some extensively metabolized drugs: lignocaine may be particularly important in this context, with potentially serious toxicity. Altered renal blood flow will naturally result in reduced glomerular filtration rate and therefore reduced clearance of drugs such as digoxin, and abnormal distribution of blood flow within the kidney may cause increased reabsorption of some drugs, and thus further diminish clearance.

DRUG INTERACTIONS

The number of possible drug interactions is astronomical, and lists of even the most important can occupy sizeable volumes. The intention of this section is to consider in a general sense possible ways in which drugs can interact with one another. Usually, but not always, these interactions are unwanted. They can be considered under three major headings: pharmaceutical, pharmacodynamic and pharmacokinetic.

Pharmaceutical interactions

These interactions occur outside the body, usually involving intravenous drugs which are incompatible with one another on the basis of chemical and physical reactions. Well-known examples include calcium salts and sodium bicarbonate, dopamine and sodium bicarbonate and amiodarone and sodium chloride. The *British National Formulary* includes a very comprehensive list

---

Box 10.2

Drugs to be avoided in severe renal impairment (glomerular filtration rate <10 ml min^{-1})

- Amiloride
- Spironolactone
- Thiazides
- Nalidixic acid
- Nitrofurantoin
- Tetracyclines (except doxycycline, minocycline)
- Methotrexate
- Pancuronium
- Chlorpropamide
- Aspirin

of permitted and incompatible intravenous mixtures and additives.

Pharmacodynamic interactions

Two main types of interaction are possible under this heading. Drugs may have an additive or even synergistic effect, or they may antagonize each other's actions. The best-known example of the first type is the action of CNS depressants, which characteristically potentiate one another, generally acting through different mechanisms. Alcohol is very frequently one of the drugs involved, while others may be antidepressants, benzodiazepines, opioids or antihistamines. This interaction is potentially very serious and even fatal in overdose. A less well-known example, potentially of importance in anaesthetics, is the enhancement of the effect of non-depolarizing muscle relaxants by aminoglycoside antibiotics. Finally, β-blockers and some calcium antagonists (notably verapamil and diltiazem) can produce bradycardia and aggravate atrioventricular block. In combination they can produce severe bradycardia, which may be associated with hypotension and heart failure. The latter might be further worsened by the negative inotropic action of both types of drug. Of all the above examples there is action at a common receptor only in the case of neuromuscular blockade.

Pharmacokinetic interactions

This can encompass many different varieties of drug interactions, most of which are listed here.

1. Drugs may interfere with each other's absorption. Well-known examples involve the tetracyclines, which chelate metal ions such as iron, aluminium and calcium. Iron supplements and antacids may therefore prevent absorption of tetracyclines, and the latter block the absorption of iron. Another example is the binding of warfarin by cholestyramine, inhibiting the former's absorption. Anticholinergics, including tricyclic antidepressants, and opiates, slow gastric emptying and, therefore, the rate of absorption of many drugs such as paracetamol, levodopa and diazepam.

2. The displacement of drugs from binding sites on plasma albumin is well known, but its importance has been greatly overemphasized. Many supposed examples actually involve changes in drug metabolism, which are discussed below. Some authentic examples include, as ever, warfarin, together with tolbutamide and salicylates. Any drug that is genuinely involved must be over 95% protein bound, in fact probably around 99%.

3. By contrast, there are many well-documented examples of alterations in drug metabolizing systems. Enzyme inducers include most of the common anticonvulsants (phenytoin, carbamazepine, primidone and phenobarbitone), rifampicin and the antifungal griseofulvin. The list of target drugs is much longer and includes these drugs themselves as well as oral anticoagulants, oral contraceptives, corticosteroids and opiates. There are many other examples. In most instances drug effects are significantly reduced.

A well-known, if specialized, case of metabolic inhibition concerns monoamine oxidase inhibitors, which prevent the breakdown of amines such as levodopa, tyramine and dopamine, potentially causing a hypertensive crisis. On the other hand, tricylic antidepressants and pethidine can cause hypotension in combination with monoamine oxidase inhibitors. Another special interaction is the prevention of alcohol breakdown by disulfiram, metronidazole and some cephalosporins. Other drugs inhibit more general drug oxidizing enzymes: for instance, cimetidine, ketoconazole, erythromycin and isoniazid. The target drugs include phenytoin, warfarin, theophylline and most benzodiazepines. As expected, this can produce drug accumulation, prolonged action and toxicity.

4. Finally, interactions can occur at the level of drug excretion. Urinary pH can alter the rate of drug clearance: alkaline urine enhances the elimination of salicylates, while acidification increases the excretion of amphetamines. There are some important examples of tubular interactions: probenecid inhibits the excretion of acidic drugs such as penicillin, salicylates and indomethacin. On the other hand, salicylates reduce the elimination of methotrexate, increasing the latter's toxicity. Finally, there is a very important and potentially lethal interaction between lithium and thiazide diuretics. The diuretics promote the excretion of sodium ions at the expense of lithium, rapidly leading to toxic plasma levels of the ion.

PHARMACOGENETICS

The genetic basis of variations in the handling of drugs, and in responses to them, is an area of growing interest. Apart from the well-investigated examples, some of which are described below, it is clear that there are many instances of more subtle but perhaps more important variations. For example, people of Chinese and Japanese origin appear to be more susceptible to the effect of β-blockers. This has far-reaching implications for drug usage, and for drug testing. For instance, Japanese licensing authorities in fact insist that clinical trials should be performed locally (though some suspect commercial motives may also play a part). This type of variability is still incompletely understood. However, most of the well-known pharmacogenetic variations are based on alterations at a single gene. One of the earliest examples, and of particular relevance to surgeons and anaesthetists, is suxamethonium apnoea. The duration of action of the muscle relaxant suxamethonium is abnormally prolonged, because the serum enzyme that hydrolyses the drug (pseudocholinesterase) is abnormal or even totally inactive. Many abnormal alleles of the gene have now been identified. Mild forms of the syndrome are relatively common and affect up to 4% of the population. The severe forms are fortunately extremely rare, with prevalence of 1 in 100 000 or less. Another well-defined genetic variation concerns the metabolism, by acetylation, of hydralazine, procainamide and isoniazid. The minority of so-called 'slow acetylators', about a third or less of the population in the UK, have a greater likelihood of developing a systemic lupus erythematosus-like syndrome. A more recently described genetic *dimorphism* (that is to say, the presence of two genetically distinct populations) involves the oxidative metabolism of certain drugs in the liver. The prototype was the antihypertensive drug debrisoquine. More clinically relevant examples include propranolol, metoprolol, phenytoin, nortryptiline and the now withdrawn hypoglycaemic drug phenformin. Poor metabolizers are more likely to develop lactic acidosis while taking phenformin. However, a given dose of these drugs may also have greater efficacy in poor metabolizers.

A much more important genetic anomaly is the sex-linked deficiency of the red cell enzyme glucose-6-phosphate dehydrogenase. This plays a vital role in the protection of the erythrocyte from oxidants, including many drugs. There are at least two major variants of this syndrome, with up to 100 rarer forms. These syndromes have a very wide geographical distribution among Africans, Chinese and several ethnic groups of the Mediterranean basin: each of these groups has one or more abnormal variants of the enzyme. The more severe, Mediterranean, forms of this syndrome have a mild chronic anaemia with severe haemolysis on drug challenge. The African variant may not cause chronic anaemia. The drugs to be avoided include aspirin, sulphonamides, chloramphenicol, nitrofurantoin and, notoriously, the Fava bean – Pythagoras seemed to be aware of this danger 2500 years ago! It is interesting that antimalarial drugs, including quinine, chloroquine and primaquine, can also precipitate haemolysis, since it is thought that the enzyme deficiency confers some protection to the red cell against malarial parasites.

Finally, a much rarer group of conditions must be mentioned, not all of them genetically determined. These are the *porphyrias*, of which the best known is the autosomal dominant acute intermittent porphyria which can cause severe abdominal pain, peripheral neuropathy, psychiatric disturbance and even death. Variegate porphyria is similar in manifestations and inheritance pattern, while a somewhat milder form may accompany acquired liver disease such as cirrhosis. The biochemical abnormalities are extremely complex and the pathogenesis of the neuropsychiatric syndromes is very poorly understood. In general, it is necessary to avoid drugs which stimulate porphyrin synthesis. This turns out to be an extensive list. Among the most important are the enzyme inducers already described, but also the short-acting barbiturates, chlordiazepoxide, chlorpropamide and tolbutamide, methyldopa, chloroquine, chloramphenicol, the contraceptive pill, and other oestrogens. It is essential to consider all potentially active drugs in patients with definite or suspected porphyria.

CONCLUSION

It is hoped that this chapter may provide a brief guide to some practical aspects of clinical pharmacology and therapeutics. There are obviously many omissions. One area which must be mentioned, however, is that of adverse drug reactions. The monitoring system in this country relies entirely on voluntary reporting to the Committee on Safety of Medicines, using the 'yellow cards'. It is therefore very susceptible to doctors' apathy, or to the feeling that a particular adverse reaction is too well known to need further reporting. Often this is quite true (amoxycillin and rashes, for instance), but it must be emphasized that all suspected adverse reactions must be reported for new drugs, marked with a black triangle in the *British National Formulary* or in *MIMS*. Even well-known reactions should be reported if they are serious or potentially life-threatening.

No references have been cited in this chapter. The size of the literature is almost incalculably large, and it is usually safe to assume that clinicians do not look up primary references outside their own specialty: that is daunting enough. Instead, there is a short list of more or less comprehensive books which deal with all the above topics, and more, in far greater detail. By the very nature of books all are out of date to some extent and become more so almost daily. Fortunately, there are many sources of information which are regularly updated. The *British National Formulary* is an obvious example, as is the *Drug and Therapeutics Bulletin*. There are also commercially published magazines (e.g. *Prescriber*) which provide valuable information on newly introduced drugs and put them in the context of existing agents. Some semi-official publications also provide data of this kind (for instance, from the Merseyside Resources

Centre, MEREC). As mentioned earlier, hospital and regional drug information centres can answer many questions relating to drug usage (while the latter exist). Finally, it is occasionally worth talking to a clinical pharmacologist, if you happen to find one.

FURTHER READING

Denham M J, George C E (eds) 1990 Drugs in old age: new perspectives. British Medical Bulletin 46 (1)

Dukes M N G 1992 Meyler's side effects of drugs, 12th edn. Elsevier, Amsterdam

Gilman A G, Rall T W, Nies A S, Taylor P 1990 Goodman and Gilman's the pharmacological basis of therapeutics, 8th edn. Pergamon Press, New York

Grahame-Smith D G, Aronson J K 1992 Oxford textbook of clinical pharmacology and drug therapy, 2nd edn. Oxford University Press, Oxford

Ritter J M, Lewis L D, Mant T G K 1995 A textbook of clinical pharmacology, 3rd edn. Edward Arnold, London

Speight T M 1987 Avery's drug treatment, 3rd edn. ADIS Press/Churchill Livingstone, Auckland/Edinburgh

Stockley I H 1994 Drug interactions, 3rd edn. Blackwell Scientific, Oxford

Wingard L B, Brody T M, Larner J, Schwartz A 1991 Human pharmacology: molecular to clinical. Wolfe, London

Preparation for surgery

11. Consent for surgical treatment

L. Doyal

For surgery to be successful, there must be a relationship of trust and confidence between surgeon and patient. Otherwise, patients will be reticent to present themselves for treatment or to divulge the detailed personal information required for recording accurate case histories and making successful diagnoses. Aside from the belief that their care will conform to a high clinical standard, the trust of patients also depends on their belief that their autonomy will be respected – that they will have the right to decide their own medical destiny, whatever anyone else may think.

Moral rights are like that. They indicate claims that individuals can legitimately make against others who have corresponding duties to respect those claims. To the degree that we believe that the right to make such a claim exists, then those on whom it is properly made must respect it and act accordingly, irrespective of their preferences. Examples of often-cited moral rights emphasize the entitlement of individuals to self-determination – to be able to pursue life choices and perceived interests in ways in which the individual has chosen – provided that others are not harmed in the process. Moral rights might or might not be backed up by the force of law. For example, the legal right of women to choose to have an abortion under certain circumstances is regarded as immoral by those who believe that a fetus has the rights of a born child. In short, our beliefs about who has a right to what inform our decisions about how we should act toward others if our actions are to be deemed morally, and perhaps legally, acceptable.

The general right of surgical patients to self-determination can be subdivided into three further rights: to informed consent, to the truth and to confidentiality. The latter two clearly follow from the first. Choices cannot be properly informed on the basis of deception and cannot be respected if what patients deem private is made public. Therefore, it is the principle of informed consent itself which is fundamental and on which both the morality and the legality of good surgical practice partly depends.

THE MORAL IMPORTANCE OF INFORMED CONSENT

The moral unacceptability of anyone exercising unlimited power over others is at the heart of many of our liberal values. It is our capacity for rational choice that differentiates humans from other creatures. Respect for this capacity – especially our right to be the informed gatekeepers of our own bodies – is an indication of the seriousness with which we respect the humanity and dignity of others.

What is informed consent?

For patients to give their informed consent to surgery – to be able to make a considered choice about what is in their personal interests – they must receive sufficient accurate information about their illness, the proposed treatment and its prognosis. For this to be more than a moral abstraction, the surgeon must complete four general tasks. Firstly, the procedure itself must be described, including information about its practical implications and probable prognosis. Secondly, the probability of specific associated risks or complications should be revealed. Thirdly, it should not be assumed that the patient already knows the risks of other aspects of the proposed surgical procedure, such as the complications that might result from a general anaesthetic, bed rest, intravenous fluids or a catheter. Finally, other surgical or medical alternatives to the proposed treatment – including non-treatment – should be outlined, along with their general advantages and disadvantages.

Ideally, the amount of such information should be that which mentally competent patients require to make their informed choice a realistic possibility. Competence should be thought of here as the ability to understand, retain and deliberate about such information and to accept its applicability to themselves. Surgeons should remember that the amount of information they are obligated to divulge may well change depending on what they should know about their patients as individuals. For example, it may not be necessary for a manual labourer to be told of an extremely small operative risk of minor stiffness in one finger. This would obviously not be true of a concert pianist, underlining the importance of recording the patient's employment in case notes and referring to it in the presentation of case histories.

Good consenting practice

As much as possible, the physical surroundings during the discussion between surgeon and patient should be conducive to easy, quiet conversation. Ideally, the place should be private and free of disturbances and interruptions by junior staff or medical students following in retinue on a busy Nightingale ward. The surgeon should not stand threateningly over a patient in bed and should avoid giving the appearance of being rushed by other duties. Empathy with the patient will be crucial.

The language with which the surgeon communicates should be as simple as possible, avoiding needless technicalities. When serious matters are being discussed, it is often helpful for a relative or friend to be present – always assuming that patients have given their permission. This is both for support and to help ensure that the patient really does understand – both at the time the information is given and later when the patient returns home. In the hospital ward, nurses with whom the patient is familiar can often fulfill this role very effectively. Appropriate leaflets or booklets can be of great help, and innovative work is also being done with audio recording of interviews with patients who are encouraged to take the recording home to discuss with others.

Having attempted to provide clear information, it is then important to try to determine whether or not the patient has actually understood it. No doubt there will be time constraints on doing both. However, it is clear that the surgeon is morally responsible for attempting to achieve both to an acceptable standard. There are a variety of ways in which this might be done – asking patients to go back over what has been said in their own terms, for example, and asking them at various times if they have any questions. The more confident surgeons become in exercising these skills, the less time it will take to obtain effective consent.

Surgeons have often limited the amount of information given to patients on the grounds of the potential distress that might result. This is unacceptable, if the long-term aim is to keep the patient in ignorance. All competent individuals have a right to decide what is and is not in their best interests, even if what they decide is not endorsed by their professional advisors. It would not be morally acceptable for a solicitor or accountant to

delude their clients on the grounds that they did not want to distress them about the possibility of losing a court action or of going bankrupt. Why should the moral obligations of the surgeon be any different?

The consent form

In principle, the consent form which patients should sign before having surgery is a public and permanent affirmation that they have indeed agreed to it. All competent patients who are 16 years or older should sign the form for all surgical procedures involving a general anaesthetic. A form should also be signed by the patient for procedures under local anaesthetic if there might be significant sequelae – for example, an excision of skin lesions. Clinicians obtaining the consent should also sign the form to indicate that, to the best of their knowledge, the patient has both been given and understands the information necessary to make a considered judgement.

This being said, two things should be remembered about the consent form. Firstly, it is not necessary for competent patients to sign it for all surgical interventions. Simple investigative procedures (e.g. sigmoidoscopy) which involve minimal risk of harm can be undertaken on the basis of a verbal explanation of what they physically entail. Explicit verbal consent should then be requested, although consent can be assumed to be implied if the patient then accepts the procedure. Secondly, the consent form is not legal proof that consent has been given – something that should always be borne in mind when there is a temptation to cut corners as regards good consenting practice. At most, it is only one piece of evidence that some attempt was made to obtain informed consent, not that it was a morally or legally satisfactory attempt.

THE LEGAL IMPORTANCE OF INFORMED CONSENT

Aside from its general moral and clinical importance, doctors also have a legal obligation to respect the patient's right to consent to treatment.

Battery

In principle, battery is a violation of the civil law which forbids intentionally touching other persons without their consent. For example, a woman won damages in the UK for this reason because she was given a sterilization to which she did not agree in the aftermath of a gynaecological operation for another problem. In Canada, a woman who made it clear that she wanted to be injected in one arm successfully sued when she received the injection in the other! The harm resulting from battery is not necessarily physical. In law, a battery can be deemed to have occurred without such harm having taken place. Here harm should be construed as the violation of the right of persons to exercise autonomous control over their own bodies.

Of course, in many situations involving minor surgical procedures or tests, it will not be possible or advisable specifically to ask for the consent of patients every time they are touched. Were this the case, surgery would become practically impossible. But it does not follow that even here the consent of patients is legally irrelevant. Rather, as we have just seen, they can be said to have given their implied consent by virtue of the fact that they have presented themselves for treatment and have accepted what is offered. A man once argued in the USA, for example, that a ship's surgeon had committed a battery because he was vaccinated without him giving specific verbal permission for the injection to be administered. He lost on the grounds that his consent was implied since he was in a queue of people who were clearly waiting to be injected and he held out his arm when his turn came!

Clearly, there will be many situations which are much less clear-cut. For example, is there a risk of battery if patients claim that had they been given more information before surgery, they would have refused it? If the patients are informed of the general nature of their conditions and the surgery proposed to try to correct them, if they are not deliberately deceived about this information, if they give no indication of desiring not to proceed by asking for more information, and if they sign the appropriate consent form then the answer is probably no. Of course, this presupposes that the surgeon has not deprived the patient of information about potential risks or discomfort that has been specifically requested, or, returning to our example of an unwanted hysterectomy, has usurped a clinical choice now commonly regarded as remaining with the patient.

Negligence

Battery is not the only legal action surgeons risk for inadequately respecting their patients' right to informed consent. In an important case, Mrs Sidaway suffered paralysis resulting from spinal surgery to relieve pressure on a nerve root without being told that the operation carried a small risk of paralysis. Here, it was judged that she had not been a victim of battery because, again, she had given her general consent to the surgery in question. However, her solicitors then claimed negligence, the legal action now recommended in such cases. The negligence concerns the professional duty of surgeons properly to advise patients not just about the proposed surgery but also about its potential hazards. In such cases, patients argue that, had they known the risks in question, they would not have proceeded with the surgery.

It would again be wrong to assume that in these circumstances surgeons are protected from such accusations by a signed consent form for treatment. Patients might still successfully argue that even though they had signed the form, they were not given enough relevant information to make an informed decision before they signed and/or that they were unaware of the significance of the form. There is no escaping the general duty of surgeons to disclose information about potentially harmful side-effects and to do so in a way that the patient can understand in principle. For example, in all cases other than those of acute emergencies, care must be taken to provide translations for non-English-speaking patients.

How are we to establish whether or not compliance with this duty has been sufficient – whether or not enough information has been disclosed about risks so that the rights of patients are respected? Legal judgments concerning negligent standards of adequate disclosure in the UK are still primarily determined by the profession itself. Suppose that expert witnesses for the defence are regarded by the court as constituting a recognized body of professional opinion. If they agree that they would have communicated the same amount of information in similar circumstances as the defendant then this should be sufficient to ensure that the plaintiff will lose the legal action. In other words, in such actions the judge does not decide which expert witnesses are right – those for the plaintiff or defendant. All that is required to exonerate the latter is for a responsible body of professional opinion to endorse the action in dispute.

Recent legal developments have underlined this 'professional standard' in the determination of what constitutes negligent informed consent. In the Sidaway case, for example, a majority of appellate judges in the House of Lords agreed with this approach to determining negligence, as have other judges since she lost. However, many have also warned of the dangers of completely equating the right of patients to information with standards set by the profession. Indeed, in the Sidaway case, one judge stated in a minority opinion that there will be some information about surgery, for example serious hazards, which any 'prudent' patient would wish to know before giving consent to proceed. A similar legal standard of negligence as regards informed consent is found in North America and is increasingly becoming accepted good practice by the medical profession in the UK.

Therefore, surgeons should not look to the law for

advice for how much information about risks and side-effects is morally required by the right of their patients to informed consent. They should ask what a prudent person would want to know under similar circumstances, especially in the context of any other personal information they have about the patient and their public and private interests. The fact that the amount of information that is required might be legally justified with reference to one representative standard of professional practice does not entail that morally it should be determined by such a standard.

The unconscious adult patient

Suppose that a surgeon in the Accident and Emergency (A&E) Department is confronted with the victim of an automobile accident who requires an immediate, life-saving operation. Here there is a clear duty to treat despite the fact that it is impossible to obtain the patient's consent, and there would be no risk of battery if surgery proceeded. This is not because the surgeon becomes the proxy of the patient and makes a substituted judgement on his behalf, one which attempts to second guess what the choice of the patient would have been. It is because it is the surgeon's moral and legal responsibility to act in the patient's best interests – to do what is 'necessary' since there is no way of knowing for certain what the patient might choose.

Indeed, no adult in the UK can legally consent to surgery on behalf of another, including close relatives. Relatives should not be asked to sign consent forms on behalf of unconscious or otherwise incompetent adults. It would be both a misrepresentation of the law and a liability risk: if the surgical outcome is poor, the relatives may inappropriately and harmfully blame themselves.

Therefore, the only circumstance that could justify surgery without consent is the dramatic need of patients coupled with their inability to give consent. Again, inconvenience will not suffice. For example, the arrest of a life-threatening haemorrhage in an otherwise healthy patient would clearly be in order, while the same could not be said of the repair of a hernia. Of course, if patients are conscious and evidently capable of rational judgement, then even in an emergency they should be advised about their condition and the proposed treatment. If it is physically possible, a patient should also sign a consent form, as would be the case in normal circumstances. Verbal consent is adequate if the patient's condition precludes giving written consent. However, in these circumstances it is advisable if possible for another health worker to act as a witness and to record the verbal consent in the notes.

Children

Ordinarily, consent for elective surgery on young children must always be obtained from someone – usually the parent – deemed competent to make informed choices about the child's best interests. This is not, however, to suggest that surgeons must always be guided solely by parental wishes. If such decisions are believed to be necessary to save the life of the child then they can be overriden. If there is time, the court should provide the appropriate order; if not, the surgeon can still proceed. If parents are proposing long-term treatment or non-treatment options which are regarded as similarly inconsistent with the best interests of the child, these wishes can again be overriden by an appropriate court order.

Generally speaking, the legal age for medical consent is 16. However, it is legally acceptable for surgeons to treat adolescents under the age of 16 years without parental consent, just as it is for GPs to prescribe contraceptives. However, if this is considered, care must be taken to ensure that the young person is competent – again, mature enough to understand, retain and deliberate about information concerning the nature of the illness, the prognosis, proposed treatment and any important associated risks. Such patients should also accept that this information applies personally to them. Equally, before proceeding without parental consent, the surgeon should encourage the young person to discuss the proposed treatment with their parents and be assured that the treatment is in the best interests of the child.

This said, treatment without parental consent should be regarded as the exception and not the rule. Unless the adolescent has specifically refused permission, attempts should be made if possible to find and consult parents who are not already on site. In the case of life-threatening illness, even young people below the age of 18 years do not have the right to reject treatment on their own which might save their lives. Only those with parental responsibility can exercise such judgement. Paradoxically, the law appears to be that the right of a competent adolescent to consent to life-saving treatment does not entail the right to refuse it. As regards elective surgery which is not life saving or will not prevent serious and permanent injury, the law is not clear. Morally, however, the wishes of the competent young person not to proceed should be and are commonly respected – even where the parent disagrees. If surgical treatment is forced upon such patients without consent then it might undermine the relationship of trust and the willingness to comply with future treatment, both of which will be important for sustained clinical success.

Certainly, quite young children often have a good grasp of their prospects and treatment, especially when they have already experienced distressing surgical therapy for an illness which they have had for some time. In such circumstances, before further surgery is undertaken, attempts should be made to consult such children about their wishes. Where there is disagreement between parent and child about the best course of action, especially in instances of potentially terminal disease, both should be counselled about what appears clinically to be in the child's best interests. Such counselling will be particularly important in situations where there is disagreement between the surgeon and parent about the most appropriate way to proceed. Again, in the unusual event that a surgeon believes parental choice dramatically conflicts with the medical interests of the child, it is always open to approach the court for a judgement.

Mental handicap and psychiatric illness

In the case of adults who are judged incompetent to choose for themselves, we have seen that no one may legally act as a proxy for this purpose. However, decisions about incompetence are complex. For example, incompetence to consent to surgery does not follow from severe psychiatric illness. Just because individuals may be incompetent in one respect due to illness does not mean that they are incompetent in all respects. People may be detained under the 1983 Mental Health Act on the grounds that, because of the seriousness of their psychiatric illness, they are a potential danger to themselves or others. As a result they may be given psychiatric treatment without their consent. However, this does not hold for ordinary surgical treatment. In such circumstances, attempts must therefore be made to obtain the patient's consent, even when communication is difficult and certainty of understanding not assured. For example, in a recent legal case in Britain, a judge accepted that a detained patient suffering from schizophrenia was competent to refuse to have a leg amputated if it became terminally gangrenous.

With the exception of specific and extreme interventions such as psychosurgery, there are circumstances where surgical treatment can be given to detained psychiatric patients who cannot consent due to extreme illness. There are two conditions: the treatment must be deemed necessary to protect life or to avoid permanent and serious disability, and patients must be diagnosed as unable to give informed consent as a direct result of their psychiatric illness. As the result of psychotic delusion, for example, they might believe that their surgeon is going to kill them and that the diagnosis of a life-threatening condition is a sinister plot. Here, necessary treatment can proceed, provided that the surgeon and the relevant psychiatric team agree that it is in the best interests of the patient. Note that this exception to the consent requirement would not ordinarily apply to elective surgical care since the assumption should be that there will be time for patients to make up their own minds when their competence to do so is no longer being impaired by their illness.

Some patients in need of surgery will suffer not from psychiatric illness but from permanent mental disability. This may severely impair their competence to give informed consent for either life-saving or elective surgery. The fact remains, however, that in such circumstances, no adult can act as a legal proxy for another as regards the provision of such consent. The only person who can make the decision that surgery is in the best interests of severely mentally handicapped patients is their surgeon in consultation with their principal carers, including close relatives. Yet great care must be taken. As regards elective surgery, responsibility for promoting the interests of mentally handicapped patients can be a heavy burden, especially if there is dispute among carers about what these actually are. The sensitivity of these issues is witnessed by the fact that the courts sometimes refuse to permit the sterilization of mentally handicapped women under the age of 16 years, even if a surgeon has agreed to perform the procedure.

TWO PRACTICAL PROBLEMS

The obligation to disclose information about both proposed surgery and its hazards is not open to debate. However, putting this moral and legal imperative into practice does involve discretion and is not always easy for two reasons.

1. Limitations on the understanding of patients

It is sometimes unclear whether or not consent has really been obtained even if the surgeon has taken care to explain the proposed procedure and its potential hazards. The comprehension of competent patients can be compromised by their illness, their educational and social background and by other aspects of their personalities which may make them overly anxious or unwilling to listen. Yet difficult as such instances of impaired autonomy can be, especially for patients facing acute and complex surgery, surgeons should still be able to show that they have disclosed adequate information for proper consent to be possible.

Practically speaking, therefore, how should surgeons demonstrate to themselves (and, if necessary, a judge) that they have done their best in this regard? Most important of all, they need to work constantly to improve their ability to communicate. Both the General Medical

Council (GMC) and the British Medical Association stress this point, and its importance is underlined by the increasing emphasis placed on communication skills within medical education. Surgeons can do no more than their best. However, it follows from the moral importance of informed consent that they should always attempt to optimize their ability to communicate well.

Furthermore, it is important to keep a written record in the case notes of the main points about treatment which have been communicated prior to the signing of the consent form. If one follows the model of the prudent patient outlined above, information should certainly be given on what will be done and why, along with significant risks of mortality and other hazards to bodily functions relevant to normal social participation: swallowing, speaking, continence, mobility, pain and sexual performance, for example. A brief indication in the notes that each of these variables has been mentioned should not be too onerous a task and will provide surgeons with evidence which could be useful if the fact is denied by the patient in a context of medicolegal dispute. This approach can be reinforced by giving patients written information about their proposed treatment and possible side-effects.

Even after they have followed good practice in obtaining consent, surgeons may conclude that patients still cannot be said properly to have given consent to treatment. Here, life-saving emergencies aside, the most appropriate choice is to postpone therapy until better communication has been achieved. This may be inconvenient, but it is necessary if the rights of patients are to be protected and if surgeons are to be able to demonstrate that they have taken their moral and legal duties to do so seriously. No reasonable person can expect more.

2. Limitations on the right of patients to consent

The right of patients to consent to surgery does not entail their right to demand and receive it. There is no professional duty to provide surgery which is requested by patients who have no need for it. The same can be said for surgery which will be futile no matter how much patients may want it. But what if patients clearly need surgery but do not want it? Here respect for the autonomy of patients may well conflict with the surgeon's other moral obligation to protect their life and health. This conflict is most acute when, in considered and unambiguous terms, patients refuse surgery which will save their lives.

The moral and legal emphasis on respect for autonomy within surgery is so strong that, even in such circumstances, treatment must not be undertaken without consent, again assuming that the patient is conscious and competent. This fact is sometimes obscured because patients who are terminally ill and do not wish further treatment are physically and emotionally unable to resist it. Where it becomes very clear, however, is in the case, say, of Jehovah's Witnesses who will only proceed with surgery on the understanding that if they haemorrhage they will not be transfused. Legally, competent patients have every right to make such a demand. A surgeon who proceeds to the contrary risks an action for battery.

It is not being suggested that surgeons have to operate on patients who place stipulations on the types of life-saving treatment which they will accept. In principle, and assuming that there is time, surgeons may refer them to others who are more sympathetic and willing to undergo the stress which such restrictions inevitably carry. Equally, we have already seen that if a patient is unconscious or incompetent for some other reason the surgeon must do what is necessary to try to save life. However, even this is changing in the face of so-called 'advance directives' or 'living wills' which are now regarded by expert opinion in the UK as having legal force. Thus any competent adult can draft a document specifying in advance which life-saving treatments they do and do not consent to if they become incompetent and contract specific types of illnesses. Ideally, an advance directive should be witnessed and should be acted upon. Such documents are common in North America and will eventually be so here.

After consultation with their surgeons, competent patients may, therefore, decide that further treatment is pointless given the irreversible and terminal character of their particular disease. It will be accepted that death and not surgery is in their best interests. Complying with such a request to omit or to stop treatment is neither actively killing nor aiding and abetting suicide. Unlike the potential suicide, competent patients may well want desperately to live but not at any cost to their quality of life. Furthermore, as we have seen, to treat them against their will constitutes a battery. What patients cannot expect is for active steps to be taken to end their lives, although they do at times request this.

Yet to go along with a patient's refusal of surgery when it is clear that the consequence will be death is a very serious moral and legal matter. Great care must be taken to ensure that the patient fully understands the implications of refusing life-saving treatment and is competent to make an informed judgement, especially if the refusal is followed by a lapse into unconsciousness. Here a mistake either about the patient's understanding or wishes cannot be corrected. Therefore, prior refusal should be respected only if it is judged to be an autonomous decision intended to apply in the circumstances that have arisen. For example, a young adult woman in the UK refused a blood transfusion on the grounds of her acceptance of the doctrine of the Jehovah's Witnesses, despite the fact that she was not a Witness herself. She lost consciousness and the court overruled her refusal on the grounds that she had been unduly influenced by her mother and that her decision was based upon a false impression of her prognosis.

INFORMED CONSENT AND SURGICAL RESEARCH

The availability of surgical options is dependent on the experimental research which makes them possible. Yet researchers must be careful. Without enthusiasm and conviction about the importance of their work, they will not have the commitment that successful research requires. However, such commitment can lead to an underestimation of the risks or discomfort of experiments. Research can either be therapeutic and to the potential benefit of participants or non-therapeutic with no such promise. Participants in the former will be patients and in the latter either patients or healthy volunteers.

Focusing for the moment on research involving patients, they have a right to informed consent for the same reasons described above. Furthermore, allowing them to make an informed evaluation for themselves is one of the best ways of regulating experimental zeal, a factor which has unquestionably led to moral abuses in the past. A clear example is the notorious and needless experiments inflicted by some Nazi doctors and surgeons on Jewish prisoners. However, there have been more recent illustrations involving patients, some of whom have died as a result of their participation in research.

The Nuremburg Code which was adopted internationally as a result declared that 'the voluntary consent of a patient is essential' in any medical research. The later Declaration of Helsinki is even more explicit. It states: 'In any research, each potential subject must be adequately informed of the aims, methods and anticipated benefits and potential hazards of the study and the discomfort it may entail'. And after this, their consent must be obtained.

The enforcement of the Helsinki Declaration in the UK is entrusted to research ethics committees. These are administered by local health authorities and are responsible for evaluating all surgical research involving humans wherever it might be undertaken. Under no circumstances should research proceed without the approval of the appropriate ethics committee, and aca-demic journals will usually not publish the results unless such approval has been given. In principle, research ethics committees are supposed to ensure that the proposed protocol makes good scientific sense and poses no further risks than those of the best available treatment. Only then should patients be asked to consent to participate, on the basis of being given appropriate information about the research which the committee has also approved.

There is, however, one significant problem concerning surgical research and informed consent which remains. As a result of differing ability and willingness to understand and to question medical authority, we have seen that patients vary in their ability to assimilate the details of clinical information. Consequently, enthusiastic researchers are in a position, wittingly or not, to manipulate patients to subject themselves to procedures that might not be proposed in ordinary treatment. Patients may be encouraged to agree to participate in the development of surgical procedures, for example, without realizing how experimental they are. Here the general guidelines concerning informed consent should be followed with extra vigilance. For example, care must be taken to identify surgical procedures that might not be regarded as standard professional practice and to proceed only when the patient gives informed and written consent with the knowledge that this is the case. When in doubt about whether or not a procedure is standard, the research ethics committee should be consulted.

In non-therapeutic research with patients or healthy volunteers, it is equally important to avoid confusing agreement to participate with informed consent to do so. The researcher must try to ensure that the moral legitimacy of the consent of the volunteer is not obtained under financial, social or professional duress. In the UK, for example, the difficulty of doing so has led to surgical research not ordinarily taking place among the prison population.

INFORMED CONSENT AND CONFIDENTIALITY

As a corollary of their right to informed consent, patients have the right to control access to information which they give to surgeons for the purposes of treatment. The GMC supports this right through the importance it attaches to the principle of confidentiality – of obtaining the permission of patients before revealing clinical information about them to others. Few acts can more quickly lead to a surgeon being professionally disciplined than a proven breach of confidence in unwarranted circumstances.

There are two types of justification for this emphasis. First, the right to be the moral gatekeeper of one's own body extends to information divulged in clinical consultations. Second, if patients are frightened that their confidence might be breached, they may not be willing to provide the honest information on which successful diagnosis depends or even to turn up for treatment at all. This can pose a severe danger to them and possibly to the general public.

But it is in the area of potential conflict between the freedom of the individual and the interest of the public that circumstances may arise in which the surgeon either must or might divulge information otherwise regarded as private. The same professional codes which stress the importance of confidentiality – the 'Blue Book' of the GMC, for example – also outline the exceptions to the rule. These fall into two general categories.

The public interest

Suppose that in a clinical consultation in A&E, a surgeon discovers that a highly agitated patient is armed, has committed a robbery and has killed a bank clerk and a customer as a result. Here, it seems straightforward that the confidence should be broken and the police informed. The patient might strike again. Indeed, it is legally mandatory to breach confidentiality where patients are suspected of involvement in terrorism within the UK or where they are found to be suffering from a highly infectious and notifiable disease.

But how serious must a risk to the public actually be to breach confidentiality legitimately? For example, should a surgeon be just as willing to turn someone in who confessed in confidence that they had stolen a badly needed winter coat? It is not always easy to balance the interests of the patient against those of the public. This can create difficult dilemmas for surgeons when the two seem in direct conflict and when, as is often the case, there is considerable professional discretion as to how morally to proceed. Debates about HIV and AIDS have recently underlined these issues.

Two things are clear. Firstly, it does not follow from a claim that the public interest demands a breach of confidence that it actually does. For example, the police have no right to disclosure or to access to clinical records which may provide evidence of a crime. A judge may issue a warrant legally authorizing such access or a subpoena demanding disclosure in court. However, even this does not make it morally mandatory. Some clinicians have felt so strongly about the immorality of breaking a patient's confidence that they have risked being charged with contempt of court for refusing to do so.

Again, the law and morality should not be conflated, even though they often do overlap.

Secondly, patients have no right to harm others through the exercise of their right to confidentiality. There is an obvious link between this right and the right of individuals to control the use of their private property. Yet just as the legitimate exercise of this property right stops at the point at which the safety of others is threatened, the same can be said about clinical information. Therefore, if a surgeon discovers that maintaining confidentiality will lead to the threat of serious harm to another known individual – just the suspicion of a general threat is not sufficient – then a breach of confidence may be warranted. For example, although the legal precedent does not apply in the UK, a psychiatrist in the USA was successfully sued for negligence for not informing a young woman that he had clearly been told by a patient that he was going to kill her. He did.

The interest of the individual patient

Breaches of confidence may not just be in the public interest. They may also be necessary in order to obtain information vital for successful treatment. Because of the physical or psychological effects of their illness, some patients are unable to communicate clearly about their medical history. Under such circumstances, relatives or friends may have to be consulted, especially in emergencies.

This said, strong attempts should still be made to obtain the patient's consent and to verify the identity of any others from whom information is sought. No more information about the patient's condition should be revealed than is necessary for the clinical purposes at hand. Knowledge about prognosis and treatment, for example, should remain confidential, remembering how its unwarranted spread might drastically affect the patient's private and public life. Certainly, clinical information should never be communicated over the phone to those not involved in treatment, unless it is with the patient's prior consent and there is a reliable way of identifying the person to whom the information is given.

The interests of patients are also served if the surgeons to whom they reveal clinical information share it with colleagues whose assistance they require. Patients are presumed to consent to such revelations by virtue of their general agreement to treatment. Given the complexity of its division of labour, surgery is an essentially cooperative exercise and its success depends on the free flow of relevant information. This said, only those professionals involved should have access to the information, something which requires caution, especially on open wards.

MORAL INDETERMINACY, INFORMED CONSENT AND OPEN COMMUNICATION

Thus far, we have examined the general principles governing informed consent which are endorsed by the profession of surgery and which are reinforced by statute and case law. Yet, clear as these are, their correct interpretation may be much more obscure in practice. Such rules do not interpret themselves: individual surgeons interpret them when faced with the complexities of specific cases.

In the majority of cases there will be a consensus among the surgical team about the most appropriate interpretation. It will be reasonably clear, for example, how much information should be communicated to knowledgeable patients about the hazards of a particular treatment and whether or not they have understood enough of it to warrant proceeding. Yet in some situations, such agreement will not exist and interpretations will conflict. Here reference to the facts of the case themselves cannot solve the problem. Their openness to conflicting interpretation is what poses it.

Suppose, for example, that despite careful attempts to communicate the considerable risks of an urgently needed operative procedure there is still disagreement among a surgical team about whether or not the patient has fully understood. Here, and against the background of the necessity to come to a quick decision, there may be no 'right' interpretation as to how ethically to proceed. Another illustration might be conflicting beliefs about whether or not urgently to operate on a Jehovah's Witness who refuses a blood transfusion but seems partly to be doing so under pressure from family or congregation.

What is crucial in such circumstances is that, despite their disagreements, individual members of the surgical team accept that the final decision about how to proceed is reached after an open and reasoned discussion where everyone has the chance to present their arguments. As a result, clinicians will be much more willing to cooperate in the search for a common view, even when it involves a degree of what they may perceive as moral compromise. Open communication does not have to conflict with the recognition that it is the senior clinician who must take responsibility for the final choice. Surgeons in authority should always try to create space for such discussions, a practice which is increasingly common in the face of taxing moral dilemmas which have to be resolved in short periods of time – for example, those concerning non-treatment.

CONCLUSION

We have argued that, in principle, patients have a right to give their informed consent to surgical treatment and that the surgeon's duty of care extends to respecting this right, just as much as it does to providing a high standard of surgery per se. What such respect generally means is clear – to allow competent patients to act as informed gatekeepers of their own bodies, even if their decisions conflict with those of their clinicians. Despite the fact that at present the law in the UK does not demand it, surgeons should provide patients with the amount of information a prudent person would require to make such an informed choice. Unless there is a clinical diagnosis of incompetence, the expressed and documented wishes of patients should not be overridden – even in serious surgical emergencies. If the patient is unconscious and incapable of choice, the necessity of the surgical intervention rather than its convenience must be the determining factor, unless there is a valid advance directive to the contrary.

It has also been argued that, in practice, gaining informed consent can be negatively affected by the education and/or receptiveness of the patient and the ability of the surgeon to communicate. As regards the latter, there is a range of opportunities for improvement which should be taken. Concerning patients, methods should be devised to ensure that they have understood as much as they are capable of and that really important information is always disclosed. Taking care to do so will reinforce the confidence of the patient and enhance the quality of the clinical relationship for all those concerned with the provision of good surgical care. Where there is disagreement about what this entails in practice, open discussion is essential. As much as possible, the importance of respecting the autonomy of patients should always extend to colleagues as well.

Acknowledgements

Many thanks to John Cochrane, Bob Cohen, Lesley Doyal, John Dickenson, Arlene Klotzko, Alastair McDonald, Rosanne Lord, Paul Lear, Norman Williams, Daniel Wilsher, Chris Wood and Richard Wood. Special thanks to Ian Kennedy.

FURTHER READING

Alderson P 1993 Children's consent to surgery. Open University Press, Buckingham
Appelbaum P, Lidz C, Meisel A 1987 Informed consent. Oxford University Press, New York

Beauchamp T, Childress J 1994 Principles of biomedical ethics. Oxford University Press, New York

Brazier M 1992 Medicine, patients and the law. Penguin, Harmondsworth

Buchanan A, Brock D 1989 Deciding for others: the ethics of surrogate decision making. Cambridge University Press, Cambridge

Davis H, Fallowfield L Counselling and communication in health care. Wiley, London p. 140

Faden R, Beauchamp T 1986 A history and theory of informed consent. Oxford University Press, Oxford

Faulder C 1985 Whose body is it? – The troubling issue of informed consent. Virago, London

Harris J 1985 The value of life. Routledge, London

Kennedy I 1988 Treat me right. Oxford University Press, Oxford

Kennedy I, Grubb A 1994 Medical law – text and materials. Butterworths, London

McLean S 1989 A patient's right to know: information disclosure, the doctor and the law. Dartmouth, Aldershot

Mason J, McCall Smith R 1994 Law and medical ethics. Butterworths, London

Skegg P 1984 Law, ethics and medicine. Oxford University Press, Oxford

Wear S 1993 Informed consent. Kluwer, Dordrecht

12. Preoperative preparation for surgery

B. R. Davidson

To obtain satisfactory results in general surgery requires a careful approach to the preoperative assessment of patients. The importance of this preparation becomes more evident as the surgical procedure performed becomes more complex. Attention to detail is the key to success.

ROUTINE PREOPERATIVE PREPARATION

Confirm that the planned operative procedure is appropriate and exclude any significant medical problems. Take a full history and carry out a clinical examination on all patients being admitted for an elective surgical procedure. Check clinical signs against the planned surgical procedure, in particular noting the side involved. Take a full drug history with specific enquiry regarding allergic responses to drugs and skin allergies. Continue medication over the perioperative period, especially drugs for hypertension, ischaemic heart disease and bronchodilators. Patients on oral steroid therapy should be given intravenous hydrocortisone and those anticoagulated with oral warfarin should have this stopped at least 48 hours preoperatively. Warfarinized patients who have had a life-threatening thrombotic episode (e.g. pulmonary embolus) within the previous 3 months should be heparinized intravenously until 6 hours prior to surgery. Stop drugs over the perioperative period which may interfere with anaesthetic agents, including monoamine oxidase inhibitors, lithium, tricyclic antidepressants and phenothiazines. If possible, stop the oral contraceptive pill 4 weeks prior to any major surgery.

If there is no history or clinical findings to suggest medical problems in a young patient, then no investigations or tests are required. Test black African patients for the presence of sickle cell anaemia and patients from Mediterranean countries to exclude thalassaemia. In older patients or those with significant medical problems, standard investigation would include a full blood count, urea and electrolytes, chest X-ray and electrocardiogram. Take blood for grouping if transfusion is possible and cross-match blood if it is likely to be needed. The number of units depend on the procedure being performed.

The operation site must be prepared by the removal of hair, if this is necessary for access, using a depilatory cream. Shaving or clipping hair from the operation site increases the risk of infection, unless the skin preparation is carried out immediately prior to surgery. Mark the operation site on the skin with an indelible marker pen. Explain to the patient or guardian the procedure and any likely complications, ask and answer any questions or clarifications, then have them sign the consent form. Antibiotic administration is guided by the surgical procedure involved and is discussed on page 142. Prophylaxis against deep vein thrombosis is considered on page 142.

THE VALUE OF PREOPERATIVE TESTS

Young and fit patients do not require any preoperative investigations. For a critical evaluation of routine preoperative investigations see Velanovich (1994).

Biochemical tests

Some abnormality is noted on routine biochemical testing in approximately 5% of patients, the majority of which relate to elevated blood sugar levels or urea. Elevated urea and creatinine levels in asymptomatic patients are mainly detected in patients over 50 years of age; under this age, therefore, it may be argued that no routine biochemical testing is necessary in asymptomatic patients, if urine analysis has excluded glycosuria.

Full blood count

This is unnecessary in young asymptomatic patients undergoing minor surgery. In other patients it is necessary to exclude anaemia and polycythaemia.

Chest X-ray

The incidence of chest X-ray abnormalities increases with age with some radiological abnormality being present in one-third of patients over 60 years of age. The majority of these abnormalities, however, are of no clinical significance. A respiratory history and clinical examination are of more importance than radiological findings in predicting perioperative respiratory complications. The preoperative chest X-ray is important in patients with new respiratory symptoms, as a baseline for those undergoing major surgery, or in the older aged patient group (>50 years).

Testing for hepatitis viral infection or HIV

Routine testing for these viral infections is not performed in the UK. Any patient with a history of jaundice should, however, have serological testing for hepatitis B and C. Patients at high risk for HIV (intravenous drug abuse, homosexuals, or patients from high-risk areas) should be asked whether or not they are willing to undergo testing. Most hospitals are progressing towards universal precautions, where all patients undergoing surgery are considered as potentially infectious. With universal precautions all operating-room staff are adequately gloved, all unnecessary sharps are avoided, instruments and sharps are not passed by hand and disposable equipment is used wherever possible.

Electrocardiogram

Patients with no history or clinical findings to suggest ischaemic heart disease who are under 40 years of age do not require a preoperative electrocardiogram (ECG). The main reasons for performing an ECG preoperatively is to detect arrthymias or conduction defects, evidence of myocardial ischaemia or previous infarction or evidence of left ventricular hypertrophy. Significant ECG abnormalities in asymptomatic patients are rare but, as would be expected, they increase with age.

THE USE OF ANTIBIOTICS

Patients with clinical infection should be treated with systemic antibiotics prior to undergoing surgery. With elective surgery antibiotic prophylaxis depends on the procedure being performed (Table 12.1). Clean procedures (e.g. varicose vein surgery) do not need anti-

Table 12.1 The risk of infection

Type of wound	Description	Incidence of infection (%)
Clean	No violation of mucosa No inflammation No drains	2
Clean–contaminated	Incision of mucosa but no spillage *or* Clean procedure in immunocompromised	10
Contaminated	Pre-existing infection Spillage of viscus contents	20–40

biotic prophylaxis. Abdominal surgery which is not associated with significant contamination (e.g. cholecystectomy) requires only a single-dose prophylaxis given on induction of anaesthesia. Procedures with a contaminated field (e.g. appendicitis) should be treated with a preoperative dose and two postoperative doses. This regime would also be satisfactory for the majority of other procedures in the gastrointestinal tract (e.g. gastric surgery and colonic surgery with prepared bowel). The choice of antibiotic prophylaxis is determined by the surgical procedure itself. Operations which may be contaminated by skin flora should have prophylaxis against staphylococcal infection with flucloxacillin 500 mg intravenously. Procedures involving the bowel require broad-spectrum cover for Gram-positive and Gram-negative organisms and anaerobes. Commonly used regimes include a cephalosporin with metronidazole. Biliary tract procedures rarely involve a flora of anaerobes, and satisfactory prophylaxis would be obtained from a cephalosporin alone. For a review of antimicrobial prophylaxis see Paluzzi (1993).

PROPHYLAXIS AGAINST DEEP VEIN THROMBOSIS AND PULMONARY EMBOLI

Pulmonary emboli are a major cause of mortality for surgical patients. In the UK it accounts for 10% of inpatient deaths. Recent surgery, immobilization and trauma was responsible for 50% of deep vein thrombosis (DVT) in a review by Cogo et al (1994), but there are other important predisposing factors (see Table 12.2). The oral contraceptive pill (when it contains a high oestrogen content) and significant obesity are also considered major risk factors. Many of the risk factors cannot be avoided, but measures should be taken to avoid propagation of any thrombosis. These measures

T hrombo
E mbolic
D eterrant
S tockings

Table 12.2   Other risk factors for deep vein thrombosis*

Risk factor	Odds ratio†	p
Age >60 years	1.61	0.0012
Male vs female	1.69	0.0004
Cancer	2.37	0.0004
Heart failure	1.79	0.03
Arteriopathy	1.90	0.04

*Adapted from Cogo et al (1994).
†Represents the increased risk associated with each factor.

include the use of pre- and postoperative subcutaneous heparin administration (heparin 5000 i.u. subcutaneously either twice or three times daily), graduated compression stockings and intraoperative intermittent pneumatic calf compression. Subcutaneous heparin may reduce the incidence of DVTs by 50%; it is generally well tolerated but very occasionally thrombocytosis may result. The systemic anticoagulation effect of low-dose subcutaneous heparin are minimal and should not produce any risk for impaired haemostasis during surgical procedures. The newly introduced low-molecular-weight heparins are as effective in preventing DVT as standard heparins and may reduce the risk of pulmonary embolism. They are more expensive. Their value has been reviewed by Jorgensen et al (1993). For discussion of risk factors for thromboembolism see also Thromboembolic Risk Factors Consensus Group (1992).

ASSESSMENT OF RISK FOR SURGERY

Unfortunately, there are few patients who have no risk factors for surgery. It is important to quantify the risks involved so they can be discussed with the patient. Risk scores may also be used to compare different forms of treatment and their effectiveness in different risk groups. The two main prognostic scoring systems which are in current use are the Acute Physiology and Chronic Health Evaluation (APACHE) II system (Knaus et al 1985) and the American Society of Anesthesiologists (ASA) system. These systems were initially introduced to predict the outcome of patients admitted to the Intensive Care Unit and have subsequently been applied to patients undergoing surgery. With the APACHE II system 12 acute physiological variables, the patients' age and their chronic health are individually scored and added to give a final figure. Many computer programs are available to instantly calculate these variables which

Table 12.3   American Society of Anesthesiologists (ASA) status

Category	Description
I	Healthy patient
II	Mild systemic disease – no functional limitations
III	Severe systemic disease – definite functional limitation
IV	Severe systemic disease that is a constant threat to life
V	Moribund patient not expected to survive 24 hours with or without surgery

are summarized in Box 12.1. The ASA assessment is very simple and has therefore been widely adopted (Table 12.3).

MANAGEMENT OF THE HIGH-RISK PATIENT

Patients with major medical problems are at a high risk from surgery and should be identified early in the

---

Box 12.1
Apache II classification
Apache II score is A + B + C

A   Acute Physiology Score (APS)
 1. Rectal temperature (°C)
 2. Mean blood pressure (mmHg)
 3. Heart rate (beats per minute)
 4. Respiratory rate (breaths per minute)
 5. Alveolar–arterial oxygen gradient if $F_IO_2 > 0.5$ or P_aO_2 if $F_IO_2 < 0.5$
 6. Arterial pH
 7. Serum Na^+ (mmol l^{-1})
 8. Serum K^+ (mmol l^{-1})
 9. Serum creatinine (mg/100 ml)
 10. Haematocrit (%)
 11. Leucocyte count (cells mm^{-3})
 12. Glasgow Coma Score (GCS)

B   Age points graded from <44 to >75 years

C   Chronic health points
 2 points for elective postoperative admission
 5 points for: emergency operation
              nonoperative admission
              immunocompromised patient
              chronic liver, cardiovascular,
              respiratory or renal disease.

preoperative period. This allows a specialist opinion to be sought and effective treatment commenced or precautions taken to minimize risk.

Assessment of cardiovascular risk

The increasingly elderly population of Western countries has resulted in large numbers of patients with cardiovascular problems presenting for surgical procedures. Ironically our ability to deal with these cardiovascular complications has resulted in patients being referred for surgery who would not previously have been considered. The major determinants of perioperative cardiac complications are recent myocardial infarction and clinical heart failure. Systemic hypertension and a history of arrhythmias may also be risk factors, but are of lesser significance. The risk of sustaining a further myocardial infarct in the perioperative period varies with the time period postinfarct. The major risk period is within the first 3 months where the risk may be of the order of 30%. The risk, however, decreases rapidly thereafter and elective surgery could be considered at 6 months postinfarct in a patient with no persisting cardiac symptoms or signs. Patients with a history suggestive of ischaemic heart disease, but no evidence of infarction on ECG, should proceed to an exercise or stress ECG which, if positive, confirms that there is significant coronary artery stenosis or occlusion. If the planned surgical procedure is essential, further information will be obtained from coronary angiography and angioplasty or coronary artery bypass grafting will be considered. Patients with a history or clinical signs to suggest congestive cardiac failure can have their left ventricular function assessed by echocardiography. Systemic hypertension is a common problem in the general population and is a significant risk factor unless satisfactorily controlled. All patients found to be hypertensive at the time of assessment for elective surgery should have their surgery delayed until they are established on antihypertensive drugs. Unnecessary delays and inappropriate investigations may be avoided by seeking the opinion of an experienced cardiologist in patients with ischaemic heart disease who require a surgical procedure.

Assessment of respiratory problems

The most common conditions found during preoperative assessment are chronic obstructive airways disease (COAD) and bronchial asthma. The severity of these conditions can largely be predicted from a careful history, but further objective evidence of the extent of their airway disease can be obtained from respiratory function tests. Commonly measured parameters are the peak expiratory flow rate (PEFR), vital capacity (VC) and forced expiratory volume in 1 second (FEV_1). The measurements can be used to assess the response to bronchodilators as well as acting as a baseline for subsequent testing in the postoperative period. Arterial blood gas analysis is also a useful baseline in patients undergoing major surgery or those expected to have significant postoperative respiratory complications. The combination of a painful incision from upper abdominal surgery and significant lung disease is of considerable concern and is best treated by the use of epidural analgesia in the intra- and postoperative period. Guidance should be given preoperatively on breathing exercises to allow expansion of the lung bases and for holding the abdominal incision to produce adequate expectoration in a less painful manner. Patients with infected sputum preoperatively are at increased risk of postoperative chest infection and should be given antibiotics guided by culture and sensitivity. The expert opinion of a chest physician may be invaluable.

Management of preoperative renal dysfunction

The most common disorder which would be diagnosed preoperatively in an elective surgical patient would be a degree of chronic renal failure as demonstrated by an elevated urea and creatinine on routine electrolyte estimations. Moderate elevation of urea and creatinine would be expected in elderly patients with significant atherosclerosis. Such patients may develop acute renal failure if exposed to a period of intraoperative hypotension. Unexplained renal impairment in a young patient should be investigated prior to any elective surgery. Patients in established renal failure on dialysis require to be dialysed prior to any surgical procedure to ensure a good fluid balance and to correct any hyperkalaemia. Patients with functioning renal transplants require to have their immunosuppression continued over the perioperative period and to avoid any periods of operative hypotension. Always consult a nephrologist to discuss perioperative management.

Nutritional assessment

There is a clear and well-established correlation between malnutrition in the preoperative period and an increased morbidity and mortality from surgery. Nutritional assessment can be based on total body weight loss, anthropomorphic measurements such as skin-fold thickness to assess the amount of subcutaneous fat, or biochemical tests which reflect protein deficiency such as the measurement of serum albumin, prealbumin or transferrin. Such preoperative nutritional assessment may detect patients in whom malnutrition is a major concern for their operative procedure, but the correction of this malnourished state, which in part reflects their underlying disease process, may be impossible in the preoperative period. Highlighting the problem, however, will allow nutritional support to be commenced at an early stage and consideration given to the insertion of a feeding enterostomy or a designated central venous feeding line at the time of surgery. Correction of a low preoperative serum albumin level with human albumin solution is an ineffective and expensive method of providing nutritional support and should not be considered unless as an adjuvant to full parenteral or enteral nutrition. For a full discussion on nutrition see Chapter 9.

Management of obesity

In many aspects, the overnourished or obese patient presents as great if not greater risks for surgery than the malnourished patient. The obese patient (greater than 30% above ideal weight) has a markedly increased risk of operative mortality from ischaemic heart disease (increased risk of approximately 40%) and almost 50% increased risk of dying from a cerebrovascular accident. In addition, there is an increased risk of deep vein thrombosis and both wound and intra-abdominal sepsis. Operative risks may be reduced by a careful search for risk factors for ischaemic heart disease and their appropriate investigation and treatment. Prophylaxis against deep vein thrombosis is vital.

Management of the diabetic patient

Diabetic patients are high-risk candidates for any surgical procedure. In addition to their susceptibility to infection and impaired wound healing, they are at risk of vascular complications due to their accelerated atherosclerosis. Careful investigation for evidence of ischaemic heart disease, peripheral vascular disease or cerebrovascular disease is essential, and careful preoperative documentation of peripheral pulses is important. The risks of surgery can be minimized by keeping the blood sugar level carefully controlled. The overall management must be tailored to the severity of the diabetes as well as the operative procedure being performed. For maturity-onset diabetics controlled by diet, or oral hypoglycaemics who are undergoing minor surgery, it is sufficient to avoid the morning dose of oral hypoglycaemics with monitoring of blood sugar levels and the recommencement of oral hypoglycaemic therapy postoperatively. For insulin-dependent diabetics under-

going major surgery, intravenous infusion of insulin and dextrose may provide the best overall control, with the infusion rate being titrated by hourly blood sugar estimations. All insulin-dependent diabetics undergoing major surgery should be discussed directly with the endocrinologist involved.

Treatment of preoperative anaemia or polycythaemia

Patients who have developed an iron-deficiency anaemia and are awaiting elective surgery may be treated by oral iron supplementation. Those requiring surgery more urgently with a haemoglobin less than $10 \, mg \, dl^{-1}$ should be transfused, but blood transfusion immediately prior to surgery (<48 hours) should be avoided as the oxygen-carrying capacity of stored blood is poor. Polycythaemia is less frequently encountered, but is a predisposing factor to postoperative deep vein thrombosis and should therefore be treated by repeated venesection until a satisfactory haemoglobin level is obtained.

Emergency surgery

The results of emergency surgery are less satisfactory than elective procedures, for a variety of reasons. The emergency nature of the surgery does not allow sufficient time for investigation and treatment of associated medical problems. The patients are commonly dehydrated, hypovolaemic and are often septic. Adequate rehydration and systemic antibiotic treatment are essential parts of initial management. The morbidity and mortality audit performed by the Royal College of Surgeons of England (Campling et al 1993) would suggest that the majority of patients with acute surgical problems are best managed by active resuscitation prior to surgery being performed on a scheduled operating list by an experienced surgeon.

PREPARATION FOR SURGERY OF SPECIFIC PATIENT GROUPS

The preoperative preparation of patients for surgery is dependent on the procedures to be performed and the stage of the underlying pathology. However, some selected patient groups are worthy of particular mention.

Large bowel surgery

Most surgeons would consider that bowel preparation of some form is essential for the reduction of sepsis. Surprisingly, several recent controlled studies have failed to support the value of bowel preparation prior to colonic

Citromag

surgery and its value is therefore open to question. For elective surgery, bowel preparation is most commonly achieved by placing the patient on a liquid diet several days prior to surgery and administering oral purgatives on the day prior to surgery (sodium picosulphate (Picolax) 10 mg morning and night, or polyethylene glycol/sodium salts (Klean Prep), 4 sachets in 4 litres of water taken 250 ml every 15 minutes. If this does not produce satisfactory cleansing of the bowel it may be combined with mechanical washouts via a rectal tube. Elderly patients may require intravenous hydration whilst undergoing bowel purgation due to associated fluid loss. In patients with an obstructing lesion, bowel preparation may not be possible. In this group of patients some have advocated on-table colonic lavage with the infusion of fluid via a caecostomy or appendicostomy with the effluent being drained by insertion of a wide-bore tube in the distal colon proximal to the obstruction. All patients undergoing bowel surgery should be warned of the possibility of colostomy formation and the most practical site for a colostomy should be marked on the abdominal wall. The site should be carefully chosen preoperatively with the patient standing and with consideration for movement of the abdominal wall fat.

Preparation of patients for upper gastrointestinal surgery

Patients presenting for upper GI surgery are often anorexic resulting in a poor nutritional state which requires correction by enteral or parenteral nutrition both pre- and post-operatively. Vomiting results in dehydration, electrolyte depletion and possible acid–base imbalance which again must be corrected preoperatively by adequate rehydration. If there is evidence of obstruction a nasogastric tube should be inserted and the stomach emptied to prevent aspiration at the time of induction of anaesthesia. Anaemia is a common feature and should be treated by blood transfusion. Vomiting may be associated with episodes of aspiration and an assessment of respiratory function from the patient's history along with a chest X-ray, respiratory function tests and blood gas analysis are helpful. Preoperative chest physiotherapy may improve gas exchange.

The jaundiced patient

The risks of surgery in patients with obstructive jaundice can be significantly reduced by careful preoperative management. Whether resolving the obstructive jaundice by preoperative insertion of a biliary endoprosthesis reduces the risk of surgery is controversial and is likely to relate to the age of the patient, the risk factors for

surgery and the nature of the underlying disease. As a general rule, preoperative drainage should be considered in elderly patients who are deeply jaundiced and all patients with biliary-tract sepsis. Jaundiced patients may be deficient in the vitamin K dependent clotting factors II, V, VII, IX and X, resulting in a bleeding tendency. Vitamin K should be given to all patients with obstructive jaundice prior to surgery (10 mg intramuscularly or intravenously). A coagulation profile should be checked, and those in whom a significant coagulopathy is present, but who require urgent surgery, should be given fresh frozen plasma at the time of surgery. Renal failure secondary to obstructive jaundice (hepatorenal syndrome) may be reduced by adequate preoperative hydration. It is essential that this patient group is not kept nil by mouth prior to surgery without intravenous fluid replacement. The value of the osmotic diuretic mannitol and the inotrope dopamine (in a dose resulting in renal vasodilatation) in preventing hepatorenal failure is unproven. Infective complications are more common in patients with obstructive jaundice, and antibiotic prophylaxis is mandatory. Patients presenting with acute cholangitis require systemic administration of fluids and antibiotics and urgent biliary tract drainage either endoscopically or percutaneously.

Thyroidectomy

Patients undergoing surgery for thyrotoxicosis should have a period of treatment to reduce thyroid activity (e.g. carbimazole 10–15 mg three times daily) and beta blockers to prevent thyrotoxic crisis (e.g. propranolol 20–40 mg, 8 hourly for 10 days preoperatively). The movement of the vocal cords should be checked prior to surgery by indirect laryngoscopy to exclude an unsuspected idopathic unilateral palsy. The extent of a retrosternal goitre can be clearly demonstrated on computed tomography.

The paediatric patient

The common surgical procedures in childhood are often performed by general surgeons with a training and interest in paediatric surgery. Complex congenital defects and surgery in neonates requires specialist surgical expertise and specific preoperative preparation. The management of all paediatric surgical cases should be carried out with the involvement of a paediatrician. Children should have surgery at the beginning of an operating list to minimize their period of fasting. If delayed intravenous fluids should be commenced, venous cannulae should be inserted using topical anaesthetic cream to reduce discomfort and fluids administered according to body weight (40–60 ml kg^{-1} per 24 hours). Heparin and antibiotics are not required for routine clean surgical procedures.

Thoracic surgery

Assessment of respiratory function is the most important aspect of preoperative preparation (see above). Active preoperative physiotherapy, treatment of any respiratory infection with antibiotics and good postoperative analgesia should minimize the risk of postoperative respiratory failure. This patient group often has associated coronary and cerebral vascular disease due to atherosclerosis, and evidence of this should be sought and a cardiologist's opinion obtained if necessary. Pulmonary emboli are well recognized after thoracic surgery, and subcutaneous heparin is routine as is antibiotic prophylaxis.

Vascular surgery

Atherosclerosis is a generalized disease and patients presenting with symptoms from vascular insufficiency (e.g. intermittent claudication) should have a careful search for cerebral, coronary and renal arterial disease. Ideally, severe ischaemic heart disease should be treated by drugs, angioplasty or coronary artery grafting prior to any surgery for peripheral vascular disease (see above). Diabetic patients with limb ischaemia should have careful diabetic control and treatment of infected skin lesions with appropriate antibiotics. Smoking is a common predisposing factor to atherosclerosis. It reduces small vessel blood flow and should therefore be stopped preoperatively. Smoking also predisposes to chronic obstructive airways disease and bronchial carcinoma. A careful history of respiratory problems should therefore be taken and a chest X-ray performed. Sputum should be sent for culture and sensitivity plus cytology.

Orthopaedic surgery

The most common orthopaedic operations are for the treatment of joint abnormalities secondary to osteoarthritis. This patient group is elderly and their preparation for surgery must include a detailed search for medical problems prevalent in this age group such as ischaemic heart disease and chronic obstructive airways disease. These should be fully investigated and treated preoperatively. Joint replacement is major surgery associated with a significant blood loss, and crossmatching of blood is essential. The increased use of prostheses in orthopaedic surgery has allowed earlier mobilization of patients but carries the risk of infection around the foreign material. Antibiotic prophylaxis should be used which covers contamination from skin commensals such as staphylococci and streptococci. Thromboembolism is a major cause of mortality in orthopaedic patients, especially those undergoing pelvic surgery and prophylaxis with standard or low-molecular-weight heparin is essential (see above).

REFERENCES

Campling E A, Devlin H B, Hoile R W, Lunn J N 1993 Report of the National Confidential Enquiry into Perioperative Deaths 1991/1992. London

Cogo A, Bernardi E, Prandoni P et al 1994 Acquired risk factors for deep vein thrombosis in symptomatic outpatients. Archives of Internal Medicine 154: 164–168

Jorgensen L N, Wille-Jorgensen P, Hauch O 1993 Prophylaxis of postoperative thromboembolism with low molecular weight heparins. British Journal of Surgery 80: 689–704

Knaus W A, Draper E A, Wagner D P et al 1985 APACHE-II: a severity of disease classification system. Critical Care Medicine 13: 818–824

Paluzzi R G 1993 Antimicrobial prophylaxis for surgery. Medical Clinics of North America 77: 427–441

Thromboembolic Risk Factors (THRIFT) Consensus Group 1992 Risk of and prophylaxis for venous thromboembolism in hospital patients. British Medical Journal 305: 567–574

Velanovich V 1994 Preoperative laboratory screening based on age, gender and concomitant medical diseases. Surgery 115: 56–61

13. Premedication and anaesthesia

M. W. Platt

M. W. Platt

PREMEDICATION

Premedication is the prescribing of drugs to be administered preoperatively. These are usually agents prescribed by the anaesthetist, at the preoperative visit, to allay anxiety, relieve pain, to dry saliva, and to maintain the dosage of intercurrent medication. After a brief discussion of intercurrent medication, the broad topic of anaesthetic premedication will be considered.

Intercurrent medication

Many patients coming to surgery have other medical problems which are treated by a variety of different drugs. Refer to the section on medical problems for detailed notes (see Ch 6).

Some patients who need special consideration include: those on antihypertensive therapy; antiarrhythmic therapy; anticoagulated patients; patients on diabetic therapy (oral hypoglycaemics or insulin); those on endocrine replacement therapy (particularly thyroxine); those on adrenocortical replacement or augmentation therapy; those patients undergoing treatment for asthma or chronic obstructive airways' disease with bronchodilators and allied treatments; and those having cardiac failure therapy and diuretics.

Because of fasting, and sometimes the surgical problem itself, it is not always possible for this medication to be continued. However, many drugs need to be continued up to the time of surgery. Sometimes, a parenteral form of the agent can be substituted.

Anaesthetic premedication

1. Anxiolysis
2. Drying secretions
3. Analgesia

Table 13.1 Anxiolytic agents in common use

Agent	Dose	Approx. duration (h)
Benzodiazepines		
Diazepam	$0.05–0.3 \text{ mg kg}^{-1}$	36–200
Temazepam	$0.15–0.5 \text{ mg kg}^{-1}$	5–20
Lorazepam	$0.015–0.06 \text{ } \mu g \text{ kg}^{-1}$	10–20
Midazolam	$0.07–0.08 \text{ mg kg}^{-1}$	0.5–2
Phenothiazines		
Promethazine	$0.2–0.5 \text{ mg kg}^{-1}$	8–12
Prochlorperazine	$0.1–0.2 \text{ mg kg}^{-1}$	

Anxiolysis (Table 13.1)

Patients attending for surgery are normally anxious about the outcome. They may have a fear of the unknown, of pain, of dying, of cancer, or non-specific fears. Although the preoperative visit by the anaesthetist does much to allay anxiety by reducing the unknown element, waiting for an operation may be unpleasant. Anxiolytics calm the patient and help to reduce time spent 'dwelling' on fears. Agents specifically used for anxiolysis are the benzodiazepines, particularly the shorter-acting agents such as temazepam, usually given orally 2 hours preoperatively. For major operations such as cardiopulmonary bypass, a long-acting drug such as lorazepam may be used. Opioid analgesics calm and sedate the patient and are often used, especially if analgesia is required (see below).

Phenothiazines may also be used, usually in combination with an opioid. Promethazine is frequently combined with pethidine. These agents are useful, especially in the elderly, since they calm the patient without too much sedation. Phenothiazines are also appropriate in atopic individuals (e.g. asthmatics), where their antihistaminic action may be useful. Prochlorperazine is used for its combined sedative and antiemetic properties.

Butyrophenones, such as droperidol, are now no

longer used for sedation since they cause dysphoria and the so-called 'locked-in syndrome'. The latter is a state of fear elicited in the patient by a feeling of not being able to communicate with the outside world, although they appear very calm. In very low doses (e.g. 0.01 mg kg^{-1} of droperidol), however, these agents are very potent antiemetics.

Drying secretions (Table 13.2)

In the days of ether anaesthesia, it was particularly important to dry oral secretions, because ether stimulates salivary secretions on induction, potentiating the possibility of laryngospasm. With modern anaesthesia it is less of a requirement, although it may be useful to dry secretions prior to dental surgery, bronchoscopy or surgery on the lung and for paediatric patients in whom salivation can be a problem. In addition to drying secretions, muscarinic receptor antagonists also prevent bradycardia, a common side-effect of general anaesthesia, especially in very young children.

Hyoscine, in contrast to atropine, contributes to the sedative properties of premedication. Glycopyrrolate does not cross the blood–brain barrier, and is a more potent inhibitor of salivary secretions, with less effect on the vagus nerve and hence on the heart rate. Atropine has also been shown to have a small antiemetic effect, presumably through inhibition of the vagus nerve, as well as a slight bronchodilator effect.

Analgesia (Table 13.3)

There are two main reasons for using opioid analgesia as part of the anaesthetic premedication, apart from the excellent sedative properties. Primarily, patients with painful conditions such as fractured hips and other types of trauma need analgesia for a comfortable transfer to theatre. Opioid analgesics are also used preoperatively to provide a continuous background of analgesia to aid the anaesthetic and extend analgesia into the postoperative period. Premedication with an opioid is usually combined with anticholinergic agents, such as glycopyrrolate, to dry secretions and (in the case of hyoscine) to potentiate sedation.

Table 13.2 Drying agents in common use

Agent	Dose (mg kg^{-1})	Approx. duration i.v.	i.m.
Atropine	0.02	15–30 min	2–4 h
Hyoscine	0.008	30–60 min	4–6 h
Glycopyrrolate	0.01	2–4 h	6–8 h

Table 13.3 Analgesic agents in common use

Agent	Dose (mg kg^{-1})	Approx. duration, i.m. (h)
Morphine	0.1–0.2	4
Papaveretum	0.2–0.4	3
Pethidine	1.0–1.5	3–4

Notes:
1. Papaveretum is a mixture of alkaloids which contains morphine (45–55% dry weight), codeine, papaverine, thebaine and noscopine. It should not be used in women of child-bearing age, because noscopine has been shown to be a gene toxin.
    Papaveretum is most commonly used as a premedication in combination with hyoscine, and comes in a premixed ampoule containing papaveretum 20 mg ml^{-1} and hyoscine 0.4 mg ml^{-1}.
2. Pethidine is often premixed with promethazine as pethidine 50 mg ml^{-1} and promethazine 25 mg ml^{-1}. Atropine is sometimes given in addition.
3. Morphine, often used alone for both its sedative and analgesic properties, is usually combined with a drying agent such as atropine (also useful to prevent bradycardia), or in combination with an antiemetic drug.

Generally speaking, the choice of premedication depends very much on the individual patient. For example, a moribund patient will not benefit, and may indeed suffer from such side-effects as respiratory or cardiovascular depression, whereas a young, fit, anxious patient could perhaps benefit from anxiolysis or sedation, besides possible analgesic requirements, especially in trauma.

GENERAL ANAESTHESIA

General anaesthesia is a reversible, drug-induced state of unresponsiveness to outside stimuli, characterized by non-awareness, analgesia and relaxation of striated muscle. Older agents such as ether need to be given in large amounts to achieve these aims, and they take a long time for induction and recovery.

With the advent of newer, more specifically acting agents such as the muscle relaxants, modern general anaesthesia is a balance between the triad of 'relaxation', 'analgesia' and 'hypnosis' (lack of awareness).

A general anaesthetic may be considered in three phases, analogous to an aircraft flight.

- 'take-off' = 'induction'
- 'cruising' = 'maintenance'
- 'landing' = 'reversal and recovery'

Each part of the triad of general anaesthesia will be

considered separately, under the heading of each phase of the anaesthetic.

Induction of anaesthesia

Hypnosis at induction of anaesthesia

In the anaesthetic room, patients are induced using one or other of several intravenous anaesthetics. In approximate order of frequency, those shown in Table 13.4 are the most commonly used agents. When drugs are taken up in the bloodstream, initial distribution is to 'vessel-rich' tissues and those taking a large fraction of the cardiac output. Thus the brain, which is vessel rich and also taking a large fraction of the cardiac output, receives a considerable portion of intravenous anaesthetic given as a bolus. Subsequently, drugs diffuse out of the brain, down a concentration gradient formed by the falling blood concentration, and are redistributed to other vessel-poor tissues. This results in an initial short redistribution half-life. The longer elimination half-life of a drug represents its metabolism and elimination from the body. In some instances, this can appear to take a long time, due to the slow leaching out of drug from vessel-poor fat tissues.

Thiopentone, a very short-acting barbiturate, was the first widely used intravenous induction agent. It was first used to great effect on casualties from the bombing of Pearl Harbor in 1942. However, the ability of thiopentone to depress the myocardium was tragically evident in the deaths of young sailors already shocked from hypovolaemia. It was soon learned to reduce the dose and only give enough thiopentone to cause sleep (a 'sleep dose'), titrating carefully with each patent – especially those with a low cardiac reserve.

Propofol has a very short half-life, and tends to be used particularly in day-case surgery, where rapid recovery is indicated. It is also used to abate the effects of procedures which occasionally cause laryngospasm, such as laryngeal mask placement and anal stretching. Propofol is sometimes infused intravenously to maintain

anaesthesia, because of its short half-life. The initial bolus of propofol sometimes causes a profound fall in blood pressure and inhibits compensatory increases in heart rate. Preinduction administration of glyco-pyrrolate or atropine may attenuate this.

Etomidate is indicated only for induction of anaesthesia. As a side-effect, it causes a reversible suppression of an enzyme in the adrenal cortex, leading to inhibition of cortisol secretion – this is especially important if it is used as an infusion. Etomidate is indicated in patients with poor cardiac reserve, or other patients in whom a fall in cardiac output could prove catastrophic, because it tends to maintain cardiac output. It is relatively long acting, and is associated with a higher incidence of postoperative nausea and vomiting.

Ketamine is used in shocked patients, because it stimulates the sympathetic nervous system and prevents a fall in cardiac output. However, patients already on full sympathetic drive will still suffer a reduction in cardiac output and blood pressure. Ketamine produces a state known as 'dissociative anaesthesia' with profound analgesia. It is structurally related to LSD.

Benzodiazepines given intravenously, particularly midazolam (the most efficacious in this respect), are occasionally used to induce or assist induction of anaesthesia.

Opioids in very high doses are used to induce anaesthesia in some situations. The most commonly used agents for this are the highly potent synthetic derivatives fentanyl, alfentanil and sufentanil. Fentanyl is used in a dosage of up to 1.0 mg kg^{-1}, particularly in cardiac anaesthesia, since it avoids hypotension and maintains cardiac output. Without other agents, awareness may occur, however, and chest rigidity, preventing adequate ventilation, occasionally occurs (easily reversed with the use of muscle relaxants).

Generally, with the exceptions outlined above, all intravenous anaesthetic agents depress the myocardium.

Relaxation at induction

On induction, muscle relaxation is necessary to facilitate (tracheal) intubation. Relaxation during maintenance of anaesthesia is discussed below.

Suxamethonium is a depolarizing relaxant used primarily for difficult intubation and crash induction. It only lasts approximately 5 minutes, after a dose of 1.5 mg kg^{-1}. Suxamethonium is essentially two acetylcholine molecules joined together. Its great similarity to acetylcholine results in activation of the receptor and depolarization of the muscle membrane. However, this depolarization lasts some 5–10 minutes, and muscles become unresponsive to acetylcholine. As it lasts some

Table 13.4 Anaesthetic agents

Drug	Dose (mg kg^{-1})	Distribution half-life (min)	Elimination half-life (h)
Thiopentone	3–5	3–14	5–17
Propofol	1–3	2–4	4–5
Etomidate	0.3	2–6	1–5
Ketamine			
i.v.	1–2	10	2–3
i.m.	5–10	15	2–3
Methohexitone	1–3	3–8	26
Midazolam	0.03–0.3	6–20	1–4

5–10 minutes, suxamethonium is useful, apart from intubation, for very short surgical procedures.

Side-effects of suxamethonium include:

1. *Histamine release*. 'Scoline rash' is very common following intravenous administration of suxamethonium. An erythematous rash is seen spreading over the upper trunk and lower neck anteriorly. Very occasionally, suxamethonium will cause bronchospasm and other more severe sequelae.

2. *Bradycardia*. This is seen particularly if a second or subsequent dose is given, especially in children. Atropine is given to prevent or reverse this effect.

3. *Generalized somatic pain*. The actual cause of this is unknown, but may be a result of widespread fleeting muscle contractions, termed 'fasciculations', caused by the depolarization of muscle fascicles.

4. *Hyperkalaemia*. Suxamethonium causes the release of potassium from muscle cells. This may be accentuated in acute denervating injuries such as spinal cord trauma or burns, and can lead to cardiac arrest.

5. *Persistent neuromuscular blockade*. Some patients may have deficient or abnormal plasma pseudo-cholinesterase, resulting in prolonged action of suxamethonium, sometimes called 'scoline apnoea'. This is genetically related. The completely silent gene is rare, occurring in approximately 1 : 7000 of the population.

6. *Malignant hyperthermia*. This is a condition occurring in some 1 : 100 000 of the population. It occurs as a reaction to certain anaesthetic drugs, of which suxamethonium and halothane are the commonest. Muscle metabolism becomes uncontrolled because of an abnormality of intracellular calcium flux. Body temperature rapidly rises at the rate of at least 2°C every 15 minutes, and $P_a\text{CO}_2$, reflecting the massively raised metabolic rate, also increases with alacrity. Treatment is with ventilation and surface cooling and intravenous dantrium given promptly before death ensues.

'Crash induction'

This consists of a rapid-sequence intravenous induction, cricoid pressure and tracheal intubation, with the aim of preventing regurgitation and aspiration of stomach contents. The patient is given a precalculated dose of thiopentone (3–5 mg kg^{-1}), immediately followed by suxamethonium (1.5 mg kg^{-1}), currently the fastest-acting muscle relaxant, acting within one circulation time. A trained assistant applies pressure to the cricoid cartilage simultaneously, compressing the oesophagus between cricoid ring and vertebral column. The trachea is intubated with a cuffed tracheal tube, and the cuff inflated. Only when the anaesthetic circuit is attached

Table 13.5 Anaesthetic volatile agents

Agent	Structure	MAC	Blood/gas partition coefficient
Diethyl ether	$CH_3CH_2\text{--}O\text{--}CH_2CH_3$	1.92	12
Halothane	$CF_3CHClBr$	0.75	2.3
Enflurane	$CHF_2O\text{--}CF_2CHFCl$	1.68	1.9
Isoflurane	$CHF_2O\text{--}CHClCF_3$	1.05	1.4

Notes:

1. MAC: the minimum alveolar concentration of a gas or vapour in oxygen required to keep 50% of the population unresponsive to a standard surgical stimulus (opening of the abdomen). MAC is expressed as a percentage concentration.

2. Blood/gas partition coefficient: indicates how rapidly a gas or vapour is taken up from the lungs. The higher the blood solubility, the longer it takes for the brain to gain adequate anaesthetic concentrations.

3. Summary of effects of modern vapours on organ systems:
   (a) *Heart*: generally cause depressed contractility: halothane > enflurane > isoflurane (halothane causes more arrhythmias)
   (b) *Blood vessels*: generally cause vasodilatation: isoflurane > enflurane > halothane
   (c) *Respiration*: depressed by all agents: enflurane > isoflurane > halothane
   (d) *Brain*: All may cause vasodilatation and raised intracranial pressure: halothane > enflurane > isoflurane (isoflurane safe up to 1 MAC)

and cuff seal confirmed, is cricoid pressure relaxed at the request of the anaesthetist.

The following patients are at risk of aspiration of stomach contents on induction of anaesthesia:

- All non-fasted patients
- Patients with a history suggestive of hiatus hernia
- Any emergency trauma patient (trauma slows stomach emptying)
- Intestinal or gastric obstruction or stasis
- Pregnancy (stomach emptying slowed and cardiac sphincter relaxed)
- Any other intra-abdominal tumours that may cause slowing of gastric emptying.

Maintenance of anaesthesia

Hypnosis during anaesthesia

Anaesthesia is usually maintained with volatile agents, which are hydrocarbons, liquid at room temperature, with high saturated vapour pressures and lipid solubility. Diethyl ether was the earliest agent used, and is still used commonly in other parts of the world. Ether is flammable and explosive. By adding fluoride and other halogens, however, the hydrocarbon molecule becomes much more stable. Modern agents are non-inflammable, non-explosive, and much more potent than ether. Being less soluble in blood (as indicated by the blood/gas partition coefficient), they also have a much faster uptake and elimination time than diethyl ether. Table 13.5 shows the most commonly used anaesthetic volatile agents (with ether as a comparison)

Halothane A hydrocarbon with fluorine, chlorine and bromine atoms. This was the first modern volatile anaesthetic agent which was not explosive or flammable. Synthesized in 1951 and first used clinically in 1956, it was the most commonly used anaesthetic agent for 30 years. Halothane is a potent anaesthetic which allows a smooth induction (which is important especially for gaseous induction of children), and relatively rapid onset of anaesthesia. In the body, up to 20% is metabolized by the liver, the majority being eliminated unchanged via the lungs. The recovery time from halothane anaesthesia is also brisk and smooth. The most common side-effects of halothane are secondary to its effects on the heart. Halothane slows the sinoatrial node, slowing heart rate and causing variations in the p–q interval. It reduces myocardial workload. Like verapamil, halothane produces these effects by blocking calcium channels in the heart. However, it also sensitizes the heart to catecholamines and may precipitate arrhythmias (which is especially important in the presence of adrenaline-supplemented local anaesthesia and if the arterial carbon dioxide tension, $P_a\text{CO}_2$, is elevated). By reducing cardiac output, halothane attenuates splanchnic blood flow, diminishing hepatic blood flow and possibly aggravating its effects on the liver. Using very fine indicators of hepatic performance, it has now been shown that even the briefest exposure to halothane will cause some degree of liver dysfunction. This is probably related to the large amount of halothane that is metabolized (up to 20%). There is also an idiosyncratic reaction which occurs after halothane exposure in some patients, known as 'halothane hepatitis'. The latter is a fulminant centrilobular necrosis of the liver which appears 2–5 days postoperatively. The incidence is 1 : 35 000 of the population (from the National Halothane Study, USA, 1966), with a mortality of over 50%. Halothane is now used in only 10% of anaesthetics given in the UK, the majority of these being for paediatric anaesthesia.

Enflurane Enflurane is an ether synthesized in 1963 and first used in 1966. It is halogenated with fluorine and chlorine atoms to render it non-explosive and non-inflammable. Enflurane is more efficacious in reducing peripheral vascular resistance and is less likely to cause cardiac arrhythmias, nor does it sensitize the heart to catecholamines. However, its pungent odour makes it unsuitable for gaseous induction in children. Enflurane causes greater respiratory depression than halothane or isoflurane, and so it is less suitable for maintaining anaesthesia in the spontaneously breathing patient. Enflurane is only slightly metabolized by the liver (up to 2.5%) and appears not to cause hepatitis.

Isoflurane. Isoflurane is the most recent volatile agent in common use. It was synthesized in 1965 and first used in 1971. It is actually a structural isomer of enflurane, but with different properties. Isoflurane tends to act on the peripheral vasculature as a calcium antagonist, causing a reduction in peripheral vascular resistance. Although it has minimal effects on the heart, isoflurane may cause 'coronary steal', a phenomenon whereby blood is diverted from stenosed coronary arteries to dilated unblocked coronary arteries, possibly compromising ischaemic areas of myocardium. This is still a controversial area, however, and isoflurane generally causes minimal depression of contractility. In the brain, isoflurane has the least effect on cerebral blood flow, causing no significant increase up to 1 MAC. Isoflurane causes least respiratory depression and is suited to the spontaneously breathing patient. Only up to 0.2% of isoflurane is metabolized by the liver and no cases of hepatitis have been reported.

New volatile agents. Desflurane was recently released for use in the UK and is proving very popular for anaesthetizing day-care patients because of its rapid recovery, and *sevoflurane* is currently being evaluated in clinical trials. Both are characterized by remarkable molecular stability, with very little hepatic metabolism. They also have a very low blood gas solubility coefficient, resulting in very rapid onset and recovery. Desflurane is more pungent than sevoflurane, the latter being potentially more useful for gaseous induction of children.

Nitrous oxide. Nitrous oxide (N_2O), unlike the volatile agents, is a gas at atmospheric pressure and room temperature. It has a MAC of 103% at sea level. The requirements of keeping the patient well oxygenated mean that it can never be relied upon to provide anaesthesia in its own right. It is, however, a very potent analgesic agent. Fifty per cent N_2O is equivalent in efficacy to approximately 10 mg morphine sulphate. It continues to enjoy popularity as the main background anaesthetic gas, usually given as 70% in oxygen. In concentrations greater than 50% it causes amnesia and contributes significantly to the overall anaesthetic.

Relaxation during anaesthesia

To allow the surgeon access to intra-abdominal contents, or to allow artificial ventilation of the patient, for example in chest surgery, muscle relaxation (paralysis) is required.

Agents used specifically to relax muscles are called

relaxants. Relaxants are agents which block acetylcholine receptors on muscle end-plates. There are two types of relaxant: depolarizing and non-depolarizing.

Depolarising muscle relaxants. Only one depolarizing relaxant is still in common use, *suxamethonium*, which is described above in relation to induction.

Non-depolarizing muscle relaxants. There are many different relaxants available today. Due to the side-effects of suxamethonium, research continues to find a non-depolarizing relaxant with a very rapid onset and very short half-life. Non-depolarizing relaxants have an onset time of the order of 2–3 minutes, and last from 20 minutes to 1 hour. They are competitive inhibitors of the acetylcholine receptors on muscle end-plates, preventing access of acetylcholine to receptor, resulting in non-transmission of nerve impulse to muscle. *Curare* was the first relaxant of this class, developed from an arrow poison used by Amazonian tribesmen to kill animals for food. Only the dextrorotatory isomer is active; the term 'tubo-' refers to the bamboo tubes in which it is carried by the Amazonian tribesmen – 'D-tubocurare'. Modern relaxants tend to be shorter acting, with fewer side-effects (Table 13.6).

Table 13.6   Non-depolarizing muscle relaxants

Agents	Dose (mg kg^{-1})	Duration of effect (min)	Side-effects
D-Tubocurare	0.5	30–60	Sympathetic ganglion blockade, histamine release, hypotension
Alcuronium	0.3	20–40	As above
Pancuronium	0.01	45–120	Vagolytic: tachycardia, increase blood pressure
Vecuronium	0.01	30–45	Bradycardia
Atracurium	0.06	15–40	Histamine release

Notes:
1. With the exception of atracurium, all these agents require renal and hepatic function for their clearance.
2. Atracurium is excreted by two mechanisms: Hoffman elimination (up to 40%) and hepatic metabolism. Hofmann elimination results in breakdown of the atracurium molecule as a result of pH and temperature. It is used in those patients with renal failure.
3. The histamine release associated with atracurium is only a quarter of that associated with tubocurare, and tends not to cause the hypotension seen with the latter agent.
4. The duration of effect with each agent varies slightly according to anaesthetic technique. The use of volatile agents, particularly enflurane and isoflurane, potentiates the effect of non-depolarizing muscle relaxants. Hypothermia also potentiates non-depolarizing relaxants.
5. The shorter-acting agents atracurium and vecuronium are often used as infusions for long cases and in intensive care.
6. Muscle relaxants have no intrinsic anaesthetic effect.

Analgesia during anaesthesia

The final part of the triad of general anaesthesia during its maintenance consists of analgesia. The anaesthetized patient derives analgesia from three potential sources: the premedication, anaesthesia supplementation with opioids, and from the analgesic properties of volatile and gaseous agents.

Premedication. Opioids used in premedication, as discussed earlier, will tend to last intraoperatively and into the postoperative period. In this way, premedication affects both the anaesthetic and postoperative analgesia.

Anaesthetic opioid supplementation. Intraoperatively, opioids are often administered to deepen the effect of the anaesthetic, or to reduce the amount of volatile agent used (often because of their side-effects such as hypotension). To limit the effects of opioids to the perioperative period, anaesthetists often use highly potent short-acting agents such as fentanyl, alfentanil or sufentanil. These agents are all much more potent than morphine, and much shorter acting (of the order 20–30 minutes). They may need to be reversed at the end of the operation, to facilitate spontaneous respiration. However, this is at the expense of analgesia. Longer acting opioids such as morphine, papaveretum, or pethidine may also be used – especially if postoperative analgesia may be a problem.

Modern non-steroidal anti-inflammatory agents, such as diclofenac and ketorolac, are increasingly used for postoperative analgesia, either on their own for minor surgery or in combination with opioid techniques to give a much better quality of analgesia. Side-effects include renal failure (prostaglandin inhibition may lead to renal shutdown), gastric ulceration and bleeding (inhibition of platelet function). Different agents have different degrees of complications, but their careful use has revolutionized the aftercare of patients, particularly after day-care surgery.

Analgesic properties of volatile agents. Modern volatile anaesthetic agents have poor analgesic properties and contribute little to this part of the anaesthetic. However, N_2O is a very good analgesic (see above) and is also used for analgesia during labour (as a 50% mixture with oxygen, known as 'Entonox').

Recovery from anaesthesia

At the end of surgery, anaesthesia is terminated. Volatile agents and nitrous oxide are turned off on the anaesthetic machine and oxygen alone administered. Anaesthetic gases and vapours diffuse down concentration gradients from the tissues to alveoli of the lungs and out via the airway.

Reversal of muscle relaxation

Competitive muscle relaxants usually need to be reversed to ensure full return of muscle power. The degree of neuromuscular blockade can be monitored with a peripheral nerve stimulator.

Neostigmine (0.05 mg kg^{-1}) or *edrophonium* (0.5 mg kg^{-1}) is given intravenously. These agents block acetylcholinesterase in the neuromuscular junction, resulting in accumulation of acetylcholine. This overcomes the competitive blockade of the relaxant molecules in favour of acetylcholine. However, both neostigmine and edrophonium cause acetylcholine accumulation at both muscarinic and nicotinic sites. Muscarinic receptors are those cholinergic receptors in the heart, gut, sweat glands etc. Therefore, to prevent bradycardia, profuse sweating, and gut overactivity, atropine (0.02 mg kg^{-1}) or glycopyrrolate (0.01 mg kg^{-1}) must be given with the anticholinesterase.

Full reversal of muscle relaxation is only apparent by appropriate neuromuscular monitoring, or when the patient is able to maintain head lifting. This aspect of recovery from anaesthesia is crucial, since full muscular control is necessary for coughing and for good control of the airway. Indeed it highlights the importance of adequate recovery facilities in the theatre suite.

REGIONAL ANAESTHESIA

Definition

Regional (local) anaesthesia is the reversible blockade of nerve conduction by regionally applied agents, for the purpose of sensory ablation, either of traumatized tissue, or to enable minor surgery. These agents are referred to as 'local anaesthetics'. Both motor and sensory nerves may be blocked, depending on the agent used and the anatomical region where the agent is applied.

Nerves may be blocked anywhere between the central nervous system and the site of required sensory loss. Local anaesthetics are used to block pain fibres as they enter the spinal cord: epidural, spinal and paravertebral techniques. They may also be blocked along their anatomical route in the neurovascular bundles: field blocks, or specific nerve blocks. Finally, local infiltration around

Table 13.7   Types of nerve fibre

Fibre	Type	Function	Conduction velocity (ms)	Diameter (μm)
A	α	Motor, proprioception	70–120	12–20
	β	Touch, pressure	30–70	5–12
	γ	Motor (spindles)	15–30	3–6
	δ	Pain, temperature, touch	12–30	2–5
B		Preganglionic autonomic	3–15	<3
C		Dorsal root: pain, reflexes	0.5–2	0.4–1.2
		Sympathetic: postganglionic	0.7–2.3	0.3–1.3

the required site may be performed (for example, skin and subcutaneous infiltration), to block conduction at the nerve endings.

Types of nerve fibre

The speed with which local anaesthetic agents are taken up by nerve fibres depends on their size and whether they are myelinated. Nerve fibres are classified according to their size and speed of conduction (Table 13.7).

Sensitivity to local anaesthetics

The smaller fibres are more sensitive to local anaesthetic agents than the larger fibres. Hence, 'C' fibres conducting pain are more sensitive than motor fibres in the 'A' group. This is why patients may still be able to move limbs, even during regional anaesthesia.

The reason for the differential is most likely due to more rapid absorption and uptake of local anaesthetic into the smaller fibres within neurovascular bundles.

Local anaesthetic agents

Drugs used as local anaesthetics all tend to have 'membrane stabilizing' properties.

Local anaesthetic agents act by inducing a blockade of nerve transmission in peripheral nerve impulses. This occurs as a result of obstruction to sodium channels in the axon membrane, preventing ingress of sodium ions necessary for propagation of an action potential.

Local anaesthetic agents belong to one of two chemical classes according to their structure, which consists of an amide or ester linkage separating an aromatic group and an amine:

Aromatic   >—<   Amine
group   Amide or ester group

Ester class

The only ester still in frequent use is *cocaine*, which is an ester of benzoic acid. It is used generally only for topical anaesthesia of mucous membranes in the nose and sinuses.

Amethocaine is still used occasionally as a topical agent, as is *benzocaine*.

Amide class (Table 13.8)

The first amide to be synthesized was *lignocaine*. This was shown to be safer than cocaine and has remained a mainstay for local anaesthetic practice. *Prilocaine* has the highest therapeutic index, and is considered the safest agent for intravenous blockade. Other amides in common usage include *bupivacaine*, *mepivacaine* and *etidocaine*. Bupivacaine is longer acting than lignocaine and is commonly used in epidural analgesia.

Clinical application

1. *Local infiltration* is used for surgery alone or in combination with general anaesthesia. Used with adrenaline, it reduces bleeding at the operative site. It also produces good postoperative analgesia. EMLA (eutectic mixture of local anaesthetics), a mixture of lignocaine and prilocaine produces good analgesia when applied topically to skin. It is useful for insertion of intravenous lines, arterial lines and removal of minor skin lesions. It needs to be applied some 2 hours before the procedure.

2. *'Field' blocks and nerve blocks* are useful for producing wider areas of anaesthesia and analgesia, for example in inguinal hernia repair, brachial plexus blockade for the upper limb and femoral and sciatic blocks of the lower limb.

3. *Spinal, epidural and paravertebral blockade* produce widespread anaesthesia and analgesia. The pain of labour and childbirth involves nerve roots of lower thoracic, lumbar and sacral regions of the spinal cord. Epidural techniques, involving the epidural placement of a catheter, allow continuous analgesia or anaesthesia, alleviating pain from all these groups of fibres. Regional anaesthesia such as this is frequently employed for urological and other surgery in the lower half of the body. It should be noted, however, that spinal and epidural techniques also block sympathetic ganglia at the appropriate levels. Hypotension will occur unless adequate precautions are taken.

Table 13.8 Amide class

Drug	Maximum dose (mg)	Side-effects
Lignocaine	300 (500 + adr.)	No unusual features. CNS excitation with toxicity
Prilocaine	600	Least toxic. Methaemoglobinaemia >600 mg
Bupivacaine	175 (225 + adr.)	Sudden cardiovascular collapse. Not indicated for intravenous blockade
Cocaine	150	Cardiac arrhythmias. CNS excitation. Topical use only

Notes:

1. The table includes only those agents currently in common use and maximal doses relate to adult size (70 kg body weight). The bracketed dosages refer to maximal doses in the presence of adrenaline.

2. All local anaesthetic agents have membrane-stabilizing properties. Their toxic effects therefore relate to this property and involve mainly the cardiovascular and central nervous systems.
Toxic effects on the central nervous system include fitting and coma, leading to death from hypoxia without adequate resuscitation. Cardiovascular effects from toxicity include hypotension, cardiac arrhythmias and acute cardiovascular collapse.
Bupivacaine has a high affinity for cardiac muscle cells – a property which is thought to be responsible for the high incidence of cardiovascular collapse associated with its use for intravenous blockade (Bier's block), for which it is no longer recommended.

3. Toxic effects may also occur with the accidental intravascular injection of drug.

4. Concentration of local anaesthetic agents varies. Bupivacaine comes as 0.5% or 0.25%, with or without adrenaline. Lignocaine generally comes as 0.5, 1.0, 2.0% concentrations, again plus or minus adrenaline. The higher concentrations obviously have lower maximum safe volumes ($1\% = 10$ mg ml^{-1}, $2\% = 20$ mg ml^{-1}).

5. Local anaesthesia techniques should always be performed where adequate resuscitation facilities are present.

6. Adrenaline and other vasoconstricting agents, such as felypressin, allow higher doses of local anaesthetic to be used, the vasoconstriction resulting in reduced absorption.

CONCLUSION

Pre-emptive analgesia has gained popularity with the recent publication of data suggesting that the administration of analgesia preoperatively, either systemically as with an opioid, or regionally as in use of local anaesthetic techniques, reduces the patient's need for analgesia postoperatively. This has been reinforced by the finding that use of epidural analgesia for 3 days prior to leg amputation produces a marked reduction in the incidence of phantom limb pain. Thus the use of regional techniques combined with general anaesthesia is becoming more popular.

The widespread development of acute pain services is enabling the continuation of regional local analgesic techniques from the operating theatre into the general wards, improving the standards of postoperative pain control and perhaps reducing the incidence of post-operative nausea and vomiting secondary to opioids.

FURTHER READING

Atkinson R S, Rushman G B, Lee A 1987 A synopsis of anaesthesia, 10th edn. Wright, London

Barash P G, Cuplen B F, Stoelting R K 1989 Clinical anaesthesia. Lippincott, Philadelphia

Gilman A G, Goodman L S, Rall T W, Murad F 1985 Goodman and Gilman's pharmacological basis of therapeutics, 7th edn. Macmillan, London

Miller R D 1990 Anesthesia, 3rd edn. Churchill Livingstone, Edinburgh, vols I–II

Nimmo W S, Smith G 1989 Anaesthesia. Blackwell Scientific, Oxford, vols I–II

Stoelting R K 1987 Pharmacology and physiology in anesthetic practice. Lippincott, Philadelphia

Vickers M D, Morgan M, Spencer P S J 1991 Drugs in anaesthetic practice, 7th edn. Butterworths, Oxford

14. Operating theatres and special equipment

M. K. H. Crumplin

OPERATING THEATRE DESIGN AND ENVIRONMENT

The operating theatre environment must provide a safe, efficient, user-friendly environment that is as free from bacterial contamination as possible. Operating theatre suites should be sited near to each other for efficient flexibility of staff movement. The theatres should preferably be situated on the first floor, away from the main hospital traffic. Ideally, operating rooms should be on the same level and adjacent to intensive care units and surgical wards. The suite should incorporate the theatre sterile supply unit. There should be minimum distance between operating rooms and the accident and emergency (A&E) unit and X-ray facilities, which will both be sited on the ground floor. All district general hospitals should now have a multidisciplinary user committee to optimize efficiency and safety. This should be composed of surgeons, anaesthetists, operating theatre and anaesthetic nurses, microbiologists, a manager and a finance officer in line with recent Department of Health recommendations. This committee should meet on a regular basis. Although there is no such entity as a standard operating theatre, an attempt was made by the Department of Health and Social Security in 1978 to introduce the nucleus concept, which at least provided hospitals with theatre suites appropriate to the average district general hospital requirements. Naturally, with orthopaedic, cardiac, neurosurgical, laser and other specialist requirements, there would have to be adjustments to the standard design, for example the Charnley tent, controlled areas for laser therapy and the provision of a pump preparation room off a cardiac bypass theatre.

The antiseptic environment

In any operating theatre suite an attempt should be made to minimize bacterial contamination, especially in the vicinity of the operating table; thus the concept of zones is useful:

- an outer zone – e.g. patient reception area
- a clean zone – the area between the reception bay and theatre suite
- an aseptic zone – the operating theatre
- a dirty zone – e.g. disposal areas and dirty corridors

To provide a minimally contaminated environment for surgeons and patients at the operating table, various principles must be employed.

Air flow

Directional air flow (laminar air flow) may be vertical or horizontal. Here, in addition to normal turbulent air flow through theatre which is necessary to maintain humidity, temperature and air circulation, an increased rate of air change is necessary to reduce the number of contaminated particles over the patient. Air is pumped into the room through filters and passed out of vents in the periphery of the operating room and does not return into the operating suite. Most theatres have 20–40 air changes per hour, but this rate may increase to 400 per hour in the vertical laminar flow system of a Charnley tent.

Wearing of disposable, non-woven fabrics

This obviously reduces dispersal of bacteria-laden particles which may emanate from the operating or nursing staff. Optimally, everybody would wear these gowns, but this might prove costly. Masks are not essential for the surgeon, but should be worn when the patient is particularly susceptible to infection, a prothesis is being inserted, or when the surgeon or nurse has an upper respiratory tract infection.

Body exhaust suits

Here personal air circulation takes place within a specially designed operating suit and helmet so that exhaust air is removed from the suit by a pipe.

The operating tent environment

There is a high vertical laminar flow within the tent, and clean air from above the table is expelled down to floor level in a funnel shape, thereby reducing contamination. By using suitable exhaust suits and such tents, infection in hip replacement may be kept as low as 0.5%.

Behaviour in theatre

It is desirable that the minimum number of people should be in the operating theatre, to provide safe and efficient management of the patient. The bacteriological count in theatre is related to the number of persons and their movement in the operating room.

Temperature and humidity control

A steady level of temperature and humidity during surgery is desirable for comfort and may be varied to suit individual preference. The temperature in the operating theatre will need to be higher for neonates, children, elderly patients and for prolonged surgery. The usual comfortable temperature range in the operating room would be 20–22°C (68–71.6°F). Temperature and humidity control should be integral to the air-conditioning system which, while maintaining a constant working milieu, will require approximately 20–40 air changes per hour. Patients will become hypothermic if the temperature is below 21°C (69.8°F) during prolonged procedures. Loss of heat may be reduced by using warming blankets placed on the sorbo-rubber table surface and by infusing warmed intravenous fluids. This is achieved by passing the blood, crystalloid or colloids through a coiled plastic infusion pipe in a heated waterbath. Postoperatively heat loss may also be minimized by wrapping the patient in aluminium foil.

OPERATING TABLES

Operating tables need to be heavy and stable, easily manoeuvrable, comfortable for the patient and highly adjustable in terms of positioning the patient correctly for a particular operative procedure. There are two basic types of operating table. First, and most common, are those which are completely mobile, thus allowing replacement if necessary. The second type of table is one which has a fixed and permanently installed column in the centre of the operating room with a variety of table tops which can be mounted on the column. These tables are usually expensive and have a remote control for their various movements. The problem is that if a fault develops with the table that theatre will be out of service. The advantage of the fixed-base system is that there is efficiency of patient handling and flexibility in operating-room scheduling using interchangeable table tops.

Essential characteristics of operating tables

It is important that the surface upon which the patient is placed is sympathetic to the contours of the patient. This is generally achieved by soft sorbo-rubber padding, which moulds to the patient to a certain degree. These pads are removable and easily cleaned. The sorbo padding will lift the patient above the metal table, for it is imperative that no part of the patient should come into contact with the metallic structure of the table. There should be easily accessible table controls, which may be motorized or hand operated. The table should be capable of two-way tilt, and breaking at its centre so that positions such as the lateral nephrectomy or jack-knife position may be used. The bottom half of the table must be easily removed so that various types of leg support and stirrups may be employed for gynaecological, urological, orthopaedic and pelvic surgery. With these leg supports it is important that joints are not overstressed and that undue pressure does not fall upon any point of the patient's lower limb. Tables for general surgery and urology should have a radiolucent section so that static X-ray films or an image intensifer may be used. A variety of arm rests, screen support bars, shoulder and pelvic supports should be available.

Safety and position on the operating table

In addition to the soft cushion support surfaces which line the hard surface of the operating table, it may be desirable to have built-in lumbar supports which are adjustable. Alternatively, partially filled intravenous fluid infusion bags can be placed under the patient's lumbar lordosis. When patient's arms are positioned either by their side, over their head or at right angles to the body, care must be taken that joints, ligaments and nerves are not overstressed. Various nerves are at risk from injury or pressure due to inappropriate positioning on the table. The brachial plexus may be stretched during arm movements, the ulnar nerve damaged at the elbow during pole insertion into the canvas sheet before transfer of a patient, and the lateral popliteal nerve may be damaged by pressure against a leg support bar. If the patient has osteoarthrosis this may be aggravated either by rough handling during transfer or excessive joint movement or distortion during the operative procedure. Should a patient have spinal or joint disorders it is perfectly reasonable to rehearse the position on the table with the patient prior to anaesthesia to make sure it is comfortable, e.g. cervical extension during thyroid surgery. Great care must be taken when moving patients on and off the operating table, and it should be ensured that no tubing attached to the patient is dislodged during transfer. Transfer of patients is best carried out using the Patslide, a tough plastic board, which acts as a bridge, on which the patient is carefully slid from trolley to table, or vice versa.

Operating table fixtures for specialist procedures

Orthopaedic surgery

There are a great variety of limb attachments to an operating table to enable circumferential access to a limb, manoeuvrability and also to allow the surgical team to use the image intensifier following fixation or reconstructive procedures.

Neurosurgical procedures

Access to the cranial cavity may be optimized by having the patient sitting up and an appropriate padded head support placed opposite the surgical field to keep the head in a comfortable and safe position.

SPECIAL EQUIPMENT IN THE OPERATING THEATRE

Diathermy

Principles and effects

Surgical diathermy involves the passage of a high-frequency alternating current (AC) through body tissue: where the current is locally concentrated (a high current density) heat is produced, resulting in temperatures up to 1000°C. Low-frequency AC such as mains electricity (50 Hz) causes stimulation of neuromuscular tissue. The severity of the 'electrocution' depends on the current (amps) and its pathway through the body. Five to ten milliamps can cause painful muscle contractions, while 80–100 mA passing through the heart will cause ventricular fibrillation. However, if the current frequency is increased there is a reduction in the neuromuscular response; at current frequencies above 50 000 Hz (50 kHz) the response disappears. Surgical diathermy involves current frequencies in the range 400 kHz to 10 MHz. Currents up to 500 mA may then be safely

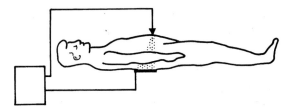

Fig. 14.1 Monopolar diathermy.

passed through the patient. Heat will be produced wherever the current is locally concentrated.

Monopolar and bipolar diathermy

Monopolar diathermy is the most common configuration (Fig. 14.1). High-frequency current from the diathermy generator (or 'machine') is delivered to an active electrode held by the surgeon. Current density is high where this electrode touches body tissue and a pronounced local heating effect occurs. Current then spreads out through the body and returns to the diathermy generator via the patient plate electrode (often incorrectly called the 'earth plate'). This plate should be in good contact with the patient over at least 70 cm² (preferably twice this or more). This ensures that the current density at the plate is so low as to cause minimal heating. Misapplication of the patient plate is by far the most common cause of inadvertent diathermy burns.

Bipolar diathermy (Fig. 14.2) avoids the need for a plate and uses considerably less power. The surgeon holds a pair of forceps connected to the diathermy generator. Diathermy current passes down one limb of the forceps through a small piece of tissue to be coagulated, and then back to the generator via the other limb of the forceps. This inherently safer system has not gained wide use for two main reasons:

1. It cannot be used for 'cutting' (see below): cutting involves a continuous arc (spark) between the active electrode and the tissue involved. In bipolar diathermy an arc could only be struck between the limbs of the forceps.

2. It will not work with the common surgical practice of holding bleeding vessels with ordinary surgical forceps and 'buzzing' them with the active diathermy electrode.

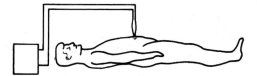

Fig. 14.2 Bipolar diathermy.

No current will pass through the tissue held by the surgical forceps. Bipolar current will only pass directly from one diathermy forceps limb to the other.

Cutting, coagulating and blend

Cutting diathermy involves the generator producing a continuous output, causing an arc to be struck between the active electrode and tissue. Temperatures up to 1000°C are produced. Cell water is instantly vapourized, causing tissue disruption with some coagulation of bleeding vessels. Coagulating diathermy involves a pulsed output. This results in desiccation and the sealing of blood vessels with the minimum of tissue disruption. Most diathermy generators have a 'blend' facility. This only functions when in cutting mode, and allows a combination of cutting and coagulation waveforms to increase the degree of haemostasis during cutting.

Earth referenced and isolated diathermy generators

Earth referenced generators. Older diathermy generators, many of which are still in everyday use, have valves and spark gaps to generate high-frequency current. These unsophisticated circuits produce a wide frequency range which includes frequencies above 1 MHz, and large earth leakage currents are unavoidable. The patient plate on these generators is earthed via a capacitor. The capacitor allows easy passage of high-frequency current such as in diathermy, but presents a large resistance to low-frequency currents such as mains electricity. (The patient is therefore not earthed for mains (50 Hz) current to reduce the risk of electrocution.)

As long as the patient plate is correctly applied, the patient is kept at earth (zero) potential for alternate sites such as electrocardiogram (ECG) electrodes or a drip stand accidentally touching the patient's skin. Unfortunately, if the patient plate is omitted, diathermy current will still flow (though a higher setting may be required) using the ECG electrodes or drip stand for the return pathway. An ECG electrode or drip stand presents skin contact of 1–5 cm², so a severe burn is inevitable.

Isolated generators. The more modern, often smaller, generators use transistors and 'solid-state' circuitry to produce the high-frequency current. Sophisticated electronics result in a much tighter frequency range (400–600 kHz) and a considerable reduction in earth leakage currents. Some of these solid-state generators (but by no means all) are designated 'isolated': the diathermy circuit is not earthed. This type of generator is inherently safer than an earth-referenced

machine. Diathermy current can only pass back to the generator via the patient plate; there is no pathway back via earth. If the plate is omitted no current will flow.

Safety

General safety. Whenever electrical equipment is to be used on patients it is vital that the equipment meets the required safety standards and is properly maintained. Everyone using the equipment should be properly trained in its use. At the very least, read the user's manual: all diathermy machines are supplied with one.

Responsibility. The thorny problem of exactly who has overall responsibility for surgical diathermy is often not considered until a diathermy disaster occurs. In many operating theatres the diathermy is set up by nurses, or ODPs, and the anaesthetist is often the only doctor present when the patient plate is applied. Few surgeons check the diathermy prior to use. The surgeon using the diathermy must realize his overall responsibility, and check the alarm wiring and patient plate before use.

Alarms. Monopolar diathermy depends on the patient plate for its safety. All diathermy machines in use will alarm when switched on if the plate is not connected to the machine (plate continuity alarm), but only a few possess any alarm system that will ensure the plate is attached to the patient. Safe practice demands rigid adherence to correct procedures: first the patient plate is connected to the patient; the return lead is connected to the plate; the diathermy machine is switched on and the plate continuity alarm will sound; only then is the return lead connected to the diathermy machine, thus silencing the continuity alarm. Never do this in the reverse order. At the end of every case all these connections must be undone and the diathermy machine switched off. If the continuity alarm fails to silence, change the patient plate and lead first, not the machine. Some modern diathermy generators (e.g. Eschmann and Valleylab) possess systems that monitor the patient–plate interface. These systems will be explained in the user's manual. Never disregard these alarms – check the patient plate contact carefully.

The patient plate. The most common cause of accidental diathermy burns is incorrect application of the patient plate. It may not be applied at all. More often there is a failure to follow guidelines. The plate should be sited close to the operation, while ensuring that diathermy current is moving away from ECG and other monitoring electrodes. The area under the plate should have a good blood supply to remove any heat generated: avoid bony prominences and scar tissue. All the plate must have good skin contact: shave hairy skin and ensure the plate is not kinked or crinkled. Do not let skin preparation fluids seep under the plate.

The patient. The second most common cause of diathermy burns is the patient touching earthed metal objects such as drip stands, uninsulated 'screens', and parts of the operating table. These small skin contacts can become alternative return pathways for the diathermy current, and the local current densities may be enough to cause a burn.

Sensible diathermy. The third most common cause of diathermy burns is careless technique. For safe diathermy:

- Check the dial settings before use.
- If a spirit-based skin preparation fluid is used, ensure it has all evaporated or been wiped away before starting or the diathermy may set it alight.
- Only the surgeon wielding the active electrode should activate the machine.
- Always replace the electrode in an insulated quiver after use.
- If diathermy performance is poor, carefully check the patient plate and lead rather than increase the dial settings.
- Beware of using diathermy on or inside the gut (intestinal gas contains hydrogen and methane and the result is often inflammable and explosive).
- Beware of using diathermy on appendages (salpinx or penis) or isolated tissue (testis). In these circumstances a high current density can persist beyond the operative site.

If a burn occurs. Diathermy burns are often poorly investigated and remain unexplained. Other skin lesions such as chemical burns from preparation solutions or pressure sores may masquerade as diathermy burns. Definite electrothermal burns are rarely due to a fault in the diathermy machine, but usually to lapses in procedure. The operating-theatre record for all patients subjected to diathermy should include the site of the patient plate, and when the plate and monitoring electrodes are removed the underlying skin should be inspected. If a possible burn is discovered at the end of a surgical case, the patient and all attached equipment should remain in the operating theatre and the electromedical safety officer summoned. If the alleged burn is discovered after the patient has left theatre, all personnel involved in the case should be contacted: the precise arrangement of equipment and patient plate should be determined. Then all electrical equipment used should be tested, including the patient plate lead. Diathermy burns are usually full thickness and will require excision. The patient should be informed of the misadventure.

Diathermy and pacemakers. There are two possible dangers:

- The high-frequency diathermy current may interact with pacemaker logic circuits to alter pacemaker function, resulting in serious arrhythmias, or even cardiac arrest.
- Diathermy close to the pacemaker box may result in current travelling down the pacemaker wire, causing a myocardial burn. The result will range from a rise in pacemaker threshold to cardiac arrest.

For safe use of diathermy with pacemakers:

- Contact a cardiologist. Information required includes the type of pacemaker, why and when it was put in, whether it is functioning properly, what is the patient's underlying rhythm (i.e. what happens if the pacemaker stops?).
- Avoid diathermy completely if possible. If not, consider bipolar diathermy.
- If monopolar diathermy has to be used, place the patient plate so that diathermy current flows away from the pacemaker system. Use only short bursts, and stop all diathermy if any arrhythmias occur.

Laparoscopic procedures. Sometimes the working space can be 'crowded', and inadvertent contact may be made between an instrument and the bowel. This may also occur when there is contact between the electrode and another metal instrument which is touching bowel. In a similar way, current can pass along an organ, which is resting against the gut, and pass out via the indifferent electrode. Insulation of instruments should be complete, and sparking between bowel wall and electrode avoided. An adequate view, CO_2 pneumoperitoneum, and using well-insulated instruments should be the aim. Careful technique, such as avoiding excessive use of the diathermy and making an effort to 'tent' structures into space before current is applied, is important. Lower voltage currents, or bipolar diathermy can be used to minimize spread of current and sparking.

Lasers

The laser is a device for producing a highly directional beam of coherent (monochromatic and in phase) electromagnetic radiation, which may or may not be visible, over a wide range of power outputs.

Laser is an acronym for Light Amplification by the Stimulated Emission of Radiation. This describes the principle of operation of a laser. Energy is pumped into the lasing medium to excite the atoms into a higher energy state to achieve a population inversion in which most of the atoms are in the excited state. A photon emitted as a result of an electron spontaneously falling from the excited to the ground state, stimulates more photons to be emitted and lasing action starts. After reflection back and forth many times from a pair of mirrors at opposite ends of the resonant optical cavity containing the lasing medium, the number of photons is amplified, i.e. the light intensity or power is increased. One of the mirrors is only partially reflecting and allows a small part of the laser light to emerge as the laser beam. The lasing medium is commonly gaseous (e.g. argon or carbon dioxide), but may be crystalline (e.g. neodymium, yttrium, aluminium, garnet (NdYAG)). It is the lasing medium which determines the wavelength emitted. It is mainly the wavelength of the laser which determines the degree of absorption in tissue. However, the surgical applications also depend on the power density, the duration of exposure being just sufficient to produce the effect required. The delivery systems are designed to allow the laser beam to be transported, aimed and focused onto the treatment site. For example, Argon and NdYAG lasers are transmitted down fibre optics to a slit lamp or into an endoscope. Carbon dioxide laser light is usually routed via a series of mirrors through an 'articulated arm', and thereafter through a micromanipulator attached to a microscope or colposcope.

Types of laser

1. Carbon dioxide infrared laser light has a wavelength of 10.6 μm. It is invisible and is rapidly absorbed by water in tissue and has very little penetration. It is therefore useful for vapourizing the surface of tissue, and water or wet drapes can be used as a safety barrier. There is a very small margin of damaged tissue and healing is rapid, with minimal scarring. Treatment is relatively pain free.

2. The NdYAG laser penetrates more deeply, to 3–5 mm. The wavelength is 1.06 μm and is in the invisible infrared light range. It is useful for coagulating larger tissue volumes and leaves behind an eschar of damaged tissue.

Both the above types require a visible guiding beam which is usually a red helium/neon beam.

3. Argon laser light is blue/green and hence absorbed by red pigment. The principal wavelengths are 0.49 and 0.51 μm. It is used principally in ophthalmology and dermatology.

Clinical applications

Gastrointestinal tract. The NdYAG laser is frequently used in the treatment of gastrointestinal problems. It can be employed for vapourizing and debulking recurrent or untreated advanced oesophageal carcinoma. Its use is predominantly in fairly short malignant strictures and may be superior to intubation. However, expanding covered metal stents may well prove an improved palliative alternative. Laser ablation is labour intensive and requires treatments every 6–8 weeks. This laser can be used for controlling gastrointestinal haemorrhage from the stomach, oesophagus and duodenum, destruction of small ampullary tumours in the duodenum and palliative resection of advanced rectal carcinomas. In the future, photosensitization may prove to be of value. The use of lasers in laparoscopic surgery is, perhaps, less frequent at present. There is a risk of carbon dioxide gas embolism.

Urology. The NdYAG laser can be used to treat low-grade, low-stage transitional cell lesions in the bladder and is suitable for treating outpatients under local anaesthetic. Here again, photosensitizing agents such as haematoporphorin (Hpd) may be used in conjunction with a laser light wavelength of 630 nm. The beam is directed at sensitized tissues which are then more easily destroyed.

Ophthalmology. The NdYAG laser can be used to destroy an opaque posterior capsule during extracapsular cataract extraction. The argon laser may be employed for trabeculoplasty, to decrease intraocular pressure in patients with open-angled glaucoma. Laser photocoagulation has become standard treatment for patients with various retinal diseases such as diabetic retinopathy, and as a prophylactic measure in patients at risk from retinal detachment. Most ophthalmic photocoagulators are argon lasers.

Otolaryngology. A carbon dioxide laser may be used for haemostasis, removal of benign tumours and premalignant conditions. The argon laser has been used in middle ear surgery.

Vascular surgery. Laser angioplasty (carbon dioxide, NdYAG and argon) has been used to vapourize atheromatous plaques. Only approximately 50% of patients benefit, and significant complications are reported (e.g. perforation of vessel wall).

Plastic surgery. Pulsed ruby lasers may be used to remove tattoos, and port wine stains selectively absorb the argon laser beam. The carbon dioxide laser may be employed to resect atretic bony plates in congenital bony coanal atresia.

Gynaecology. There are several uses in gynaecology. Perhaps the most frequent is the treatment with a carbon dioxide laser of cervical and vulval precancerous lesions which are identified by colposcopy.

Classification

Lasers are classified according to the degree of hazard.

Class 1 (low risk). These are of low power and are safe. The maximum permissible exposure (MPE) can not be exceeded.

Class 2 (low risk). These are of low power, emitting visible radiation. They have a maximum power level of 1 mW. Safety is normally afforded by natural aversion responses, e.g. the blink reflex.

Class 3a (low risk). These emit visible radiation, with an output of up to 5 mW. Eye protection is afforded by natural aversion. There may be a hazard if the beam is focused to a point, e.g. through an optical system.

Class 3b (medium risk). These emit in any part of the spectrum and have a maximum output of 0.5 W. Direct viewing may be dangerous.

Class 4 (high risk). These are high-power devices with output in any part of the spectrum. A diffusely reflected beam may be dangerous and there is also a potential fire hazard. Their use requires caution. Most medical lasers are in this class.

Hazards

The manufacturers are required to classify and label the product according to hazard level.

1. *Patient hazard*: inevitably, burning of normal tissue or perforation of a hollow viscus may occur with increasing depth of treatment (e.g. perforation of oesophagus) or damage to trachea or lungs during ear, nose and throat (ENT) procedures.

2. *Operator hazard*: usually the operator is not exposed to laser beams, but should accidental exposure occur it is frequently the eyes or skin that are damaged. Eye protection is important as some laser beams will penetrate and be focused on the retina. Also corneal burns or cataract formation have occurred with less penetrating beams.

Safety measures

1. There should be a laser protection advisor (LPA) to consult on the use of the instruments throughout the hospital and to draft local rules.

2. A laser safety officer (LSO) should be appointed from the staff of the appropriate department using each laser. This person may well be, for example, a senior nurse and will have custody of the laser key.

3. All persons using the laser should be adequately trained in its use and be fully cognizant with all safety precautions.

4. There should be a list of nominated users.

5. A laser controlled area (LCA) should be established around the laser while it is in use. There should be control of personnel allowed to enter that area and the entrance should be marked with an appropriate warning sign, usually incorporating a light which illuminates while the laser is functioning.

6. While in the laser controlled area adequate eye protection should be worn. This must be appropriate to the type of laser used. The laser should not be fired until it is aimed at a target, and usually there will be an audible signal during laser firing.

7. The laser should be labelled according to its classification. Lasers in classes 3a, 3b and 4 should be fitted with a key switch and the key should be kept by a specified person. The panels which constitute the side of the laser unit should have an interlocking device so that the laser cannot be used if the panels are damaged.

There are various safety features which are required by way of shutter devices and emergency shut-off switches. Foot-operated pedals should be shrouded to prevent accidental activation. Medical lasers require a visible low-power aiming beam which may be an attenuated beam of the main laser, should this be visible, or a separate class 1 or 2 laser, e.g. helium/neon. The laser must be regularly maintained and calibrated.

8. Environment: reflective surfaces should be avoided in the laser controlled area. However, matt-black surfaces are not necessary. Adequate ventilation must be provided and should include an extraction system to vent the fumes produced. These fumes are known as the 'laser plume'.

Attention should be paid to the avoidance of fire as class 4 lasers will cause dry material (e.g. drapes or swabs) to ignite. Thus, damp drapes will provide an effective stop (e.g. for a carbon dioxide laser beam).

Fibre optics in theatre

Flexible instruments

The advent of fibre optics has undoubtedly made an immense impact on the management of patients. There is little evidence, however, that the use of instruments which incorporate fibre optics necessarily reduces mortality. Hollow viscera may be carefully inspected, and both diagnostic and therapeutic procedures can be performed under clear vision. Fibre-optic instruments are

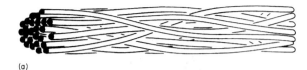

(a)

(b)

Fig. 14.3 (a) Non-coherent fibre bundles for light transmission. (b) Coherent fibre bundles for viewing. Reproduced from Ravenscroft & Swan (1984) by permission of Chapman & Hall.

integral to the development of minimal access surgery (e.g. ureteric or bile duct stone retrieval).

In the 1950s, Professor Harold Hopkins of Reading University, UK, developed the earlier work of John Logie Baird (the inventor of television) to further the design of fibre-optic bundles which not only could transmit a powerful light beam but also, when suitably arranged, deliver an accurate image to the viewer. In the 1960s, urological instruments were developed incorporating multiple flexible glass-fibre rods. Each fine fibre rod is constructed of high-quality optical glass and transmits the image (or light beam) by the process of total internal reflection. This principle allows light to travel around bends in the fibre. Each fibre is small (8–10 μm in diameter), and to achieve the principle of total internal reflection must be covered by a coating of glass of low refractive index to prevent light dispersion. Many such coated fibres are bound together in bundles which can bend. For light transmission, fibres may be arranged in a haphazard manner (non-coherent) but for clear-image transmission the fibres must be arranged in a coaxial way (coherent) (Fig. 14.3). The following are examples of currently available flexible endoscopes utilizing fibre-optic light bundles:

- Oblique (for endoscopic, retrograde, cholangio-pancreatography (ERCP) and end-viewing gastro-scopes
- Laryngoscope
- Bronchoscope
- Fibre-optic sigmoidoscope and colonoscope
- Cystoscope (pyeloscope)
- Choledochoscope
- Arterioscope.

Each instrument has similar design principles incorporating the following:

- Coherent fibre bundles for high-quality visual image transmission
- Non-coherent fibre-optic bundles for light transmission
- A lens system at a tip and near the eyepiece of the instrument
- A proximal control system to manoeuvre the tip of the instrument and also to control suction and air/water flow
- Channels for blowing air or carbon dioxide and water down the instrument, and for suction – the latter doubles as a biopsy channel
- A wire guide incorporated to control tip movement, which takes place in four directions, each usually allowing a deformity of greater than 180° movement
- A cladding, consisting of a flexible, jointed construction, covered by a tough outer vinyl sheath.

Figures 14.4 and 14.5 show the basic structure of a typical endoscope, and Figure 14.6 shows the tip of an instrument, illustrating the lenses for light transmission and viewing, a suction channel (which should be large for use in the presence of gastrointestinal haemorrhage)

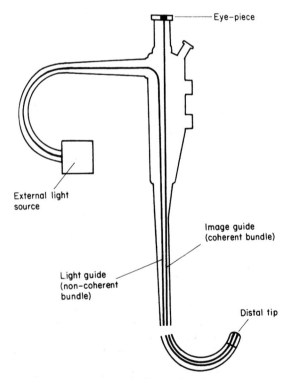

Fig. 14.4 Basic design of a fibre-optic endoscope. Reproduced from Ravenscroft & Swan (1984) by permission of Chapman & Hall.

and a small nipple directed over the lens, to enable the wash solution to clear the lens of debris.

Light sources should emit a powerful beam and the intensity is usually 150 W. Many light sources employ a halogen bulb, which needs to be fan cooled.

Rigid endoscopes

Optical systems in rigid endoscopes also employ the principle of total internal reflection, but there are several lens systems in addition. The objective lens systems are nearest the image and the relay lens systems nearer the eyepiece of the rigid instrument, through which the observer views a rectified and magnified image. A light cable (non-coherent fibres or liquid electrolyte solution) is employed and the fibres direct the light coaxially with the lens systems in the rigid tube. Some of the longer lenses are made of high-quality optical glass and act as a single large optical fibre for image transmission. Examples of rigid instruments are:

- Cystoscope, urethroscope, pyeloscope, ureteroscope
- Choledochoscope
- Laparoscopes.

The lenses at the far end of the instruments will vary to allow differing fields of view and minimize peripheral field distortion.

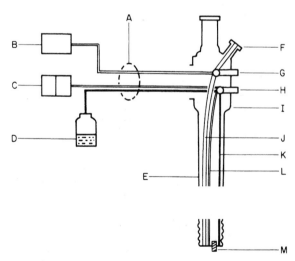

Fig. 14.5 Further details of the basic design of a fibre-optic endoscope. A, endoscopic 'umbilicus'; B, suction pump; C, air pump; D, water reservoir; E, endoscopic insertion tube; F, biopsy port; G, suction button; H, air/wash button; I, endoscope control head; J, combined suction biopsy channel; K, water channel; L, air channel; M, combined air/water port. Reproduced from Ravenscroft & Swan (1984) by permission of Chapman & Hall.

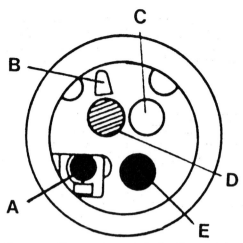

Fig. 14.6 The top of an end-viewing fibre-optic instrument. A, forceps raiser; B, wash jet; C, image guide; D, light guide; E, biopsy/suction channel. Reproduced from Ravenscroft & Swan (1984) by permission of Chapman & Hall.

Care of fibre-optic instruments

1. Instruments must be properly cleaned and disinfected before use. Debris may block channels and make suction and insufflation of air and liquid difficult. After use, the instruments should be cleaned internally by utilizing one of several automatic cleansing machines and externally with a suitable detergent solution. 'Q-tips' may be employed to clean lenses. Instruments should be soaked for at least 5–10 minutes between patients and a 2% gluteraldehyde solution is frequently used, though 70% alcohol and low-molecular-weight providone–iodine are alternatives.

2. Avoidance of damage to the instrument: in most district hospitals endoscopies are performed in dedicated units where the care is certainly superior. When a variety of people handle and clean the instrument, damage is more likely to occur. Forcible distortion, dropping and, particularly, crushing of the instruments (e.g. by patients' teeth) must be prevented. In the latter instance, biting may be prevented by insertion of a suitable mouth gag. Individual fibres may break and become opaque, appearing as black dots down the instrument.

Cryosurgery (syn. cryotherapy or cryocautery)

Cryosurgery is the freezing of tissue to destruction. Although cells are destroyed at −20°C they may recover at higher temperatures than this. After freezing, the destroyed tissue sloughs off and reveals a clean, granulating base. The treatment is relatively pain free and minimizes blood loss. The object is to destroy abnormal

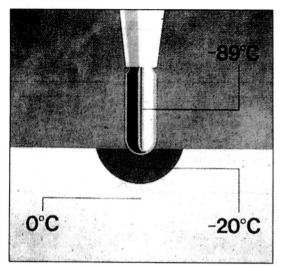

Fig. 14.7   An ice ball at the tip of a cryoprobe. Reproduced by permission of Eugene A. Felmar, Santa Monica Hospital Medical Center, USA.

tissue growth and preserve adjacent, healthy areas. This is achieved by the production of an ice ball at the tip of a cryoprobe (Fig. 14.7). To control the volume of tissue destroyed the size of the ice ball produced may be watched. The size of the lesion produced by cryosurgery depends on the temperature at the tip of the ice probe, the size of the tip and the number of freeze–thaw sequences. The size of the iceball will increase until the heat loss at the edge of the iceball is too small to permit further freezing of adjacent tissues. The size of an iceball and the extent of destruction can then be increased by a further freezing sequence. It is usually recommended to allow spread of the iceball 2–3 mm into healthy tissue to ensure adequate destruction of the diseased area. Inevitably, freezing a wart on the sole of the foot is less critical than reattaching a retina, and for all the tasks demanded of cryosurgery there are various probe tips available.

Principles of therapy

The Joule–Thompson principle is that when gas expands heat is absorbed from the surrounding matter. The simplest example of this is spraying ethyl chloride on skin, which subsequently freezes. With a cryoprobe, however, the liquid gas (usually nitrogen or carbon dioxide) is sprayed against the inside of a hollow metal probe. The gas then expands in the tip and freezes the tissue on contact (Fig. 14.8).

Cell injury with cryotherapy

1. *Immediate phase*: rupture of the cell membrane caused by formation of ice crystals in the cell (most effective with rapid freezing (e.g. greater than $5°C\ s^{-1}$)).

2. *Intracellular dehydration*: this will result in increased and toxic levels of intracellular electrolytes.

3. *Protein denaturation*: this occurs to the liporotein structure of the cell membrane, nucleus and mitochondria.

4. *Cellular hypometabolism*: this results in enzyme inhibition.

Later in the course of injury there is also a loss of blood supply which causes tissue necrosis, and the resultant slough, before separation, will protect the tissues deeper to the injury so that when the slough separates it will leave a clean ulcer.

As nerve endings are susceptible to cold injury, painful lesions can be rendered insensitive. Also, the treatment is not particularly painful to the patient, and local analgesia is usually unnecessary. Adjacent neurovascular structures are relatively safe as collagen and elastic tissue resist freezing. Thus, the advantages of cryotherapy are that it is a relatively pain-free and simple method of destroying tissue, usually leaving clean wounds, often with a reasonable scar.

The disadvantages of the technique are that frozen tissue cannot be analysed histologically, and thus this method of treatment is unsuitable for any lesion requir-

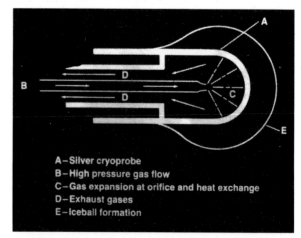

A–Silver cryoprobe
B–High pressure gas flow
C–Gas expansion at orifice and heat exchange
D–Exhaust gases
E–Iceball formation

Fig. 14.8   Cross-section of a cryoprobe tip, illustrating the Joule–Thompson principle. Reproduced by permission of Eugene A. Felmar, Santa Monica Hospital Medical Center, USA.

ing microscopic examination. It may sometimes be difficult to gauge the exact penetration in the depth of the tissues treated. Thus, its use may be limited in curative treatment of malignancy, but obviously is of value in palliation. There may also occasionally be some bleeding and discharge after the slough separates (e.g. in the cryosurgical treatment of haemorrhoids).

Clinical applications

Given the various shapes of probe tips, a reasonable variety of therapeutic applications is available. When placing the probe tip, freezing must occur through a wet contact to ensure proper thermal conductivity. Two to three freeze–thaw cycles may be applied with overlap of areas treated if necessary.

Examples. Examples of the clinical application of cryosurgery include the following:

- Proctology: haemorrhoids and warts
- Gynaecology: cervical erosions and warts
- Dermatology: warts, low-grade skin cancers, herpetic lesions
- ENT: pharyngeal tonsillar remnants, carcinoma of the trachea, hypophysectomy
- Ophthalmology: cataract extraction, glaucoma, detached retina
- Neurosurgery: Parkinson's disease and cerebral tumours.

Ultrasound in the operating theatre

Ultrasound probes are employed during surgery to identify tumour deposits and anatomical landmarks such as blood vessels. In this way, clear guidance may be obtained as to the resectability of tumours or the presence of clinically undetected metastatic deposits. Not only may hand-held ultrasound probes be employed at open operations, but small laparoscopic instruments are also used for staging and anatomical purposes. At open surgery, for example, small islet cell tumours of the pancreas may be located accurately. During laparoscopic cholecystectomy, a probe may not only identify structures, but also locate common bile duct stones.

Ultrasonic surgical aspirator

There are various ways in which the liver parenchyma may be dissected, with minimal blood loss. One of the most widely used, and efficient, is the CUSA (Cavitron UltraSonic Aspirator). The operating titanium tip of the instrument vibrates longitudinally at 23 000 oscillations per second (23 kHz). The way the instrument works is

that electromagnetic energy is converted to mechanical movements. An electrical coil wrapped around metal laminations sets up a magnetic field, thus causing the metal to vibrate. The fine hollow tip of the instrument disrupts solid parenchyma by its fine vibrations and the heat generated. When debris is shed, it is mixed with fluid jetting from the instrument and the mixture is sucked away. More solid and fibrous structures, such as ducts and blood vessels, are not disrupted, and may then be clipped or ligated. Not only may this instrument be useful for open, solid parenchymal dissection, but it may also be used during laparoscopic dissection of the gallbladder or mobilization of the colon.

X-rays in theatre

Preoperative work-up

Normally completed prior to surgery, the preoperative work-up should address details of diagnosis and, where appropriate, anatomical or physiological factors which could affect the conduct or outcome of surgery. It should go without saying that appropriately labelled radiographs must be available in theatre at the time of operation.

The preoperative chest X-ray is generally unhelpful in the absence of cardiothoracic symptoms and should be reserved for older patients or those with specific indications.

Perioperative procedures performed in X-ray

Example: needle localization for impalpable breast lesions. Coordination between the surgeon and radiologist is vital, and both need to understand what the other is doing. Premedication can make the procedure very difficult; for example, the patient may faint while sitting upright for mammography. It is imperative for the surgeon to inspect the postlocalization mammogram for the relationship between the wire and the suspected abnormality. Remember that mammograms are performed with the patient sitting and the breast subsequently compressed. The breast usually adopts a different configuration when supine. The excised specimen should be radiographed to confirm a satisfactory biopsy before the patient is wakened.

Example: retrograde pyelogram. This examination can be performed in theatre at the time of cystoscopy using fluoroscopy, or subsequently in the X-ray department where the radiologist has the advantage of being able to turn the patient and obtain films.

Intraoperative procedures

These fall into two categories. The first is purely diagnostic.

Example: on-table cholangiography. Use sufficiently dilute contrast medium to allow one to 'see through' the common bile duct on the film. The biliary tree should be adequately filled to show the main intrahepatic ducts as well as the common bile duct. Contrast medium is heavier than bile and tends to gravitate to dependent ducts. If the ampulla is patent, contrast medium flows into the duodenum, which is clearly recognizable by its mucosal pattern. Remember to put a 20° lateral tilt on the table to eliminate the overlap of contrast on the vertebral column.

Example: intraoperative angiography. Films may be exposed following a steady intra-arterial injection in theatre and adequate results obtained. Adverse reactions to modern contrast media while under general anaesthetic are very rare.

The second category consists of procedures where imaging is used to facilitate a therapeutic procedure. They require fluoroscopy and range from simple procedures such as reducing fractures to the sophisticated techniques of interventional uroradiology. Many of these techniques can be performed either in the operating room or in the X-ray department, but it is fair to say that facilities for fluoroscopy are usually better in X-ray while asepsis is better in theatre. X-ray machines are difficult to clean and a potential source of cross-infection. Specialist centres may have dedicated complex X-ray rooms which are organized in a fashion similar to operating theatres (or vice versa).

Equipment

This may be static or mobile, and it is the latter which is usually found in the operating theatre. Image intensification allows 'screening' without having to dark-adapt your eyes first! A mobile image intensifier for use in theatre will be mounted on a small 'C' arm. The table top must be radiolucent and there must be space under as well as over the table for the X-ray tube and the image intensifier. If films only are required, the table top will need a 'tunnel' to admit the X-ray cassette under the patient. Alternatively, the cassette may be draped in sterile towels. This would be necessary, for example, if intraoperative mesenteric angiography was to be performed on bowel lifted out of the abdomen at laparotomy. For a small field, the X-ray cassette can be placed on the image intensifier itself, and film obtained.

Some modern machines can produce dry silver images directly from the TV monitor.

Biplane screening is a luxury not usually available in the operating theatre. The mobile 'C' arm is, nevertheless, quite versatile and the effect of 'parallax' can help to judge 'depth'.

Mobile X-ray sets operate from designated 13 A sockets which are on a separate ring main from other essential equipment. Modern mobile sets use 'sparkless' switching and should not therefore ignite inflammable gases. It is desirable to keep the mobile X-ray machine in the operating suite.

X-rays and the law

X-rays (and scalpels) can be weapons of assault if not used with care and a prospect of benefit to the patient. Medical staff clinically directing examinations employing ionizing radiation are required to have obtained a certificate demonstrating that they have received some training in radiation protection. It is hoped that eventually this will be included in the undergraduate curriculum. Staff physically directing exposure must be either a radiologist, radiographer, or hold an approved qualification.

Equipment must be regularly serviced and calibrated, and 'local rules' applied. The radiation protection supervisor in the hospital is the point of contact if in any doubt.

Safety

Look after yourself, other staff in the theatre and the patient. Use the lead aprons. Remember that the patient 'scatters' the X-ray beam. The inverse square law applies, so staff should not be unnecessarily close. Be aware of the screening time and record it.

The abdomen of pregnant patients should be X-rayed only if absolutely necessary. The last menstrual period should be established before the patient is anaesthetized.

Sundry points

1. Maintain a close relationship with the department of radiology.

2. Discuss problems before surgery. Radiologists (generally) will want to know the outcome. Remember that this includes anatomical details as well as the diagnosis.

3. Give the radiographer as much notice as possible.

4. Dim the theatre lights when using fluoroscopy and use viewing boxes to view films.

5. Take an interest in imaging, as 'a picture is worth a thousand words'.

Microscopes in the operating theatre

Microcsopes have been introduced very gradually to the operating theatre; however, they have now become indispensable in a wide variety of surgical fields.

Advantages

The microscope offers an improved view of the surgical field, more precision, greater flexibility and less trauma to delicate tissues. It provides good stereoscopic appreciation of depth, through a narrow surgical approach, much smaller than the unaided surgeon's own interpupillary distance would allow.

Historical

Spectacles have been available for nearly 700 years and the compound microscope for about 300 years, but it was only 70 years ago that a microscope was used in theatre and only 30 years ago that its usage became more widespread.

A Swedish otolaryngologist, Nylen, introduced his monocular microscope in the surgical treatment of otosclerosis in 1921. A year later his chief, Professor Holmgren, used a binocular microscope for the same condition. In 1925, Hinselman used a microscope for colposcopy, but aside from this for three decades only otolaryngologists continued to use microscopes. In Chicago, Perritt used a microscope for ophthalmic surgery in 1950, Zeiss started to mass produce their MiI surgical microscope in 1953. Clinical applications then expanded: Jacobson in vascular surgery in 1960; Kurle in neurosurgery and Burke in plastic surgery in 1962.

Features of an operating microscope

Eyepieces. There is an adjustment for interpupillary distance and each eyepiece has a range of 5 dioptres.

Binocular tube. This can be straight or inclined.

Beam splitter. This is for connection of extra viewing tubes for observation and assistance. It also makes the use of still and video cameras possible as teaching aids.

Magnification system. Magnification is available as a Galilean system, variable in steps (e.g. ×6, ×10, ×25, ×40), or as a zoom system.

Objective lens. This affects working distance by changing lenses with variable focal lengths. For example:

$f = 150, 175, 200$	for opthalmology and plastic surgery
$f = 250$	for otology and vascular surgery
$f = 250$ or 300	for tubal surgery (gynaecology)
$f = 300$ or 400	for neurosurgery
$f = 400$	for laryngoscopy

Depth of field. The stereoscopic depth of field is less at higher magnification. It is best to focus at higher magnification first, then to reduce to working magnification so as to have the best focus at the centre of the depth of field.

Light. A powerful coaxial halogen light is incorporated in the body of the microscope. Oblique light is available for eye surgery.

Instruments used with microscopes

Each specialty has developed microsurgical instruments for its own needs. However, the following basic instruments are common to many specialities.

Spring-handled needle holder. Needle holders such as Borraquer or Castrovieso, ophthalmic, are available.

Spring-handled microscissors. These can be straight or curved. The straight are for cutting vessels and the curved for cutting tissue and thread.

Jewellers' or watchmakers' forceps. A wide variety of these are available.

Microsurgical clips. Scoville–Lewis microsurgical clips or fine Heifetzs neurosurgical clips can be used for vessel anastomosis.

Microelectrode. Monopolar or bipolar cautery is necessary.

Suture material. (a) Blood vessel anastomosis: 9.0 or 10.0 nylon on a 3–6 mm needle with a tapered end. (b) Nerve anastamosis: as above, but the needle needs a cutting point. (c) Fallopian tube work: no. 7.0 or 8.0 absorbable non-reactive suture with a 4 mm or 6 mm reverse cutting needle.

Sterilization. Sterile rubber cups or drapes are available to cover the controls.

Adjustment. Versatility in position needs several interlocking arms, counterbalanced vertical movement as well as a geared angled coupling between the microscope carriage arm and body. This will enable the microscope to swing from side to side while mounted in an oblique axis.

Mounting. This can be on a solid, well-balanced mobile floor stand, or a fixed ceiling mounting. Wall-mounted microscopes are also available.

Control of tremor

Counteracting surgical tremor is of vital importance. The key is that the instrument or the limb on which it is held must be firmly supported as close to the point of work as possible.

The future

The combination of the laser with a micromanipulator to the objective lens of the microscope will enhance the use of both instruments in the future.

ACKNOWLEDGEMENTS

I am deeply grateful for help with writing this chapter to: Mr John Bancroft for the diathermy section; Dr David Parker for the section on X-rays in theatre; Mr Derry Coakley for the section on microscopes; and to my wife for her help in the section on lasers. I should also like to thank Miss Sharon Langford for typing the manuscript.

REFERENCES

Brigdem R J 1988 Operating theatre technique, 5th edn. Churchill Livingstone, Edinburgh

Douglas D M (ed) 1972 Surgical departments in hospitals: the surgeons's view. Butterworth, London

Johnston I D A, Hunter A R (eds) 1984 The design and utilization of operating theatres. Edward Arnold, London

Diathermy

Dobbie A K 1974 Accidental lesions in the operating theatre. NAT News December

Earnshaw J J, Keene T K 1989 Gastric explosion: a cautionary tale. British Medical Journal 293: 93–94

Editorial 1979 Surgical diathermy is still not foolproof. British Medical Journal 12: 755–758

Pearce J A 1986 Electrosurgery. Chapman & Hall, London

Lasers

1982 General guidance on lasers in hospitals. Medical physics and bioengineering working group. Welsh Scientific Advisory Committee (WSAC)

1983 Guidance on the safe use of lasers in medical practice. HMSO, London

Murray A, Mitchell D C, Wood R F M 1992 Lasers in surgery – a review. British Journal of Surgery 79: 21–26

Fibre optics

Ravenscroft M M, Swan C M J 1984 Gastrointestinal endoscopy and related procedures – a handbook for nurses and assistants. Chapman & Hall, London

X-rays

Ionizing Radiation Regulations 1985, 1988

Mound R F Radiation protection in hospitals (Medical Sciences Series), Adam Hilger, Bristol

Microscopes

Taylor S 1977 Microscopy. Recent advances in surgery. Churchill Livingstone, Edinburgh, ch 8

15. Adjuncts to surgery

A. L. G. Peel

In health service economics an operating suite requires large capital and revenue budgets and this is favourably influenced by careful management of utilities. Good care of quality instruments ensures their long use, appropriate ordering and stocking means the shelf-life of equipment is not exceeded, wastage due to change in practice is reduced to a minimum and storage space is efficiently used. The avoidance of an unnecessarily wide range of equipment and materials allows better use of capital.

From the medicolegal aspect, the establishment of simple protocols aids efficient management within the theatre complex and helps to reduce errors, such as breakdowns in sterility or retention of swabs or instruments in patients.

A practical example of the rapidly changing scene in surgical practice is illustrated by orthopaedic surgery, where considerable expansion has occurred, particularly in prosthetic joint replacement, and in this field infection can result in very costly failure in terms of patient morbidity and financial implications to the health service.

In the attempt to 'abolish' infection to elective orthopaedic surgery the following factors are considered important.

Patient screening for occult infection

This is especially important with regard to urinary tract infection in females. Patients with positive carrier status should be rejected until the infection is corrected.

Theatre management

Orthopaedics theatre. A theatre should be dedicated to orthopaedics in which no dirty or contaminated orthopaedic surgery and no general surgery whatsoever is carried out.

Clean air enclosures. The routine use of clean air enclosures has resulted in the infection rate in prosthetic joint surgery (hip and knee) falling from 1.5% in the conventionally ventilated theatre to 0.6% (Lidwell et al 1982). Unidirectional air systems, especially with a downflow direction, reduces bacteria-carrying particles from 400–500 m^{-3} to 30–40 m^{-3}. Power tools produce additional problems since they produce an aerosol spray which effectively disseminates bacteria and viral particles.

Theatre gowns. Airborne bacterial dispersion can be further reduced by the use of appropriate fabric clothing. It is not widely appreciated that, in either conventional or unidirectional airflow theatres, the use of disposable fabric gowns alone in lieu of cotton gowns has not achieved a significant reduction in bacteria-carrying particles. The drawbacks to conventional sterile cotton clothing and gowns are not always appreciated and they fail to prevent:

- Bacteria being pumped by air through or out of the clothing into the room air
- Bacteria being drawn through the clothing by capillary action when wet and thence, by contact transfer, to the wound
- Contamination of the surgical team with the patient's fluids.

In addition to fabric gowns the following garments are currently available:

- Charnley total-body exhaust gowns
- Disposable, non-woven clothing
- Breathable, plastic membrane fabrics
- Close-woven polyester or polycotton fabrics.

Of these, the use of the first is well established in clean orthopaedic surgery; the second, Sonta (manufactured by Du Pont Ltd), has been shown to be effective; the third requires seals at the neck and trouser opening, with the result that the wearer soon becomes hot and uncomfortable. The fourth option is expensive, but represents a significant improvement over conventional garments. Although the cost is high, this must be equated with the significant costs of morbidity due to infection.

It has been stated that pharmaceutical manufacturing areas would be closed down if they used clothing currently worn in the majority of operating rooms (Whyte 1991).

Theatre technique

1. Ensure appropriate disinfection of hands in scrubbing up.
2. Closed gloving: apply your gloves over the cuffs of your theatre gown before pushing your hands through into the gloves. In this way your hands are not exposed and cannot be contaminated.
3. Double gloving: this is used routinely for joint replacement and when using power tools, wire saws, chisels, etc.
4. Antiobiotics: prophylactic antibiotics may be given when anaesthesia is induced. They may also be incorporated into the cement before fixing metal prostheses.
5. Dressings: occlusive dressings are applied to orthopaedic wounds, and are not disturbed until the wound is healed. Transparent dressings allow for the inspection of wounds.

INSTRUMENTS

Surgeons and instrument makers have combined to produce a wide range of instruments. Some, such as certain scissors, forceps and retractors, may be used in several different fields of surgery. Others are more specific; for instance, those used in anal surgery (Park's anal retractor and Lockhart–Mummery fistula probes). You should consider your requirements for instruments and appreciate the range and potential of different instruments. One advantage of a training rotation scheme is that it allows experience to be gained in a number of surgical disciplines and permits you to observe the use of instruments in different surgical disciplines. This knowledge can be reapplied to particular problems in whatever field you subsequently work.

Instruments are a sound investment and, whenever possible, use those of the highest quality. Of equal importance is the investment in maintenance care, not forgetting the basics of mechanical and chemical cleansing, particularly of hinge joints, adjustment of misalignment and regular sharpening of cutting instruments. In this context you have a very important role in avoiding damage to the instruments by not dropping them or using them inappropriately.

Sterilization

The majority of instruments are autoclaved (moist heat under pressure for a prescribed time) and this process needs constant monitoring, with care in the packing of the autoclave and verification that the temperature, pressure and time are correct. Where standard autoclaving is impracticable and may cause damage, alternatives include:

1. Formaldehyde autoclaving.
2. Ethylene oxide gas sterilization.
3. Prolonged immersion in 2% glutaraldehyde (avoid skin contact and ensure there is adequate ventilation). Replacements are currently being researched and an expensive alternative, Steris (Rimmer Bros.), is under evaluation.
4. γ-Irradiation is widely used commercially for nonmetallic utilities.

Instrument sets

It is of considerable advantage to have the instruments required for a particular surgical procedure packed and sterilized in a single set. Within this set, as far as possible, each type of instrument should be in multiples of five. Thus each separate design or size of artery forceps may be grouped in separate fives or tens, whereas scissors of differing size and design are grouped in fives, etc. A standardized typed list of contents and numbers for each particular tray is routinely retained in the sterilized set. This reduces the number of single packed instruments that need to be opened and, more importantly, simplifies the instrument count at the beginning and end of each procedure.

A close liaison between the Central Sterile Supply Department (CSSD) and theatre management is vital in the provision of adequate supplies of trays to meet the demand of a full schedule of operating lists, particularly when many minor procedures with a quick turnover are carried out.

LIGATURES, SUTURES, STAPLES AND CLIPS

When selecting a ligature or suture, consider several factors with regard to the material itself:

- Whether the material is to be absorbed
- The tensile strength
- The thickness
- The handling and knotting properties
- The intensity of the body's inflammatory reaction to the material.

A fine, absorbable suture is frequently selected for anastomoses in the gastrointestinal tract, and cat gut is being replaced by the more reliable and less reactive synthetic monofilament polydioxanone (PDS or PDS II) or polyglactin 910 (coated Vicryl – the coating comprising glycolide, lactide and calcium stearate). When longer-lasting tensile strength is required, polymers, such as polyamide (Nylon), polypropylene (Prolene) or polytetrafluoroethylene (PTFE, Goretex) have proved to be of considerable value in, for example, abdominal wound closure and vascular anastomoses.

Metal clips are valuable alternatives to ligatures where access is difficult. They were originally made of stainless steel and were frequently used to demarcate an area for subsequent radiotherapy, or to assess by radiology the response of a neoplasm to treatment by radiotherapy or chemotherapy. They may produce a stellate shadow, obscuring detail in computed tomography (CT) scans, so they are now made from titanium.

The majority of sutures are now atraumatic, which facilitates passage through the tissues and also relieves the scrub nurse of the arduous and tedious job of threading needles. The older practice of adding a half-hitch at the needle eye to prevent unthreading of the suture is especially traumatic to tissues. Having considered the suture material, make your choice of needle according to:

1. *Shape*: straight or curved and, if the latter, decide the extent of the circle.
2. *Tip*: a round-bodied needle is suitable for suturing viscera or fascia, cutting for skin suture, or a taper cut for the penetration of a considerable thickness of tissue or for tissues of different density (e.g. the approximation of intestine and skin at the time of the creation of an ileostomy). Blunt taper pointed needles, attached to polypropylene, polydioxanone or polyglactin, reduce the risk of finger stick injuries and thus the risk of viral transmission.
3. *Size and thickness*: a knowledge of the requirement is important – a slim-blade needle is suitable for subcuticular sutures, but delicate needles may break when suturing more fibrous tissue (e.g. breast).

Steristrips and staples may be used in skin closure. Staples were originally made of stainless steel wire but are now made from titanium wire and so do not interfere with CT scanning. Staples are relatively expensive. Subcuticular sutures may be valuable, especially if the wound will be subsequently encased in an orthopaedic splint. The introduction of a variety of staples for use in visceral tissues has also involved a number of changes in practice. You need to be aware of the range, the indications and contraindications for each type of instrument, including staple size, and the differences in design

between manufacturers. Remember that surgical technique may need to be adapted as compared with the standard suture procedure. However, staple techniques are not as versatile as suturing and, as a trainee, you should concentrate on mastering the traditional method of uniting tissues. I believe staples should be used in preference to sutures only when:

1. The procedure can be carried out with greater immediate safety (e.g. avoiding anastomotic leak), and with no significant increase in later postoperative complications such as stenosis.
2. The procedure can be performed more quickly but with equal or greater safety and you consider that the time factor is of clinical importance (e.g. in the elderly patient undergoing a major procedure).

SWABS AND PACKS

All cotton or fabric swabs and packs used during surgery must have radio-opaque marking. The size must be appropriate to the procedure and the purpose must be defined, e.g. small 'patty' swabs for neurosurgical procedures, narrow swabs for tonsillar surgery, large packs or gauze rolls for keeping abdominal viscera out of the operative field, for limiting gross contamination or for haemostatic control of raw surfaces.

Although haemostasis is usually achieved by electro-coagulation, ligation, undersewing or the use of clips, it is invaluable in certain situations to use certain manufactured haemostatic agents in the presence of a slow ooze. There is a choice between Surgicel, Oxycel or Sterispon, and again experience of the particular properties of each of the above is important. The application of Surgicel to the gallbladder bed with overlying pressure from a warm, moist swab controls a slow persistent ooze. When the overlying swab is removed, the haemostatic agent remains undisturbed. In neurosurgery the more delicate Sterispon may be preferred.

DISPOSABLE ACCESSORIES

Included in this category are accessories that remain on the surface of the body, skin or epithelial lining, or those that attain access to the interior of the body, usually for a limited period. Remember that they cause tissue irritation and create a break in the body's defence system. Disposable accessories include:

1. Vascular cannulae and catheters for the administration of intravenous fluids and drugs, central venous and arterial access lines for use in pressure monitoring or biochemical analysis, and parenteral feeding catheters;

adjuncts to arterial surgery, such as Fogarty embolectomy catheters.

2. Urological catheters and stents.

3. Oesophageal stents for strictures; nasogastric and the less commonly used intestinal decompression tubes; fine-bore enteral feeding tubes and hepato–biliary–pancreatic tubes and stents.

4. Stoma appliances.

5. Neurological valved shunts.

6. Drains are most frequently manufactured from polyvinyl chloride. They are designed to transmit fluid from the operative area, or a body cavity or compartment to the exterior, either as an open system, which is liable to bacterial contamination, or a closed system with a reduced pressure within the container, which not only encourages effective drainage but also reduces contamination (see Ch. 27).

ENDOSCOPES

The development of endoscopes and their application in diagnosis and therapy continues. Instruments can be passed in the upper and lower respiratory tracts, the upper and lower alimentary tracts (including the biliary tree and pancreas), the upper and lower urinary tracts, the female genital tract, and into joints, the peritoneal cavity and along blood vessels. Design modifications have resulted in a wide range of instruments with considerable therapeutic capabilities, often with the use of specialized accessories. They must be stored carefully, and maintained, cleaned, decontaminated and disinfected expertly, otherwise there is a risk of transmitting infection, particularly viral infection such as hepatitis B and C and human immunodeficiency virus (HIV).

Flexible instruments are usually disinfected by immersing them in a buffered 2% solution of gluteraldehyde for 20 minutes. Modern cystoscopes, for instance, may now be autoclaved.

Do not neglect, however, to master the use of simple instruments, such as a proctoscope and anal retractor, such as Park's or Eisenheimer's retractors for anorectal endoscopy.

IMPLANT MATERIALS

Prosthetic surgery continues to expand, and perhaps the greatest impact has been in orthopaedic surgery where successful joint replacement is well established in the hip, knee and interphalangeal joints and to a more limited extent in the shoulder and elbow joints. Prosthetic implants are also used widely in general, vascular, cardiac, urological, plastic and other branches of surgery, and there is wide variation in the materials used.

Basic considerations and principles apply:

1. Ease and reliability of manufacture and cost.

2. Appropriate tensile strength and durability, e.g. some joint replacements need revision after a number of years due to wear and tear, causing fragmentation.

3. Reaction between prosthetic materials themselves of the body tissues, e.g. the metal and plastic components of certain artificial hip replacements or between the joint prosthesis, cement and the bone.

4. Platelet aggregation and plasma protein precipitation that occur around intravascular prostheses.

5. The degree of incorporation into the body. Both metallic and silicone implants are surrounded by a collagen capsule but PTFE (Goretex) allows the ingrowth of fibroblasts.

Implant materials in orthopaedic surgery

1. Surgical-grade stainless steel is used for joint replacement bearing surfaces, plates, screws and wires.

2. Alloys, including Vitallium, are also used in joint replacement surfaces, wires and, less frequently now owing to the preference for compression steel plating for internal fixation, in plates.

3. High-density polyethylene (ultra-high molecular weight) is used for joint replacement bearing surfaces to articulate with steel or Vitallium.

4. Silicone is used for hinge-type joint replacement, but not in bearing surfaces where debris produces a synovitis. It has been used very successfully in metacarpophalangeal and proximal interphalangeal joints.

5. Dacron and PTFE are materials that can be used under tension (e.g. synthetic ligament repair). Carbon fibre has been abandoned due to fragmentation and foreign body reaction.

The risk of infection

This is one of the most serious complications of prosthetic surgery, and the following risk factors must be considered:

- Immune compromised host
- Active infection present elsewhere in the host or in contacts
- Positive carrier state in patient or staff
- Cross-infection in hospital
- Failure of sterilization and/or packaging
- Inadequate air ventilation in the operating theatre and ineffectual operating theatre clothing
- Poor operative technique with contamination, poor haemostasis or ischaemic tissue
- Inadequate antimicrobial prophylaxis

The time-scale of presentation is of significance, and this is one of the areas where late infection up to a year or more after surgery may occur, particularly with the deep insertion of a prosthesis. The implant itself can be of significance: whereas a smooth surface is bacteriostatic and non-wettable, a textured surface allows the entrapment of blood, serum, particles and bacteria in the crevices.

In deep infection occurring late around implants (e.g. hip) the bacteria may produce changes: *Staphylococcus aureus* produces a thickening of the capsule and *Staphylococcus epidermidis* produces a polysaccharide slime. The prosthesis becomes loose, causes pain and may need removal.

Do not use an implant unless there is no natural alternative. Thus, in vascular surgery use vein grafts for lower limb arterial bypass surgery such as infrainguinal bypass and especially for below-knee femoropopliteal bypass. Synthetic materials, Dacron (collagen-coated knitted Dacron) or Goretex (PTFE) may be used, particularly where large vessels need to be bypassed or replaced.

Tissue response to foreign material

Tissue reaction varies according to the material and the roughness of the surface. Marked inflammatory response, with microabscess formation, occurs around a buried silk or linen knot. By comparison, minimal response occurs around polypropylene, with not only a reduced likelihood of bacterial infection but also increased tensile strength, depending on the material used, and a lack of surrounding tissue inflammatory infiltrate.

Silicone forms a capsule. Fibroblasts orientate themselves to the surface of the foreign material and the collagen is formed in mirror image to the specific surface. As collagen matures it contracts. Fibroblasts cease to secrete collagen when they are in contact with other fibroblasts, but not when in contact with other cells. Thus over a smooth surface sheets of collagen are produced with increased contractile force of the capsule. Gradually, fibroblastic activity on the free surface subsides, collagen deposition is completed and moulding takes place, producing a mature capsule at approximately 3 months after surgery. Collagen production against the smooth inner capsular surface continues because the fibroblasts are not in contact with each other and, as a result, the cavity diameter decreases and the contractile force increases. By comparison, roughened surfaces allow fibroblasts to conform to the crevices; the fibres of collagen are then orientated at random with counteracting contractile forces and the fibroblasts lie in different planes and directions, allowing a greater chance of contact with each other, thus reducing the collagen deposition and resulting in a thinner capsule. Silicone particles are found in phagocytes in the capsule wall adjacent to lymphatic vessels, in the outer layer of capsules, and may reach the lumen of lymphatic vessels since they are found in regional lymph nodes.

Metal-on-metal joint replacement produces small particulate debris which is incorporated into the synovium, producing foreign-body giant cells.

Acrylic cement (polymethylmethacrylate), used in the fixation of prostheses, becomes encapsulated by fibrous tissue, the inner layer of which is sometimes hyaline and acellular and sometimes contains histiocytes and multinucleate giant cells. There is no evidence for malignant transformation or chronic inflammatory reaction with sinus formation (Charnley 1970). Revisional surgery of the cemented prosthesis is difficult. Alternatives under trial are based on isoelastic or mesh coating of the prosthesis to allow fibrous tissue to grow in.

The controversy over the safety of silicone mammary prostheses

In 1992 in the USA a moratorium was placed on the use of silicone gel breast implants because of the possible association with connective tissue disorders. In the UK, an independent expert advisory group reported to the Department of Health in 1993 that there was no evidence of an increased risk in implanted patients (Park et al 1993). In 1994, the Medical Devices Directory supported the Chief Medical Officer in stating that there was no evidence for a change in policy:

1. Selective reporting and bias was found in some articles.
2. There was confusion with the effects of the polyurethane coating of implants.
3. Difficulty was encountered in interpreting the psychological effects of breast implants.
4. Since the incidence of connective tissue disorders in the population is low and the latent period is long, large numbers and prolonged follow-up are needed.
5. Silicone, like any foreign body, may initiate an antibody, cell-mediated and inflammatory response, but this is not in itself suggestive of an adverse effect on the immune system.

Thus, there is currently no evidence that breast-implanted patients have an enhanced risk of developing either autoimmune connective tissue disease or mammary carcinoma. Silicone implants do, however, reduce the value of mammography. Newer tryglyceridefilled prostheses may be preferred; the shell is still silicone but mammography is satisfactory.

TISSUE GLUES

Research into new methods of surgical tissue repair has yielded the prospect of using tissue glues. One such method is fibrin adhesion, based on the conversion of fibrinogen into fibrin on a tissue surface by the action of thrombin. The fibrin is then cross-linked by factor XIIIA to create a firm stable fibrin network with good adhesive properties.

The addition of aprotinin prevents premature dissolution of the fibrin clot by plasmin. In the presence of heavy bleeding the fibrin glue tends to be washed away before sufficient polymerization of the fibrin has occurred. The use of collagen mesh sheet with fibrin glue dispersed over the surface has been of considerable practical value. Note that the sheet should be kept in contact with the surface by gentle pressure for 3–5 minutes.

The indications are for tissue adhesion, haemostasis and suture support. In general and abdominal surgery it may be used in patients where there has been trauma or surgical resection of either the liver, spleen or pancreas, after cholecystectomy to aid haemostasis and healing of the gallbladder bed, to support difficult anastomoses such as pancreaticojejunostomy after Whipple's operation (pancreaticoduodenectomy) and anastomoses of the small and large bowel.

In the specialities it has been particularly useful in neurosurgery for the repair of dural tears, thus sealing leakage of cerebrospinal fluid, and in securing haemostasis when there is bleeding from the cerebral surface. It is also useful in peripheral neural anastomoses.

In orthopaedic and trauma surgery it is useful for reattachment of osteochondral fragments, in acetabuloplasty when using cement-free hip joint prostheses and in certain tendon and ligament repairs.

In cardiovascular surgery it has also proved useful for sealing anastomotic suture lines and in the placement of patches, in bypass surgery, valve replacement surgery and prosthetic implantation. It has been used with success in sealing accidental injury to the thoracic duct, biliary and pancreatic fistula. When used to seal air leaks in pulmonary surgery, fibrin glue is combined with a collagen mesh sheet.

Fibrin glue is also applicable in ophthalmic surgery, in cataract operations and in ear, nose and throat surgery, again for sealing cerebrospinal fluid leaks, and in plastic operations on the tympanic membrane. It is undergoing assessment in urology for suture support and also for haemostasis, particularly after transurethral resection of the prostate. In plastic surgery it has found considerable application in securing skin grafts.

There has been concern that the use of human fibrinogen and factor XIII might allow the transmission of viral agents such as hepatitis B, hepatitis C or HIV. Commercial inactiviation of a virus is achieved by pasteurization with purification of the proteins and then heating the solution for 10 hours at 60°C. Laboratory studies have demonstrated that this process not only inactivates the hepatitis B and HIV viruses, but also herpes simplex virus and cytomegalovirus. Particular care is taken to use human fibrinogen from hepatitis B antigen negative, anti-HIV-negative and anti-hepatitis-C-negative plasma of healthy donors.

Marked arterial or venous bleeding renders the system ineffective. Hypersensitivity reactions have been described. The process is under evaluation in the UK.

ACKNOWLEDGEMENTS

My gratitude to Sister J. Knott, RCN, for extracting current data relating to usage and costs, and to Mr John Stothard, FRCS, for his help with regard to orthopaedic surgery.

REFERENCES

Charnley J 1970 Acrylic cement in orthopaedic surgery. E and S Livingstone, Edinburgh
Lidwell O H, Lowbury E J L, Whyte W et al 1982 Effect of ultraclean air in operating rooms in deep sepsis in the joint after total hip or knee replacement: a randomised study. British Medical Journal 285: 10–14
Park A J, Black R J, Watson A C H 1993. Silicone gel breast implants, breast cancer and connective tissue disorder. British Journal of Surgery 80: 1097–1100
Whyte W 1991 Operating theatre clothing: a review. Surgical Infection 3: 14–17

16. Asepsis and antisepsis

A. M. Emmerson

THEATRE CLOTHING

Gowns

When conventional cotton theatre wear is used in a theatre in which the air is ventilated in a conventional way, i.e. high-level input, the airborne counts depend on the number of people present and their degree of activity. Normal cotton clothing does little to prevent the passage of bacteria, especially when present on large skin scales, as the diameter of the holes at the interstices of the cloth is normally greater than 80 μm. Materials are available which reduce the dispersion of skin scales and bacteria, but these may be restrictive in nature. A surgeon who is comfortably dressed in light, cool theatre clothing is less likely to make an error of judgement than one who is perspiring in a heavy, airless gown. A compromise has to be reached and clothing made from disposable non-woven fabric, e.g. Sontara (Fabric 450) is suitable. However, these disposable materials are expensive, especially since the whole team has to wear them to reap the benefit. Special attention has to be made to the design of the clothing so that bacteria are not discharged or 'pumped out' at the neck or at the ankles. Breathable membrane fabrics are available, e.g. Goretex, which consists of a fabric in which a layer of polytetrafluoroethylene (PTFE) is laminated to one or two layers of a polyester; other materials such as tightly woven washable polycottons are also effective, but require careful laundering. The most effective reduction of airborne bacteria is obtained by using the Charnley exhaust gown. However, to obtain maximum benefit this protective barrier has to be used in conjunction with a unidirectional high-efficiency particulate air (filter) air flow system and, owing to its restrictive nature, this is rarely used by general surgeons.

In a conventional operating theatre, air is prefiltered and delivered to the theatre in a turbulent fashion but is free of known pathogens such as *Staphylococcus aureus* and *Clostridium perfringens*. Almost all the airborne bacteria present in theatres are derived from people in the room; airborne contamination can be decreased by restricting the entry of non-essential personnel. Once the surgical operation has commenced, movements (excessive activity) should be controlled. This kind of discipline is still required, even when ultraclean air systems are used. Such systems are expensive to install in existing theatres and may only be of significant value in clean implant surgery (Lidwell et al 1982). However, it must be borne in mind that low infection rates can also be achieved by good surgical technique, theatre discipline, purpose-designed occlusive clothing (Whyte et al 1990) and the propitious use of single-dose prophylactic antibiotics.

Masks

Face masks are worn for many and varied procedures, but their use is seriously questioned. Few bacteria are dispersed from the mouth during normal breathing and quiet conversation, and it is argued that for general abdominal operations masks are not required. They are certainly not required for members of staff not directly assisting in the operating theatre. If it is decided that masks should be worn, e.g. in implant surgery, then a fresh mask should be worn for each operation and discarded with care at the end of each operation. Re-use or manipulation of the mask during use will simply contaminate the outside of the mask and the hands with skin commensals, which include staphylococci.

An efficient mask must be capable of arresting low-momentum droplets which contaminate the front of the operator's gown, gloves and subsequently the wound. Paper masks have no place in operating theatres as they become wet within a few minutes and lose their barrier qualities. As with clothing, the frequency of wet 'strike-through' correlates well with the length of operation and the degree of wetness. Disposable masks made of synthetic fibres are tolerable and contain filters made of polyester (e.g. Bard Vigilon) or polypropylene (e.g. Filtron). Surgical anti-fog masks with flexible nosebands are available which follow facial contours and yet retain a high efficiency of filtration.

Eye protection

Masks and protective eyewear or face shields should be worn during procedures that are likely to generate droplets of blood or other body fluids, to prevent exposure of mucous membranes of the mouth, nose and eyes. A variety of anti-fog goggles, wraparound spectacles and face shields are now available which are efficient, easy to wear and pleasant in appearance. They are lightweight, adjustable and do not obstruct vision. An educational programme is necessary to introduce surgeons to these new barriers.

Hair/beard cover

All members of staff entering the theatre area should wear their hair in a neat style. Long hair should be tied back in such a way that when the head is bent forward hair does not fall forward, occlude vision or, at worst, fall into a surgical wound. Hair must be completely covered by a close-fitting cap made of synthetic material. Once the head cover is in place it must not be adjusted or manipulated as this facilitates the dispersal of many bacteria-carrying particles. Beards should be fully covered by a mask and a hood of the balaclava type which is tied securely at the neck.

Footwear

There is little evidence to show that the floor plays a significant role in the spread of infection in hospital, and expensive efforts to minimize bacterial contamination of feet are unnecessary. Staff should wear clean, comfortable, antislip and antistatic shoes. If there is a real risk of fluid spillage, e.g. in genitourinary surgery, then ankle-length antistatic boots should be worn. These should be cleaned, when required, with warm soapy water and stored dry. A variety of styles of shoes and clogs are available which allows choice with style. They should fit snugly and must not be allowed to produce a bellows effect. If sufficient shoes or half-wellingtons are not available then freshly laundered socks should be provided as hygienic inserts.

Gloves

It is now commonplace for all surgeons to wear gloves in order to reduce the risk of contaminating operation wounds. Nowadays, it is equally important to wear gloves in order to prevent the transmission of blood-borne viruses (e.g. hepatitis B (HBV) and human immunodeficiency virus (HIV)) from surgeon to patient and patient to surgeon. However, it is a sobering thought that between 20% and 30% of gloves develop holes during surgery through which bacteria can escape. Often, the wearer of the glove is unaware of the fact that the glove has been punctured. Worse still, many gloves have been found to have pre-existing holes prior to use as a result of poor manufacture and inadequate quality-control procedures.

Some surgeons have attempted double gloving; additional protection is achieved, but at the expense of possible discomfort, reduced sensitivity and dexterity. Others have tried covering the first pair of gloves with glutaraldehyde cream and then covering the cream with a second pair of gloves. Unfortunately, even this sandwich technique will not stop a determined assistant from puncturing the latex gloves. It is important to purchase sterilized (by irradiation) single-use, surgical rubber gloves from a reputable source and bearing the kite mark (BS 4005: 1984).

Surgical gloves made from natural rubber (latex) are increasingly reported to cause cutaneous and systemic hypersensitivity reactions. Non-latex gloves without glove powder are available.

Protective clothing

There are occasions when operations have to be performed on patients known to be carriers of, or infected with, notifiable diseases. Under these circumstances, and where it is known that heavy aerial dispersal of microorganisms is inevitable and blood soak through is commonplace, protective clothing is required. Some gowns are made entirely of impermeable materials (double-layered polyester fabric or laminated plastic films), while others have these materials in key areas such as in the front and on the sleeves. Surgical staff may get uncomfortably hot in gowns made only of these materials unless the room temperature is lowered or ventilation turnover is increased. If these costly fabrics are not available then disposable long-sleeve gowns can be used together with disposable plastic aprons. All skin must be covered, including the face, eyes and hair.

PREPARATION OF THE SURGEON

In Sweden it is considered unethical to perform high-risk surgery without preoperative whole-body disinfection with chlorhexidine. The microbiologist who made this statement was in fact referring to the preoperative preparation of the patient. What about the preoperative preparation of the surgeon? Surgeons have to be physically fit to sustain the rigours of surgical activities. Some operations last hours and require intense concentration and intricate surgery, while others are short, physical and crude. Theatres are not the place for the faint hearted and the below-par surgeon. Surgeons should not operate when they are suffering from a skin infection or are in the prodromal period of a viral infection. Most theatre-acquired infections are of endogenous origin, but a surgeon who is disseminating staphylococci from active skin lesions is a menace.

Surgeons should begin the day with socially clean hands; they should scrub dirt from the nails and hands with a nail-brush before entering the operating department in the morning.

Showering

The Swedish experience points to the benefits obtained by patients using 4% chlorhexidine gluconate soap solution (Hibiscrub) during two preoperative whole-body showers. These results have been challenged by a European Working Party on the Control of Hospital Infection, but there is sufficient evidence to show that showering is preferable to bathing in terms of removal of skin bacteria, and chlorhexidine has a greater effect than non-medicated soap. It would seem reasonable that surgeons could safely shower between long operations or between sessions using Hibiscrub followed by non-perfumed body oils to all accessible skin. The benefits of a refreshing top-to-toe shower outweigh any theoretical disadvantages.

Scrubbing up

Repeated hand disinfection with scrubbing brushes between operations results in skin abrasions and result in more bacteria being brought to the surface. A surgeon's hands should be socially clean before he or she enters the operating theatre. If scrubbing brushes are used at all they should be sterile, single-use and made of polypropylene. Wooden brushes with bristles should not be used. An initial scrub of 3–5 minutes at the beginning of an operating list is all that is required; modern-day skin antiseptics act rapidly and often show a cumulative effect. Repeated scrubbing is counterproductive, but the term 'scrubbing up' is unlikely to disappear from surgical practice; 'washing up' does not have the same impact or mystique! Hexachlorophane (pHisoHex) is effective against Gram-positive bacteria only and has slow action, but has a cumulative effect, even under rubber gloves. Povidone–iodine (Betadine/Disadine) acts more rapidly than hexachlorophane and has a broader spectrum but does not have a prolonged effect.

Chlorhexidine gluconate 4% w/v (Hibiscrub) is rapidly active, broad spectrum and persists. It is easy to use but requires constant running water to wash off the detergent-like effect. Patients allergic to chlorhexidine can use either povidone–iodine or hexachlorophane.

Hands should be thoroughly dried using single-use sterile towels. Hot-air drying machines are not recommended for this purpose. Disinfection of the surgeon's hands is important because gloves, which often develop small holes during use, are an imperfect barrier against contamination of operation wounds.

PREPARATION OF THE PATIENT

The longer the patient stays in hospital before an operation, the greater is the likelihood of a subsequent wound infection (Cruse & Foord 1980). The hospital stay before the operation should be as short as possible; in particular, tests and therapeutic measures that may prolong the preoperative stay beyond 1 day should be performed in the outpatient department where possible. Cultures from postoperative wound infections often suggest that organisms are transferred from other areas of the patient to the operative site (endogenous transfer), despite the use of antiseptics. A preoperative shower using hexachlorophane for washing has value in reducing wound infection. The programme practised in Sweden for whole-body disinfection involves three top-to-toe (including the hair) sessions on the day before admission, one the evening before the operation and one on the operative day. Hibiscrub is used. Not all countries in Europe practise this procedure.

All signs of skin infection in the patient should be identified and pretreated or covered with waterproof dressings.

Shaving

Hair adjacent to the operative site is often removed to prevent the wound from becoming entangled with hair during the operation. However, hair removal often causes injury to the skin and wound infection rates have been shown to be higher when skin is shaved. If hair removal is necessary, clippers should be used and it should be performed as near to the time of the operation as possible, preferably by the surgeon. If clippers are not available, depilatory cream can be used.

Preoperative screening

Preoperative screening of nasal or skin areas is of little value and is not cost-effective. In general, the mere presence of potentially pathogenic bacteria is not commensurate with subsequent infections.

Transport of the patient to theatre

After the patient has been prepared for operation and has been changed into a clean operating gown he or she can be transferred directly from the ward to the operating room in a bed, provided ward blankets are removed before entering the theatre. There is little advantage in having a transfer area and changing trolleys or porters putting on plastic overshoes. Trolleys are exposed to some degree of contamination during the journeys to and from the wards and require cleaning on a daily basis. Passing the trolley wheels over a sticky mat has doubtful benefits and the cost does not justify their use.

Preparation of the patient's skin

The area around and including the operative site should be scrubbed with a detergent-impregnated sponge or swab. No benefit is to be gained by preparing the skin the night before operation, as was performed with povidone–iodine for lower limb amputations. After the skin has been cleaned and degreased, antiseptic solutions should be used. Application of alcohol or of an alcoholic solution of chlorhexidine or povidone–iodine gives better disinfection when the antiseptic is rubbed on until the skin is dry. This can be achieved by using a double-gloved hand or sponge forceps. To obtain maximum reduction of transient skin flora, the alcohol must be allowed to dry. Care must be taken when using alcoholic solutions with diathermy; alcohol should not be allowed to pool in the umbilicus or under the perineum. For vaginal and perineal disinfection it is advised that a solution of chlorhexidine and cetrimide (Savlon) should be used.

Drapes

Part of the ritual of preparing the patient for surgery includes protecting the periphery of the proposed incisional site with sterilized cotton drapes. Because these cotton drapes become wet very quickly and their protective properties are diminished, the use of incisional plastic drapes has been advocated. Early work by Cruse & Foord (1980) demonstrated that wound infections are not decreased by applying adhesive plastic skin drapes to the operative area. More recent work has confirmed this finding in a study of caeserian section.

STERILIZATION

This is a process usually defined as the complete destruction or removal of all viable microorganisms, which includes spores and viruses. In practice this is difficult to establish and the definition is often couched in the probability of a single viable organism surviving on one million items. This definition meets the requirement of the *European Pharmacopoeia* and complies with the EEC directive.

The term 'sterilization' is applied to inanimate objects (e.g. instruments and equipment) but not to the skin, as the process is a tissue-damaging one.

Sterilization by steam

Steam under pressure attains a temperature higher than boiling water and the final temperature is directly related to pressure. Instruments can be sterilized reliably by steam under pressure using autoclaves. Steam transfers its latent heat to microorganisms on the surface of previously cleaned instruments. Both vegetative bacteria (including tuberculosis (TB) bacteria), viruses (e.g. HBV and HIV) and heat-resistant spores (e.g. *Clostridium tetani* and *Clostridium perfringens*) treated in steam pressure vessels are rendered non-infectious and non-viable (i.e. killed).

The recommended combination of time and temperature varies, and for instruments which can withstand moist heat under pressure the following cycles are recommended:

- 134°C (30 lb in.$^{-2}$) for a hold time of 3 minutes
- 121°C (15 lb in.$^{-2}$) for a hold time of 15 minutes.

The higher temperature of 134°C for 3 minutes is preferred. It is important to remember that these times are the hold time at the stated temperature and that the entire cycle time, i.e. heating up/cooling down, is much longer; the cycle time at 134°C is approximately 30 minutes. In the past, flash autoclaves operating at 147°C (40 lb in.$^{-2}$) were used, but these are no longer recommended or available, for safety reasons.

All steam sterilizers should comply with the requirements of BS 3970: British Standard 1990 Sterilizing and Disinfecting Equipment for Medical Products. All sterilizers should have a preset automatic cycle which cannot be interrupted until the cycle is completed. Most large autoclaves are centralized in specialized units (e.g. the sterile service department (SSD) or theatre sterile service unit (TSSU)) and are subject to close scrutiny and maintenance by highly trained personnel.

Wrapped instruments/packs

All pre-packed materials/instruments are processed through a porous load autoclave which incorporates a prevacuum cycle, necessary to extract air. Unless the trapped air is removed, dry saturated steam cannot penetrate efficiently and the sterilization process will be hindered.

Unwrapped instruments

A convenient method of sterilizing small numbers of surgical instruments is to use a portable steam sterilizer (e.g. Little Sister II). Instruments should be thoroughly cleaned and dried and placed on a perforated stainless steel tray that slides into the autoclave. When the autoclave cycle is completed, the instruments should be left to cool down (often down to 80°C) and can be used straight away or stored dry on a trolley laid with sterile paper (BS 6255: 1994). This is a convenient way to deal with dropped (or thrown!) instruments.

Monitoring

The sterilizer must be maintained according to the manufacturer's instructions. In addition, maintenance requirements and routine and commissioning performance tests are strictly controlled according to the Health Technical Memorandum (HTM2010: 1994).

Porous load autoclaves are checked daily using the steam penetration test (e.g. Bowie-Dick test), and cycle performance is recorded on a temperature chart. Biological indicators are not appropriate, but there is a limited role for chemical indicators (e.g. Brownes tubes No. II) which provide visual indication that a particular time–temperature relationship has been achieved. Bowel and instrument autoclaves employ fixed automatic cycles and tend not to have temperature chart recorders attached. Brownes tubes No. I can be used to verify that the cycle is completed.

Much reliance is placed on process control, and autoclaving at high temperatures (e.g. 134°C) will usually meet the required standard with a very large safety margin.

Sterilization of fluids

Fluids for parenteral or topical use are generally prepared by industry or by specialized pharmacy production units. Fluids are prepared aseptically and appropriately labelled in sealed containers (bags or bottles) and sterilized in bottle autoclaves at 121°C for 15 minutes or 115°C for 30 minutes.

Sterilization by hot air

The efficiency of dry heat sterilization depends on the initial moisture of the microbial cells, but all microorganisms are killed at 160°C for a hold time of not less than 2 hours. Compared with moist steam sterilization, dry heat sterilization is inefficient.

The main advantages of dry heat sterilization are its ability to treat solids, non-aqueous liquids, grease/ointments and to process closed (airtight) containers. Lack of corrosion is important in the sterilization of non-stainless metals and surgical instruments with fine cutting edges (e.g. ophthalmic instruments).

The process is not to be used for aqueous fluids or materials that are denatured or damaged at 160°C for 2 hours (e.g. rubber, plastics and intravenous fluids).

It is essential that all items are thoroughly cleaned, dried and packed before they are placed inside a hot-air oven. The chamber must be fitted with perforated shelves and the oven must be fitted with an electrical heater and fan unit with an independent adjustable thermostat.

Hot-air ovens should meet the specification for Performance of Electrically Heated Sterilizing Ovens in BS 3421. It is not appropriate to use converted catering equipment! Door seals must be maintained routinely and all instrumentation and charts checked.

Monitoring

The duration of the sterilization cycle is governed mainly by the penetration and holding times. Temperatures are checked using thermocouples.

Biological indicators such as spores are not used routinely. Chemical indicators (e.g. Brownes tubes No. III) may be used to demonstrate that the packages have been processed.

Sterilization by ethylene oxide

Ethylene oxide (EO) is a highly penetrative, non-corrosive agent which has a broad-spectrum cidal action against vegetative bacteria, spores and viruses under optimal conditions of concentration, relative humidity, temperature and exposure time. At ambient temperatures and pressures, EO vapourizes rapidly and is flammable in mixtures containing more than 3% vapour in air. It is also toxic, irritant, mutagenic and potentially carcinogenic. Nevertheless, under strictly controlled conditions it is an extremely valuable sterilization process. It is not to be used where heat sterilization of an item is possible.

Preferred uses

Sterilization by EO is restricted to wrapped and unwrapped heat-sensitive materials. It is ideal for delicate items such as electrical equipment, flexible-fibre endoscopes, photographic equipment and for reuse or resterilization of single-use items (e.g. cardiac catheters); this latter practice is not condoned by the Department of Health but it is recognized that recycling occurs.

EO sterilization is predominantly an industrial process used, for example, for single-use medical devices constructed of plastics. Limited NHS regional units process predominantly cardiovascular items.

The process is not recommended for ventilatory and respiratory equipment and is inappropriate for soiled items. Organic debris, oil, serum, etc., exhibit a marked adverse effect. The preferred wrapping is spun-bodied polyotefin (Tyvek) or sterilization paper (BS 6255: 1994).

EO sterilization is usually carried out within the temperature range 20–60°C and with operating cycles of 2–24 hours.

High-pressure sterilizers (6 bar) operate with a mixture of inert gases, such as carbon dioxide which greatly reduces the risk of flammability but increases the risk of leaks. Gas cylinders require replacement after one to four cycles, which makes the process expensive. The cycle time is 1.5–2.5 hours.

Subatmospheric sterilizers are operated by single-shot canisters which are situated inside the chamber and punctured automatically during the cycle. Pure EO is used to maintain an optimal concentration. The chamber capacity is small (115 litres) and the cycle time long (3.5–5 hours).

Monitoring

It is imperative that the purpose-designed cabinet is operated according to the manufacturer's instructions. Physical parameters such as humidity, pressure, temperature and EO concentration are monitored. Since these measurements do not guarantee sterility, rigorous monitoring by biological indicators (e.g. *Bacillus subtilis* var. *niger* spore strips) and chemical indicators is essential.

EO sterilization is an expensive and potentially dangerous process and must be carefully controlled. A major disadvantage is that the gas takes a long time to elute. Prolonged aeration requirements make for long turnaround times for processed items. This means that contaminated items (e.g. endoscopes) may not be returned to the user (owner) for 5–7 days. However, the Health and Safety Commission have taken a particular interest in EO usage and it is unlikely that short-cuts in safety measures will be taken.

Sterilization by low-temperature steam and formaldehyde (LTSF)

This is a physicochemical method which uses a combination of dry saturated steam and formaldehyde to kill vegetative bacteria, bacterial spores and most viruses. The main advantage of this process is that sterilization is achieved at a low temperature (73°C) and the method is thus suitable for heat-sensitive materials and items of equipment with integral plastic components susceptible to damage by other processes.

LTSF sterilization is not recommended for sealed, oily or greasy items or those with retained air. Other items are excluded where chemical reactions between the steam/chemical atmosphere and the material/object concerned may produce damage. Reversible absorption by some plastics and fabrics may lead to delayed elution of formaldehyde and subsequent hypersensitivity. All items contaminated with body fluids are excluded because hardened fixed protein deposits will be produced by this process. Narrow-bore tubing is likely to contain condensed water with trapped formaldehyde which will be hazardous to patients. This consideration excludes endoscopes as well as tubing.

LTSF sterilization is carried out in a purpose-built sterilizer and undergoes an automatic control system similar to that of other sterilizers. The cycle includes air removal and the introduction of dry saturated steam at 73°C (under vacuum) into which formaldehyde is introduced in a pulsing fashion. Prior to removal of sterilized objects all formaldehyde must be removed to provide a dry, sterile, formalin-free load.

Monitoring

Monitoring requires the recording of process time, temperature and steam pressure, the amounts of formaldehyde introduced into the chamber, and the duration of the various stages. In addition, biological indicators are used to confirm the effectiveness of the process. These are standard test objects bearing a known number of the spores of *Bacillus stearothermophilus* NCTC 10003. The Line Pickerill helix is employed as a standard test carrier for these biological monitors.

Sterilization by irradiation

Sterilization by irradiation employs γ-rays or accelerated electrons. Sterilization by ionizing radiation is an industrial process and is unsuited to the constraints of the

NHS. It is particularly suited to the sterilization of large batches of similar products (e.g. single-use items such as catheters, syringes and intravenous . . . .).

The delivery of an irradiation dose in excess of 25 kGy (2.5 Mrad) is accepted as providing adequate sterility assurance. When packaging of any sterile product has been damaged, the sterility of the contents cannot be guaranteed.

Monitoring

The dose delivered at any point within a product container can be measured by the use of dosimeters. The validation and routine monitoring of sterilization by irradiation is under the control of the UK Panel on Gamma and Electron Irradiation.

N.B: Irradiation can cause serious physical deterioration of materials, and therefore the resterilization of γ-irradiated items by any other method may further damage the item and jeopardize its function.

DISPOSAL BY INCINERATION

This is the preferred method of disposal for all combustible material of an infectious nature (e.g. contaminated needles, plastic syringes and clinical waste). In purpose-designed incinerators immediate combustion occurs in furnaces with a secondary combustion zone exit-gas temperature in excess of 850°C. This temperature should exceed 1000°C if cytotoxic drugs are in the waste stream.

Careful separation of clinical waste must occur before colour coded (e.g. yellow) plastic bags and boxes are incinerated. This process is not to be used for metal instruments or equipment. Disposable linen and infected protective clothing and drapes should be incinerated. There is no need to incinerate equipment, instruments or reusable linen as advice on the decontamination of such materials does not include incineration.

DISINFECTION

Disinfection is a process used to reduce the number of viable microorganisms but may not necessarily inactivate some viruses and bacterial spores. *Cleaning* is a process which physically removes contamination but does not necessarily destroy microorganisms. The reduction of microbial contamination cannot be defined and will depend on many factors, including the efficiency of the cleaning process and the initial bioburden. Cleaning is a necessary prerequisite of equipment decontamination to ensure effective disinfection or sterilization.

Disinfection with low-temperature steam (LTS)

This disinfection pasteurizing process kills most vegetative microorganisms and viruses by exposure to moist heat.

Typical conditions are exposure to dry saturated steam at a temperature of 73°C for a period of 20 minutes at below atmospheric pressure. Items and materials not damaged by the conditions of the process are suitable, provided that air removal and subsequent steam penetration are assured. This is a useful process which can be used to render it safe to handle dirty returns from operating theatres and clinics which may be contaminated with protein from bodily secretions and microorganisms. Following LTS disinfection, instruments can be readily cleaned as the coagulated protein residues are readily removable, unlike the baked-on residues produced following autoclaving. The process requires a disinfector, which is most likely kept in the TSSU. Instruments can be replaced on the tray on the set-up trolley or can be transferred to the TSSU in impermeable plastic bags and transported in leak-proof polypropylene or metal boxes. These boxes can subsequently be cleaned and disinfected.

Disinfection with boiling water

Boiling water is an efficient disinfection process which kills vegetative bacteria (including TB bacteria), some viruses (including HBV and HIV) and some spores. It is not a sterilizing process. Water is non-toxic, but at high temperature causes tissue damage. Soft water at 100°C at normal pressure for 5 minutes or more forms the disinfection cycle. All items for disinfection should be thoroughly cleaned and totally immersed in boiling water in a safe manner. Suitable items include metal instruments such as speculae, proctoscopes and sigmoidoscopes. Care should be taken to ensure that air is not trapped in tubing, etc.

A purpose-designed water boiler should be used which should be electrically heated and incorporate an overheating cut-out. The machine should have a hinged lid and a perforated tray with a raising/lowering lever. The unit should be designed to operate at temperatures such that the contained water will continue to boil when instruments are lowered into it.

Monitoring

It is not possible to monitor this process satisfactorily. A temperature gauge is fitted but a record is not kept. A time-lock should be fitted to prevent cycle disruption.

A major disadvantage of the process is that it leaves

the article wet and unfit for storage. Items should be stored dry and covered prior to use.

Disinfection with formaldehyde

Formaldehyde gas is a broad-spectrum antimicrobial agent which under optimal conditions of concentration, exposure time and relative humidity can be used as a disinfecting agent. This process is quite distinct from LTSF sterilization. At atmospheric pressure and temperatures up to 50°C the gas has limited sporicidal action.

The formaldehyde cabinet comprises a large airtight cabinet and a control console which automatically dispenses and circulates gaseous formaldehyde up to 50°C. Following an appropriate exposure time for disinfection, ammonia gas is released to neutralize residual formaldehyde. The cabinet and its contents are flushed through with fresh air.

Formaldehyde is a hazardous substance; it is a flammable and explosive gas, irritant to the eyes, respiratory tract and skin. Such properties require careful control and monitoring of the process and consideration of possible adverse effects to staff, equipment and patients.

This process can be used to provide terminal disinfection of large thermolabile items such as ventilators, suction pumps and incubators. If ventilators can be protected by bacterial filters this process is not required. Paper, rubber and some plastic materials are excluded from this process because formaldehyde residues may persist or be trapped within the product.

Two main types of formaldehyde cabinet are currently used in the UK:

- The Draeger Aseptor Unit offers a short cycle (3.5 hours) or a long cycle (10 hours)
- The Vickers Formalaire is a smaller machine and can accommodate only a single item; the cycle time is 3 hours.

Monitoring

There is limited process control directly monitoring the item to be processed. Formaldehyde-sensitive indicator paper may be used to indicate that the gas has reached a particular part in the load but will not confirm disinfection. Biological indicators for this process are available but require careful evaluation as to their applicability to the process.

Disinfectants

Where heat cannot be used for sterilization or decontamination, chemical disinfection may be used. The choice and methods of use are set out in the PHLS booklet on Chemical Disinfection in Hospitals (Ayliffe et al 1993).

DECONTAMINATION OF ENDOSCOPES

Immersion in a suitable liquid chemical disinfectant is the most widely used procedure for the decontamination of flexible endoscopes due to the heat-sensitive nature of many of the components. The most widely used agent at present is 2% freshly activated alkaline glutaraldehyde.

Glutaraldehyde is rapidly active against most vegetative bacteria and viruses, include HIV and HBV, and slowly effective against TB and spores. Glutaraldehyde is a hazardous substance and is recognized as toxic, irritant and allergenic. An assessment of procedures involving glutaraldehyde is required by the COSHH regulations (1989, HMSO).

SPILLAGES

It is essential to remove body fluid spillages promptly. Protective clothing should be worn (e.g. gloves, plastic apron and goggles) and the spillage contained by covering blood and other body fluids with absorbent paper towels. For a spillage involving a patient with a known or suspected infection (e.g. HIV or HBV) refer to the local disinfection policy or PHLS booklet (Chemical Disinfection in Hospitals) (Ayliffe et al 1993) for the relevant disinfectants (e.g. 10 000 ppm freshly made hypochlorite).

FURTHER READING

1990 Guidance for clinical care workers: protection against infection with HIV and hepatitis viruses. HMSO, London

Ayliffe G A J, Collins B J, Taylor L J 1990 Hospital-acquired infection: principles and prevention, 2nd edn. Wright, London

British Medical Association 1989 A code of practice for sterilization of instruments and control of cross infection. BMA, London

British Medical Association 1990 A code of practice for the safe use and disposal of sharps. BMA, London

REFERENCES

Ayliffe G A J, Coates D, Hoffman P N 1993 Chemical

disinfection in hospitals. PHLS Blackmore Press, Shaftesbury

Cruse P J E, Foord R 1980 The epidemiology of wound infection: a 10-year prospective study of 62,939 wounds. Surgical Clinics of North America 60: 1

Lidwell O M, Lowbury E J L, Whyte W, Blowers R, Stanley S J, Lowe D 1982 Effects of ultra clean air in operating rooms on deep sepsis in the joints after total hip or knee replacement: a randomized study. British Medical Journal 285: 10–14

Whyte W, Hamblen D L, Kelly I G, Hambraeus A, Laurell G 1990 An investigation of occlusive polyester surgical clothing. Journal of Hospital Infection 15: 363–374

17. The risks to surgeons of nosocomial virus transmission

C. Wastell

Since the inspirational work of Semmelweis we have become progressively more aware of the dangers of transmission of microorganisms from patient to patient, patient to surgeon and surgeon to patient. Jenner was perhaps the first experimental worker, however, to manipulate the pox virus, with his classical studies on the prevention of smallpox by means of immunization. With this eighteenth and nineteenth century background and all the great works of the microbiologists, it appears extraordinary that practising surgeons in the late twentieth century accept both contamination of themselves by the blood and body fluids of their patients and the contamination of patients with their own blood when a 'sharps' injury occurs during an invasive procedure. It is perhaps the advent of the human immunodeficiency virus (HIV) that has resulted in a sharpened perception of the dangers inherent in this contamination. In the UK, the majority of surgeons still insist on wearing linen gowns, which offer absolutely no protection against anything at all, except perhaps the sensibilities surrounding nakedness.

This chapter considers briefly the main viruses which may be transmitted either way, that is from surgeon to patient or patient to surgeon, and then provides guidelines for a safe system of practice.

VIRAL HEPATITIS

Hepatitis A

The precise prevalence of hepatitis A is unknown but it is likely to be almost universally present in most countries. It is likely that the incidence is decreasing in industrialized and developed countries. Infection is generally via the faecal–oral route and the incubation period is between 3 and 5 weeks. There is no known carrier state and subclinical and subjaundice infections are common. Although transmission of the virus can occur by means of sharps injuries this is unusual, and the presence of hepatitis A virus cannot be demonstrated by immune electron microscopy in the stool after the first week of illness.

Hepatitis B

The hepatitis B virus (HBV) may be transmitted by inoculation via sharps injuries from blood or products derived from blood, by droplet transmission, for example in association with open systems of renal dialysis, and also by sexual and oral contact. The prevalence of the virus is much higher in less well-developed countries including those of Eastern Europe, the Middle East, Asia and South America. In the UK, the prevalence is relatively low, being only between 1% and 2% except for certain selected groups of workers, and these include health-care workers, particularly those involved in invasive procedures, those working in geriatric and psychiatric institutions, dentists and personnel employed in pathology laboratories. The incubation period of HBV is between 6 weeks and 6 months, although it may occasionally be longer. Between 5% and 10% of infected patients will develop a carrier state and awareness of this possibility is important for surgeons. The onset of the clinical disease may be insidious, but in a small proportion of those infected fulminant hepatitis may develop. Also in a small proportion of patients hepatitis B carrier state is associated with chronic active hepatitis and, eventually, cirrhosis.

There are a number of antigen–antibody systems relating to HBV.

HBsAg

Detection of the surface antigen to hepatitis B is the first manifestation of infection before other evidence of liver disease. The surface antigen persists throughout the clinical disease, and the majority of those infected will develop an antibody to this surface antigen. The demonstration of the antibody to HBs is associated with protection from infection from further inoculations of the virus and non-infectivity from the patient.

HBcAg

The c antigen is detected by the development of an antibody to it which appears shortly after the surface antigen to hepatitis B is detected. It may persist for between 1 and 2 years. Its significance is that in donors infectivity has been demonstrated where HBsAg has been negative but HBc antigen is present. With the development of antibodies, infectivity becomes absent.

HBeAg

The e antigen is found only in HBsAg-positive sera and appears during the incubation period. The importance of this antigen is that it is an index of infectivity. Carriers with a persistence of this antigen are many times more likely to infect others. Surgeons have been shown to infect their patients during operative procedures, particularly in the pelvis when they have carried this antigen (Welch et al 1989).

DNA polymerase

DNA polymerase activity is first detectable in serum when the titre for HBsAg is rising. It is suggested that this enzyme indicates the presence of virions in the serum and is associated with viral replication. Its presence is usually transient but it may persist for years in the patient who is a carrier and it may therefore be associated with continuing infectivity.

Delta agent

This is a defective viral RNA genome and has only been demonstrated in association with hepatitis B infection. It has only been demonstrated in the presence of HBsAg. It is usually associated with more severe forms of HBV infections and has been reported to be present in half those patients who develop fulminant hepatitis.

Hepatitis C

The hepatitis C virus appears to be responsible for the majority of hepatitis infections occurring as a result of contaminated transfusion. It would seem likely that vertical transmission is a possibility.

Other viral causes of hepatitis

Hepatitis may be associated with infection with the Epstein–Barr virus and the cytomegalovirus.

Treatment

Hepatitis A

Human normal immunoglobulin is available which protects if given during the incubation period. It should be given to all close personal contacts of patients who are known to have developed hepatitis A and to persons who are travelling to areas of high endemicity (all countries except northern Europe, North America, New Zealand and Australia) and will protect for a period of up to 5 months.

Hepatitis B

1. Hyperimmune globulin may protect an infected individual if given within 7 days of exposure. A second dose is required 21–23 days later and is recommended for individuals who are at risk of having received contamination via mucous membranes or implantation. In addition, vaccination with the hepatitis B vaccine should be commenced at the same time.

2. Hepatitis B vaccine is now available from a monoclonal source and is appropriate for individuals who are HBsAg and HBcAg negative. It should be given to individuals at high risk of developing the infection, and these include patients on renal dialysis, renal dialysis technicians, patients receiving repeated transfusions, the partners of HBsAg-positive patients, male homosexuals and the neonates of HBsAg-positive mothers. All individuals entering nursing or the medical professions, depending upon the indications above, should receive immunization against hepatitis B. The development of a fulminant hepatitis or a carrier state is no longer an acceptable risk. If a surgeon becomes HBeAg positive he will be unable to perform invasive procedures until such time as this state can be reversed.

HUMAN IMMUNODEFICIENCY VIRUS (HIV)

The first report in the world implicating the virus was in 1981 by Gottlieb et al, who reported five patients with pneumocystis pneumonia who also had profound depression of cellular immunity. Since that time the virus has been identified as being a retrovirus containing a reverse transcriptase. Certain antiretroviral drugs acting by the inhibition of this enzyme system have been developed, such as Zidovudine (AZT), Didanosine (DDI) and Zalcitabine (DDC). The use of AZT when used in combination with DDI or DDC even in the asymptomatic but infected patient has been shown both to reduce morbidity and to prolong survival. However, acquisition of HIV in the vast majority of patients eventually results in death from profound depression of cellular immunity.

The virus is acquired sexually, most commonly by sexual intercourse between men but to an increasing degree during heterosexual intercourse, by implantation of the virus following contamination with the blood, body fluids or transplanted tissues of an infected person, and by babies from infected mothers which may occur in utero or, possibly, during delivery (European Collaborative Study 1992). There is good evidence to suggest that a combination of infection with HIV and another ulcerative genital tract disease facilitates the transmission of HIV during heterosexual intercourse. It is this observation that explains the rapid heterosexual spread of disease in sub-Saharan Africa. From this may be derived a list of groups of high-risk individuals:

- Homosexual males
- Intravenous drug abusers
- Haemophiliacs before October 1985
- Residents from areas of high endemicity
- Sexual partners of the above
- Children of infective mothers

Following infection with the virus there is a period of up to 6–12 weeks during which no detectable antibody response occurs, but there is a rising titre of antigen and the patient is presumably capable of passing on the infection. At 12 weeks approximately 85% of patients have mounted an antibody response that is detectable in serum, the antigenaemia falls to undetectable levels and, though HIV antibody positive, the patient is not infective. There are a small number of individuals in whom an antibody response takes longer to develop, and the period for this to occur has even been reported as taking 2 years. The second stage of the infection is not associated with any symptoms at all and is detectable only by antibody testing. At some time, usually between 3 and 12 years, the antibody response diminishes, antigen becomes detectable in serum and body fluids, and the patient moves into the next stage of the disease process and eventually to acquired immune deficiency syndrome (AIDS). The virus has been isolated from blood, semen, saliva, tears, urine and cervical secretion. Up until July 1995 there were 24 444 people in the UK who had HIV antibodies; 11 051 cases of AIDS had been reported, of whom 7571 were known to have died (Communicable Disease Report 1995). The greatest risk of HIV acquisition for the health-care worker relates to lifestyle. However, there are currently reports of 214 health-care workers who would appear to have acquired

HIV by virtue of their occupation, and these are summarized in Table 17.1.

The majority of occupationally acquired HIV infection occurs as a result of a sharps injury. Since there is only one report of transmission due to injury by a 'solid sharp' it is clear that such an injury from a hollow needle carries a much greater risk, particularly where the source of the infection is a patient with AIDS rather than the 'pre-AIDS' state. The risk of transmission following a sharps injury was reviewed by Gill et al (1991), who found that of 2475 percutaneous exposures 9 resulted in seroconversion, giving a transmission rate of 0.36%.

Contamination of the surface of the skin is more common in more junior grades of surgeons and in operations where larger quantities of blood are lost. Since it is known that it is possible to become infected with HBV by contamination of the conjunctiva, great anxiety has been expressed about blood-droplet aerosol created by power tools such as used by orthopaedic and ear, nose and throat (ENT) surgeons. However, to date no case of seroconversion has occurred by this route.

Treatment

The question as to what should be done following either a needle-stick injury, mucosal or contamination of non-intact skin surface from a high-risk patient has been considered exhaustively. There would seem to be no good evidence that postexposure chemoprophylaxis with Zidovudine is effective. There are of course enormous pressures on physicians expert in this area to treat a health-care worker who has been hazarded in this way, but there is really no evidence for the efficacy of Zidovudine. Hospitals have tended to develop their own policies and to offer the health-care worker this drug with appropriate speed; that is, within a period of 6 hours and at an appropriate dose. Unfortunately, symptoms of nausea, malaise and fatigue, headache and vomiting have been reported in a high proportion of people taking the drug.

HERPES VIRUSES

Herpes simplex types 1 and 2

These members of this group of DNA viruses are mainly important because of the possibility in the health-care worker of greater contact with direct cutaneous or mucocutaneous lesions produced by the virus. These herpetic sores may become widespread and extragenital, for example affecting the anal canal in patients who are immunosuppressed.

Table 17.1 The number of health-care workers who are HIV positive as a result of occupationally transmitted infection (Report of the Working Party of the Royal College of Pathology July 1995)

	USA	Europe	UK	Rest of world	Total
Documented seroconversion after specific occupational exposure	43	21	4	5	73
Possible occupationally acquired infection	91	34	7	9	141
Total	134	55	11	14	214

Treatment

Several drugs are effective in inhibiting replication of herpes viruses and these include acyclovir, which may be given intravenously (15 mg kg^{-1} per 24 hours) and is effective in symptomatic primary genital infections and in disseminating herpetic mucocutaneous lesions in patients with AIDS. In addition, oral acyclovir (200 mg five times daily) can also be effective. Topical acyclovir in a 5% concentration will help to reduce viral shedding.

Cytomegalovirus

This is the human herpes virus 5 and is acquired by mucocutaneous contact. It is present in up to one-quarter of healthy individuals and in up to 95% of homosexual men, in whom it is sexually transmitted.

Because of its ubiquitous nature it is not especially important in relation to the transmission of the disease from patient to surgeon, or vice versa. In patients with AIDS it can produce a wide variety of symptoms, but amongst the most troublesome is retinitis, for which treatment with gancyclovir or foscarnet may be required.

PAPILLOMA VIRUSES

There are over 40 types of human papilloma virus and their importance, apart from the enormous clinical load that is provided by cutaneous juvenile warts, relates to their ability to stimulate neoplasia. Types 6, 16 and 18 are associated with uterine and cervical carcinomas. Fifty per cent of all surgical referrals in patients who are HIV1 positive are for anorectal complaints. Of these, anogenital warts form a high proportion. Ninety per cent of patients presenting to a rectal clinic with warts were found to be in a high-risk group.

The significance to surgeons treating anogenital warts is that the smoke resulting from laser destruction has been shown to contain viable virus particles. These particles can become implanted in the nasopharynx of the surgeon.

PREVENTION OF INFECTION

The principles of the prevention of infection of health-care workers from virus diseases in patients are to maintain an effective barrier between patient and surgeon and to ensure that all the usual measures to prevent cross-infection are undertaken.

Identification of high-risk patients

The term 'high-risk patient' means a patient who is at a high risk of being HIV or HBV positive. It is possible that a patient who is so infected may also harbour the human papilloma virus and types 1 and 2 herpes virus. Debate exists as to whether detection of high-risk patients is either desirable or possible. However, many surgeons feel that if they know they are operating on high-risk patients their technique is modified so as to avoid sharps injuries.

The history is helpful and, if skilfully taken, often provides knowledge as to risk behaviour. Identification of the significant physical signs is also important; for example, the multiple injection marks associated with drug addiction or the likely association between anogenital warts and homosexuality.

Testing for HIV and HBV

If it appears that a patient may be in a high-risk category the patient is advised to accept antibody testing for the above viruses. This is always only carried out with the express permission of the patient, and after counselling in the case of the HIV test. It is important even in asymptomatic patients to know the HIV antibody status, since current evidence would suggest that AZT with either DDI or DDC even in the asymptomatic patient is effective in prolonging life. This can then be added to the benefit to the surgeon of knowing the HIV antibody status of the patient.

All patients

The operating theatre

The provisions necessary within the operating theatre are those necessary to prevent cross-infection. The table top is covered with an impervious sheet so that the mattress is not contaminated with blood or body fluids. The surgeon scrubs up in the normal way and wears a completely impervious gown. Currently it is sometimes necessary to wear a plastic apron beneath the gown, particularly if heavy contamination is expected. A particular area of risk is the forearm, and contamination tends to seep between the top of the glove and the elasticated cuff. The bottom of the gown should be lower than the top of impervious footwear. A mask is worn, and this should be a special impervious mask if warts are being treated by either diathermy or laser.

The skin of the patient is cleaned in the usual way and impervious drapes are used so that neither blood nor fluid seeps around the patient's body.

During the operative procedure no sharps are passed hand to hand between the scrub person and the surgeon. Knives and needles are conveyed from one to the other in a transit dish. After use, all sharps are disposed of in a self-locking disposal carrier or an appropriate bin which is not filled to more than half its capacity. In no circumstances is the finger used as a guide for a needle, particularly in body cavities such as the pelvis.

High-risk patients

Before operation

High-risk patients are not placed at the end of the operating list unless this is appropriate for other reasons. Such placement is discriminatory if it occurs and is associated with a greater tendency for cancellation because of lack of time. The patient is transported to the anaesthetic room in the normal manner and the anaesthetic is induced in the usual way before transfer to the operating room. Anaesthetists should wear gloves and eye protection.

The operating theatre

The procedures are exactly similar to those outlined above and used for all patients.

Recovery room

By the time the patient leaves the operating theatre all wounds should be dressed and not leaking. Any spills of blood or tissue fluids are covered with a suitable antiseptic such as hyperchlorite solution. The disposable drapes and the gowns are placed in a yellow viscose bag for incineration.

The patient is recovered in the usual way in the recovery room.

Extra precautions to be taken for high-risk patients

1. Double gloving: two pairs of gloves are worn as there is good evidence to show that the likelihood of glove perforation is reduced by this practice. It is usual to wear the inner glove a half-size larger than the surgeon's usual size.

2. Eye protection: eye protection should be worn at all times when power tools are being employed, but should also be used by the surgeon and those immediately around the operating table when high-risk patients are being operated on. Splash contamination of the conjunctiva is not uncommon and should be avoided, particularly from the point of view of transmission of HBV.

3. Overshoes: these are worn to prevent contamination of footwear.

CONCLUSION

It is impossible to know accurately the existence or otherwise of HBV and/or HIV in all patients. In principle anyhow, we should assume that all patients may contain a potentially dangerous infective organism. Therefore, when handling all patients much stricter attention must be paid to the barrier that should exist between patient and surgeon. This barrier, though in fact mechanical and composed of impervious materials of one sort or another, is also the barrier of good practice.

It is important to identify so far as is possible those patients who carry a higher risk of harbouring the hepatitis virus or HIV. Obviously when operations are carried out on these patients the precautions dictated by good practice and an impervious barrier must also be employed, but these must be added to by the use of double gloves, eye protection and overshoes. Unfortunately, no satisfactory treatment or prophylaxis exists for HIV or hepatitis C virus but there is now absolutely no excuse for health-care personnel not to be immunized and protected against HBV.

REFERENCES

Communicable Disease Report, 5, 140, July 1995
European Collaborative Study 1992 Risk factors for mother-to-child transmission of HIV1. Lancet 339: 1007–1012
Gill O N, Heptonstall J, Porter K 1991 Occupational transmission of HIV: summary of published report to September. Internal publication of the Public Health Laboratory Service

Gottlieb M S, Schanker H M, Fann P F et al 1981 Pneumocystis pneumonia: Los Angeles. Morbidity and Mortality Weekly Report 30: 250–252
Report of the Working Party of the Royal College of Pathologists July 1995 HIV and the Practice of Pathology
Welch J, Webster M, Tolsey A J, Noah N D, Banatvala J E 1989. Hepatitis B infections after surgery. Lancet i: 205–207

Operation

18. Good surgical practice

J. L. Dawson

Good surgical practice will provide effective control of clinical practice as well as protecting you from legal pitfalls which await the unwary. Good surgical practice is a hard taskmaster. It demands self-discipline at all times in order to organize yourself and your commitments and combine this with honesty to your patients, your colleagues and, not least, yourself.

It is important to develop the right surgical working habits from the very beginning of training, especially

- time keeping
- note keeping

Your day should be organized so that all inpatients have been seen and assessed before the first fixed commitment. Always be on time for ward rounds, outpatients, operating lists and clinical meetings.

The essential discipline of writing concise clear contemporaneous notes cannot be overemphasized. They should contain an objective account of the history and clinical findings. Avoid judgmental or flippant comments. The notes may, for a few patients, be used as a legal record of the patient's care and progress.

The organization of modern hospital practice has led to a serious erosion of the continuity of care by one doctor for an individual patient. The notes now provide the written record of what was previously carried in the mind of the attending resident. A Duty Doctor is now regularly called to see patients who are under the care of a different firm. Accurate and comprehensive notes are essential for a proper assessment to be made in the event of such an emergency call. There is no doubt that the number of complaints about clinical management and clinical care is increasing: accurate clinical records are an essential safeguard to rebut any inappropriate or vexatious complaints.

Emotional neutrality

It is essential that all surgeons, of whatever grade, maintain a completely neutral stance and do not get into any sort of emotional conflict with patients, relatives or indeed professional colleagues who are responsible for patient care. Emotional conflict clouds judgement and should be avoided at all costs. Always resist responding to provocation, however tempting it may be.

Surgical team

The organization of the delivery of surgical care and training is centred around a unit or firm, usually consisting of two to three consultants plus junior staff. With the shortening of the period of surgical training, firm timetables are being adjusted to allow space for continuing surgical education. The basis of this includes a regular audit meeting at which the patient's notes are scrutinized. The basic surgical trainees are usually responsible for producing the clinical information for these audit meetings. One consultant member of the team is usually designated as the trainer responsible for a particular trainee's education. Loyalty to the firm and good rapport with your trainer are the hallmarks of a successful training programme.

Many surgical patients require imaging of one sort or another to make or confirm the diagnosis or to monitor progress after surgical treatment. Regular meetings with the Radiology Department are now the norm in most hospitals, but you should develop the habit of calling in to the X-ray Department to arrange urgent investigations personally; in this way you will find you enjoy maximum cooperation which contributes enormously to the smooth running of the treatment of patients under your care.

Patient's understanding

Before proceeding to operate you must ensure that both the patient and relatives understand the aim of the operation and that their expectations of the outcome are realistic (see Ch. 11). In addition, the patient should be in the best possible mental and physical condition and all appropriate prophylactic measures should have been taken to minimize complications.

Informed consent

The fact that the patient signs a consent form will not be accepted as evidence that he or she has received an adequate explanation of the operative procedure. In principle, the explanation of the operative procedure should be given by the person undertaking the operation. With more complicated procedures resulting in serious permanent changes, such as mastectomy or establishing a stoma, more than one consultation is necessary with the patient, and preferably with a spouse or relative present as well as a Nurse Counsellor. This is important so that the patient does not feel rushed into making a decision which later may be regretted. There is now widespread use of printed leaflets explaining the common procedures.

Emergency admissions

History and physical examination remain the basis for diagnosis in the majority of surgical patients. However, clinical assessment of emergency referrals may be much more difficult. The patient and relatives are more anxious and there is a degree of urgency to make a diagnosis and decide upon action. It will be rapidly apparent to you that the florid abdominal signs elicited in the Casualty Department may later, after a period of warmth and security in a hospital bed, have largely disappeared. Reassessment and re-examination is an essential part of the process of evaluating a patient referred as an emergency. It follows that the signs and symptoms of each examination should be carefully recorded in the notes, together with the time and also the results of any emergency investigations undertaken.

For emergency patients difficulties do arise when the patient is too ill or too young to understand the implications of what is proposed. In these circumstances it is highly desirable to speak to close relatives or other responsible persons to explain what is proposed. However, the guiding principle is that you should always act in the best interests of the child or adult, and very occasionally this may require recourse to making an application to the court.

Avoidance of errors

The surgeon responsible for the operation should also mark the lesion to be operated upon before any premedication is given. Once an operating list has been agreed and published any change to the order is best avoided. If it is necessary, alert the theatre staff and the anaesthetist so that no error can occur.

Prophylactic measures

The established and accepted prophylactic measures taken in elective surgery are easily overlooked in the emergency case, especially prophylaxis against venous thrombosis, which is especially important in those patients who are taking a contraceptive pill.

Operation notes

At the completion of any operation, write up the notes personally. These should include a clear and accurate account of the pathology found and also a description of precisely what procedure was done and what was the state of affairs on completion. Record any intraoperative testing (e.g. anastomoses or blood flow following revascularization procedures). The importance of these notes cannot be overemphasized.

Delegation

The surgeon in training is the responsibility of the trainer. The delegation of any operative procedure must take place only when there is adequate supervision either by assisting, watching or being readily available for advice. Avoid embarking on any procedure which you regard as beyond your capability. Increasing specialization and expertise together with the introduction of new techniques (e.g. minimal access surgery) has focused patients' (and lawyers') attention on the matter of professional competence. The rapid expansion of workshops devoted to instructing the trainee in new techniques using simulation material are an essential part of surgical training and experience.

Day surgery

Day surgery presents special problems. Make sure you see all patients before undertaking the list to confirm what is to be done and carry out any necessary marking. At the end of the day, before the patient is discharged home, check that the patient is fully recovered and that there are no untoward symptoms or signs. Make proper arrangements for the patient's further care. Give an adequate and legible discharge note for the GP's information, and an emergency call number for the patient, so that advice is available should anxieties arise in the hours after returning home.

Postoperative course

You learn the variations which may occur from patient to patient during normal recovery only from assiduously looking after large numbers of patients. Experience at the bedside is of paramount importance. It is almost impossible to learn these things from a textbook. Over time the expected pattern of recovery becomes second nature, and deviation from this pattern instinctively prompts appropriate and expeditous action. The decision to re-explore a patient is always difficult, but early evacuation of blood clot or arrest of continued bleeding may prevent serious complications later on (e.g. infection of a haematoma within the peritoneum leading to prolonged and life-threatening sepsis).

Daily note making in the postoperative period helps to imprint on your mind the variation in recovery patterns.

Surgical audit and continuing medical education

Carefully audit and self-review outcomes throughout your professional career as an essential part of maintaining surgical standards. For individual surgical teams this is ideally done on a weekly basis. Only in this way can the head of the team maintain an overall view of precisely what is happening.

Delegation of audit to a hospital audit department does not remove responsibility from individual surgeons for producing accurate data about the service provided. If an accurate weekly record is kept it is no great burden to produce monthly and annual figures on the activities of the firm. Although most surgical teams do this for inpatients, the activities in the day surgery unit and outpatient department may receive less careful scrutiny. Control of what happens in the outpatient department is particularly difficult, especially when locums are employed. Unless there is some form of audit a patient attending an outpatient clinic can often be subjected to various procedures and investigations and even be put on the waiting list for operative treatment without the consultant having any knowledge. Regular audit meetings also provide a forum to discuss policy change and encourage a cohesive team approach. They are an excellent and essential basis for the continuing surgical education of all grades of surgeon.

19. Surgical access, incisions and the management of wounds

D. J. Leaper

There are records describing successful wound management from as long ago as the time of the Assyrians and the ancient Egyptian empire. Techniques using sutures and threads, linen adhesive strips and skin 'clips' of soldier ant heads have all been described historically. Dressings have been equally diverse, their value often being based on erroneous principles, but in the last 30 years there has been increasing interest resulting in many tailor-made and improved types of dressing.

The scourge of successful wound healing is infection, which was well recognized by Hippocrates and Galen, although some of their remedies were far from adequate. Microscopic confirmation of Celsian hypotheses and observations (the calor, rubor, tumor et dolor of acute inflammation) was slow in coming, but the understanding of the physiology of wound healing has advanced greatly over the last two to three decades and is continuing to do so. The correct concepts and control of infection became established with the introduction of antisepsis through Semmelweis and Lister, associated with the work of Pasteur. Aseptic techniques were adopted at the turn of this century. Antibiotics are now an integral part of surgical management, particularly in prophylaxis, and again we have seen continuing advances since the days of Ehrlich, Fleming, and Florey and Chain.

In retrospect, our surgical repertoire seems to have found no bounds or restrictions. Operative surgery and anaesthesia allow procedures such as heart–lung transplantation to be undertaken safely. Our forebears would not believe what is now possible, but the natural processes of wound healing must not be forgotten. The aphorism of 'cut well, sew well, get well' depends on a knowledge of these wound-healing mechanisms and the adverse effects that may influence them.

SURGICAL ACCESS AND INCISIONS

Hair removal

Body hair is conventionally removed from a proposed operative field the day before surgery. This is done for aesthetic reasons and also to allow painless removal of dressings, particularly the currently popular polymeric transparent sheet dressings (such as Opsite or Bioclusive) which were introduced as incise drapes. It has been shown, however, that the time of shaving is critical: when performed over 12 hours before surgery clean wound sepsis rates increase from 1–2% up to more than 5%. Inexpert or unsupervised shaving by patients worsens these rates. Minor skin abrasions and cuts which are exuding by the time of surgery allow emergence of skin commensals to the surface and colonization by pathogens.

Clipping of hair or the use of depilatory creams which are messy, reduces infection rates to a tenth of those following shaving. Shaving, if it is necessary, should be undertaken shortly prior to surgery. Avoidance of shaving altogether does not increase wound infection rates.

Operative drapes

Following skin preparation, usually with 0.5% chlorhexidine or 10% povidone–iodine (1% available iodine) in 70% alcohol, the operative field needs to be delineated with operative drapes. Conventionally these are resterilized double-thickness linen sheets which are held with towel clips. These need substantial care for further use: as well as the need for steam sterilization, and they have the drawback of allowing permeation related to the weave.

Disposable fabrics do not allow penetration by body fluids and their waterproofing is a benefit when operating in the face of contamination or when there is a risk of human immunodeficiency virus (HIV) or hepatitis infections. They are expensive. Incise drapes of adhesive polyurethane film were introduced over 30 years ago. They are widely used in prosthetic or vascular surgery when there is an increased risk of opportunist infection by skin organisms such as *Staphylococcus epidermidis*.

There is no definite indication that they reduce infection, and in fact the wound bacterial count at the skin surface increases during their use.

Antiseptic impregnation has little protective effect. However, in general surgical operations incise drapes avoid the need for towel clips and can isolate stomas or an infected nearby focus (such as an infected separate wound). Wound guards can be placed into the wound but do not reduce the risk of wound infection, although they reduce bacterial contamination during open viscus surgery.

General principles of access incisions

The overriding consideration is *access*. Never forget that in order to carry out a surgical procedure safely you must be able to see and control your actions. There are many aspects such as cosmetic, avoidance of damage to structures in or near the line of incision, the blood supply, ease of closure and functional result, that enter into the decision of access incisions.

Fortunately, our predecessors have laid down standard approaches to structures such as joints, blood vessels, nerves, and individual organs. Remember, though, that disease processes may alter the anatomy.

LAPAROTOMY INCISIONS

Laparotomy incisions reflect the requirements for any type of operative approach. To be useful they must allow adequate access or allow extension if necessary for an operative procedure or a full staging assessment, for example. Most abdominal incisions can be planned for a specific operation as surgical diagnosis is usually near to perfect, particularly with the availability of modalities such as computed tomography (CT) scanning and ultrasound. An upper right transverse abdominal incision allows access to explore the common bile duct and a Lanz incision allows appendicectomy, but neither wound allows a full laparotomy. It is unusual, except occasionally in management of the acute abdomen, to need an exploratory midline or right paramedian (the 'registrar's incision') to make or confirm a presumptive diagnosis (Fig. 19.1).

There must be no wound failures on closing an incision. Insecurity following an abdominal incision may result in burst abdomen or incisional hernia. Complications such as infection (including knots and wound sinuses) must be minimal. Finally, patients expect an acceptable cosmetic appearance of their healed wounds, without excessive or persistent pain.

The requirements of a laparotomy incision are as follows:

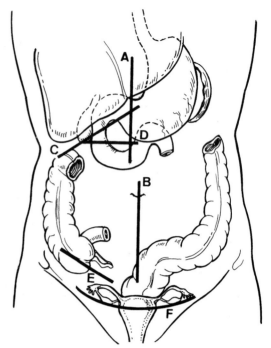

Fig. 19.1   Favoured laparotomy incisions: **A**, paramedian; **B**, midline; **C**, Kocher; **D**, transverse; **E**, Lanz; **F**, Pfannenstiel.

- Allow access
- Be secure
- Low complication rate
- Be pain free
- Cosmetic appearance.

Types of laparotomy incision

Laparotomy incisions can be broadly categorized as vertical or transverse, or as muscle cutting or muscle splitting. Many incisions used in the past with eponymous names have disappeared from modern use and there is a trend to use incisions placed cosmetically in Langer's lines which are usually transverse in type. There will never be a replacement for midline incisions, nor paramedian, particularly the lateral paramedian which is associated with a low wound failure rate.

Vertical incisions

Midline incisions allow rapid access to the abdominal cavity and are easily extended when necessary. When placed accurately through the linea alba they are associated with minimal bleeding and are quickly closed in a single layer using a mass technique. The peritoneum does not require closure. The skin incision may be placed through the umbilicus or curved around the umbilicus (banana incision). Undercutting the peri-umbilical skin should be avoided as it makes cosmetic closure more difficult.

Paramedian incisions are time honoured and have been recently popularized as a lateral variant which appears to give sound wounds and a low incisional hernia rate relating to the shutter mechanism (Fig. 19.2). They take longer to make and to close, and blood loss is more than in midline incisions, although probably not appreciably so.

Transverse incisions

These may be muscle cutting in type (e.g. the Kocher incision for cholecystectomy) or muscle splitting (e.g. the Lanz incision for appendicectomy). There is some evidence that they are associated with wound failures and less postoperative pain. Muscle-cutting incisions take more time to make and close, with more blood loss than midline incisions.

Complex incisions

These incisions afford access to specific sites for major procedures. They may be muscle cutting (the gable or roof-top incision for pancreatic operations), be extended into the chest (the left abdominothoracic incision for lower-third oesophagectomy) or be partly muscle split-ting (the extraperitoneal approach to the infrarenal abdominal aorta).

Retraction

Retraction must be adequate during laparotomy. Con-ventional retractors in abdominal surgery are the Deavers, Dyballs and Morris types, or the St Marks retractor for pelvic dissection, which require extra skilled assistants for most benefit. Specialized ring retractors (favoured for gynaecological and pelvic surgery) and sternal retractors (for mediastinal approaches to the heart) allow hands to be free. Self-retaining retractors are useful in more superficial surgery, such as the Joll for thyroid surgery, or the many types of clawed retrac-tor, such as the Travers, for inguinal surgery.

Lighting

Theatre lighting based on ceiling mounts offers focused, well-directed light for all procedures, particularly when experienced operating department assistants are avail-able. Sterile handles allow placement of satellite lighting by the operating surgeon. Head lighting or cold light sources are necessary for procedures when access is limited.

PRECAUTIONS AGAINST LOSS OF INSTRUMENTS OR SWABS

The following precautionary measures are essential:

1. Correctly organize instrument trays, limiting the number of individually packed instruments as far as possible.

2. Arrange swabs and packs in 'fives' bound together with red cotton or, if small, carefully packaged (e.g. on a safety pin).

3. Check the number of instruments on trays against printed lists incorporated in each pack.

4. Record all sutures, swabs, packs, needles and extras clearly and legibly on a board in the theatre.

5. Use of special swab racks, including the modern disposable wallets, which facilitate counting at the end of a long complex operation during which many swabs are used.

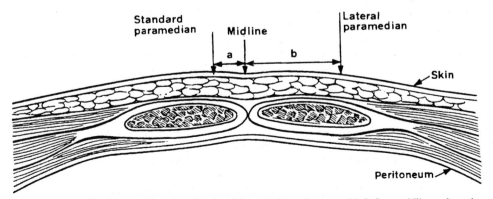

Fig. 19.2   Lateral and standard paramedian incisions *a* = 2 cm; *b* = two-thirds from midline to lateral rectus sheath.

6. Mark radio-opaque non-implantable non-metallic equipment such as drains and the laparomat.

7. The theatre record book must be signed by the scrubbed and assistant nurses.

8. You should record and sign that the count was correct at the end of the operation note in the patient's records.

The way to reduce errors is to establish a simple, well-disciplined routine of accountability, including a permanent and accurately maintained record.

LAPAROTOMY CLOSURE

The success of laparotomy closure depends on adequate technique, materials and avoidance of adverse factors, particularly infection. The closure of the musculoaponeurotic layers is traditionally performed in layers. Such closure is still necessary for closing paramedian incisions, and some surgeons prefer it for transverse incisions, but it is unnecessary (and not easily performed) for closing midline incisions.

Mass closure has been shown to have a low incidence of burst abdomen and can be undertaken for all midline and transverse incisions, but there appears to be no benefit in reducing the incidence of incisional hernia. The earliest described mass closures employed a far-and-near or figure-of-eight technique using interrupted sutures but simple over-and-over continuous sutures are easier to place, avoid excessive numbers of knots and are secure (Figs. 19.3 and 19.4).

Jenkins has shown that a wound length/suture length ratio of 1 : 4 should avoid wound dehiscence. This allows for the increased tension and increased effective length of vertical abdominal incisions during healing. This requires sutures to be placed 1 cm apart with at least 1 cm tissue bites, but is not so easy to achieve in layered closure without risking entering the peritoneal cavity with a second layer and the risk of damage to underlying viscera.

Using mass closure the viscera can be seen and protected with the non-dominant hand during suture. Cadaveric studies have reinforced that 1 cm bites are secure. There is also biochemical evidence that a 1 cm bite affords security because there is a zone of activity around a wound where collagen lysis prior to repair reduces the tissue integrity. Sutures placed within this zone (which widens with infection) are insecure. The tightness of abdominal wall closure has been shown to be important: too much risks later incisional hernias; too little risks burst abdomen.

Tension sutures cause cosmetically unacceptable scars and make the siting of stomas difficult. There is some

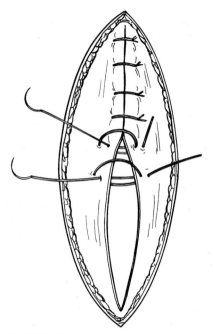

Fig. 19.3   Interrupted far and near mass closure: 1 cm bites, 1 cm apart.

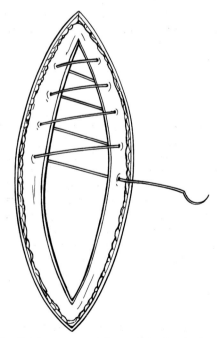

Fig. 19.4   Continuous over-and-over mass closure: 1 cm bites, 1 cm apart.

evidence that they are associated with more pain, but no evidence that wound closure is more secure with their use.

SKIN CLOSURE

Skin closure should be cosmetically acceptable, with avoidance of inversion of the edges, and should avoid infection, hypertrophic scars or keloid formation. Several techniques are available: continuous or interrupted, simple or mattress and subcuticular. All are acceptable, but the latter gives the best results.

Tape closure and clip sutures are associated with a low infection rate and also give good cosmetic results. The use of a polyurethane adhesive sheet dressing (Bioclusive, Opsite) over a sutured wound acts as a large tape closure, allowing easy inspection.

Cyanoacrylate skin adhesives are expensive and demand near-perfect haemostasis. There is no definite evidence that reducing dead space with subcuticular sutures or drains is either effective or prevents wound infection.

Undue tension must be avoided to allow postoperative swelling.

Sutures require removal at, as a working rule, 3–5 days (head and neck), 7 days (inguinal and upper limb), 10 days (other abdominal incisions, lower limb) and up to 14 days for dorsal incisions. Knots placed well to the side of the incision facilitate removal. Special instruments allow painless removal of clips (rapidly if necessary after thyroidectomy).

Langer's lines

These are low-tension lines in the skin and correspond to natural skin creases. If an incision crosses them at right angles then there is a risk that resultant scars become hypertrophic and cosmetically unacceptable. Whenever possible, therefore, Langer's lines should be followed for incisions. When these lines have to be crossed for surgical access, particularly in operations on small joints, for example, then skin crease lines should be crossed obliquely or incisions employing Z-plasties or an S-shape should be planned.

Plantar of Finger Oblique

Hypertrophic skin scars

These show a proliferation of scar tissue, but this stays within the boundaries of the wound and not beyond it as keloids do. They tend to occur in scars around joints and in areas of skin tension. With the passage of time they become avascular and may regress to form a white, stretched, widened scar.

Contractures

These should not be confused with the normal process of wound contraction. Contractures follow delayed wound healing and occur after infection and inadequate treatment of burns in particular. Deep burns which are not excised are prone to contracture. Established contractures can be released by plasty incisions, excised and covered with split-thickness grafts or with transposition flaps.

Keloids

These are formed by abnormal collagen metabolism and result in a proliferation of scar tissue beyond the boundaries of the original wound. They occur in dorsal areas of the body and over the face and deltopectoral region. Keloids occur in dark-skinned people and may be encouraged to form as a cultural body decoration.

Excision of keloids is almost always followed by a more exuberant recurrence. X-rays have been used but topical steroid creams or steroid injections are more definitely effective. Pressure on an excised keloid can prevent recurrence, a useful example being the use of a clip or peg on an earlobe that has developed a keloid after piercing for earrings.

CHEST INCISIONS

There are three principal routes into the chest.

Lateral thoracotomy

This may be anterior or posterior in approach or a combination. An anterior approach, through the 4th rib space, allows access for transaxillary sympathectomy, and a posterior approach, through the 6th rib space, allows access to the lung; a combination gives access to the whole pleural cavity for pulmonary or on the left-side oesophageal surgery. This latter incision is made in the 6th or 7th rib interspace or the rib bed starting medial to the nipple, passing 2–3 cm under the scapula, then turning superiorly between the scapula and midline. Muscles are divided using diathermy, the pectoralis major anteriorly then latissimus dorsi, serratus anterior and the rhomboids. Once the scapula is raised the periosteum of the selected rib can be incised with diathermy, then elevated. There is no need to remove the rib, but division at the neck facilitates insertion of a rib-spreader to give access.

Chest closure requires pleural drainage with an apical chest drain connected to an underwater seal. A basal drain may be added. Drains should be removed as soon as the pneumothorax is evacuated (after transaxillary sympathectomy) or after a few days, depending on the amount of drainage or need to ensure pleurodesis. Chest closure is effected in layers using a rib approximator using 00 non-absorbable polypropylene (Prolene) or absorbable polyglactin (Vicryl) material. The inter-costals are approximated and the serratus anterior and latissimus dorsi are closed separately. Skin closure is the same as for laparotomy closure.

Thoracoabdominal incision

This is used when access is needed urgently following trauma, and electively for wide exposure of the liver and kidney (on the right) or spleen, oesophagogastric junction and kidney (on the left). Access may be allowed to the great vessels between chest and abdomen. The incision runs obliquely from the midline in the epi-gastrium in line with the 9th or 10th rib. The incision is muscle cutting in the abdomen, the muscles being divided over the ribs, and is extended to the anterior or midaxillary line.

Median sternotomy

This allows access to the pericardium, the heart and great vessels in the chest. It is made strictly in the midline from the suprasternal notch to the xiphoid. The sternal periosteum is divided with diathermy and the rectus muscles split in the midline before inserting a finger into the mediastinum, above and below, and behind the sternum. The anaesthetist should keep the lungs in expiration while the sternum is divided using a power or Gigli saw.

Closure requires strong monofilament non-absorb-able sutures (stainless steel wire or Nylon) together with drainage of the pericardium and deep to the sternum.

SURGICAL DRESSINGS

The last 30 years have seen an increased depth of under-standing of wound-healing processes and many dress-ings are being manufactured to provide the requirements of the ideal wound environment. There is no clear-cut evidence, however, that wounds should be left open with a dry surface and a fibrinous coagulum, which seals the wound, or whether they should be covered (and hidden from view). Exuding wounds are at risk of secondary infection and may not be protected by a dressing. If covered by an absorptive dressing, pathogenic organisms

---

> **Box 19.1**
> The ideal surgical dressing (which does not exist)
>
> - Absorbent and able to remove excess exudate
> - Maintain moist environment and aid own tissues to debride necrotic material and promote healing
> - Prevent trauma to underlying healing granulation tissue or to prevent shed of foreign particles into the wound
> - Be leakproof and prevent strike-through and sec-ondary infection
> - Maintain temperature and gaseous change
> - Allow simple dressing changes, easy, less frequent application and removal, and be pain free
> - Be odourless, cosmetically acceptable and comfor-table
> - Not be expensive

can track through a soiled wet dressing from its surface (strike-through). The requirements of an ideal surgical dressing are listed in Box 19.1. Some of their require-ments are theoretical, but many are based on sound experimental evidence. The armamentarium of modern surgical dressings is mainly directed at management of chronic open wounds such as venous leg ulcers.

Polyurethane incise drapes have become popularized as a primary wound dressing for sutured wounds and skin donor sites. They maintain moisture which enhances epithelial closure, and allow easy inspection and aspiration of excessive exudate. On donor sites they are claimed to relieve pain. They are gas and water-vapour permeable but excessive maceration risks sec-ondary infection, although the dressings are imper-meable to organisms. More traditional wound dressings include Melolin or non-adherent sheet dressings which require a secondary pad dressing if there is excessive exudate.

For open wounds such as a healing pilonidal sinus cavity or a superficially dehisced, infected abdominal wound we are spoilt for choice. The moulded polymeric Silastic form dressing is ideal, allowing pain-free wound care, by the patient if necessary. Other bead and powder dressings may be equally useful; they absorb exudate and maintain the moist environment (examples are Debrisan, Iodosorb and Intrasite). Sheet polymeric dressings are reserved for more superficial open wounds. They may be fully occlusive (Comfeel Ulcer Dressing or Granuflex) or semiocclusive (Geliperm) or with a biological source (the alginates Kaltostat or Sorbsan). The list of dressings increases, and satisfactory trials are required to show their merit and comparative relative worth.

PRINCIPLES OF WOUND MANAGEMENT

An operation is a responsibility to be undertaken with informed consent of the patient and should be performed in the most optimal circumstances. This should be tailored with management of the intercurrent illness, nutrition, the need for resuscitation and prophylaxis against infection and phlebothrombosis. Surgery is based on ritual and it is difficult to measure the quality of operative surgery, although we achieve much through audit, and morbidity and mortality meetings.

Lord Moynihan taught that an operation should start with a clean sweep of the knife. Techniques of aseptic procedures and swab and instrument counts are easy to teach. Gentle handling of tissues is more difficult to learn – some surgeons in training find it comes naturally, whereas others take time to be able to oppose cut tissues perfectly without undue suture tension. It is logical to secure haemostasis in surgical wounds; it is poor technique that leads to a wound needing resuture or evacuation of a haematoma. Excessive use of diathermy or the failure to avoid dead space are signs of poor surgery, but evidence to show impaired healing or increased infection risk is hard to prove. The use of drains to evacuate dead space, 'protect' against the consequences of an anastomotic leak or to remove fluid collections or body fluids effectively is a classical example of an ingrained surgical technique which again still needs clear scientific evidence that it works.

FURTHER READING

Anonymous 1986 Dressings for ulcers. Drug and Therapeutics Bulletin 24: 9–12

Cox P J, Ausobsky J R, Ellis H, Pollock A V 1986 Towards no incisional hernias: lateral paramedian versus midline incisions. Journal of the Royal Society of Medicine 79: 711–712

Harland R N L, Irving M H 1988 Surgical drains. Surgery 1: 1360–1362

Jenkins T P N 1976 The burst abdominal wound: a mechanical approach. British Journal of Surgery 63: 873–876

Leaper D J 1985 Laparotomy closure. British Journal of Hospital Medicine 33: 317–322

Leaper D J 1992 Local effects of trauma and wound healing. In: Burnand K G, Young A E (eds) Ian Aird's companion to surgical studies. Churchill Livingstone, Edinburgh, ch 2, p 27–35

Leaper D J 1992 Surgical factors influencing infection. In: Taylor E W (ed) Infection in surgical practice. Oxford University Press, Oxford, ch 3, p 18–27

Leaper D J, Foster M E 1990 Wound healing and abdominal wound closure. In: Taylor I (ed) Progress in surgery. Churchill Livingstone, Edinburgh, vol 3, ch 2, p 19–31

Lucarotti M E, Billings P J, Leaper D J 1991 Laparotomy, wound closure and repair of incisional hernia. Surgery. 10: 1–6

Wadstrom J, Gerdin B 1990 Closure of the abdominal wall: how and why. Acta Chirurgica Scandinavica 156: 75–82

20. Minimal access surgery

A. Darzi   C. Fowler

'Diseases that harm call for treatments that harm less.'
William Osler

Minimal access surgery is a marriage of modern technology and surgical innovation which aims to accomplish surgical therapeutic goals with minimal somatic and psychological trauma. Technology is often blamed by those who claim to detect a deterioration in the doctor–patient relationship and is frequently cited as a major cause of the upward spiral of health-care costs. Although these are valid concerns, the properly controlled development of minimal access surgery with well-considered pre- and postoperative management offers benefits, including cost benefits, without sacrificing the quality of care of the patient as a whole individual. Minimal access techniques are less invasive, less disabling and less disfiguring. With increasing experience it offers cost-effectiveness to both health services and employers by shortening operating times, shortening hospital stays and allowing faster recuperation. State of the art video recording can help communication, bring the patient and family closer to the process, improve clinical decision-making and enhance rapport.

NOMENCLATURE

The urologists Wickham and Fitzpatrick (1990) who were instrumental in highlighting the need for techniques which reduced therapeutic and surgical trauma advocated the term 'minimally invasive therapy', but there remains much debate about the most accurate title for this new discipline (Box 20.1). Cuschieri (1992), argues that this terminology is inappropriate because it inaccurately implies increased safety, a connotation which is fallacious because there is no correlation between invasiveness and risk. The most important argument against the use of this terminology is that it fails to emphasize the essential attribute of the approach which is the reduction of surgical trauma. The alter-

---

Box 20.1
Minimal access surgery: nomenclature

- Endoscopic surgery
- Laparoscopic surgery
- Keyhole surgery
- Minimally invasive surgery
- Minimal access surgery

---

native terminology minimal access surgery (MAS) is more accurate and descriptive (Cuschieri 1992).

Technology has effectively miniaturized our eyes and extended our hands to perform microscopic and macroscopic operations in places which formerly could be reached only with large incisions. It has also provided new ways to look at tissues, using light, sound waves and magnetic fields which can detect disease and guide therapy (Darzi et al 1993). These same technologies, more highly focused and used at much higher power, can also be used to give highly controlled resection and tissue destruction. It is vital that surgeons understand the principles of these devices so that they can help to shape the future development of minimal access surgery and not become the servants of the machines they use.

BOUNDARIES OF MINIMAL ACCESS SURGERY

Minimal access surgery has crossed all traditional boundaries of specialities and disciplines. Shared, borrowed and overlapping technologies and information are encouraging a multidisciplinary approach which serves the whole patient rather than a specific organ system. Broadly speaking, minimal access techniques can be categorized as follows:

Laparoscopy. A rigid endoscope is introduced through a metal sleeve into the peritoneal cavity which has been inflated with a carbon dioxide pneumoperitoneum. There is little doubt that laparoscopic cholecystectomy has revolutionized the surgical man-agement of cholelithiasis and has become the mainstay of management of uncomplicated gallstone disease. With improved instruments and more experience, it is likely that other advanced procedures, currently regarded as controversial, will also become fully accepted.

Thoracoscopy. A rigid endoscope is introduced through an incision in the chest to gain access to the thoracic contents. Many feel that the benefits of thoracoscopy will prove to be even greater than those of laparoscopy.

Endoluminal endoscopy. Flexible or rigid endo-scopes are introduced into hollow organs or systems, such as the urinary tract, upper or lower gastrointestinal tract, respiratory and vascular systems.

Perivisceral endoscopy. Body planes can be accessed even in the absence of a natural cavity. Examples are mediastinoscopy, retroperitoneoscopy and retroperitoneal approaches to the kidney, aorta and lumbar sympathetic chain. Other more recent examples include subfascial ligation of incompetent perforators in varicose vein surgery.

Arthroscopy and intra-articular joint surgery. Orthopaedic surgeons have long used arthroscopic access to the knee and have now moved their attention to other joints, including the shoulder, wrist, elbow and hip.

Combined approach. The diseased organ is vis-ualized and treated using an assortment of endoluminal and extraluminal endoscopes and other imaging devices.

SURGICAL TRAUMA IN OPEN AND LAPAROSCOPIC SURGERY

Most of the trauma of an open procedure is inflicted because the surgeon must have a wound large enough to give adequate exposure for safe dissection at the target site. The wound is often the cause of morbidity, including infection, dehiscence, bleeding, herniation and nerve entrapment. The pain of the wound prolongs recovery time and by reducing mobility, contributes to an increased incidence of pulmonary collapse, chest infection and deep venous thrombosis.

Mechanical and human retractors cause additional trauma. Body wall retractors tend to inflict localized damage which may be as painful as the wound itself. By contrast, during laparoscopy, the body wall is retracted by the low pressure pneumoperitoneum giving a diffuse force applied gently and evenly over the whole body wall, causing minimal trauma.

Exposure of any body cavity to the atmosphere also causes morbidity through cooling and fluid loss by the evaporation of body fluid. There is also evidence from the literature to suggest that the incidence of postsurgical adhesions have been reduced by the use of the lapa-roscope because there is less damage to delicate serosal coverings. In handling intestinal loops the surgeon and assistant disturb the peristaltic activity of the gut and provoke adynamic ileus.

In minimal access surgery the trauma of access and exposure are reduced, while visualization is magnified and improved.

DISADVANTAGES OF MINIMAL ACCESS SURGERY

To perform minimal access surgery with safety, the surgeon must operate remote from the surgical field using an imaging system which provides a two-dimen-sional representation of the operative site. The endo-scope offers a whole new anatomical landscape which the surgeon must learn to navigate without the usual cues which make it easy to judge depth. The instruments are longer and sometimes more complex to use than those common in open surgery. The result of all this is that the beginner in minimal access surgery is faced with significant problems of hand–eye coordination. Stereo-scopic imaging for laparoscopy is still in its infancy. Future improvements in these systems will greatly enhance manipulative ability in critical procedures such as knot tying and dissection of closely underlying tissues. There are, however, some drawbacks, such as reduced display brightness and interference with normal vision due to the need to wear glasses. It is probable that brighter projection displays will be developed, at increased cost. However, the need to wear glasses will not be easily overcome. Looking further to the future, it is evident that the continuing reduction in costs of elaborate image-processing techniques will make a wide range of transformed presentations available. It will ulti-mately be possible for a surgeon to call up any view of the operative region that is accessible to a camera and present it stereoscopically in any size or orientation, superimposed on past images taken in other modalities. It is for the medical community to decide which of these many imaginative possibilities will contribute most to effective surgical procedures.

Another problem occurs when there is intraoperative arterial bleeding. Haemostasis may be very difficult to achieve endoscopically because blood obscures the field of vision and there is a significant reduction of the image quality due to light absorption.

Some of the procedures performed by this new approach are more technically demanding and are slower to perform. Indeed, on occasions a minimally invasive operation is so technically demanding that both patent and surgeon are better served by conversion to an open procedure. Unfortunately, there seems to be a sense of embarrassment or humiliation associated with conversion, which is quite unjustified. It is vital for surgeons and patients to appreciate that the decision to go for an open operation is not a complication, but rather usually implies sound surgical judgement.

Another disadvantage of laparoscopic surgery is the loss of tactile feedback. Laparoscopic ultrasonography might substitute the need 'to feel' in intraoperative decision-making. Although ultrasonography has progressed significantly in the past several years, laparoscopic ultrasound remains in its infancy. The rapid progress in advanced laparoscopic techniques, including biliary tract exploration and surgery for malignancies, has provided a strong impetus for the development of laparoscopic ultrasound. Although incompletely developed, laparoscopic ultrasound already offers advantages that far outweigh its disadvantages (Box 20.2).

In more advanced techniques the large piece of resected tissue, such as the lung or colon, has to be extracted from the body cavity (Monson et al 1992). Occasionally, the extirpated tissue may be removed through a nearby natural orifice, such as the rectum or the mouth. At other times a novel route may be employed. For instance, a benign colonic specimen may be extracted through an incision in the vault of the vagina. Although tissue 'morcellators, mincers and liquidizers' could be used in some circumstances, this has the disadvantage of reducing the amount of information available to the pathologist. Recent reports of tumour implantation in the sites of portholes has raised important questions about the future of the laparoscopic treatment of malignancy.

There is growing need for improvement in dissection techniques in laparoscopic surgery, and specifically of improving the safe use of electrocautery and lasers. Ultrasonic dissection and tissue removal has been utilized by a growing number of specialities for several years. The adaptation of the technology to laparoscopic surgery grew out of the search for alternative, possibly safer, methods of dissection. The current units combine the functions of three or four separate instruments, reducing the need for instrument exchanges during a procedure. This flexibility, combined with the ability to provide a clean, smoke-free field, improves safety while shortening operating times.

Although dramatic cost savings are possible with laparoscopic cholecystectomy the position is less clear-cut with other procedures. There is another factor which may complicate the computation of cost versus benefit. A significant rise in the rate of cholecystectomy followed the introduction of the laparoscopic approach as the threshold for referring patients for surgery lowered. The increase in the number of procedures performed has led to an overall increase in the cost of treating symptomatic gallstones.

TRAINING FOR MINIMAL ACCESS SURGERY

It is probably true to say that no previous surgical innovation has aroused so much public questioning of how surgeons are trained. While the pioneers of a new technique are inevitably self-trained, there comes a time when patients rightly demand that all those who offer a new technique have had proper training to perform it safely and effectively. This is particularly so in laparoscopic surgery, which employs skills that are not commonly used in everyday life.

The importance of training in minimal access surgery has been recognized with the establishment of several training centres dedicated to teaching the fundamentals of safe minimal access surgery. These centres, including the Minimal Access Therapy Training Unit (MATTU) at The Royal College of Surgeons of England, are working to develop training methods using various forms of simulation which will allow surgeons to complete a significant part of their skills training before they begin to operate on patients. The sophistication of these simulation techniques seems likely to increase with the development of virtual-reality machines, which will generate an artificial environment in which the surgeon can practise with complete safety.

Box 20.2
Advantages of laparoscopic ultrasound

- Substitutes for the sense of touch
- Allows visualization through tubular fluid-filled and solid organs as well as vascular structures
- Permits differentiation of solid and cystic masses
- Allows evaluation of the wall layers of hollow viscera
- Allows evaluation of the dimensions, infiltration and dissemination of tumours for better staging
- Helps formulate an optimal surgical plan
- Avoids unnecessary tissue dissection
- Allows guided biopsies
- Easily performed, safe, and economic
- Does not use ionizing radiation or contrast media
- Can be employed at any time during surgery
- Can be used during pregnancy
- Has no contraindications

THE FUTURE

Although there is no doubt that minimal access surgery has changed the practice of surgeons, it has not changed the nature of disease. The basic principles of good surgery still apply, including appropriate case selection, excellent exposure, adequate retraction and a high level of technical expertise. If a procedure makes no sense with conventional access, it will make no sense with a minimal access approach.

Improvements in instrumentation and the development of structured training programmes are the key to the future of minimal access surgery. It is certain that there is much that is new in minimal access surgery. Time will tell how much of what is new is truly better.

'The cleaner and gentler the act of operation, the less the patient suffers, the smoother and quicker his convalescence, the more exquisite his healed wound.'

Lord Moynihan of Leeds

REFERENCES

Cuschieri A 1992 A rose by any other name: minimal access or minimally invasive surgery. Surgical Endoscopy 6: 214

Darzi A, Goldin R, Guillou P J, Monson J R T 1993 Extracorporeal shock wave thermotherapy. new antitumour option. Surgical Oncology 2: 197–204

Monson J R T, Darzi A, Carey P D, Guillou P J 1992 Prospective evaluation of laparoscopic assisted colectomy in an unselected group of patients. Lancet 340: 831–833

Nduka C, Monson J R T, Darzi A 1994 Abdominal wall metastases following laparoscopic surgery. British Journal of Surgery 81: 648–652

Nduka C, Super P, Monson J R T, Darzi A 1994 Cause and prevention of electrosurgical injury in laparoscopic surgery. Journal of the American College of Surgeons 179: 161–179

Wickham J, Fitzpatrick J M 1990 Minimally invasive surgery [editorial] British Journal of Surgery 77: 721

21. Principles of skin cover

D. Davies

Wound healing is the restoration of anatomic integrity and function of an injured tissue. In humans, regeneration of normal cellular elements is limited to epithelium and liver and most wound healing and repair results in scarring. You should understand the basic science and physiology of wound healing. The cellular sequences of repair and their controlling factors are not discussed in this chapter.

If a wound is debrided (originally meaning 'unbridling' or 'releasing', but now meaning 'excision') of nonviable tissue and repaired in a physiological manner, normal phases of wound healing should proceed without difficulty. Disturbances of wound healing can be attributed to the patient and/or the surgeon. Often the disturbances that prevent ideal wound healing are due to the surgical techniques used in wound repair and not to the patient. There can, however, be both systemic and local causes for delayed wound healing.

When you are faced with the closure of a wound you should return to first principles. Take a history from the patient, not only of how and when the wound occurred, as to whether it is a clean incised wound or contaminated and crushed, but also enquire about the general condition of the patient. Is their diabetes well controlled, are they malnourished or taking cytotoxic or anti-inflammatory agents?

Examine not only the local wound to ascertain the viability of local tissues, but also take into account damage to other structures. In particular, in the face area detect whether there is a fracture of the underlying facial bones, damage to vital structures such as the eye, facial nerve and also the parotid duct. These often can only be diagnosed preoperatively and not at the time of exploration. Lastly, carry out investigations, including wound swabs, where indicated, X-rays for bony fractures, proceeding occasionally to CT scans.

PRINCIPLES OF WOUND MANAGEMENT

Evaluate any wound considered for closure for the level of necrotic tissue, debris and bacterial contamination. Necrotic tissue requires sharp debridement. Irrigation will aid in the removal of foreign bodies, and pulsating jet lavage is an improved modification. Bacterial contamination can be measured by taking a wound biopsy and bacterial quantities exceeding 100 000 organisms per gram of tissue in general prevent the take of skin grafts and primary wound healing. Manage such contamination by excision/debridement, with or without topical antibacterial agents. Systemic antibiotics have little local effect when dead tissue persists or if there is excessive thick granulation.

Surgical debridement is the poorest performed operation by junior hospital doctors, but it is the key to reaching bacterial balance. If there is any doubt about the viability of tissue then a second-look policy should be undertaken 24–48 hours later. This can be repeated several times until there is absolutely no doubt that what is left in the wound is alive and viable and not seriously contaminated by bacteria. Only when this is achieved can effective wound closure be obtained.

Closure of acute wounds may be divided into primary, delayed primary, secondary and tertiary. In *primary healing* the wound is usually closed by direct approximation of the wound edges without tension. Larger defects may be closed by skin grafts or flaps. In general, traumatic injuries should be closed primarily, if appropriate.

In *secondary healing* the wound is left open and allowed to heal spontaneously. Spontaneous wound closure is a process of wound contraction and epithelialization from the edges. Usually, granulation tissue develops in the middle of this which consists usually of inflammatory cells, bacteria and the proliferation of capillaries in a fibrous network. There are a number of options allowing the closure of this granulating wound. You may simply allow healing by second intention to continue, or scrape off the granulation and cover it with a split thickness skin graft.

Tertiary or delayed wound healing is closure of the wound by active intervention after a delay of several days to weeks, but obviously only wounds that are in bacterial balance should be closed in this way.

If a wound is left open then topical agents and dressings may be required. An open contaminated wound may benefit from a topical antimicrobial agent, but once a wound is closed topical antimicrobial agents will have no function and may lead to topical sensitivity. A dressing serves to protect the wound from additional bacterial contamination and further injury. An absorptive gauze allows exudate to be trapped in the gauze away from the skin, and occlusive dressings prevent dehydration of the wound, thus enhancing epithelialization. Lastly, a well-executed dressing will be more psychologically impressive to the patient and observers.

PRIMARY CLOSURE

Wound edges should be accurately opposed to permit healing. There should be no skin edge step off and they should not be so tightly approximated that oedema causes further ischaemia to the edges of the wound. The major strength in the skin is in the dermis and the collagen fibres in the dermis will give the wound its tensile strength. Good approximation of the dermis is therefore vital. Sutures placed in fat generally cause necrosis and serve as a foreign body and a nidus for infection. The fascia has sufficient collagen to permit approximation with sutures, but underlying muscle will not support sutures. Thus the best closure of a wound extending through muscle includes good approximation of the fascia and dermis. A buried dermal closure with an inverted suture will place the knot in the depth of the wound and minimize the likelihood of its erosion to the surface and the formation of a stitch abscess. Except in the face where accurate epidermal skin edge approximation is required, interrupted cutaneous sutures are very rarely indicated.

The epidermis in the face can be approximated with a non-absorbable suture such as nylon which will best approximate the wound edges accurately. These sutures should be removed prior to invasion by epithelium into the suture holes. The density of the dermal appendages in the area will determine the timing of the suture removal.

In areas such as the face, which has a high density of dermal appendages, suture track marks may occur when the stitches are left in place for as little as 4 days. Areas such as the palmar and plantar surfaces have such a low density of dermal appendages that the sutures may be left in place for as long as 3 weeks.

If there is loss of skin then it may not be possible to approximate the wound edges, even if the skin is undermined for a short distance. Reconstruction of the skin cover will therefore be required and a ladder of reconstruction is presented. The second rung of the ladder following primary suture is skin grafting.

SKIN GRAFTS

A skin graft is the transfer of a segment of skin which has been totally separated from its blood supply. All skin grafts initially adhere to the recipient bed by fibrin, which must be vascular enough to support the metabolism of the graft. The thinner the graft the less nutrition it requires and the more likely it is to take. Within 48 hours capillaries will grow in from the underlying bed into the graft, a process known as *inosculation*, and the graft becomes vascularized.

Skin grafts are of two types. The workhorses of reconstruction are split thickness skin grafts, but on the face in particular, where a more cosmetic reconstruction is required, full thickness skin grafts are often employed. Remember that a donor site for a partial thickness skin graft will always leave a cosmetic abnormality and thus, particularly in a young patient, skin should be taken from the buttock whenever practical rather than the thigh.

Since a graft must derive its new vascularity from the recipient bed, some general observations may be made.

1. Skin grafts should do well on well vascularized non-infected wounds, clean granulation tissue or wounds created following the excision of tissue. Irregular or less well vascularized surfaces such as fat are less predictable.

2. Grafts do not require pressure, but they do require immobilization and thus patient cooperation is required.

3. The best results are accomplished when the donor tissue matches the recipient bed in texture and colour.

4. Avascular wounds such as bone without periosteal cover, tendon without peritenon, denuded cartilage and irradiated wounds are incapable of nourishing a graft.

5. Heavy contamination by microorganisms is an important cause of graft loss. Usually this is because the fibrin is degraded by the fibrinolytic cascade initiated by the presence of large amount of bacteria and quantities exceeding 100 000 organisms per gram of tissue frequently results in the non-take of grafts.

6. Grafts can survive on plasma through which oxygen and nutrients can diffuse, but grafts cannot survive on blood clot. Pressure may help prevent seroma/haematoma formation and will also help immobilize

the graft. Immobilizing some areas of the body is notoriously difficult (e.g. the back), and in such areas graft failure is common.

If the patient is cooperative, if the wound is appropriate for a graft, if the wound has been properly prepared, if the grafting is performed accurately and if the postoperative management is conducted well, then a skin graft will always take. Every surgeon should be capable of harvesting a partial thickness skin graft, either by a dermatome, or using a protected skin graft blade (e.g. a Humby knife or later modifications by Watson and Cobett). Acquire this skill by practising on a cadaver. Also be aware of the fact that in many instances meshing the skin graft will allow both expansion of the graft and also an increased chance of take by allowing seroma to escape between the perforations.

Be aware of the long-term management of a skin graft. Provide external support to a graft on the lower limb by using Tubigrip and apply creams for dry, pruritic donor sites and grafts. Later, prevent hypertrophic scarring by the use of Jobst pressure garments.

Full thickness skin grafts are used commonly on the head and neck area, particularly the eyelids and nose. The principles that apply for the successful take of a partial thickness skin graft apply even more to a full thickness skin graft, as the metabolic requirements of a full thickness skin graft are relatively greater. Postoperatively, a full thickness skin graft usually provides a better cosmetic match and is less likely to contract.

SKIN FLAPS

If a wound bed is avascular, such that it is unlikely to be able to support a skin graft, then skin that retains its blood supply has to be used to cover a wound. This is the definition of a skin flap.

Random pattern flaps

One of the several functions of skin is temperature regulation and thus skin has a blood supply many times in excess of its metabolic requirements. Skin can be designed as a flap and survives being nourished through its base or pedicle. In a random pattern flap there is no specific blood vessel in the pedicle, the flap being nourished by the dermal plexus. Experience shows that, provided the length of the flap is not greater than 1.5–2 times the width of its base, then it should survive. Random flaps are not new – Sushruta in the Samhita in India used such flaps for nasal reconstruction in about 600 BC. Random flaps can be based on the geometry of 2 : 1 and can be used to fill a local defect, either by

rotation, advancement, transposition, V–Y advancement or Z-plasty.

This geometric design obviously presented limitations in covering larger skin defects, which could only be covered by using a tube pedicle. A tube pedicle was a method of designing a much larger flap which in fact was two random pattern flaps joined together in the middle. One end of the tube was then divided and attached to the wrist and by a process of 'delay' which encouraged the blood supply to develop from the other end of the flap, the flap could be waltzed round the body attached to the wrist. Unfortunately, in general it took 6 months to complete the procedure, and 50% of flaps never completely covered the defect they were designed for.

Axial

Towards the end of the 1960s, McGregor and his colleagues in Glasgow questioned why flaps in the groin area and forehead could be safely designed 4–5 times as long as the base and commonly survive. They found that the skin in the groin area is supplied by a specific blood vessel (the superficial circumflex iliac artery) and, provided this artery with its accompanying venae commitans is included in the base of the flap and not damaged, then a skin flap can be raised on a very narrow pedicle right out over the most lateral part of the iliac crest. The groin flap was introduced into reconstructive surgery in the early 1970s and was a major breakthrough. It was soon recognized, however, that there were only a few other axial pattern flaps in the body, e.g. the deltopectoral flap (on the chest) based on the perforating vessels of the internal mammary artery, and the forehead flap based on the anterior branch of the superficial temporal artery.

Myocutaneous flaps

Following further investigations in the postmortem room it became apparent that skin in large areas of the body is supplied by blood vessels which come through from the underlying muscles. The rediscovery of the latissimus dorsi myocutaneous flap by Olivari in Germany and the further discovery of other myocutaneous and muscle flaps (the important ones being the latissimus dorsi, pectoralis major, rectus abdominus, tensor fascia lata, gluteus maximus, and gastrocnemius) allowed a vast expansion in reconstruction.

The principle of a myocutaneous flap is that the skin overlying a muscle will survive provided the pedicle to the muscle, which is usually a dominant vessel at one end, is not divided. Thus a paddle of muscle with overlying skin can be rotated over an arc of 360° to cover a local skin defect.

Fascial flaps

Further investigations into the blood supply of skin, particularly in the limbs where the muscles tend to be long and narrow, show that perforating vessels come between the muscles and supply a vascular plexus just superficial to the deep fascia. Thus if the fascia is included together with the perforating vessel in the skin flap, then long flaps, much greater than the original random patterned 2 : 1 can safely be raised. These are fasciocutaneous flaps, and are of particular importance in repairing skin defects on the lower limb, where they can be based either proximally or even distally.

Free flaps

Despite the wealth of flaps available, two problem areas remain for the closure of large wounds. These are the top of the head and the lower third of the leg. In the late 1970s, microvascular surgery (i.e. the repair of small blood vessels below 1–2 mm in diameter) became a practical proposition, although Carrel had been able to undertake successful anastomoses of small blood vessels experimentally in the early part of this century. This ability to join blood vessels, however, allows the pedicle of axial and myocutaneous flaps to be divided and the vessels reanastomosed to local blood vessels, adjacent to the wound on the head or lower leg. This is the basis of so-called 'free flaps' and is the top rung of our ladder of reconstruction.

SUMMARY

When confronted with a skin wound, take a history, examine the wound and institute appropriate investigations before considering closure. The surgical principles are straightforward:

1. A dirty wound must be converted first into a clean wound. The scalpel is mightier than any antibiotic. Once there is gross contamination by bacteria, wound closure cannot be safely obtained until the balance of the wound is improved.

2. Convert a clean open wound to a closed wound by using the surgical ladder of reconstruction. Start with the simplest method (either primary or delayed primary closure). Where there is skin loss or excessive tension, a skin graft should be employed. However, when the bed is avascular and will not support a skin graft, skin flips will have to be used, starting with the simplest random pattern flap through to larger and safer axial and myocutaneous flaps, and lastly, in the very occasional difficult wound, a free flap.

22. Transplantation

P. McMaster   L. J. Buist

BASIC PRINCIPLES

Early Christian legends attest to the attempts by man to replace diseased or destroyed organs or tissues by the transfer from another individual. The father of modern surgery, John Hunter, carried out extensive experiments on the transposition of tissues and concluded what he thought were successful experiments on the transposition of teeth! However, it was not until the dawn of the twentieth century that the practical technical realities of organ transfer were combined with sufficient understanding of the immunological mechanisms involved to allow transplantation to become a practical reality.

While it had long been recognized that successful blood transfusion was in large measure dependent on matching donor and recipient cells, it was only in the 1950s that Mitchison (1953) demonstrated that, while cell-mediated immunity was responsible for early destruction and rejection, it was the humoral mechanism with cytotoxic antibodies that was primarily involved in the host response to foreign tissue. It became increasingly recognized that all tissue and fluid transfer was governed by basic immunomechanisms (Box 22.1).

The need in the Second World War to find improved ways of treating badly burned pilots led Gibson & Medawar (1943) to carry out a series of classic experiments on skin transplantation. They were able to conclude that the transfer of skin from one part of the body to another in the same individual (an *autograft*), survived indefinitely, whereas the transfer of skin from another individual (an *allograft*) was in due course destroyed and that the recipient retained memory of the donor tissue and further transfers or allografts were destroyed in an accelerated mechanism. Thus the wider recognition of the universal acceptance of autografts became realized, whereas the failure of an allograft was recognized as part of an immune response. An alternative source of organs is, of course, the animal world, and the transfer from another species is known as a *xenograft*.

FIRST CLINICAL PROGRAMMES

The recognition that an autograft would be universally acceptable led to the first successful attempts at organ grafting in man. In the early 1950s, Murray et al (1955) at the Peter Bent Brigham Hospital in Boston, were able to demonstrate the successful transfer of a kidney graft from an identical twin with acceptance and successful function, and to develop a programme of renal transplantation between monozygotic twins. Living related organ transfer continues to be the most successful form of grafting without the need to alter the recipient's immune mechanism, as it fails to recognize the donor tissue as foreign.

Some of the recipients of kidney transplants from identical twins remained well more than 30 years after grafting. However, grafts between unrelated living individuals performed by this same group invariably failed, although not as quickly as experimental studies might have suggested.

RESPONSE

The other major human source of organs, other than from living relatives, is from individuals who have died as a result of road traffic accidents or cerebral injuries. Cadaveric organ grafting from non-related individuals is now the major source of organs. Within Europe, more than 90% of all organs transplanted are from brain-dead donors.

Thus, although technical considerations presented the initial formidable barrier to organ transfer, it was increasingly the understanding of the immune response causing organ destruction by rejection which led to clinical schedules permitting practical transplantation services to be established. The body's immune response to destroy the invading organ we now recognize as *rejection*.

REJECTION

Early experimental studies involving tissue transfer suggested genetic regulation of the rejection process. It was suggested in the 1930s that rejection was a response to specific foreign antigens (alloantigens) and that they were similar to blood groups of other species. The development of inbred lines of experimental animal models allowed the demonstration of antigens present on red blood cells and the concept of histocompatability. This suggestion of an immunological theory of tissue transplantation stimulated Medawar's (1944) work in rabbits and later in mice, and led to similar studies in man with the discovery of the human leucocyte antigen (HLA) system.

Further experimental studies defined the concept of rejection into three primary categories: *hyperacute rejection*, which can occur in a matter of hours due to preformed antibodies in a sensitized recipient; *acute rejection*, which takes place in a few days or weeks and is usually caused by cellular mechanisms; and *chronic rejection*, which occurs over months or years and remains largely undefined, but involves primarily humoral antibodies. A detailed review of experimental and modern transplantation biology is quite beyond the scope of this chapter, but increasing understanding of this area will allow more refined changes in rejection management and increasingly successful organ grafting.

AVOIDING REJECTION

The degree of disparity between donor and recipient is an important key element in the severity of the immune rejection response. In xenografting (transfer between species) the presence of preformed antibodies leads to rapid endothelial damage, causing vascular thrombosis, gross interstitial swelling and necrosis of the graft, all within a matter, usually, of hours.

Similarly, when transfer occurs between human beings, the degree of compatibility between donor and recipient is important to the success, or otherwise, of the graft.

As indicated earlier, transfer between identical twins is associated with universal success, without the need to modulate the immune mechanism. However, transfer between non-identical relatives or using cadaveric organs produces the recognition of non-self by the recipient and the mounting of an immune response. It is the avoidance or modification of this immune response which has been the main target over the last 25 years and the avoidance of overwhelming rejection has been a prime goal.

Two approaches have been taken to the problem: tissue typing, and reduction of immune response.

Tissue typing

In the attempt to match the donor and recipient more closely, the concept of typing has become widely developed. Early work demonstrating that blood transfusion was dependent on matching between donor and recipient was extended into experimental and then clinical transplantation studies in the 1960s and 1970s.

The human chromosome 6 contains the genetically determined major histocompatability complex (MHC), i.e. the HLA-A, HLA-B, HLA-C (class 1) and HLA-DR (D-related; class 2) loci. A whole series of additional genetic regions have been linked to the HLA complex, although in clinical terms these are probably less significant.

Thus it has become increasingly possible, using serological studies, to genetically map an individual on the basis of the HLA region of this chromosome. Since one chromosome is inherited from each parent and each individual has two HLA haplotypes, there is a 25% chance that two siblings will share both haplotypes (i.e. identical) and, by standard and Mendelian inheritance, a 50% chance that they will share one haplotype. Thus in first-degree relatives when the donor and recipient are matched for HLA-A and B antigens there is an excellent likelihood of graft success, whereas because of the complexity of the MHC allele, the wide diverence of antigens and random cadaveric donors, even if matched for one or two antigens, there may still be very substantial disparity.

Thus, in order to avoid rejection, the concept of tissue typing trying to match more accurately the donor and the recipient has gained wide acceptance. Serological methods allow class 1 HLA antigens to be defined using typed serum obtained from nulliparous women. Using a microcytotoxicity assay, multiple antisera against HLA-A, B, C and DR antigens are provided on Terasaki trays and then frozen until needed. When needed, the trays are thawed and the donor lymphocyte cells are added to the wells containing complement and the antisera against specific HLA types. If the antibody causes the cells to lyse, acridine orange (a dye) enters the damaged cell and appears orange under fluorescence microscopy. Thus by using microcytotoxicity tests it is possible to identify quite rapidly the HLA class 1 antigens present in a donor.

Until recently, class 2 antigen typing required a mixed leukocyte reaction to determine individual constituents, but more recent techniques have avoided this laborious investigation. From the clinical standpoint the practical importance of identification of the degree of compatibility between donor and recipient is clearly defined in many organ-grafting systems. Cadaveric grafting can only achieve this level when beneficially matched donor and recipient pairs, in which all major class 1 and class 2 antigens are identical, are grafted. This so-called 'full house' HLA match can give 1 year cadaveric graft survival approaching 90%. However, this is only when combined with chemical non-specific immunosuppression.

When grafts are transferred between donor and recipient with a complete mismatch an additional 20–25% of grafts will be lost over the ensuing 5 years. Thus, in cadaveric grafting the degree of matching has an important role in determining the severity of the immune response and the ultimate success, or otherwise, of the graft.

Nevertheless, no matter how good the matching is in cadaveric situations, modulation of the immune response continues to be necessary to ensure graft survival.

Reduction of immune response

Reduction in the immune response occurs frequently in clinical practice in such situations as uraemia, profound jaundice and in patients with advanced malignancy and acquired immunodeficiency syndrome (AIDS). The controlled reduction of an immune response to foreign antigen on graft requires careful clinical judgement. Initial attempts using widespread radiation produced severe depletion of not just lymphocytes but also a pancytopenia, and although skin grafts and other organs were readily accepted immunologically by the recipients, the majority of patients quickly died from overwhelming infection.

A refinement of this technique in which partial lymphocyte irradiation was used has been successful both experimentally and in clinical practice, depleting the immune response so that grafts can be accepted.

Chemical immunosuppression

Since the mid-1950s the primary mode of immunomodulation has been the administration of chemical agents. A demonstration by Hitchings & Elion (1959) over 40 years ago that 6-mercaptopurine had immunosuppressive potential allowed Schwartz & Dameschek (1959) to treat rabbits stimulated by foreign antigen. The treated animals did not produce antibodies to the antigen stimulation, and work by Calne in 1960 showed that 6-mercaptopurine could also inhibit the immune response in dogs. A number of other agents were studied at that time and those found to be of clear benefit were steroids, reducing the cellular response, and eventually azothioprine, which showed improved results when compared to 6-mercaptopurine.

For more than 20 years chemical immunomodulation with the combination of steroids (prednisolone) and azothioprine was to be the main non-specific immunosuppressant used. They inhibited the immune response largely by depressing circulating T cells.

The production of antilymphocytic globulin by sensitization in animals was also demonstrated to inhibit the immune response, although variability and efficacy limited its clinical use.

Cyclosporin. Clearly the ultimate goal of selectively inhibiting the recipient's immune response remains a long way off, and in clinical practice non-specific agents continue to be used. In 1976, Borel working in Sandoz laboratories assessed the potent immunosuppressive properties of cyclosporin A, a cyclical peptide with 11 amino acids. The demonstration of both the in vitro and in vivo immunosuppressive activity was quickly followed by extended clinical studies. It was clearly demonstrated that cyclosporin could suppress both antibody production and cell-mediated immunity, exhibiting a selective inhibitory effect on T-cell-dependent responses. Of critical importance was the observation that the drug was neither profoundly lympho- nor myelotoxic and had no influence on the viability of the mature T cells or the antibody-producing B cells. Further agents have recently been introduced to clinical practice, perhaps resulting in less rejection still (FK506 or Tacrolimus).

CURRENT CLINICAL IMMUNOSUPPRESSIVE USE

For nearly 25 years the mainstay of clinical immunosuppression was the combined use of steroids and azothioprine. With increasing clinical experience it

---

Box 22.2   Side-effects of steroids and azothioprine

Steroids
- Avascular necrosis of bones
- Diabetes
- Obesity
- Cushing's syndrome
- Pancreatitis
- Cataract
- Skin problems
- Psychosis

Azothioprine
- Bone marrow suppression
- Polycythaemia
- Hepatotoxicity

---

became possible to adjust the dosage of these agents so that in many individuals it was possible to maintain immunosuppression and thus prevent rejection, while minimizing the risk to the recipient of over-immunomodulation, a delicate balance which requires considerable clinical skill.

Patients receiving steroids and azothioprine required careful, meticulous monitoring for signs of early infection and the presence of organ rejection. Progressive reduction in haemopoietic production leads to thrombocytopenia and leucopenia, with the attendant risk of infection (bacterial, fungal and viral). The major complications of long-term steroid and azothioprine immunosuppression are outlined in Box 22.2.

Thus considerable clinical skill was needed to avoid the risks of infection, and in cadaveric grafting, when the degree of matching between donor and recipient was often less than optimal, death from infection was the commonest cause of death in the first 3 months after grafting. In addition, the need to administer steroids continually became a major limiting factor, particularly in children where the complications of steroids can be so crippling (Box 22.3).

The results of organ grafting using prednisolone and azothioprine left much to be desired, and so the intro-duction of cyclosporin into clinical trials in the early 1980s was an important step forward in the more selective use of immunomodulation. Not only could steroids be minimized or avoided in some individuals, but pancytopaenia was rarely encountered. Nevertheless, cyclosporin was rapidly found to have its own attendant problems and difficulties and nephrotoxicity remains a persistent problem (Box 22.4).

With increasing clinical experience, however, many of these toxic effects can now be minimized such that excellent rehabilitation can be achieved and organs can now be grafted which previously would have been unsuccessful in the prednisolone and azotioprine era. The overall results of cyclosporin will be outlined in the individual sections, but there have been no clinical series in which the results of cyclosporin have been inferior to the treatment with azothioprine and prednisolone, and for the most part an improved benefit of between 15% and 20% of graft survival at 1 year has been reported.

Postoperative monitoring of all patients with transplanted organs involves regulation of the immunosuppressive regime, detection of the development of organ rejection and constant vigilance for signs of infection.

CADAVERIC ORGAN DONATION

The concept of the diagnosis of brain death and increased awareness by both the public and doctors alike of the need for organ donation have improved the supply of cadaveric organs for grafting. In the UK, about a third of patients who become organ donors have died from spontaneous intracranial haemorrhage, although head injuries and road traffic accidents also provide a significant number.

Box 22.3   Side-effects of steroids in children

- Growth retardation
- Cushingoid appearance
- Diabetes
- Obesity

Box 22.4   Side-effects of cyclosporin

- Nephrotoxicity
- Hepatotoxicity
- Tremors, convulsions
- Skin problems
- Gingival hypertrophy
- Haemolytic anaemia
- Hypertension
- Malignant change

SPECIFIC ORGAN TRANSPLANTATION

KIDNEY

Kidney transplantation is now well established as the most effective way of helping patients with end-stage renal failure. Despite a significant expansion in the number of kidney transplants, long waiting lists exist for those on dialysis awaiting treatment. In the UK an integrated approach has shown a steady increase in the proportion of patients treated by transplantation, such that nearly 50% of patients now have a functioning transplant.

Patient selection

With kidney transplantation affording the optimal quality of rehabilitation, few patients will be denied the prospect, although the patient's age and underlying real condition may need to be taken into account.

Age

In general, children do very well after transplantation, although infants below the age of 5 years present a more controversial issue because of the difficulty of management of immunosuppressive agents. The newer immunosuppressive regimes, however, allow adequate growth and physical development. The goal for children must be the establishment of normal renal function before maturity and to take full advantage of the growth spurt that occurs at puberty.

While in the early days patients over the age of 55 years were frequently denied transplantation, many centres now offer renal transplantation to patients over 65 or 70 years. Patient and graft survival has been very satisfactory in this group, but immunosuppressive schedules frequently need to be reduced in the elderly to ensure that overwhelming infection does not occur.

Renal disease

Renal transplantation is now offered for many primary and secondary renal conditions resulting in chronic renal failure, including glomerulonephritis, pyelonephritis and polycystic disease. Some types of autoimmune glomerulonephritis antibodies have been demonstrated to cause damage to the transplanted kidney, but this is not a contraindication to transplantation since probably less than 10% of grafts will be seriously injured.

Assessment of potential recipient

Careful review of both the physical and psychological status of the patient is needed prior to transplantation and factors which may increase the hazards of surgery or immunosuppressive management require evaluation. Patients in renal failure frequently suffer from cardiovascular problems (hypertension with left ventricular hypertrophy, and coronary artery disease) and the symptoms are increased by anaemia. There is a high incidence of peptic ulceration in uraemic patients and of metabolic bone disease, causing renal osteodystrophy. All these associated conditions must be optimally treated or controlled prior to transplantation surgery. Sources of underlying or potential infection such as an infected urinary tract or peritoneal cavity from peritoneal dialysis must be irradicated or treated and the patient's status for viruses such as hepatitis B, HIV and cytomegalovirus must be known to minimize activation following immunosuppression. Careful surgical review related to previous abdominal operations, peripheral vascular ischaemia, or the presence of ileal conduits following previous urogenital surgery needs also to be carefully taken into account and a surgical plan initiated.

Careful counselling and support are also needed to ensure that the patient understands and is prepared for transplantation.

Surgical technique

The technique of renal implantation has remained unchanged now for nearly 40 years, with the donor kidney being implanted extraperitoneally in one of the iliac fossae. The renal artery is anastomosed to either the internal or external iliac artery and the renal vein to the recipient's external iliac vein. The donor ureter is then implanted into the recipient's bladder. Over 100 000 kidney grafts have been performed around the world, but total transplantation rates vary significantly from one country to another.

Postoperative problems

Monitoring of the kidney allograft is required to detect signs of rejection, suggested by a reduction in urinary output and an elevation in serum creatinine, and then confirmed by biopsy or aspiration cytology. This allows the prompt recognition of acute rejection crisis and its treatment by steroids.

With increased clinical experience the hurdles of acute rejection and infectious complications can usually be overcome, and patient survival at 1 year is in excess of 95% in many programmes, with over 85% of kidney grafts functioning well. However, a steady attrition of renal grafts will occur over the next 10 years, so that only just half of all renal transplants will be functioning well at 10 years, with many having been lost from the slow process of chronic rejection.

Rehabilitation can be spectacular, allowing patients the freedom to eat without restriction on salt, protein or potassium, the resolution of anaemia and infertility and an improvement in their overall sense of well-being.

Renal transplantation in the diabetic patient can be combined with pancreas transplantation, with implantation of the whole organ and drainage of the pancreatic duct into the gastrointestinal tract or the urinary bladder. Transplantation of isolated pancreatic islets is in its infancy.

HEART

While the patient afflicted by renal disease has the benefit of chronic haemodialysis, the individual with progressive cardiac problems has no life-support system and death invariably ensues unless cardiac transplantation is undertaken. Initial efforts in the late 1960s by Barnard (1967) led to a progressive expansion of increasingly successful programmes. The majority of patients will suffer from cardiomyopathy, terminal ischaemic cardiac disease or, more rarely, some congenital form of cardiac disease. Donor selection must be rigorous because immediate life-sustaining function is required of the graft.

Orthotopic replacement of the diseased heart has been the most frequently undertaken procedure, although the heterotopic placement of auxiliary cardiac implants has been undertaken. The donor atria are anastomosed to the posterior walls of the corresponding chambers of the recipient prior to joining the pulmonary artery and the aorta.

Postoperative cardiac function is monitored and endomyocardial biopsy allows histological examination of heart muscle for ventricular cellular infiltration indicative of acute rejection. While the early attempts at cardiac grafting resulted in poor overall survival, the situation has improved remarkably. A 1-year survival of over 85% and a 5-year survival of 60% of patients with excellent quality of rehabilitation is most encouraging.

This solid foundation of cardiac grafting inevitably led to an extension to combined heart and lung transplantation, primarily for those suffering from pulmonary hypertension, or for some terminal lung diseases, such as cystic fibrosis or emphysema. If the recipient has lung disease but a good functioning heart on receipt of a combined heart–lung graft, the heart from the first recipient can be implanted into a second cardiac patient – the domino procedure. As a result of technical advances, transplantation of single lung is now possible. Because of the risk of infection in the implanted lungs immunosuppressive management is critical. Sputum cytology and even lung biopsy may be needed to differentiate infection from rejection. In spite of this, the Stanford University Series now reports 2-year survival of over 60% in heart–lung recipients.

LIVER

Although the first attempts at liver transplantation were made in the early 1960s, the formidable technical, preservation, immunological and organ availability difficulties meant that it was only in the early 1980s that successful programmes were established. The majority of adult patients coming to liver grafting have extensive cirrhosis (primary biliary cirrhosis, chronic active hepatitis and hepatitis B) or, less frequently, primary liver cancer. In the paediatric group the most common indication for liver transplantation is biliary atresia.

The liver is particularly susceptible to ischaemic injury and the ability to harvest and store livers for only a few hours led to an extremely complex surgical procedure, undertaken often in the most difficult emergency situations.

The liver is placed orthotopically after removal of the diseased organ, and to reduce the physiological changes during the anhepatic phase venovenous bypass is employed. Improvements in organ preservation (principally the introduction of the University of Wisconsin solution) mean that livers can now be stored for 12–14 hours and transferred from one country to another. The evidence that tissue matching is important in liver grafting has yet to be fully established, but as in other forms of transplantation this may prove to be the case.

Patients coming to liver grafting are frequently critically ill with multisystem failure, and the complexity of the operation inevitably has meant that technical failures have been frequent. In spite of this, results have continued to improve, and with nearly 7000 liver transplants performed in Europe alone and 1-year survival of over 75%, liver transplantation is increasingly being established as one of the most effective modalities of treatment for liver disease. In some groups the results have shown even more impressive improvement. Infants and children with biliary atresia undergoing grafting stand a greater than 90% chance of 1-year survival, with the majority going on for many years. The longest survivor is now over 20 years after transplantation.

The major limiting factor in liver grafting now is donor availability and, while in the UK some 550 grafts were performed in 1994, the need is probably double that. The most acute shortage is of paediatric organs, and often a larger liver has to be divided and only part transplanted into a child.

ETHICAL ISSUES

The development of transplantation in the 1950s and 1960s caught not just the imagination of the medical profession but the public as well, and led to the reappraisal of fundamental beliefs in many areas. The concept of death was challenged from the traditional one of the cessation of the heart beat to that of the concept of brain-stem death, and wide public and professional debates ensued. Death, the great taboo of the twentieth century, was addressed in a new fundamental way. The majority of countries enacted legislation or medical guidelines identifying new criteria which would allow more effective recognition of an individual's incapacity to regain essential and vital functions. Some of these issues were challenged in courts of law and were often widely reported in the media.

Thus ethical and moral issues were raised from the very outset of organ grafting. With the increasing success of organ transplantation these pressures have grown. The rights of the individual to dispose of his or her own organs as they wish has been a matter of debate, and the profession has loudly condemned the commercialism which is in danger of entering clinical practice. The purchase or sale or organs is now condemned by almost all international transplantation organizations.

Should a living individual during his lifetime voluntarily donate an organ to another? The first successful grafts between identical twins from within a family were clearly perceived to be an act of great charity and compassion. Living-kidney grafting in the USA accounts for more than a third of all grafts, but should such altruism be permitted between non-family members, or those in whom a loving and caring bond does not exist? These new issues continue to be addressed by society.

One other issue has particularly focused on cardiac and liver transplantation and this relates to the consumption of economic resources for an individual. In the UK the cost of renal transplantation in total is approximately £8000–10 000, whereas the cost of dialysis per year per patient approaches £15 000. While renal transplantation is clearly the most cost-effective way of dealing with renal failure compared with some other forms of medical and surgical treatment and perhaps health-care initiative, it is seen as being expensive. Cardiac and liver transplantation can equally be seen to consume an inappropriate amount of the health resources available in some areas, and indeed the State of Oregon has now withdrawn financial support from liver transplantation programmes, giving them a very low priority compared with their other health schedules.

Each new development in science and clinical medicine raises its own issues which need to be addressed, and as these modalities of treatment spread to other countries different cultural approaches may be required. It will be for the individual community to decide whether such treatments are appropriate for its fellow human beings and what extent of resources can be made available.

Clinical organ transplantation has evolved rapidly over the last 25 years, affording treatment to many thousands of patients who would otherwise be dead or enduring an existence of chronic illness. Further advances are sought in the fight against the recipient immune response and to procure donor organs of the highest quality, thus enabling even more patients to experience the increasing benefits of transplantation.

REFERENCES

Barnard C N 1967 The operation. A human cardiac transplant: an interim report of a successful operation performed at Groote Schuur Hospital, Cape Town. South African Medical Journal 41: 1271–1274

Borel J F, Feurer C, Gubler H U, Stahelin A 1976 Biological effects of cyclosporin A: a new antilymphocytic agent. Agents and Actions 6: 468–475

Calne R Y 1960 The rejection of renal homografts: inhibition in dogs by 6-mercaptopurine. Lancet i: 417–418

Gibson T, Medawar P B 1943 The fate of skin homografts in man. Journal of Anatomy 77: 299–309

Hitchings G H, Elion G B 1959 Activity of heterocyclic derivatives of 6-mercaptopurine and 6-thioguanine in adenocarcinoma 755. Proceedings of the American Association for Cancer Research 3: 27

Medawar P B 1944 Behaviour and fate of skin autografts and skin homografts in rabbits. Journal of Anatomy 78: 176–199

Mitchison N A 1953 Passive transfer of transplantation immunity. Nature 171: 267–268

Murray J E, Merrill J P, Harrison J H 1955 Renal homotransplantation in identical twins. Surgery Forum 6: 423–426

Schwartz R, Dameschek W 1959 Drug induced immunological tolerance. Nature 183: 1682–1683

Malignant disease

23. Principles of surgery for malignant disease

P. J. Guillou

In 1989, malignant disease accounted for just under a quarter of all deaths in the UK, being second only to cardiovascular disease (45.9% of all deaths) in the league of individual causes of death (OPCS Monitor 1991). Table 23.1 indicates the contribution of different types of malignant disease to the total figure. Lung cancer constitutes the greatest overall number of cancer deaths, although amongst women carcinoma of the breast is more common. Cancer arising in the gastrointestinal tract constitutes 26.5% of all cancer deaths. Surgery has mainly a diagnostic and staging role in the management of the most common cancer, lung cancer. Surgeons most frequently contribute to the therapeutic management of patients suffering from malignant disease of the breast and gastrointestinal tract, although similar principles apply to malignant disease managed by urologists

Table 23.1 Causes of death

	1987	1988	1989
All causes	556 994	571 408	576 872
Cardiovascular disease	271 061	267 927	264 600
(% of all causes)	47.8%	46.9%	45.9%
All malignant neoplasms	140 768	142 540	143 439
(% of all causes)	24.8%	24.95%	24.86%
Numbers of deaths from individual tumour sites			
Bronchus/lung	35 138	35 302	34 581
Lip/oral cavity	1 689	1 687	1 716
Oesophagus	4 770	4 884	5 108
Stomach	9 509	9 425	9 062
Small bowel	204	242	220
Colon	11 378	11 494	11 626
Rectum/anus	5 675	5 755	5 756
Pancreas	6 065	6 009	6 116
Primary liver	666	674	676
Genitourinary	22 188	22 527	24 145
Carcinoma of female breast	13 751	13 723	14 008
Lymphoma	9 489	9 718	9 913

(bladder, kidney, testis and prostate), head and neck surgeons, etc. The nature of modern cancer therapy demands considerable familiarity with the pathological basis of malignancy.

PATHOLOGICAL BASIS OF THE ORIGINS AND SPREAD OF MALIGNANT DISEASE

A tumour results when an individual cell or group of cells escapes from the constraints which control normal cell replication. Controlled proliferation occurs during embryogenesis, hypertrophy, healing, regeneration, repair, and during the metabolic response to trauma and sepsis. Controlled cellular replication is mediated by small peptide growth factors which bind to their specific receptors on the cell surface. Growth factors may be *autocrine* (i.e. bind to receptors on the cell which produces them), *paracrine* (i.e. bind to receptors on a cell adjacent to the cell of origin), or classically *endocrine* (i.e. bind to receptors on a cell at some distance from the cell of origin, usually being transferred via the circulation). Once a growth factor binds to its cell surface receptor, intracellular signals are induced which, amongst other things, activate the nucleus and promote the cell to enter the cell cycle. Within the nucleus nucleoproteins ensure accurate DNA replication, DNA repair, and DNA transcription via messenger RNA (mRNA). Clearly the growth factors, their receptors, the enzymes which their binding activates and the nucleoproteins (e.g. DNA polymerase) which regulate DNA synthesis and repair are all coded for by codons within the human genome. They are therefore susceptible to modifications of their structure, either by mutations, deletions or amplifications of their corresponding genes or by errors of transcription of the code into the mature protein. Mutations occur either spontaneously or as result of the reaction of chemical carcinogens with DNA.

Tumours rarely grow simply because their cell cycle times or proportion of proliferating cells (growth fraction) are greater than those in normal tissues.

Tumours grow because, unlike normal tissues, where in general a cell divides only in order to replace one which has been lost, there is failure to respond to the constraints which regulate normal growth, irrespective of cell loss. This is not to say that tumours do not also shed cells. It has been estimated that 50% of tumour cells are lost as a consequence of exfoliation, hypoxia, non-viability, metastasis and host defences. Tumour size therefore depends on three factors: the cell cycle time, the growth fraction and the numbers lost from the tumour surface. A tumour will become clinically palpable when it consists of 10^9 or more cells, but most tumours contain far more cells than this when they first present. Even the smallest radiologically detectable mammary carcinoma contains 10^7–10^8 cells and patients usually die before a size of 10^{12} cells has been achieved. In rapidly proliferating tumours the cells dedifferentiate and increasingly less resemble the parent cells. Failure to be inhibited by contact with neighbouring cells is an important characteristic of tumours, but two further properties of this uncontrolled replication distinguish the malignant from the non-malignant tumour. These are the capacity to invade and destroy adjacent normal structures, and the ability to invade lymphatic and venous vessels and produce metastases.

Oncogenes, growth factors and the multistep hypothesis of tumour progression

The concept has evolved that cancers proceed through multiple stages before reaching the point of invasive malignancy. This may involve the inheritance of a genetic change which provides susceptibility to the development of malignancy (e.g. the retinoblastoma (Rb) or familial polyposis (FAP) gene deletions on chromosomes 13 and 5 respectively), or exposure to environmental carcinogens which activate particular genes which, if dominant, will induce cellular proliferation. The resultant increase in cellular proliferation results in an increase in the frequency of mistakes in DNA synthesis which, if unrepaired, become permanent mutations. If a critical suppressor gene (e.g. the P53 gene which is coded for on chromosome 17p) is lost or mutated then the last molecular constraint over controlled cell growth disappears and further mutation leads to the development of cells with the capacity for invasion and metastasis. Thus the multistep hypothesis suggests that although a single activated gene or, perhaps more importantly, a lost suppressor gene may be necessary, it alone is insufficient to produce the complete malignant phenotype. Although the fine molecular details have not been fully elucidated, this is considered to be the basis

of, for example, the well-known polyp–cancer sequence of carcinoma of the colon.

Many of these abnormalities involve genetic sequences known as oncogenes, which were originally identified as the genes within certain tumour-forming RNA viruses that were responsible for tumour formation, hence the expression v-*onc* (oncogene) to describe them when they are isolated from the virus in question. In fact it would appear that the viruses acquired the genes from the human genome during viral excision, and thus when identified in mammalian cells the sequences are given the prefix c-, as shown in Table 23.2. Cellular (c-) oncogenes or proto-oncogenes are normal genes which code for proteins (oncoproteins) that are implicated in normal cellular proliferation. They are expressed at certain stages in embryogenesis and during regeneration, healing, etc. Since oncoproteins are important components of the process of regulated cell division, their involvement in carcinogenesis is best understood by categorizing them as dominant oncogenes or recessive/suppressor oncogenes, but this needs to be combined with a knowledge of the site and function (if known) of their oncoproteins. Box 23.1 represents one such classification, but it is important to reiterate that oncogenes and their corresponding oncoproteins are *normal components of cellular molecular physiology*. They become implicated in carcinogenesis when their encoded proteins become overexpressed, truncated (mutated) or otherwise modified so that their function is constitutively expressed rather than declared in a regulated fashion as in the normal cell. Hence 60–70% of colorectal cancers possess a mutated Kirsten (K-) *ras* oncogene. Similarly, the P53 oncoprotein, which is a normal suppressor of cell division and which prevents entry of the cell into S-phase, has been found to exist in mutated forms in at least 50% of tumours of the breast, colon, lung, bladder and hepatomas. The mutated forms can bind to and inactivate the 'wild-type' normal P53 and inactivate it, resulting in uncontrolled cellular replication.

The c-*erb*B2 oncogene product is overexpressed in 20% of breast cancers and correlates with increasing tumour grade, but is independent of oestrogen receptor status, nodal involvement or any other risk factor for recurrence of breast cancer. It appears to have considerable prognostic significance independently of the aforementioned parameters, even in those patients who are node negative.

It is this unregulated expression or neo-expression of deregulated genes that may also be responsible for the capacity of certain tumours to secrete proteins into the circulation which may be used to detect or monitor for the recurrence of certain tumours, e.g. carcino-

Table 23.2 Oncoproteins and their functions

Dominant oncogene products				
Growth factors	*Plasmalemmal*	*Cytoplasmic*	*Nuclear*	
Ligands	Membrane receptors	Signal transducers	Transcription factors	Cell cycle factors
c-*sis* (platelet + derived growth factor, PDGF)	EGF-receptor c-*erb*B2 c-*kit* PDGF-receptor c-*fms*	GTP-binding c-Ha-*ras* c-Ki-*ras* C-N-*ras* c-*src*	c-*fos* c-*jun* c-*erb*A (thyroid hormone receptor)	c-*myc* c-*myb*

embryonic antigen (CEA) for gastrointestinal, particularly colorectal, cancer or α-fetoprotein (AFP) for hepatomas.

The concepts of early cancer, invasion and metastasis

A number of conditions are recognized which, although not being malignant per se, have the potential to become so and are categorized as *premalignant*. In the gastrointestinal tract these include leukoplakia of the oral mucosa, Barratt's columnar-lined oesophagus, certain types of severe gastric dysplasia, Peutz–Jehger syndrome and ulcerative colitis. However, in these conditions malignant cells may be present but they have not yet invaded the basement membrane. This defines *carcinoma in situ*, which may be encountered in the breast (ductal carcinoma in situ), the cervix, the oral mucosa and a number of other sites. Depending on its site, carcinoma in situ may be treated by local resection, although in the breast removal of all breast tissue has been advocated because of the multicentricity of the condition. In the gastrointestinal tract it is necessary to distinguish carcinoma in situ from so-called 'early'

lesions such as early gastric cancer and colorectal cancer of stage A in the Dukes' classification. 'Early cancer' of the digestive tract is therefore defined as frankly invasive cancer which has not yet breached the muscular layer of the intestine. Under these circumstances major resectional surgery is often curative but simple locally destructive approaches are inadequate.

The concept of early malignancy is also applied to malignant melanoma, where two main criteria are employed to express the invasiveness of the tumours. These are the thickness of the lesion (Breslow) and the histological level of invasion (Clark's level). Tumour thickness correlates well with overall prognosis, the so-called 'thin' melanomas (<0.85 mm thick) rarely metastasizing following excision with a 1–2 cm clear margin. In contrast, the 5-year survival rate of patients with melanomas thicker than 3.5 mm is only 38%.

Occasionally, primary malignancy in an organ is seen which is pathologically 'early' (e.g. has not yet invaded the muscularis mucosae of the gastrointestinal tract) but is associated with the presence of lymph node deposits. This is a scenario sometimes seen with gastric carcinoma or with a Duke's 'A' carcinoma which is accompanied by hepatic metastases, and these examples indicate the

---

Box 23.1 Suppressor/recessive oncogene products display a normal phenotype despite the inheritance of one abnormal parental gene but not if one is inherited from each parent, e.g.:

1. The retinoblastoma (Rb) gene
Only when the normal gene (13q14) undergoes spontaneous mutation in the eye and a homozygous genotype is present does retinoblastoma develop. Of course retinoblastoma will develop if the child inherits the Rb gene from both parents

2. The P53 oncogene
Normally prevents malignant transformation unless mutated. Mutated P53 protein binds to normal (wild-type) P53 protein and inactivates it

3. Wilms tumour gene
The molecular genetics of this gene is similar to that of the Rb gene

biological complexity of the process of metastasis. The mechanisms which underlie the development of metastasis have yet to be fully elucidated.

Metastasis occurs via three distinct routes:

- Via the lymphatic drainage
- Via the venous drainage of the organ containing the tumour
- Via the body cavities (e.g. transcoelomic metastasis).

Rarely, metastasis may occur transluminally, as for example with the implantation of exfoliated viable colorectal cancer cells into distal healing sites such as haemorrhoidectomy wounds or anastomoses.

These routes are surgically important. Because most common tumours spread via the lymphatics, and since lymphatic vessels and their associated lymph nodes commonly accompany the arterial supply to an organ, in many instances the surgery of malignant disease is based on the anatomy of the arterial supply to the organ containing the primary tumour. Similarly, the venous drainage of an organ is an important determinant of the haematogenous pattern of distribution of metastases from tumours arising from that organ.

The capacity of tumour cells to form a metastasis is a function of a complex sequence of events which involves direct invasion of a venous radical or lymphatic vessel by such processes as adhesion to the vascular endothelium and digestion of the basement membrane of the vessel in which the tumour cell has been arrested. These events relate to tumour cell receptors for the laminin of basement membrane and the release of enzymes such as collagenase which facilitate the invasion of tissue parenchyma. Also involved are host factors such as platelet–tumour cell aggregates, thrombosis, ischaemia and the further release of tumour cells into a growth-factor-rich environment.

The organ distribution of metastases is determined by factors which are not necessarily related to the proportion of the cardiac output received by the organ. The 'soil' for metastatic implantation must be conducive to the growth of the metastatic 'seed'. However, anatomical considerations such as venous and lymphatic drainage cause metastatic disease to follow identifiable and predictable patterns, e.g. liver metastases from colorectal cancer, pulmonary metastases from renal cell cancer and malignant melanoma, and lymphatic metastases from early gastric and breast cancers. Secondary metastatic sites such as the liver may in turn serve as a source of metastases such as from the liver to the lungs and from the lungs to the bones, adrenals, brain, etc. The surgeon should appreciate these patterns of metastasis for individual tumours because: (1) modern management demands that patients be appropriately

screened for recurrent disease which may be amenable to further excisional surgery (e.g. 'second-look' surgery following colorectal cancer excision, or lymphadenectomy after excision of a limb melanoma); (2) the introduction of adjuvant therapies targeted at organs where recurrence is likely or where surgery cannot completely guarantee the eradication of micrometastatic disease (e.g. radiotherapy to the breast and axilla following local excision and node sampling for carcinoma of the breast; and (3) for monitoring those patients whose primary treatment modality may not be surgical but in whom subsequent recurrent disease may lead to the use of radical surgical excision as the next line of therapy (e.g. following radiotherapy to laryngeal carcinoma or bladder carcinoma).

Tumour staging and grading

Pathological tumour staging and grading have an impact on the choice of therapy, which increasingly is being individually tailored to the patient. Tumour grade mainly refers to the degree of differentiation of a particular tumour on histological examination using well-characterized criteria, such as the degree of nuclear polymorphism, capacity to resemble the parent histiotype, number of mitoses, etc. Tumours are generally described as well, moderately or poorly differentiated, this being the best available separation obtainable by even the most experienced of pathologists. Unfortunately, most tumours contain mixed elements of these grading systems and it is conventional to grade a tumour according to its worst area of differentiation. While poorly differentiated tumours tend to be more aggressive than well-differentiated lesions, the prognostic correlation with degree of differentiation is rather weak for most tumours.

Staging systems attempt to quantify the tumour mass in a manner which has clinical value for prognostic, therapeutic and comparative purposes. Most systems are based on an assessment of the size of the primary tumour (T), the presence of lymphatic metastases in lymph nodes (N) and the existence of distant metastases (M). For some tumours it is possible to make a clinical estimate of the state of a tumour, as for example the clinical staging of carcinoma of the breast. However, for the purposes of comparing prognosis and the results of adjuvant therapy between different centres and therapeutic protocols, the TNM system based on pathological data is preferable. It provides prognostic guidelines and aids enormously in the decision for or against administering adjuvant therapy to an individual patient. However, clinical staging (e.g. for breast cancer) is of importance because of the possibility of treating the primary lesion with chemotherapy and/or radiotherapy in an attempt to reduce the tumour bulk before attempts are made to surgically resect the primary lesion. This so-called 'neo-adjuvant' therapy is currently being utilized in the management of patients with oesophageal and breast cancers, but may become part of the future management of patients with pancreatic or even gastric cancer.

In general, nodal status plays a dominant role in determining prognosis, but with certain tumours other factors may carry equal weight. For example, in the schema devised by the Japanese Society for the Study of Gastric Cancer, serosal involvement represents a major prognostic indicator with the albeit rare but interesting paradox of serosa-negative/node-positive tumours enjoying a better prognosis than those who are serosa positive but node negative, provided of course that radical lymphadenectomy is conducted during the course of the gastrectomy. In contrast, nodal status remains the strongest independent prognostic indicator in patients with operable carcinoma of the breast and this influences therapeutic strategies in the management of such patients.

Because lymphatics tend to accompany the main arterial supply to the organ in question, radical resectional surgery for malignant disease tends to be the surgery of blood vessels. For carcinoma of the stomach radical resection with lymphadenectomy can be achieved only by division of the left gastric artery at its origin, the right gastric artery at its origin, the splenic artery in the lesser sac and the right gastroepiploic artery at its origin, etc. These vessels are removed along with all their accompanying lymphoid tissue, including that along the hepatic artery and hilum of the liver, together with the pre-and paraaortic lymphatic tissue in the retroperitoneum. This inevitably necessitates removal of the body and tail of the pancreas. Of course such an extensive dissection is accompanied by greater morbidity and mortality than the somewhat less radical lymphatic resections more commonly undertaken for gastric carcinoma in the UK. This surgical risk is perhaps worthwhile if it is offset by a significant increase in disease-free interval and survival. Whereas this is true for gastric cancer in the Japanese it is as yet uncertain whether this is also the case in European patients, whose disease tends on the whole to be rather advanced at presentation. Nevertheless, the pathological staging of gastric cancer has led the Japanese Society for Gastric Cancer to devise a logical plan for the surgical treatment of gastric cancer.

Modern developments in cellular and molecular biology have also contributed to more accurate definition of prognosis for an individual patient. For example, in addition to the dominant influence of axillary lymph node status, it has now been determined that the expression of receptors for epidermal growth factor (EGF-r) and the c-*erb*B2 oncoprotein are also implicated as risk factors for metastatic breast cancer. The presence of nuclear oestrogen receptors is a good prognostic factor in such patients and is inversely related to the expression of EGF-r. The expression of EGF-r is second only to nodal status as an indicator of prognosis in breast cancer and further serves to discriminate a poor prognostic group in those who are node negative. It is likely that the identification of this latter marker will enter routine practice for the decision for administration or otherwise of adjuvant therapy for primary breast cancer. This is an important example of the incorporation of progress in molecular and cellular biology into the clinical arena which will undoubtedly be paralleled in the management of other tumour types. Other examples already exist, including, for example, the finding that the degree of amplification of the c-*myc* oncogene (N-*myc*) in childhood neuroblastoma correlates inversely with the disease-free interval following resection and also appears to render the tumour cells more resistant to chemotherapy.

It is obviously desirable that the patient be accurately staged before surgical intervention is applied. With certain tumours (e.g. carcinoma of the breast) this can be performed quite accurately. With many others, however, even with sophisticated imaging techniques such as ultrasound, computed tomography (CT) scans, magnetic resonance imaging (MRI) scans, positron emission tomography (PET) scans, various isotope scanning procedures and the more recent advent of scanning with radiolabelled monoclonal antibodies, the final decision as to the nature of the surgery to be undertaken and the necessity for surgical adjuvant therapy must await the operative findings and final pathological staging.

POPULATION SCREENING FOR MALIGNANT DISEASE

The assumed relationship between detectability and cure rate shown in Figure 23.1 has resulted in the development of screening programmes for the more common malignant tumours. Routine endoscopic screening of the whole population has significantly improved the detection rate for early gastric cancer in Japan, where the disease is almost endemic. However, in countries such as the UK where the incidence is 11 000 new cases annually, a whole population endoscopic screening programme would not be cost-effective (see Ch. 38).

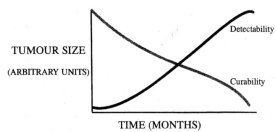

Fig. 23.1   Relationship between detectability and curability

The role of tumour markers in screening and follow-up after surgical excision

Genetic abnormalities are almost certainly responsible for the capacity of tumours to secrete certain proteins, which are not normally secreted in great quantities, into body fluids. Mostly these are normally detected in the plasma, and measurement of these 'tumour markers' is used predominantly for the monitoring of response to therapy or detection of recurrent disease following surgical excision of a primary or secondary tumour (see Ch. 26).

SYMPTOMS, SIGNS AND DIAGNOSIS OF MALIGNANT DISEASE

Space does not permit a full description of all the symptoms to be expected with malignant disease of every organ. However, the symptoms and signs with which cancer commonly presents may be categorized as follows.

1. As a palpable swelling. This is most often painless until local structures are invaded. Occasionally, as with inflammatory carcinoma of the breast, the swelling may be 'inflamed', but more usually it is not detected until ulceration and secondary infection supervene.

2. With the symptoms of obstruction. In tubular structures this is a most important and sinister group of symptoms. Examples are:

- dysphagia in carcinoma of the oesophagus
- the vomiting and succession splash of gastric outflow obstruction due to gastric cancer
- obstructive jaundice
- small bowel colic
- large bowel colic
- spurious diarrhoea
- the bladder outflow symptoms associated with carcinoma of the prostate.

3. With symptoms resulting from haemorrhage. Anaemia, haemoptysis, haematuria, haematemesis, rectal bleeding, etc. Cutaneous lesions which itch and bleed should be viewed as highly suspicious.

4. With symptoms due to local compression or invasion of local structures. For example, caval compression, gastric or colonic outflow obstruction, nerve root pain, etc.

5. With the symptoms and signs of metastatic spread. Pleural effusion, ascites, hepatomegaly, isolated lymphadenopathy, anorexia and weight loss, pathological fractures, grand mal fits from cerebral metastases, etc.

6. Asymptomatic incidental findings. It should not be forgotten that cancer may be totally asymptomatic even when it is quite advanced (e.g. the silent pulmonary metastases discovered on a routine chest X-ray, or asymptomatic axillary or groin metastases). The investigation and final diagnosis of a patient with malignant disease will of course be determined by the site of the lesion and the symptoms which it produces, but again certain principles apply. Firstly, it is rare that treatment of a particular tumour can be rationally prescribed without first obtaining a histological diagnosis. It is a tragedy for unnecessary major ablative surgery, irradiation or chemotherapy to be given to a patient who is suffering from a benign condition. A histological diagnosis is, in the vast majority of instances, an absolute requirement for planning treatment. Secondly, all investigations should aim not only to confirm the histological diagnosis but also to stage the tumour preoperatively as far as is possible. This is important not only to decide whether or not other treatments should also be administered preoperatively (e.g. neo-adjuvant therapy for carcinoma of the breast, or radiotherapy for oesophageal cancer or rectal cancer), but also to avoid surgery where it is inappropriate. It is futile to undertake major resectional surgery for oesophageal cancer in the presence of extensive liver metastases. In contrast, the presence of a solitary liver metastasis or even more advanced disease should not necessarily deter the surgeon from resecting an obstructing primary colorectal carcinoma.

In general, the principles of investigation of a patient suffering from malignancy involves the following procedures:

1. Endoscopic. The roles of oesophagogastroscopy, endoscopic retrograde cholangiopancreatography (ERCP), proctoscopy, sigmoidoscopy, colonoscopy and bronchoscopy are all widely appreciated. All abdominal surgeons involved in the management of patients with malignant disease should be able to perform a laparoscopy as part of the staging process. The 'open and close' laparotomy should rarely, if ever, be performed in this era of modern imaging technology.

2. Radiological. Most readers will be familiar with the principles of contrast radiology, particularly in relation to tubular structures such as the gastrointestinal and urological systems. Plain radiology still has a role in the evaluation of the patient with malignant disease, especially of the bones. Chest X-ray should never be omitted. Ultrasound remains the most sensitive pre-operative modality for detecting tumours within the liver, with a sensitivity of around 75%. Ultrasound also affords an opportunity to obtain an ultrasound-guided biopsy of the lesion. Other information provided by ultrasound is that it can detect masses in the pancreas, kidneys, etc., and also detects the dilated biliary tree. Unfortunately ultrasound is not a terribly useful method for following the progress of a liver lesion which is being treated non-surgically, because it is very operator dependent and measurements of tumours can be quite difficult to make using ultrasound unless the same radiologist is available on every occasion. CAT scanning is much more useful in this regard, especially when combined with the administration of intravenous contrast, either as a 'CT portogram' or as a delayed CT scan after intravenous contrast injection.

It is now simply not enough to detect the presence of tumours within the liver. Their size, number and precise anatomical localization in relation to the anatomical segments of the liver must be determined. At the very worst this has a bearing on prognosis but may also enable surgical treatment for metastases to be adequately conducted. MRI may possess the advantage over contrast-enhanced CT scanning for the purposes of imaging the liver because it now permits visualization of the portal veins and hepatic artery and veins for the purpose of planning the type of surgery to be conducted.

Other radiological investigations include of course the use of other isotopes as, for example, bone scans using radioactive technetium, or the detection of cold non-functioning nodules within the thyroid using radio-iodine. However, a modern development of isotope scanning is the conjugation of a radioisotope to a monoclonal antibody which specifically identifies an epitope expressed on the surface of the tumour cell. Isotope-conjugated monoclonal antibodies to antigens related to the CEA molecule allow, in some cases, quite accurate determination of the localization of metastatic deposits from colorectal cancer. Monoclonal antibodies to antigens present on breast cancer, ovarian cancer and prostatic cancer have been developed and are being employed in a similar fashion.

3. Pathology in the investigation of the patient with malignant disease. The necessity of having an accurate histological diagnosis prior to initiating treatment in a patient with malignant disease cannot be overemphasized. This may be obtained in a number of ways:

1. Via a fine needle: fine needle aspiration cytology (FNAC) can be performed on an outpatient basis and provides rapid diagnosis in the investigation of squamous tumours of the head and neck, tissue thyroid, breast, subcutaneous nodules, enlarged lymph nodes and within a variety of other scenarios including at CT scanning and endoscopy where the use of needles of wider bore than 19 to 21 gauge in relatively inaccessible sites might be hazardous. The false-positive rate for carcinoma of the breast is less than 1%, but the false-negative rate is somewhat higher and is dependent on the skills of both the clinician performing the aspirate and the cytologist who reads it. However, further levels of refinement may be added with the use of monoclonal antibodies to particular antigens. Both the sensitivity and specificity of cytology for carcinoma of the breast are now so highly developed in most institutions that confidence in this particular mode of investigation enables the surgeon to proceed to definitive therapy without necessarily having histological proof via a needle biopsy or frozen section.

2. Needle biopsy: this should be distinguished from FNAC because it provides a core of tissue which is treated as a histological preparation and not a cytological one. It is used less frequently nowadays, having been largely replaced by FNAC. However, there are specific instances such as liver biopsy where it remains the procedure of choice and it is used when FNAC has failed to provide a definitive diagnosis.

3. Wedge biopsy: this is rarely used these days except perhaps at open operation on the liver. It is rarely indicated for skin lesions, where excisional biopsy is more appropriate.

4. Excision biopsy with a wide margin: this is the procedure most often performed for cutaneous lesions such as malignant melanoma.

Although the use of standard histological stains such as haematoxylin and eosin frequently provide definitive diagnostic information, difficulties occasionally arise in distinguishing the organ of origin of certain malignancies, particularly when they are poorly differentiated. Here, again, the use of a panel of monoclonal antibodies may facilitate diagnosis. For example, positive staining with an antibody to the common leukocyte antigen permits a diagnosis of lymphoma to be made when standard histological preparations may be unable to distinguish the lesion from anaplastic carcinoma. Clearly such a distinction is important because of the relatively successful treatment which can be applied to lymphoma compared with that available for anaplastic carcinoma. Use of the S-100 antibody may also categorize an undifferentiated lesion as malignant melanoma rather than a carcinoma, again with therapeutic implications.

Errors in histological or cytological diagnosis usually relate to sampling errors rather than errors of interpretation. The endoscopic biopsy forceps may have failed to take a bite from the tumour tissue and this may mistakenly be categorized as normal. Aspirates are occasionally unsuitable for cytodiagnosis because of insufficient material. Errors of interpretation occasionally occur, particularly where severe dysplasia occurs in a tissue known to have malignant potential. For example, many pathologists will differ on the classification of severe dysplasia in gastric biopsies. The presence of severe dysplasia in biopsies of a large polyp of the colon or rectum should always arouse clinical suspicion that this is in fact a carcinoma.

PRINCIPLES OF SURGICAL TREATMENT OF MALIGNANT DISEASE

Sight must not be lost of the fact that the treatment of malignant disease is nowadays often based on a multi-modality approach. The surgeon may play a central role in initiating treatment but also must coordinate the close teamwork between a group of clinicians, which often includes radiotherapists and medical oncologists.

Curative surgery for primary malignant disease

The modes of extension of malignant disease exert a dominant influence on the design of curative surgical procedures for cancer. Lymph nodes and their vessels lie along the major arterial supply to an organ and surgical excision involves not only the vascular isolation of the organ in question for the purpose of safety of its excision but also the removal, as far as is feasible, of any tumour-containing lymphoid organs. In addition, it must not be forgotten that tumours also spread directly to invade contiguous structures as well as into laterally placed tissues and longitudinally along tubular organs. Thus in squamous carcinoma of the oesophagus involvement of the trachea or bronchus renders the tumour inoperable but, because of its propensity to spread submucosally, it is considered that total oesophagectomy is the procedure of choice for curative surgery for this condition. Orointestinal continuity is restored by full gastric mobilization and transthoracic routing of the gastric tube to form a neo-oesophagus which is anastomosed to the residual cervical oesophagus in the neck. Similarly, although it was previously considered that a longitudinal margin of clearance of 5 cm was essential for curative surgery for carcinoma of the rectum, it is now recognized that clear lateral margins are of equal, if not greater, importance in avoiding local

recurrence of rectal carcinoma. The recognition of the surgical significance of the lymphatic vessels present in the pelvic mesorectum has also contributed to the reduction of the incidence of local recurrence of rectal carcinoma. The slightly diminished importance of wide longitudinal margins of clearance of rectal carcinoma from 5 to 3 cm may also have permitted the more frequent performance of restorative (low anterior resection) rather than ablative (abdominoperineal excision) rectal excision, these low anastomoses also being facilitated by the use of intestinal stapling devices.

A further important principle in performing curative surgery for malignant disease is the avoidance of transecting lymphatic vessels en route to the regional lymph nodes. Thus whenever axillary dissection is performed during segmentectomy or mastectomy for breast cancer then this should be performed 'en bloc' with the main operative specimen to avoid local spillage of any metastatic tumour cells which may be in transit to the regional nodes, the aim being to minimize the risk of this causing a local recurrence. A similar principle is applied during the conduct of an R3 gastrectomy in which the body and tail of the pancreas, spleen and retroperitoneal lymph nodes are excised 'en bloc' together with the stomach.

Curative surgery for secondary malignant disease

The development of local or locoregional recurrence of malignant disease should not necessarily be an occasion for surgical despair. Regional lymph node metastases following earlier excision of a malignant melanoma from the limb or trunk should be treated initially by a block dissection of the regional lymph nodes, provided that distant metastases are excluded by CT scanning. The 5-year survival rates following this procedure are, as described earlier, dependent on the characteristics of the primary lesion, but overall figures of 20–25% may be expected. A policy of 'second-look' surgery is also appropriate for recurrent colorectal malignant disease, which should be detected through regular monitoring with plasma CEA levels and liver ultrasound. Local recurrence of colorectal cancer is rarely amenable to curative resectional surgery, but useful palliation can sometimes be achieved by further resection. In contrast, the detection of liver metastases from colorectal surgery should always lead to consideration for liver resection. Approximately 10% of all such patients will ultimately prove to have disease which is suitable for resection, and if there are fewer than four metastases confined to fewer than two anatomical segments of the liver, then a 5-year survival rate of 35% may be accomplished following liver resection. Of course the presence of extrahepatic disease should be excluded as far as possible before this is undertaken.

Reconstructive surgery for malignant disease

The ablative nature of radical surgery for malignant disease means that there is often a need for reconstructive or restorative surgery. The basis of reconstructive surgery is a sound knowledge of the vascular supply to the tissues to be used to reconstruct the defect which has been created. For example, the use of the stomach to restore intestinal continuity following total oesophagectomy is based on the fact that, provided the left gastric artery is divided at its origin from the coeliac axis, the stomach can be supplied totally by the right gastric and gastroepiploic arteries. By dividing the short gastric arteries and mobilizing the duodenum the gastric fundus can be made to reach almost to the base of the skull and can be used to replace the pharynx and oesphagus even following full pharyngolaryngo-oesophagectomy.

Similarly, the use of the rectus abdominis flap to reconstitute the breast following mastectomy is based on the anastomosis between the superior and inferior epigastric arteries. Another major myocutaneous flap commonly used for breast reconstruction is the latissimus dorsi flap which is based on the thoracodorsal vessels for its integrity. A number of other myocutaneous flaps such as the pectoralis flap are available for head and neck reconstruction, but several technological advances have been introduced which have greatly facilitated superficial reconstructive surgery. These are the use of subcutaneous tissue expanders to increase the amount of skin available to replace a defect and the advent of microvascular surgery to enable the transposition of large islands of tissue as free grafts.

Palliative surgery for malignant disease

It is self-evident that surgery for malignant disease cannot always be curative because either the primary or the secondary disease cannot be totally eradicated by surgical means. However, there are many circumstances under which surgical procedures may be employed to alleviate symptoms. These may be variously categorized as follows:

1. *For the alleviation of obstructive symptoms.* Obstruction by tumours of the oesophagus, stomach, periampullary region, small bowel and colon can all be alleviated by appropriate bypass surgery if resectional surgery (even if palliative) is not feasible. However, for certain conditions less invasive intervention enables obstructive symptoms to be overcome. The endoscopic insertion of an Atkinson tube through an inoperable carcinoma of the oesophagus has largely replaced the perioperative insertion of a Mousseau–Barbin tube. However, modern technology has now intervened to permit the endoscopic use of a laser beam to burn a lumen through the tumour. Although this is never curative it at least facilitates swallowing but carries the disadvantage of having to be repeated at intervals. Similarly, the insertion of stents through unresectable malignant strictures of the periampullary region, common bile duct and common, right and left hepatic ducts can be procured via ERCP, the transhepatic route or a combination of the two. Unfortunately, even with sophisticated scanning modalities it is often difficult to be certain that a stricture within the biliary tree is inoperable, and one should not lose sight of the fact that even with pancreatic cancer the 5-year survival rate after resection is 5%, and with carcinoma of the ampulla 35% of patients will survive 5 years after a pancreaticoduodenectomy. The subject of bypass surgery versus stenting for obstructive jaundice is currently the subject of considerable controversy, partly because of the difficulty in deciding which lesions are inoperable preoperatively and partly because of the frequency with which stents tend to block, compared with the relatively complication-free, though invasive, surgical bypass procedures.

2. *For the diminution of transfusion requirements.* Ulcerated lesions of the stomach or colon may not necessarily be curable by surgical resection but their existence may result in chronic anaemia as a consequence of chronic occult haemorrhage. Even in those deemed incurable at operation, resection may alleviate the symptoms of anaemia suffered by these unfortunate patients.

3. *For the relief of pain.* Pain, other than that of intestinal colic, is seldom relieved by surgical resection of a locally invasive tumour. Occasionally, neurectomy may be of help but this may also cause a degree of motor loss. For the deep infiltrating pain of conditions such as unresectable pancreatic cancer a coeliac axis block may be preferable to systemic analgesia.

OTHER MODALITIES OF CLINICAL ONCOTHERAPY

It is unfortunate that for many tumours in which the surgeon plays a central management role alternative treatments are seldom successful in providing a cure once surgery is no longer an appropriate therapeutic option. There are three types of non-surgical treatment for malignant disease. These are readily categorized into radiotherapy, chemotherapy and biological response modification.

Radiotherapy

A detailed description of the way in which radiotherapy works is beyond the scope of this chapter (see Ch 24). The principles of radiation therapy are well established, but it is important to appreciate that there is no consistent difference between the radiosensitivity of normal and tumour tissue within a particular organ. The unit of absorbed radiation dose is the gray, 1 Gy being equivalent to 1 J of energy per kilogram. Cells in mitosis are those which are most susceptible to the lethal effects of irradiation, but cells in the late S phase when the nuclear material has been duplicated are more resistant. Nonetheless, such is the level of expertise with fractionated radiotherapy that not only is this modality used as palliative therapy for certain unresectable or metastatic lesions, but it is now also employed as adjunctive to surgery, as for example following wide local excision of T1–T2 breast carcinoma or following excision of a rectal carcinoma. Unfortunately, a disappointingly large number of tumours remain relatively radioresistant, as for example those arising in the adult kidney, adenocarcinomas of the stomach and malignant melanoma.

Irradiation depopulates a tumour of its malignant cells mainly via direct effects during mitosis, and thus the efficacy of fractionated irradiation is determined by the number of clonogenic cells which the tumour contains, its intrinsic radiosensitivity and the mitotic rate. Since irradiation damage becomes manifest during mitosis it follows that the normal tissues and tumour cells with a high cellular turnover such as the bone marrow and enterocytes will show evidence of damage within a few hours of irradiation. Conversely it may be many weeks or months before the maximum effect of radiotherapy is apparent in more slowly proliferating tumours such as basal cell carcinoma of the skin. A more detailed description of the scope and clinical application of radiotherapy is given by Duncan (1988).

Chemotherapy

As with radiotherapy, more sophisticated application of chemotherapeutic regimens, coupled in many instances with reduced systemic toxicity, has led chemotherapy from a palliative role to that of a surgical adjunct and, occasionally, the sole curative therapy for some tumours (see Ch 25). It may be used as an adjunct prior to surgery (so-called 'neo-adjuvant therapy'), as in the treatment of locally advanced breast or oesophageal cancer, or postoperatively as in premenopausal women. Thus the scope of chemotherapy has broadened enormously in recent years. Cytotoxic drugs interfere with cell division, irrespective of whether the cell is normal or malignant.

This means that the success of chemotherapy is dependent on the intrinsic resistance of the tumour cell to the drug and the dose-limiting toxicity of the drug against the normal tissues. In general, four main groups of anticancer drugs are categorized. These are as follows:

1. *Alkylating agents* such as the nitrosoureas and epoxide groups (cyclophosphamide, melphalan, chlorambucil, etc.). These compounds contain an alkyl group (.e.g. CH_3) which combines with other intracellular molecules such as nucleic acids, proteins (especially enzymes) and cell membranes. Damage to the enzymes which link DNA strands thus impairs mitosis during the S phase of the cell cycle.

2. *Antimetabolites* have a similar chemical structure to the compounds required for the elaboration of nucleic acids. They therefore disrupt the sequence of DNA by being incorporated instead of the normal nucleotide or irreversibly bind to the constituting enzyme and render it ineffective. This class of drugs includes methotrexate, 5-fluorouracil, cytosine arabinoside and 6-mercaptopurine.

3. *Vinca alkaloids* bind to intracellular tubulin and inhibit microtubule formation which constitutes the spindle during mitosis. Thus mitosis is arrested at metaphase. The components of this group are vincristine, vinblastine and vindesine.

4. *Antimitotic antibiotics* are a large group of agents which includes adriamycin, epirubicin, actinomycin D, mitomycin C and bleomycin. The first two drugs act in a variety of ways, including intercalation between opposing DNA strands leading to disturbed DNA function. Actinomycin D and mitomycin C impair DNA and RNA synthesis and generate harmful toxic free oxygen radicals.

There also exists a further miscellaneous group of agents whose mechanisms of action are varied or unknown. Cisplatin and its less toxic derivative carboplatin react with the guanine in DNA and form cross-linkages along the DNA chain as well as between DNA strands. Other agents such as etoposide are tubular poisons derived from podophyllotoxin.

Clinically, many of these agents are used in varying combinations which have been developed to maximize therapeutic efficacy without excessively augmenting toxicity. However, their effects on normal proliferating cells cause them to be especially toxic to bone marrow and intestinal cells.

Biological response modifiers

These are a miscellaneous group of compounds, many of which have been developed by recombinant DNA technology. Some, such as the interferons and tumour necrosis factor (TNF), act directly on tumour cells to produce cytostasis or cell death through as yet obscure mechanisms. Others act directly by augmenting endogenous host responses to the tumour, as for example interleukin-2, which activates cytotoxic T-lymphocytes in patients with malignant melanoma. A further group of agents, the colony-stimulating factors, are finding an important role in preventing the bone marrow suppression and septicaemic episodes commonly associated with high-dose chemotherapy. Whether this results in higher clinical response rates as a consequence of higher and more protracted chemotherapeutic dosages remains to be seen.

It seems reasonable to include endocrine manipulation under the heading of biological response modifiers. The concept that the trophic or stimulatory effects of a hormone can be abrogated by agents which block the activity of a receptor for that hormone is an important one in the management of patients with breast cancer, where tamoxifen is employed to block the binding of oestrogen to its receptor. The discovery of receptors for autocrine hormones on tumour cells, as described at the beginning of this chapter, will undoubtedly lead to the construction of synthetic analogues of these autocrine growth factors, so that their administration can be used to block the receptor binding sites for therapeutic purposes in the future.

As with surgery, the cost/benefit ratio of these various treatments must be considered carefully before they are administered to a particular patient. It is quite unreasonable to impair the quality of life of a patient in the terminal stages of disease by administering a toxic therapy or the physical assault of surgery unless this is going to prolong life considerably, or relieve symptoms. This is one of the most difficult judgements which the oncologist has to make and the trainee must learn how to enter into a careful, informed and sympathetic discussion with the patient in order to reach a joint conclusion as to the desirability or otherwise of a therapeutic course of action.

ACKNOWLEDGEMENTS

I am grateful to Miss V. France for her expert typographical assistance in the preparation of this chapter.

FURTHER READING

Duncan W 1988 Ionising radiation and radiotherapy. In: Cuschieri A, Giles G R, Moosa A R (eds) Essential surgical practice, 2nd edn. Wright, London, p 190–202
Guillou P J 1990 Biological response modifiers in the treatment of cancer. Clinical Oncology 2: 347–353
McArdle C 1990 Surgical oncology. Butterworth, Oxford
Priestman T J 1989 Cancer chemotherapy: an introduction, 3rd edn. Springer, Berlin

24. The principles of radiotherapy

R. A. Huddart   J. R. Yarnold

SOURCES OF IONIZING RADIATION

Radiotherapy is the therapeutic use of ionizing radiation for the treatment of malignant disorders. Natural sources of radiation include radioactive isotopes which decay with the production of a β-particles (electrons) and γ-rays (a form of electromagnetic radiation). Originally radium was used, but over the last 20 years this has been replaced by safer artificial isotopes such as cobalt-60, caesium-137 and iridium-192, which are generated in nuclear reactors. Isotopes are used mainly as sources implanted directly into tissues (e.g. iridium needles in the treatment of carcinoma of the tongue) or inserted into a cavity (e.g. caesium sources inserted into the uterus and vagina for the treatment of carcinoma of the cervix). Radioactive isotopes may also be given systemically (e.g. iodine-131 in the treatment of thyroid cancer).

External beam radiotherapy was revolutionized in the 1950s by the advent of megavoltage treatment machines; initially cobalt machines and later linear accelerators. The linear accelerator generates a stream of electrons which is accelerated to high speed by microwave energy before hitting a tungsten target. This interaction results in the emission of high-energy X-rays. The high-energy X-ray beam produced by a linear accelerator has several properties which make it well suited for present day radiotherapy:

1. The greater penetration of the γ-rays means that a high proportion of the dose applied to the body surface reaches the tumour.

2. All X-ray beams have a fuzzy edge (the *penumbra*) due to the reflection and scattering of the beam by tissues. High-energy X-rays suffer relatively little sideways scatter as they pass through tissues, and this helps to keep the edge of the beam sharp.

3. The forward scattering effect is also indirectly responsible for the point of maximum dose being 1–2 cm below the skin surface (Fig. 24.1). The skin therefore receives a low dose and is spared from radiation

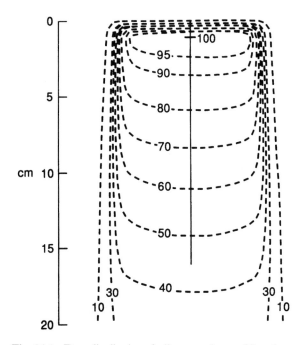

Fig. 24.1 Dose distribution of a linear accelerator. Note the maximum dose is below the skin surface and 65% of the applied dose is present at 10 cm.

reactions. It was the high skin doses associated with low-energy X-ray machines that in the past caused the uncomfortable skin reactions and limited treatments of deep-seated tumours.

In addition, cyclotrons can be used to produce ionizing beams of heavier particles such as neutrons or protons. However, these machines are yet to find a place in routine clinical practice.

ACTIONS OF IONIZING RADIATION

X-rays (from linear accelerators) and γ-rays (from isotopes) are both forms of electromagnetic radiation and are biologically indistinguishable. High-energy X-rays consist of packets of energy (photons) which interact with the molecules of body tissues to cause ionization and release electrons of high kinetic energy. These electrons cause secondary damage to adjacent molecules, including DNA via an oxygen-dependent mechanism. The resultant DNA damage is mostly repaired by enzymes in a matter of hours, but certain DNA lesions are irreparable. Non-repairable DNA damage causes a variety of chromosomal abnormalities which prevent normal mitosis from occurring. It may also trigger programmed cell death in some normal cell lineages (e.g. lymphoid, myeloid and germ cells). When the cell tries to divide it dies in the attempt. This DNA damage, however, does not stop most cells from performing their normal physiological functions effectively. Thus damage is expressed only if the cell attempts mitosis, and in fully differentiated cells incapable of further division (e.g. muscle cells) this damage may never be expressed. Hence:

- Tissues may be severely damaged by irradiation but appear essentially normal; damaged cells may be expressed only if they are stimulated to divide
- Response to radiotherapy by tumours may be delayed, especially in tumours with slow rates of growth (e.g. pituitary tumours).

There are many data on the respective effects of radiotherapy on normal tissues and tumours. It appears that tumour cells may not differ greatly from the cell of origin in response to single doses of radiotherapy, although there may be differences in the ability of tumours and normal tissues to recover from the effects of cell damage. For example, normal tissues have a greater ability to respond to radiation-induced cell depletion by accelerated repopulation, an ability which seems to be less developed in tumours. To eradicate a tumour within the limits of tolerance of surrounding normal tissues, radiotherapy must exploit these and other subtle differences in DNA repair and regrowth of normal tissues.

In external beam treatments, therapeutic advantage is generally achieved by dividing the total dose of radiotherapy into small parts over several weeks, a practice called *fractionation*. A full discussion of the effects of fractionation is not possible in this chapter but generally:

1. Reducing the dose per fraction allows certain critical normal tissues such as the nervous system, the lungs and other slowly proliferating tissues to repair damage more effectively than tumours.

2. Fractionation over a period of several days or weeks gives rapidly proliferating normal tissues such as skin and gut a chance to repopulate and hence recover from

radiotherapy-induced damage faster than tumours.

3. Many tumours contain hypoxic areas. As the major effect of radiotherapy is by an oxygen-dependent mechanism, these areas are relatively resistant to radiotherapy. Each fraction of radiotherapy reduces the number of tumour cells and allows some hypoxic areas to become better oxygenated. Fractionation allows this process of reoxygenation which may take hours or days to occur and is thought to make tumours more radiocurable.

The above comments help to explain the empirical finding that radiotherapy is most effective when given daily over several weeks. A comparable effect to fractionation is seen with interstitial and intracavity treatments where a continuous low exposure over several days is biologically equivalent to multiple small fractions.

The ability to a cure a tumour probably depends on being able to eliminate every clonogenic tumour cell from the target volume. This is influenced by a variety of factors: size of tumour, radiosensitivity of tumour cells and tolerance of normal tissues.

Size of tumour

In theory, successive doses of radiotherapy will eliminate equal fractions of the tumour cells. The larger the tumour the greater the number of cells present and hence a larger number of fractions will be necessary to have a high probability of eliminating the last clonogenic tumour cell. For example, the majority of 2 cm carcinomas can be controlled by 60 Gy, whereas a 4 cm carcinoma needs 80 Gy for similar control rates. As discussed above, large tumours may also contain large hypoxic areas which are relatively radioresistant and thus reduce the chance of cure. Large tumours usually need a larger treatment volume than small tumours. This usually increases the volume of normal tissue irradiated; the greater the volume of normal tissue the higher the chance that a part of that tissue is damaged by the radiotherapy and hence the normal tissue complication rate rises. To reduce this complication rate a dose reduction is often necessary, with a corresponding reduction in the chance of cure.

Radiosensitivity of tumour cells

The commonest histological types of tumour have cells of similar radiosensitivities (e.g. squamous carcinoma cells and adenocarcinoma cells). Differences in tumour cure between these common histological types probably relate more to differences in tumour bulk, oxygenation and proliferation. There are exceptions, with the cells of some tumours being more radiosensitive (e.g. seminoma and lymphoma) and others being more radioresistant (e.g. melanoma, glioma and sarcomas). The reasons for these differences are not clear. Radiosensitive tumours may be more sensitive due to a greater tendency to undergo apoptosis in response to DNA damage, but there is evidence, at least in vitro, that a variety of other mechanisms may have a role (e.g. melanoma seems to be more resistant to radiotherapy due to an increased ability to repair DNA damage).

Tolerance of normal tissues

The total dose which can be applied to a tumour is limited by the tolerance of the surrounding normal tissue. This varies greatly between tissues. If the tumour lies close to a sensitive organ (e.g. the spinal cord), then the total dose that can be safely delivered is much less than if the tumour lies within muscle or bone, for example. Hence the chance of cure may be reduced. The dose that can be applied will also depend on the volume needed to be irradiated. A good example of this is the lung. The tolerance dose for whole lung to be able to function after treatment is in the region of 20 Gy in 10 fractions of 2 Gy. Therefore, if the whole lung or large sections need to be treated (e.g. selected cases of Hodgkin's disease) this is the maximal fractionated tolerated dose. However, doses as high as 60 Gy can be given to portions of a lung, such as the lobe, because small areas of permanent damage are acceptable and have little overall effect on lung function.

RADIOTHERAPY PLANNING

The major principle of radiotherapy is to give the maximum possible dose to the smallest volume which will encompass all the tumour. This volume, termed the *target volume*, consists of:

1. The macroscopic tumour volume determined from clinical findings, imaging (X-rays, computed tomography (CT) scans, radioisotope scans, etc.) and operative findings.
2. A biological margin (often 0.5–1 cm) which allows for microscopic tumour spread beyond the visible tumour. It may also include allowance for nodal spread.
3. A technical margin, usually 0.5 cm to allow for errors and variability in daily set-up (e.g. due to respiratory movements of the patient). Minimizing these errors and improving quality assurance is an area of active research. Techniques such as megavoltage imaging (in which an X-ray image of the patient is produced as the treatment beam passes through the tumour, showing how well the area actually treated cor-

responds to the treatment plan) may enter clinical practice in the future.

Localizing the tumour in the patient accurately is essential to the success of radiotherapy. In most cases the tumour cannot be visualized directly and localization depends on physical examination, imaging and operative notes. The importance of accurate and detailed operative records cannot be overemphasized. An operation is a unique opportunity to visualize the tumour directly, and full advantage of this opportunity must be taken to describe the extent of disease and acquire as much additional information as possible about local pathology. Limited information invariably leads to larger target volumes, increased radiotherapy morbidity and reduced cure rates.

Once the radiotherapist has determined the exact size, shape and location of the target volume the aim is to encompass the target volume with a radiation dose distributed as homogeneously as possible. A variation of under 10% is aimed for and achieved. Single fields are usually inadequate in this respect, except for superficial tumours. Opposing two fields at 180° to each other treats intervening tissue homogeneously. This arrangement is very simple to plan and is suitable for most low-dose palliative and a few radical treatments. Two opposed fields usually include more normal tissue in the high-dose volume than is strictly necessary (Fig. 24.2). Therefore, more complex multifield arrangements are normal for curative treatments to confine the high dose volume more closely to the target. These arrangements are planned either by drawing the target volume on orthogonal anteroposterior and lateral X-ray films of the patient or, more usually, by taking the cross-sectional target volume directly from CT scans of the patient in the treatment position.

Directing several beams of radiation accurately to intersect across the target volume does not necessarily guarantee an even dose distribution because the X-rays have to pass through different amounts of tissue on the way from the entry point on the skin to the target volume. In addition, lung absorbs less energy than other tissues because of the air it contains. These potential sources of dose inhomogeneity throughout the target volume must be calculated and compensated for using a number of measures that alter the beam shape and profile (e.g. different weightings on each X-ray beam and the introduction of wedge-shaped filters which absorb different amounts of energy across the beam) (Fig. 24.3). Production of homogeneous dose distributions has been greatly facilitated by the introduction of planning computers and CT planning which can visualize and allow for tissue inhomogeneities directly. This area continues

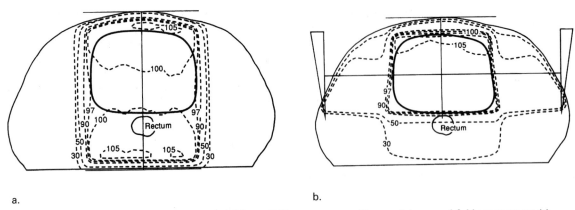

a.   b.

Fig. 24.2   Comparison of the dose distribution of different field arrangements. The parallel opposed field arrangement (a) adequately treats the target volume (the bladder) but gives a high rectal dose. A three-field arrangement (b) covers the target volume with a much reduced rectal dose and is therefore preferable.

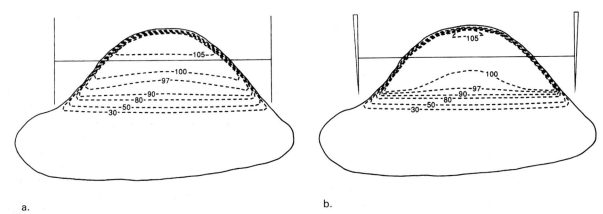

a.   b.

Fig. 24.3   Treating the breast without compensation for breast curvature produces an inhomogeneous dose distribution (a). When this is compensated for by a wedge filter (b) the dose distribution is improved.

to develop rapidly, and in the future more sophisticated means of compensating for potential sources of uneven dose distribution will come into routine practice, as will more advanced beam-defining devices.

Once satisfactory dose distribution and treatment plans have been produced and checked, treatment of the patient can begin. It is important that treatment is applied in a reproducible fashion. The patient must be positioned, lying in a recorded position, with appropriate supports to maintain stability. Lasers are frequently used to help establish and monitor patient alignment. If extra accuracy is desirable (especially in the head and neck region) a light plastic shell may be used to immobilize the patient. The machine is then positioned according to skin markings and recorded settings determined during planning, and treatment is commenced.

RADIOTHERAPY: THE FUTURE

In recent years several new techniques have improved the therapeutic ratio in selected circumstances.

Accelerated radiotherapy

This involves giving multiple daily treatments of the same size as used in conventional fractionation but given to shorten the overall treatment time from 6 weeks to less than 3 weeks. Recent research suggests that clonogenic tumour cells can proliferate significantly during a treatment course of 6 weeks and this could, theoretically, reduce the chance of tumour control. Reducing the overall treatment time could make an important difference, allowing less time for proliferation and leaving fewer tumour cells to kill. However, reducing treatment time also gives normal tissues less time to recover. Enhanced early skin and mucosal reactions may limit this approach.

Hyperfractionation

This delivers two or three smaller fractions a day over the conventional treatment period (i.e. the number of treatment days remains the same but the number of fractions is increased). Reducing fraction size reduces late tissue damage, with relatively less effect on tumour control. Theoretically, this allows dose escalation, with an increased chance of cure.

CHART

This stands for 'continuous hyperfractionated accelerated radiotherapy'. This new regime aims to combine the advantages of accelerated and hyperfractionated radiotherapy by giving three treatments a day over a 12-day period, with no gaps (including no breaks for weekends and bank holidays). Preliminary results from a multicentre trial has shown that CHART improved survival in patients with localized lung cancer and, to a lesser extent, local control and survival in patients with head and neck cancer.

Neutrons and heavy ion therapy

Heavy ions, including neutrons, can be produced by cyclotrons which can now be used in the therapeutic situation. They damage DNA by a non-oxygen-dependent mechanism. Therefore, hypoxic areas in tumours are not protected from the lethal effects of this form of ionizing radiation. Recent work, however, suggests that hypoxic areas are not as important as was previously thought, and it is also now recognized that neutron-induced damage is less well repaired by normal tissues. This means that, though increased local control has been demonstrated in selected tumours (e.g. salivary gland tumours), an increase in late morbidity is observed. Neutrons therefore have, to date, no role in common tumours.

Conformal therapy

Conventional therapy uses rectangular fields to encompass the target volume. As tumours are not cubes, an unnecessary amount of normal tissue is included in the treated volume. This causes increased morbidity and limits the doses that can be given (e.g. for pelvic tumours the dose given is limited by the amount of small bowel included in the target volume). Conformal therapy uses new engineering and computer technology to generate irregularly shaped fields so that tumours can be encompassed by high dose volumes which correspond more precisely to the tumour's shape. The hope is that the same cure rate can be achieved with reduced morbidity, or that dose escalation can occur with increased cure rates for the same morbidity.

ROLE OF RADIOTHERAPY

Radiotherapy may be used in the management of malignant disorders in the following ways:

- As primary treatment
- As adjuvant treatment prior to or following primary surgery (or chemotherapy)
- For palliation of symptoms
- As a systemic treatment, either in the form of external beam total body irradiation or systemic administration of a radioactive isotope.

Radiotherapy as primary treatment

When radiotherapy is used as the primary treatment the aim is to effect cure with the minimum of side-effects. It is an alternative modality of local control to surgery (Table 24.1). Radiotherapy, like surgery, is most effective at controlling small, well-localized and defined tumours, but has the advantage of preserving normal function. For many cancers, surgery and radiotherapy are equally effective modes of treatment and close liaison between surgeons and radiotherapists is essential if the appropriate modality of treatment is to be chosen for any given patient. This choice may vary between patients and depends on a variety of tumour (including site, stage and histology) and patient (including age and performance status) factors. Choice of modality of treatment is not restricted just to either surgery alone or radiotherapy alone; a policy of initial radiotherapy followed by planned salvage surgery if this fails (as in many head and neck tumours) or initial combination therapy may best serve the patient.

Radiotherapy may be indicated as the initial treatment by a variety of circumstances, including:

1. Sites where surgery and radiotherapy are equally effective but radiotherapy gives better functional or cosmetic results (e.g. in bladder cancer where radical radiotherapy gives good results and avoids the necessity of cystectomy and ileal conduit, or laryngeal cancer where radiotherapy gives equal results to surgery but allows preservation of the voice).

2. Very radiosensitive tumours such as lymph node

Table 24.1   Results of curative radiotherapy

Site	Stage	Survival (5 years)	Comment
Skin	All	90–95%	Equivalent to surgery. Choice depends on site
Head and neck			
Tongue	T1	91%	50–60% for all stages
Glottis	T1	90%	
Other sites	All	30–80%	Local control rates with salvage surgery used for local relapse
Gastrointestinal tract			
Oesophagus	All	9%	Equivalent to surgery
Anal canal	All	66%	Better results than ano-perineal resection
Urology			
Bladder	T2/3	34%	Salvage cystectomy for local relapse. Surgery only 28% 5-year survival
Prostate	T1/2	80%	Equivalent to surgery
	T3	60%	
Penile	All	75%	Over 90% cure for stage 1 tumours
Gynaecology			
Cervix	1B	85–90%	Equivalent to surgery in randomized studies
	2A/B	61–85%	
Endometrium	All	60–65%	For patients unfit for surgery only
Vagina	Stage 1	75%	

metastases from testicular cancers or early Hodgkin's disease.

3. Inoperable tumours. Occasionally radiotherapy can be used for attempted cure (e.g. brain-stem gliomas or pelvic sarcomas).

4. At sites where operations carry a high morbidity/mortality and equivalent results are gained by radiotherapy (e.g. carcinoma of upper or mid-oesophagus).

5. In patients unfit for radical surgery when surgery is otherwise the treatment of choice (e.g. patients with bronchial cancer and chronic airways disease).

All cases, however, need to be carefully assessed to decide the appropriate treatment option. In some cases where radiotherapy would normally be indicated other factors may make surgery preferable in that patient. For instance, it may not be possible to apply a radical dose because of an adjacent sensitive structure (e.g. if small bowel is adherent to the bladder, giving a full radical dose may be impossible without a risk of severe morbidity and cystectomy may be indicated). Alternatively, bone or cartilage involvement by tumour may have occurred (especially in head and neck cancer). In such cases the risk of osteoradionecrosis following radical radiotherapy is greatly increased, making surgery the preferred option.

Adjuvant radiotherapy

For some tumours preoperative or postoperative radiotherapy may improve local control. Adjuvant radiotherapy (Table 24.2) achieves this by controlling microscopic spread beyond resection margins, tumour spilled at operation or lymph node metastases. The low tumour burden means that lower doses than those normally used in radical treatments can be employed with a resultant reduced morbidity while obtaining a high rate of local control. If local control is an important determinant of survival then this may equate with an improvement in overall survival. Even if metastases limit survival, adjuvant radiotherapy often has a valuable role in improving locoregional control and quality of life. This may be especially important if symptoms of relapse cannot be easily controlled (e.g. rectal cancer).

Adjuvant treatment may be given to (a) the site of primary disease to reduce local recurrence or (b) sites of potential metastatic spread.

Postoperative radiotherapy has the advantages of the radiotherapist having details of surgical and pathological findings available in addition to clinical and radiological assessment. This allows for accurate staging and selection of those cases which would most benefit from radiotherapy.

However, the planning of postoperative radiotherapy can be more difficult, as the radiotherapist can no longer

Table 24.2   Role of adjuvant radiotherapy (RT)

Site	Stage	Criteria	Results No RT	RT	Comment
Breast	T1/2 N0	LC	63%	88%	NSABP randomized trial of conservative
	T1/2 N +	LC	57%	94%	surgery/radiotherapy
Central nervous system					
Astrocytomas	Gd 1	S	25%	58%	
Oligodendrogliomas	All	10 year S	27%	50%	
Pituitary	All	10 year LC	10%	90%	RMH data
Craniopharyngioma	Incomplete excision	S	35%	90%	70% Survival for complete excision
Gastrointestinal tract					
Pancreas	Operable tumour	2 year S surv.	15%	42%	GITSG trial NO RT V RT with 5-fluorouracil
Rectum	Dukes' C	LC	65%	90%	MRC 3rd trial survival advantage in some series
Cholangiocarcinoma	Operable tumour	Median surv.	5 mo.	11 mo.	Non-randomized data
Gynaecology					
Endometrium	Stage 1	LC	88%	99%	
	Stage 1	S	64%	81%	
	Stage 2	S	20%	56%	
Parotid					
Carcinomas	All	LC	62%	87%	
Pleomorphic adenomas	Incomplete excision	LC	76%	98%	
Bladder	T2/T3B	S	28%	45%	Non-randomized data

LC, 5-year local control rate.
S, 5-year survival.
NSABP: National Surgical Adjuvant Breast and Bowel Project.

GITSG: Gastrointestinal Tumor Study Group.
MRC: Medical Research Council.

directly image the tumour. Accurate operation notes greatly aid localization of treatment, as does marking the tumour bed with clips. If the need for postoperative radiotherapy is anticipated prior to operation it is often helpful for the radiotherapist to see the patient pre-operatively (e.g. prior to wide local excision of a small breast cancer). Postoperative radiotherapy is of proven value in reducing local recurrence at many sites, some of which are discussed below. At most sites postoperative radiotherapy is of no proven benefit in prolonging survival after complete resection of the primary tumour.

In selected circumstances, preoperative radiotherapy may be of value. Preoperative radiotherapy has the potential advantage of a downstaging effect which may allow an easier or less extensive operation to be performed (e.g. in rectal cancer or limb sarcomas). It may also reduce the risk of seeding at the time of operation and control microscopic disease at the edges of the tumour. Certain problems have limited the usefulness of this approach; foremost is the fear that radiotherapy increases the surgical morbidity. However, it is now thought that, as long as the operation is performed

within 4 weeks of radiotherapy, this increase is minimal with doses of radiotherapy up to 40 Gy. A further problem is that the downstaging effect of the radiotherapy makes interpretation of the subsequent surgical specimen and pathological staging difficult. This also causes difficulties in comparing different series of patients, assessing prognosis and giving advice on further treatment. It is therefore a less established form of treatment, but is used particularly in bladder cancer and sarcomas and, less often, in the treatment of rectal, oesophageal and endometrial cancers.

Radiotherapy to sites of lymph node spread has been used in the treatment of many cancers, especially when it was thought that blood-borne spread followed lymph node invasion. Increasingly, studies suggest that lymph node metastasis may be a marker of synchronous blood-borne metastasis and at several sites prophylactic lymph node irradiation has been shown to be of little value in survival terms (e.g. bladder and prostatic cancer). Despite this, in a variety of cancers, lymph node irradiation is of value when initial spread is to lymph nodes and is an important determinant of survival (e.g.

head and neck cancers) or relapse-free survival (e.g. seminoma). Prophylactic lymph node irradiation is also justified in reducing the risk of macroscopic nodal disease when symptomatic relapse is difficult to salvage. An example of this is supraclavicular fossa irradiation in axillary lymph-node-positive breast cancer. Node relapse at this site is difficult to salvage and has a high morbidity in terms of lymphoedema and brachial plexus neuropathy. The risk of such relapse is markedly reduced by applying adjuvant radiotherapy.

In a similar fashion, craniospinal irradiation improves prognosis when central nervous system (CNS) spread is common (e.g. medulloblastoma and ependymomas). Chemotherapy only poorly penetrates the CNS, and for some otherwise chemosensitive tumours the CNS may act as a sanctuary site (e.g. acute lymphoblastic leukaemia (ALL) and small cell lung cancer). If cerebrospinal fluid (CSF) metastases are common, cranial or craniospinal irradiation is a highly successful form of prophylaxis. For example, following the introduction of irradiation the incidence of CNS relapse was reduced from 67% to 4% in patients.

Palliation

Of all modalities used to treat advanced cancer, radiotherapy is the most useful for the palliation of symptoms either from advanced primary or metastatic disease. The criteria of success must be in terms of quality of life rather than survival. The aim is therefore to give sufficient treatment to relieve symptoms without short-term side-effects for as long as the patient is expected to survive. High-dose prolonged palliative courses are necessary in certain circumstances, especially if prognosis is relatively good and substantial growth delay is necessary (e.g. recurrent chest wall breast cancer or pelvic recurrences of rectal cancers). Nevertheless, the trend is towards short courses delivering a few large fractions of radiotherapy, thereby achieving maximum symptom relief with minimal interference in the patient's life. Frequently, a single large fraction of radiotherapy is all that is necessary to palliate symptoms. Palliative radiotherapy may be used for symptomatic incurable primary cancer or locally recurrent disease. For example, most patients with lung cancer present with disease too advanced for any radical treatment. Such patients are frequently symptomatic with, for example, haemoptysis, dyspnoea, pain or cough. They are usually well controlled with one or two fractions of radiotherapy. At other sites, particularly in pelvic tumours, longer fractionated courses to higher doses are necessary to offer a good chance of sustained symptom relief. In addition, palliative radiotherapy may be used for relief of

symptoms due to metastases. The treatments of different types of metastasis are considered below.

Bone metastasis

Symptomatic bone metastases effect approximately 20% of patients at some stage during their illness. Radiotherapy is a highly effective means of controlling local pain due to such bone involvement. Recent work has shown that a single 8 Gy fraction of radiotherapy will relieve pain partially or completely in 80% of patients 4 weeks after treatment. Lesions with substantial cortical bone erosion should, however, be considered for orthopaedic fixation followed by radiotherapy to prevent fracture. Patients with extensive bone metastases (as frequently see in prostate cancer) obtain good palliation from wide-field hemibody irradiation given as a single treatment. The other half-body can be treated 4–6 weeks later and 67% of patients obtain good pain relief. An alternative approach is to use a radioactive isotope (strontium-89) which is taken up by bone metastases. It is given as a simple intravenous injection and may be repeated. In randomized studies (in prostate cancer) strontium-89 produced pain relief equivalent to local or hemibody irradiation, with the advantage of lower toxicity and the appearance of fewer new sites of pain on subsequent follow-up.

Spinal cord compression

This is an emergency which can cause devastating motor, sensory and sphincter disturbances. Metastatic disease can cause cord compression by direct extension from vertebral disease, epidural deposits or, rarely, intramedullary disease. There has been no trial of radiotherapy versus surgery in the treatment of this disorder, but it is generally considered that neurosurgical decompression gives the most rapid relief and should be considered for fit patients with short, single blocks. This should be followed by postoperative radiotherapy. Patients not fit for surgery (including patients with multiple levels of compression, anterior tumours and poor performance status) should receive urgent radiotherapy. Over 70% of patients will achieve good pain relief and 50% a useful response if treated before a major neurological deficit develops. Some patients will regain the ability to walk, but only 10% of total paraplegics regain useful function.

Brain metastases

This is a frequent complication of advanced cancer and is associated with a high morbidity. They are especially common in lung cancer, breast cancer (10% of all patients at some stage), melanoma, kidney and colon carcinomas. They are usually multiple and the prognosis is poor, with the median survival if untreated being 6 weeks. A 50% symptomatic response rate to radiotherapy and dexamethasone is expected, the radiosensitive tumours such as small cell lung, breast and colon cancers responding better than average. A good response to dexamethasone and good performance status also predict for good outcome. Frail patients with poor performance status tend to gain little and treatment may not be indicated in such patients. Short courses of treatment seem to be as effective as longer courses and a current study organized by the Royal College of Radiologists is comparing 12 Gy in two fractions with a conventional course of 30 Gy in 10 fractions. Patients with a single metastasis have a better outlook, with a median survival of 4–6 months, and 30% of patients with breast cancer survive over 1 year. There is some evidence that surgical resection followed by whole-brain irradiation is better than whole-brain irradiation only (in selected patients fit for surgery). It is unclear whether whole-brain irradiation with a local boost to the tumour would do equally well.

Superior venal caval obstruction (SVCO)

SVCO is caused by enlarged right-sided mediastinal lymph nodes or tumours (especially lung cancers). It causes engorgement of veins to the neck, cyanosis, facial oedema and dyspnoea. Seventy per cent of patients gain relief within 14 days following mediastinal radiotherapy.

Other indications

Some other indications for palliative radiotherapy are retinal metastases, skin metastases and lymph node metastases.

Radiotherapy for the treatment of systemic disease

Radiotherapy is generally used to treat local disease. There are, however, two areas where radiotherapy is used to treat systemic disease: total body irradiation and radioactive isotopes.

Total body irradiation

A total body dose of >4 Gy will result in bone marrow failure. This has limited the usefulness of the technique for the treatment of malignant disease until the onset of bone marrow transplantation. Total body irradiation using a dose of 8–10 Gy as a single dose or a higher fractionated dose is a highly effective conditioning regimen for the treatment of leukaemias. It is also being examined in trials in the treatment of other radiosensitive tumours such as lymphomas.

Radioactive isotopes

This technique uses radioactive isotopes which emit short-range β-particles and/or γ-rays. If the tumour concentrates the isotope compared to the surrounding tissues it will be preferentially irradiated. The best example is the use of iodine-131 in the treatment of follicular and papillary thyroid cancer. The malignant tissue takes up and concentrates iodine, and hence residual tumour is irradiated to a high dose. Using this technique, lung and sometimes bone metastases can be eliminated. Other examples are the use of phosphorus-32 in polycythaemia rubra vera, strontium-89 in metastatic prostate cancer (see above) and m-iodo-benzylguanidine (MIBG) in neuroblastoma.

COMPLICATIONS

Normal tissue side-effects are due to cellular damage inflicted at the time of irradiation. This damage is largely expressed at the time of mitosis, so the sensitivity to and the expression of this damage depend on the proliferative characteristics of each tissue.

In some tissues, such as the epidermal layers of the skin, the small intestine and bone marrow stem cells, turnover is rapid and damage is expressed early. Skin is the classic example of such a tissue. Stem cells in the basal layer of the skin divide; the daughter cells differentiate and move to the surface over a 2-week period to replace shed cells. After irradiation, production of replacement cells is reduced or halted. The epidermis gradually thins and, if sufficient damage has occurred, epidermal integrity is lost and desquamation occurs. Recovery will occur over a period of days or weeks after the end of treatment by surviving stem cells producing enough daughter cells to cover the deficient area.

It can be seen that:

- The time to onset of side-effects is determined by the skin turnover time, i.e. 2 weeks for skin but 5 days for small intestine
- The severity and length of time to recovery depend on the amount of damage to the stem cells and hence on radiation dose
- Provided there is a certain number of clonogenic cells surviving, recovery is likely to be complete.

Although this mechanism is responsible for most acute reactions the clinical effect will vary from site to site. For example, in the upper gastrointestinal tract acute reactions cause inflammation and discomfort (mucositis and oesophagitis, while small or large bowel damage by similar mechanisms causes vomiting, diarrhoea or, more rarely, ulceration and bleeding.

Other acute reactions, however, may operate by different mechanisms and are less well understood (e.g. somnolence after cranial irradiation).

Stem cell damage, as described above, usually recovers completely but, if severe, long-lasting effects can occur. The most important example of this is gonadal damage. Oocytes are particularly radiosensitive and even moderate doses of a few grays of radiation precipitate premature menopause. Spermatogenesis is also sensitive to radiotherapy. Doses in the region of 3 Gy cause oligospermia or azoospermia which may last 6 months to 1 year, but higher doses (>6 Gy) cause permanent sterility. In many tissues the parenchymal cells turn over very slowly (e.g. hepatocytes). As radiation damage is expressed at mitosis, lethal damage will not be expressed until cells divide weeks, months or even years later. In such tissues damage can be due to depletion of parenchymal or connective tissues, or to vascular damage.

Depletion of parenchymal or connective tissues

Irradiation of the thyroid gland, for example, leads to gradual depletion of thyroid follicular cells and can cause hypothyroidism over a period of many years. Likewise, renal irradiation causes depletion of renal tubular cells and renal impairment over a period of years.

Vascular damage

Damage to the vasculature is a common mechanism of damage, especially in tissues which never replicate (e.g. neurons or cardiac muscle) or which replicate only very slowly (e.g. fibroblasts). Radiation has a wide range of pathological effects on the vasculature due to damage to both endothelial cells and to connective tissue. This leads to impairment of the fine vasculature, often in a patchy fashion. The damage can result in poor wound healing, tissue atrophy, ulceration, strictures and formation of telangectasia.

The precise clinical effect depends on the organ involved. For example, in the bladder the telangectasia can cause haematuria, while fibrosis, ulceration and tissue atrophy can cause a constricted fibrotic bladder which causes frequency and nocturia. Similar changes in the gastrointestinal tract may cause bowel obstruction by stricturing of the viscous or by peritoneal adhesions.

At other sites vascular damage is manifest differently.

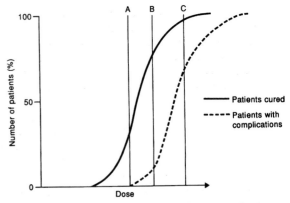

Fig. 24.4 The relationship between cure and complications. A dose may be chosen with a very low risk of observable side-effects, but this may mean a very low chance of tumour cure as well (A). On the other hand, a high tumour cure rate may be associated with an unacceptable rate of complications (C) – forcing an intermediate dose to be chosen as optimal under a particular set of clinical circumstances (B).

In the CNS glial tissues are depleted as a direct effect of radiation and via vascular effects, causing secondary demyelination and neuronal loss. Damage to the cardiac vasculature may result in early ischaemic heart disease if the dose is high enough, with myocardial infarction being an increasingly recognized cause of late morbidity and mortality in a minority of patients 15 years after internal mammary irradiation for breast cancer.

High-dose radiotherapy can also damage lymphatic vessels, leading to reduced drainage and limb lymphoedema. The risk is increased if there has been previous or successive surgery. For example, radiotherapy to the axilla after complete axillary dissection for early-stage breast cancer carries a much higher risk of arm lymphoedema than either modality alone.

The incidence and severity of late damage tend to increase with time, but provided the treatment schedule has been carefully selected, planned and delivered, organs function normally for the remainder of the patient's life. Increasing the dose increases the risk of damage and this damage becomes clinically relevant at an earlier stage.

Late effects are usually irrecoverable and show a dose response. Low doses are less likely to cause damage, while progressively higher doses have a greater chance of causing complications. The radiation dose therefore has to be chosen carefully, taking into account normal tissue tolerance as well as predicted tumour cure dose. The actual dose chosen depends on a variety of factors. For each site an acceptable level of damage must first be decided and balanced against the chance of tumour control (Fig. 24.4). Damage to the spinal cord has such disastrous consequences that no morbidity can be accepted. A lower dose than that used at many other sites has to be accepted, even at the expense of tumour cure probability. Damage to other soft tissues (e.g. muscle and fat) is undesirable but of lesser importance and a higher dose and higher risk are accepted. As mentioned previously, the volume treated is important; the larger the volume the greater the risk of damage and the lower the tolerable dose (e.g. for the spinal cord a short length of cord can be treated to 50 Gy, but long segments, i.e. over 10 cm, will not tolerate over 40 Gy). Other factors affecting tolerance include age (children and the elderly being less tolerant), pre-existing vascular disease and previous surgery.

In addition to specific organ complications the problem of secondary malignancies is being increasingly recognized. This has been best studied in Hodgkin's disease, where an increased incidence of acute leukaemias are seen 3–10 years after irradiation, with a smaller increased risk of solid tumours following. The precise risk is difficult to quantify, but data give an overall risk of leukaemia of approximately 1–2% at 15 years. The risk is greatest if radiotherapy is given in conjunction with or is followed by chemotherapy (especially chemotherapy with alkylating agents, e.g. cyclophosphamide or mustine), being 0.2% if no chemotherapy is used and 8.1% if the patient receives multiple courses. Similar increased incidence of leukaemia has been seen in other cohorts of patients, including those with ankylosing spondylitis who have received spinal irradiation. The risk of solid malignancy is being increasingly recognized, estimates rising to 10% of patients surviving Hodgkin's disease 15–20 years following radiotherapy, though a disease-related phenomenon could also be responsible. The overall risk of secondary malignancy is, however, more than outweighed by the risks of dying from the primary disease in most cancer sufferers.

In conclusion, radiotherapy is set to remain the chief curative modality in patients with non-surgical cancer. As screening and other early detection methods diagnose an increasing percentage of individuals with truly localized disease its importance is likely to increase. This continued role in the curative treatment of cancer patients continues to stimulate research into the technical and biological basis of radiotherapy. In future years, further improvements in the efficacy and safety of radiotherapy should be expected to result from this research.

FURTHER READING

Dobbs J, Barrett A 1985 Practical radiotherapy planning: Royal Marsden Hospital practice. Edward Arnold, London

Horwich A 1995 Oncology: a multidisciplinary textbook. Chapman & Hall, London

Steel G G 1993 Basic clinical radiobiology for radiation oncologists. Edward Arnold, London

25. Chemotherapy – principles, practice, complications and value

C. A. E. Coulter

Localized tumours may be treated successfully by surgery or radiotherapy, but metastases can only be cured by systemic treatment, which will normally be chemotherapy.

The combination of chemotherapy with surgery and/or radiotherapy may also increase local tumour control. Chemotherapy given after surgery or radiotherapy has been used to control the primary disease is called *adjuvant chemotherapy*.

Neo-adjuvant chemotherapy or *primary chemotherapy* describes the use of chemotherapy as an initial treatment for patients who present with localized but extensive cancer (such as large primary breast tumours) where the local control may be improved by combining two modalities of treatment.

Chemotherapy may be given as primary treatment for patients with widespread disease and is then called *induction chemotherapy*.

The word 'chemotherapy' was first used by Paul Ehrlich. He used rodent models to develop antibiotics and this led George Clowes in the early 1900s to work on rodents which could carry transplanted tumours. The modern chemotherapeutic agents were alkylating agents and their use followed the observation that seamen who were exposed to mustard gas had marrow and lymphoid hypoplasia. This led in the 1940s to the use of nitrogen mustard in humans with Hodgkin's disease and other lymphomas. The demonstration of successful regression of advanced cancer with these chemicals caused much excitement. Subsequent to this work at Yale, Sidney Farber's observations on the treatment of children with leukaemia and the successful treatment of children with Wilm's tumour led to a rapid increase in the number of cytotoxic drugs available and a rapid increase in the range of tumours in which they were used.

BASIC PRINCIPLES

The aim of chemotherapy is to selectively destroy tumour cells while sparing normal tissues. Growth

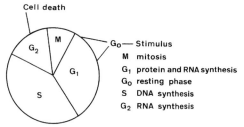

Fig. 25.1 Growth characteristics of tumour cells.

characteristics of tumour cells allow selective tumour cell destruction and relative sparing of normal cells (Fig. 25.1).

Kinetic classification of anticancer drugs

Non-phase-dependent drugs kill cells exponentially with increasing dose and are equally toxic for cells in cycle and in G_0.

Phase-dependent drugs kill cells at lower doses but reach a plateau kill if given at high doses because they can only kill cells in a specific part of the cell cycle.

Predominantly phase-dependent drugs:
- Etoposide
- Methotrexate
- Procarbazine
- Vinca alkaloids

Non-phase-dependent drugs:
- Alkylating agents
- Actinomycin D
- 5-Fluorouracil
- Anthracyclines.

Growth characteristics of tumours

The rate of proliferation during the lifetime of a tumour is not constant. In the early stages of tumour growth the growth fraction is high, but as the tumour enlarges the growth fraction is lower. The growth fraction peaks when the tumour is about 37% of its maximum size.

As the tumour enlarges the growth fraction falls and the growth rate slows. Chemotherapy will be less effective in larger tumours because the growth fraction is smaller and the number of cells killed by a therapeutic dose of chemotherapy will be smaller.

Skipper et al (1964) formulated principles of tumour cell kill by drugs by using L1210 leukaemia in mice. They showed that the survival of the animal is inversely related to the tumour burden and that for most drugs there was a clear relationship between the dose of drug and the eradication of tumour cells. A given dose of drugs kills a constant fraction of cells, not a constant number. This means that cell destruction by drugs follows first-order kinetics and a treatment reducing a population from one million to 10 cells should reduce a population of 100 000 to one cell. The implication of the fractional cell killing is that to eradicate a tumour population effectively it is necessary either to increase the dose of the drug or drugs within limits tolerated by the host, or to start treatment when the number of cells is small enough to allow tumour destruction at reasonably tolerated doses. The implication is not, as has sometimes been stated, that eradication of the last neoplastic cell is not possible with chemotherapy, but that the toxic effects on normal cells may be a limiting factor.

Development of new cytotoxic drugs

Phase I:
- Maximum tolerated dose
- Toxic effects
- Pharmacology

Phase II:
- Evaluation of anticancer action.

If the drug has an objective response rate in a specific tumour type of 25% or more it may then proceed to phase III testing.

Phase III:
- Controlled clinical trials.

Pharmacology of cytotoxic drugs

Alkylating agents. These compounds produce their effects by linking an alkyl group (R–CH–) covalently to chemical moieties in protein and nucleic acids.

Antimetabolites. Antimetabolites are agents that by virtue of their structural similarity with physiological intermediates are accepted as substrates for vital biochemical reactions and thus interfere with the required cell process.

Antitumour antibiotics. These drugs produce their effect by binding to DNA and intercalating between the base pair.

Plant-derived agents. These are mitotic spindle poisons that bind to tubulin, which is a protein of the cellular microtubules.

Biological agents. Biological therapy utilizes biological reagents to elicit tumour regression.

Hormonal therapy. Hormones are used in the management of patients with metastatic or locally advanced breast or prostatic cancers.

USE OF CYTOTOXIC AGENTS (Table 25.1)

Alkylating agents

Cyclophosphamide. Breast cancer, small cell lung cancer, non-Hodgkin's lymphoma, leukaemia and sarcomas.

Chlorambucil. Low-grade non-Hodgkin's lymphoma, ovarian and breast cancer.

Dacarbazine. Melanoma and soft tissue sarcoma.

Cisplatin. Testicular teratoma and seminoma, ovarian cancer, bladder cancer, small cell cancer of the lung, and head and neck cancer.

Procarbazine. Hodgkin's disease and brain tumours.

Antimetabolites

Methotrexate. Acute leukaemia, non-Hodgkin's lymphoma, breast cancer and sarcomas.

5-Fluorouracil. Breast and gastrointestinal cancer.

Antitumour antibiotics

Doxorubicin. Breast cancer, lymphomas, small cell lung cancer, ovarian cancer and bladder cancer.

Mitozantrone. Leukaemia, lymphomas and breast cancer.

Bleomycin. Testicular tumours, head and neck cancers and lymphoma.

Actinomycin D. Teratomas, Wilm's tumour and paediatric sarcomas.

Vincristine. Lymphomas, leukaemia, small cell lung cancer and breast cancer.

Vinblastine. Testicular tumours and lymphomas.

Vindesine. Melanoma.

Paclitaxel. Ovarian and breast cancer.

Etoposide. Testicular tumours, lymphomas, leukaemia, small cell lung cancer and Ewing's sarcoma.

Biological therapy

The pharmacopoeia includes recombinant cytokines which have immunomodulator activity and antitumour activity. These include interleukin and α-interferon.

Interleukin-2 (IL-2) is a T-cell growth factor that is central to T-cell mediated immune responses. IL-2 has been approved for treatment of metastatic renal cell carcinoma. Response rates of 20–30% have been observed. IL-2 has also demonstrated activity against malignant melanoma and the response rate approaches 20%.

Other recombinant cytokines, termed colony stimulating factors (CSFs), exert effects on haematopoiesis and immune functions. They do not have an antitumour effect but reduce chemotherapy-induced haematological toxicity and are useful adjuvants in high-dose chemotherapy and bone marrow transplants. They are *erythropoietin* and *granulocyte CSF (filograstin)*.

Additional anticancer biological reagents including IL-2, IL-4, IL-6, IL-7 and IL-12 are currently being evaluated.

α-Interferon (α-IFN) has demonstrated activity against

Table 25.1   Major cytotoxic agents

Class	Route	Dose (guidelines only)	Acute toxicity		Nausea/ vomiting	Other toxicity
			Plasma WBC	Platelets		
Alkylating agents						
Cyclophosphamide	i.v./p.o.	50 mg to 1.5 g	Marked	Mild	Moderate	Cystitis/alopecia
Chlorambucil	p.o.	10 mg	Moderate	Moderate	Mild	Leukaemia
Melphalan	p.o.	10 mg	Moderate	Moderate	Mild	Leukaemia
Dacarbazine	i.v.	500 mg	Mild	Mild	Marked	Flu-like syndrome, painful arm
Cisplatinum	i.v.	150 mg	Moderate	Moderate	Severe	Neuropathy Otoxicity Nephropathy
Carboplatin	i.v.	600 mg	Mild	Moderate	Mild	
Procarbazine	p.o.	150 mg	Moderate	Moderate	Mild	Incompatible with cheese and alcohol
Antimetabolites						
Methotrexate	i.v./p.o/i.t.	50 mg to several grams (folinic acid given if dose greater than 50 mg m^{-2})	Mild	Mild	Moderate	Renal and liver dysfunction Mucositis
5-Fluorouracil	i.v.	500 mg	Mild	Mild	Minimal	Diarrhoea Conjunctivitis Cerebellar syndrome Hand–foot syndrome
Antitumour antibiotics						
Doxorubicin	i.v.	40 mg	Marked	Marked	Marked	Alopecia Cardiomyopathy
Mitozantrone	i.v.	20 mg	Moderate	Moderate	Moderate	Mild alopecia
Bleomycin	i.v./i.m./i.p.	30 mg	Minimal	Minimal	Minimal	Flu-like illnesses Discolouration and thickening of skin over joints (Pulmonary fibrosis)
Actinomycin D	i.v.	1 mg	Marked	Marked	Minimal	Alopecia Mucositis
Plant-derived agents						
Vincristine	i.v.	2 mg	Mild	Mild	Mild	Peripheral neuropathy
Vinblastine	i.v.	10 mg	Marked	Marked	Mild	Mucositis
Vindesine	i.v.	5 mg	Marked	Marked	Mild	Neuropathy
Etoposide	i.v./p.o.	150 mg	Moderate	Moderate	Mild/moderate	Neuropathy
Paclitaxel	i.v.	175 mg m^{-2}	Marked	Mild	Mild	Neuropathy Alopecia

many solid and haematogenous malignancies. A response rate of 80–90% has been observed among patients with hairy cell leukaemia. Survival appears to be prolonged compared with historical controls. Patients with chronic myeloid leukaemia respond to α-IFN, but no survival benefit has been demonstrated. α-IFN has been approved for use in Kaposi's sarcoma. There is a 30% response rate. Liposomal doxorubicin is also licensed throughout Europe.

Hormonal therapy

As oestrogen and androgen are necessary to maintain the growth of some breast and prostatic cancers; these diseases may be controlled but not cured by the removal or addition of hormones. Oestrogen receptors (ER) and progestogen receptors (PgR) may be assayed in primary breast tumours. If the tumour is ER positive 60% of patients will respond to hormone manipulation. PgR is made as a result of oestrogen action through functional ER; if no PgR is present the probability of response to hormone therapy is reduced. If PgR and ER are both positive there is an 80% chance of response to hormone therapy. Agents used for treatment are as follows.

Breast cancer:
Premenopausal patient:
● Oophorectomy
● LHRH agonist
● Tamoxifen

Postmenopausal patient:
● Tamoxifen
● Progestin
● Aminoglutethimide
 or
● Formestane

Prostate cancer:
● LHRH agonists
● Antiandrogen (e.g. flutamide)
 or
● Orchidectomy
 or
● Diethylstilboestrol

PHARMACOLOGY

The susceptibility of a tumour cell to a drug depends on the sensitivity of the cell to the action of the drug, to the cycling of the tumour cell and to the concentration delivered to the tumour.

There is evidence of a dose–response relationship for some cytotoxic drugs and in breast cancer adriamycin has been shown to confer greater therapeutic benefit at high dose. Very high dose chemotherapy with autologous bone marrow or stem cell support is a technique used for treatment in acute leukaemia or as second-line therapy in lymphomas. The same technique is under trial as treatment for women with high-risk breast cancer.

The dose of an anticancer drug is limited by its toxic effect on normal tissues. The cells which normally turn over rapidly are the usual sites of dose-limiting toxicity. The bone marrow and intestinal epithelium are therefore problem sites. The dose given is usually calculated on the basis of milligrams or grams per metre of the surface area of the patient's body. Dose schedules are also affected by the function of major organs such as the liver and kidneys.

Liver

The liver is the principal site for metabolism and excretion of some drugs, and when the serum bilirubin is elevated doxorubicin, mitozantrone and the vinca alkaloids should be used with caution and the dose of the drugs reduced.

Kidneys

Drugs which are cleared by the kidney may cause increased toxicity if the patient has impaired renal function. When certain drugs are given, renal function must be checked carefully before each course of chemotherapy. The important drugs to note are cisplatin, cyclophosphamide, methotrexate, ifosfamide and procarbazine. When these drugs are given the patient should be well hydrated.

Carboplatin, which is similar in use to cisplatin, may be given, with a low creatinine clearance.

COMBINATION CHEMOTHERAPY

The potential circumvention of resistance to treatment has historically been the most important factor prompting studies of drug combinations. Human tumours present with a greatly reduced percentage of cells in the proliferation pool. Effective chemotherapy has in most cases to be repeated over long intervals, and under these circumstances exposure of tumour cells to chemicals can lead to chemical resistance. Because of this, combinations of drugs have been used to reduce resistance.

The major principles of combination chemotherapy are that all drugs included in the combination would be active against the tumour when used alone, that they should have different mechanisms of action and that they should have minimally overlapping toxicities.

MODES OF ADMINISTRATION

Drugs may be given orally, intramuscularly, intravenously or intrathecally. Venous access devices may be required for convenience, or because of poor veins or for infusion chemotherapy. Long-term catheters may be inserted into the right atrium; usually, double-lumen catheters (Hickman or Groschong) are used. Implanted venous access ports may be placed subcutaneously against the chest wall.

An implanted pump may be placed into the common hepatic artery to infuse chemotherapy continuously into the liver. This technique is being evaluated in patients with liver metastases from the colon and rectum.

COMPLICATIONS

Acute toxicity

Local toxicity

Doxorubicin and vinca alkaloids cause tissue destruction when extravasated. This devastating toxicity can be avoided by ensuring that the needle is within the vein and that the vein is tested using a non-vesicant substance before the injection of vesicant drugs is started.

Bone marrow toxicity

For most drugs bone marrow toxicity is a dose-limiting factor. It is mandatory that a full blood count is taken on the day of the treatment so that dose modifications or postponement of treatment can be considered.

Patients with granulocyte counts of less than 1.0×10^9 per litre should receive oral ciproxin. If patients have a fever and a granulocyte count of less than 0.5×10^9 per litre they should receive intravenous antibiotics and cytokines such as granulocyte colony simulating factor (GCSF).

Bleeding does not usually occur until the platelet count falls to 20×10^9 per litre, but patients with low counts should be checked for signs of haemorrhage. Platelet support should be given if the count falls below 20×10^9 per litre.

Gastrointestinal toxicity

Nausea and vomiting are caused by cisplatin, cyclophosphamide, doxorubicin and actinomycin C. This is probably due to a combination of stimuli from the chemoreceptor trigger zone, the gut and cerebral cortex.

Patients receiving less-toxic combinations of chemotherapy will respond to treatment to metoclopramide or domperidone and dexamethasone. For patients receiving highly emetogenic drugs such as cisplatin, treatment with a 5-hydroxytryptamine antagonist such as ondansetron or granisetron should be given prophylactically together with dexamethasone. Oral premedication with lorazepam will help the patient to relax before treatment.

Methotrexate may cause mucositis, and oral hygiene should be given particular attention.

Vincristine may cause constipation and paralytic ileus. Treatment with laxatives is sometimes required.

5-Fluorouracil and cyclophosphamide may cause diarrhoea, and prophylactic codeine may be given.

Alopecia

Doxorubicin, cyclophosphamide, etoposide, vincristine and paclitaxel cause alopecia. Hair loss due to doxorubicin may be much reduced by scalp cooling. All hair loss is temporary and patients can be reassured that there will be hair regrowth after treatment has been completed. Wigs are available and should be provided for patients before hair loss occurs. Hair loss will start at 18–21 days after the first injection of these drugs.

Long-term toxicity

Carcinogenesis

Long-term treatment with alkylating agents such as chlorambucil and melphalan is associated with the development of acute leukaemia. The risk is directly related to the total dose of the drugs give. This is an important reason for reducing the length of treatment and, therefore, the cumulative dose of these agents. The risk of developing a second solid tumour due to chemotherapy appears very low.

Gonodal damage

Alkylating agents are the drugs most commonly implicated in causing sterility. After combination chemotherapy for Hodgkin's disease the majority of men are azoospermic. This is due to a combination of chlorambucil and procarbazine. Sperm banking is available, but unfortunately many patients are very ill with their lymphoma and have a poor sperm count at that time. However, with modern assisted reproductive techniques it is possible to achieve ovum fertilization with a very low sperm count and sperm storage should always be done. Men do not need hormone replacement therapy.

For women over 30 years of age there is a very high risk of permanent amenorrhoea when they have received combination chemotherapy for Hodgkin's disease. It is now possible, but time consuming and expensive, to hyperstimulate the ovaries before chemotherapy to obtain ova which can be fertilized and frozen. Female patients will need hormone replacement therapy.

Patients receiving chemotherapy must receive counselling about the risk of long-term infertility and the inadvisability of pregnancy during chemotherapy. Men who receive treatment with cisplatin for germ cell tumours usually retain fertility, as do women who have received chemotherapy for choriocarcinoma.

VALUE

Chemotherapy can cure some patients with advanced cancers. Cure is possible in the following tumours, which constitute about 12% of cancers:

Advanced tumours which are potentially curable
- Acute lymphoblastic leukaemia
- Germ cell tumours
- Choriocarcinoma
- Ewing's sarcoma
- Wilm's tumour
- Diffuse large cell lymphoma
- ? Ovarian cancer

Tumours which are potentially curable by local treatment and adjuvant chemotherapy
- Breast cancer
- Osteogenic sarcoma

Tumours which have a response rate which leads to prolonged survival
- Ovarian cancer
- Lymphoma
- Osteogenic sarcoma

- Breast cancer
- Acute myeloid leukaemia
- Small cell lung cancer

Tumours which have an overall response rate of 50% but no definite survival benefit
- Head and neck cancer
- Bladder cancer

Tumours which are poorly responsive to chemotherapy
- Pancreatic cancer
- Melanoma
- Soft tissue sarcoma
- Colorectal cancer
- Renal cancer
- Thyroid cancer
- Gasric cancer
- Cervical cancer

FURTHER READING

Carmo-Pereira J, Costa F O, Henriques E et al 1987 A comparison of two doses of adriamycin in the primary chemotherapy of advanced breast cancer. British Journal of Cancer 56: 471–475

DeVita V T 1978 The evolution of therapeutic research in cancer. New England Journal of Medicine 298: 907–910

Kaye S B, Cumming J, Kerr D 1985 How much does liver disease affect the pharmacokinetics of adriamycin? European Journal of Cancer 21: 893–895

Marshall E K 1964 Historical perspectives in chemotherapy. In: Goldin A, Hawking I F (eds) Advances in chemotherapy. Academic Press, New York, vol 1, p 1–8

Skipper H E, Schabel F M, Wilcox W S 1964 Experimental evaluation of potential anticancer agents. Cancer Chemotherapy Reports 35: 1–11

26. Tumour markers

G. J. S. Rustin   H. D. C. Mitchell

Tumour markers are substances present in the body in a concentration which is related to the presence of a tumour. A tumour marker does not have to be tumour specific. It may be a substance secreted or shed into blood and other body fluids or expressed at the cell surface in larger quantities by malignant cells than by their non-malignant counterparts. Tumour markers can be detected either by measuring the concentration of the marker in body fluids (usually by immunoassay) or by detecting the presence of the marker on the cell surface in paraffin sections or fresh biopsies (by immunohistochemistry). Although the association between human chorionic gonadotrophin (hCG) and trophoblastic tumours was identified more than 60 years ago, measurement of tumour markers has, until recently, been confined to a small number of specialized laboratories. However, the development of monoclonal antibody technology and automation of commercial assays has led to tumour marker estimation becoming widely available. This chapter examines critically those situations where estimation of circulating tumour marker levels may be of clinical value. The terms used to describe the usefulness of a tumour marker measurement are first defined, and the potential applications of tumour marker measurement are discussed. The role of tumour marker measurements in the management of patients with specific tumour types is then outlined.

DEFINITIONS

The terms most commonly used to describe the usefulness of a tumour marker are defined in Box 26.1. Sensitivity is a measure of how commonly a tumour marker level is elevated in the presence of that particular tumour. Specificity measures the proportion of patients without tumour who have normal marker levels, and are therefore the true negatives. The positive predictive value is the percentage of positive results (i.e. elevated marker levels) which are true positives. An ideal tumour marker would have 100% sensitivity, thus detecting all

Box 26.1

	Present	Absent
Assay positive	TP	FP
Assay negative	FN	TN

$$\text{Sensitivity} = \frac{\text{TP}}{\text{TP} + \text{FN}} \times 100$$

$$\text{Specificity} = \frac{\text{TN}}{\text{FP} + \text{TN}} \times 100$$

$$\text{Positive predictive value} = \frac{\text{TP}}{\text{TP} + \text{FP}} \times 100$$

$$\text{Negative predictive value} = \frac{\text{TN}}{\text{FN} + \text{TN}} \times 100$$

TP, true positive; FP, false positive; FN, false negative; TN, true negative.

cases of a particular tumour, and 100% specificity, being elevated only in the presence of that tumour and not in any other situations.

POTENTIAL USES OF TUMOUR MARKERS

The potential clinical uses of tumour marker estimation are:

- Screening
- Diagnosis
- Prognostic indicator
- Monitoring therapy
- Early diagnosis of relapse.

An ideal tumour marker would be sensitive enough to detect a tumour in a large proportion of cases before it became clinically apparent, and specific enough to be rarely elevated in patients without cancer. Such a tumour marker assay could thus be used for screening, either of the whole population or at least of selected high-risk groups. In addition, the detection of an elevated marker level would allow a diagnosis of tumour to be made without further investigations having to be performed. Unfortunately, such an ideal situation does not exist and, despite many claims, there is no marker that can be used as a general screen for cancer. The closest to the ideal marker is measurement of hCG in patients with gestational trophoblastic disease. Tumour markers are being recognized as important prognostic factors due to their relationship with tumour bulk and invasiveness. Prognosis may be related to the presence or absence of a marker, its absolute level at diagnosis or at certain time points during therapy, or to its rate of disappearance or half-life following therapy.

The most common current use of tumour marker estimation is to monitor the response of a tumour to treatment. Such measurements are essential in the management of patients with germ cell tumours and gestational trophoblastic disease, where treatment is undertaken with curative intent, and where the detection of the development of drug resistance can lead to a change to an alternative, effective therapy. Although information on response to treatment can also be deduced from serial tumour marker estimation in some of the more common solid tumours such as colorectal and ovarian tumours, a change in treatment is less likely to lead to an improved outcome. Nevertheless, early detection of resistance to treatment can lead to the cessation of ineffective, costly and potentially toxic treatment.

Another potential function of a tumour marker is to provide early evidence of tumour recurrence, before it becomes clinically apparent. Once again, this is of greatest use in those tumours where prompt detection of recurrence can lead to effective treatment. It is far from clear whether serial tumour marker estimations leading to the earlier diagnosis of recurrence of the commoner solid tumours such as colorectal, ovarian or breast cancers, where treatment on relapse is usually only palliative in nature, is actually of any benefit to the patient. Indeed, there are potential drawbacks to the early detection of asymptomatic, incurable recurrences, which may easily lead to anxiety for patients at a time when they would otherwise feel perfectly well.

Finally, although they will not be discussed in any further detail in this chapter, a number of clinical trials have attempted to exploit the existence of cell surface tumour markers to localize a tumour either for imaging purposes, using a radiolabelled antibody, or as a treatment modality, using antibodies to carry radioactivity or toxins selectively to the tumour.

REVIEW OF THE USE OF TUMOUR MARKER ESTIMATION IN THE MANAGEMENT OF PARTICULAR TUMOURS

Gestational trophoblastic tumours

The role of human chorionic gonadotrophin (HCG) in the management of GTT is discussed in detail as it becomes closest to the ideal use of a tumour marker. HCG is a glycoprotein produced by trophoblast cells. The a-subunit is identical to that of follicle-stimulating hormone (FSH), luteinizing hormone (LH) and thyroid-stimulating hormone (TSH), but the C-terminal end of the β-subunit is unique to hCG and provides the basis of the specific immunoassay. There are many different assays for HCG available. It is essential to know whether the assay in use locally recognizes just the β-subunit or the intact complete HCG molecule, as they can give quite different results.

Diagnosis and screening

Elevated levels of hCG are found with as few as 10^5 trophoblast cells, while the smallest number of cells detectable by clinical examination is over 10^9, and even computed tomography (CT) scanning can only detect about 10^7 cells. However, although hCG is a highly sensitive marker for gestational trophoblastic tumour (GTT) it is not specific. Elevated serum hCG levels are also found in normal pregnancy, in ectopic pregnancy, in patients with germ cell tumours and, occasionally, in patients with non-germ-cell tumours. Pelvic ultrasound examination therefore remains the best method for diagnosing hydatidiform mole. The great sensitivity of hCG, however, allows it to be used to screen a high-risk population. The first national screening programme for any cancer was set up in 1972 by the Royal College of Obstetricians and Gynaecologists in the UK. Following a diagnosis of hydatidiform mole, all patients are centrally registered at Charing Cross Hospital, Sheffield or Dundee. Patients are then followed using serial hCG measurements to detect any evidence of recurrence for varying lengths of time, depending on the initial rate of fall to normal. Although most hydatidiform moles die out spontaneously after evacuation, approximately 8% of patients require chemotherapy. This screening allows these patients with persistent trophoblastic disease after evacuation of hydatidiform mole to be detected on the basis of plateauing or rising tumour markers before any clinical evidence of disease develops (Bagshawe et al 1986).

Prognosis/monitoring response to treatment

Since hCG levels in patients with GTT reflect the total body burden of viable tumour they constitute a significant prognostic factor, with high values contributing to high-risk status. In patients with GTT, serial hCG estimation is used to monitor response to chemotherapy and to detect the development of drug resistance. The hCG value may initially increase after starting treatment. This initial surge in hCG has been attributed to either tumour lysis or to increased syncytial differentiation induced by the therapy. The hCG level then falls at a rate which is a function of metabolic clearance and the rate of synthesis. Plateauing of hCG values or rising values during the course of chemotherapy indicate the development of drug resistance. The early detection of the development of drug resistance is particularly useful in GTT because, unlike many more common tumours, change to an effective second-line chemotherapy is still very likely to result in cure (Newlands 1991).

Detection of recurrence

Serial measurement of hCG will detect any recurrence of GTT with 100% sensitivity. The accurate measurement of HCG in urine, which is stable in the post, increases the ease of monitoring and obviates the need for frequent hospital visits. A rise in hCG is not, however, diagnostic of recurrent disease, and a new pregnancy must always be considered and ruled out by ultrasound examination. Patients who have had a hydatidiform mole have a slightly increased risk of choriocarcinoma after any subsequent pregnancy and should have further hCG estimations at 4 and 12 weeks post-partum.

Germ cell tumours

Tumour marker measurement is essential for the correct management of patients with germ cell tumours of the testis or ovary. α-Fetoprotein (AFP) and hCG are elevated, either singly or in combination, in more than 80% of patients with disseminated non-seminomatous germ cell tumours (NSGCT) and in approximately 60% of patients with localized, stage I disease (Kohn & Ragavan 1981). Other markers of use in patients with germ cell tumours include lactate dehydrogenase (LDH), but many laboratories only measure hydroxybutyrate dehydrogenase (HBD) which is mostly isoenzyme 1 and 2 of LDH. Placental alkaline phosphatase (PLAP), although elevated in about 50% of patients with seminomas and in smokers, adds little to clinical management as it is rarely greatly elevated and usually falls

to normal so quickly on therapy that it adds little to monitoring (Nielsen et al 1990).

Diagnosis and staging

All patients who are suspected of having a germ cell tumour should have serum sent for tumour marker estimation before excision of the primary tumour. None of the markers mentioned above are sufficiently specific to be used alone to diagnose a germ cell tumour. However, patients whose clinical status could be compromised by a biopsy (e.g. a patient with severe dyspnoea due to extensive lung metastases) should be considered to have an NSGCT if the distribution of the disease is compatible with such a tumour and there is significant elevation of either hCG or AFP. Measurement of hCG and AFP can also be a helpful adjunct to histological examination in the differential diagnosis of seminoma and NSGCT. Elevated hCG is associated with the presence of trophoblastic elements in an NSGCT, and can be produced by syncytial giant cells in a pure seminoma. However, any patient with a histologically pure seminoma but a substantially elevated hCG should be treated as if they had an NSGCT (Bosl et al 1981). AFP, a glycoprotein with a molecular weight of 63–70 kDa, is secreted by the yolk sac element of an NSGCT, and a patient with an elevated AFP should never be considered to have a pure seminoma, regardless of the histological findings.

An additional reason for preoperative estimation of tumour markers in all patients with suspected germ cell tumours is the use of tumour marker measurement in initial staging and in the follow-up of patients with stage I disease. Failure of tumour marker levels to fall to normal postoperatively indicates the presence of occult metastatic disease, even if all other staging investigations are normal. One further situation in which hCG estimation may be of diagnostic value is in the detection of brain metastases. A pretreatment cerebrospinal fluid hCG level that is more than one-sixtieth the serum hCG level indicates the presence of brain metastases; the normal ratio, however, does not exclude brain metastases (Bagshawe & Harland 1976).

Prognosis

Initial tumour marker levels are now recognized as the single best predictor of failure to achieve complete response following chemotherapy. An international collaborative group has recently proposed a prognostic classification (Table 26.1) based on an analysis of 3433 patients which found tumour marker levels and the presence or absence of mediastinal and non-pulmonary,

Table 26.1 Tumour markers in prognostic classification of germ cell tumours

	Marker		
	AFP (ng ml^{-1})	HCG* (ng ml^{-1})	LDH† (× N)
Good	<1000	and <1000	and <1.5 N
Intermediate	1000–10 000	or 1000–10 000	or 1.5 N–10 N
Poor	>10 000	or >10 000	or >10 N

*For HCG, 1 ng ml^{-1} is approximately equal to 5 iu l^{-1}.
†N, upper limit of normal.

non-nodal visceral metastases as the important risk factors (Mead et al 1995).

Monitoring response to treatment

In patients with elevated hCG or AFP, these markers are the most sensitive method for assessing response to treatment. Although, in general, successful chemotherapy is invariably accompanied by a fall in serial hCG and AFP levels, there are two situations in which this may not occur. Firstly, an initial rise in tumour marker levels may occur soon after starting the first course of chemotherapy due to tumour lysis. The second situation is a plateau or even a rise in AFP levels, despite evidence of response from all other investigations (Coppack et al 1983). This is thought to be due to AFP production by the liver in response to toxicity and appears to be more common in those patients receiving hepatotoxic drugs such as methotrexate and ifosfamide. The only situation where falling marker levels are not associated with a decreasing germ cell tumour mass is when there is enlargement of cystic differentiated teratoma. These masses require resection before they become inoperable.

Early detection of recurrence

The great sensitivity of hCG, and to a lesser extent of AFP, means that a rise in values is often the first indication of relapse. All patients with germ cell tumours should continue to have serial tumour marker estimation after completion of chemotherapy. Although most patients who enter complete remission will already be cured, early detection of relapse is of great importance since, unlike the situation with most other solid tumours, second-line treatment can still result in cure in a substantial proportion of cases.

The other situation in which serial marker estimation is invaluable in early detection of disease is in surveillance of patients with stage I disease following orchidectomy. In this situation, where there is no evidence of residual tumour on scans or marker measurement after orchidectomy, almost 75% of patients with NSGCT will never relapse. Close follow-up clinical examination, tumour markers, chest X-ray and at least one CT scan 3 months after orchidectomy will detect relapse early in the 25–30% of those in whom the disease is destined to recur and, with adequate treatment, virtually all patients will be cured. In view of the potential for tumour markers to double rapidly, it is important that markers are measured frequently, with one recent study suggesting 2-weekly markers for the first 6 months of surveillance (Seckl et al 1990).

Gastrointestinal tumours

There are a number of antibodies currently available which detect antigens expressed by gastrointestinal tumours. The most widely used are the antibodies which react with carcinoembryonic antigen (CEA), a 200 kDa glycoprotein first described by Gold & Freedman in 1965. Assays dependent on monoclonal antibodies include CA 19.9, an antigen derived from a human colon adenocarcinoma cell line with an epitope structurally identical to the sialylated Lewis A antigen, and CA 50, which is similar but not identical to CA 19.9. Elevated levels of several other markers such as CA 72-4 have also been found.

Diagnosis and screening

Serum CEA is elevated in fewer than 5% of patients with Dukes' grade A colorectal cancer, about 25% of Dukes' grade B, 44% of Dukes' grade C and about 65% of patients with distant metastases (Begent & Rustin 1989). CEA can be elevated not only in cancers of the gastrointestinal tract but also in a variety of other conditions, including: severe benign liver disease; inflammatory lesions, especially of the gastrointestinal tract; trauma; infection; collagen disease; renal impairment; and smoking. The low incidence of high serum CEA levels in early disease and its poor specificity explain its lack of value in screening normal populations for colorectal cancer. The low sensitivity precludes its being useful even for screening patients with ulcerative colitis or familial polyposis coli; although these patients are at high risk of developing colorectal cancer, both conditions may cause raised serum CEA in the absence of malignancy. No tumour markers currently available are sensitive enough to screen for oesophageal, gastric or pancreatic cancers. Although CA 19.9 is elevated in 75–90% of patients with pancreatic carcinomas, by the time the marker is elevated the tumour is already incurable by surgery in the vast majority of cases.

Prognosis/monitoring treatment

Although a raised preoperative CEA level has been shown to be associated with a poorer prognosis, this is in large part due to the fact that CEA level reflects tumour burden. The value of preoperative CEA as an independent prognostic factor is unclear. Serum CEA levels should fall to normal within 4–6 weeks of complete resection of a colorectal carcinoma, the mean half-life being about 10 days. Levels usually rise with disease and fall with response to chemotherapy or radiotherapy. Failure of CEA to fall during radiotherapy usually indicates the presence of tumour outside the radiation field. Several studies have shown that survival is longer in patients who have a fall in serum CEA level during chemotherapy than in those in whom there is no change or an increased level (Allen-Mersh et al 1987).

Follow-up and detection of relapse

In approximately two-thirds of patients with recurrent colorectal cancer, a rise in serial serum CEA values predicts recurrence on average 11 months before it becomes clinically apparent (Begent & Rustin 1989, Lennon et al 1994). Surgical resection of isolated metastases of colorectal cancer has been advocated. Unfortunately, a randomized, multicentre trial under the auspices of the Cancer Research Campaign has failed to show any survival benefit from surgery after early detection of recurrence by rising CEA levels. However, further work is required to determine whether such patients would benefit from chemotherapy.

Ovarian cancer

The site and pattern of spread of ovarian cancer make it very difficult to detect and monitor using conventional clinical and radiological techniques, so a circulating tumour marker is potentially very valuable. CA 125 is the most commonly used tumour marker for ovarian cancer. The CA 125 antigen was originally defined by its reactivity with a murine monoclonal antibody (OC 125), which was raised by immunization with a human cell line derived from a serous cystadenocarcinoma of the ovary. CA 125 is found in derivatives of coelomic epithelium, including pleura, pericardium and peritoneum, but is not detected in normal ovarian tissue.

Diagnosis

CA 125 is elevated in over 95% of patients with advanced (stage III or IV) ovarian cancer, but in less than 50% of patients with stage I disease (Bast et al 1983). However, an elevated CA 125 is not diagnostic of ovarian cancer. Levels above 30 iu ml^{-1} are frequently seen during the first trimester of pregnancy, in patients with endometriosis or with cirrhosis, especially if ascites is present, and in 1% of healthy controls. In addition, over 40% of patients with advanced non-ovarian intra-abdominal malignancies have elevated CA 125 levels. Nonetheless, in a patient suspected of having ovarian cancer, the presence of an elevated CA 125 should prompt the surgeon either to refer the patient to a gynaecological oncologist or to perform the surgery through a more extensive midline incision to allow adequate debulking of tumour.

Screening

Despite the low sensitivity of CA 125 for potentially curable stage I tumours, large screening studies have been performed. One study at the Royal London Hospital measured serum CA 125 in 22 000 postmenopausal well women. Those women who had CA 125 levels above 30 U ml^{-1} underwent pelvic ultrasound, and if that was positive a laparotomy was performed. In all there were 11 confirmed cases of epithelial ovarian cancer (true positives) and 11 cases in whom laparotomy did not reveal an ovarian tumour (false positives). Of note, however, is the fact that only 3 of the 11 patients with screen-detected ovarian cancers had stage I disease (Jacobs et al 1993). These findings led the UK Coordinating Committee on Cancer Research to recommend in 1989 that screening for ovarian cancer should not yet be offered to women outside a clinical trial. A randomized trial run by Dr Jacobs is currently investigating the value of serial CA 125 and OVX1 levels.

Assessing completeness of excision

In order to decide optimum postoperative management, it is important to know whether one is dealing with a patient with completely excised, stage I disease, or whether the patient has residual tumour after surgery. A persistently elevated CA 125 after oophorectomy for suspected stage I disease is definite evidence of residual tumour. Such patients are candidates for chemotherapy rather than surveillance.

Prognosis and response to treatment

Very high CA 125 levels prior to surgery are associated with a worse prognosis, but knowledge of this is unlikely to lead to any alteration in management. Similarly, the fact that a patient with a CA 125 level above 250 U ml^{-1} prior to starting chemotherapy has a poor prognosis is unlikely to prevent a trial of treatment. Several groups have shown that the CA 125 level after one, two or three courses of chemotherapy, a long half-life or greater than seven-fold fall are the most important prognostic factors for survival. Prognostic information based on CA 125 should not be used to decide therapy, as in nearly 20% of cases where CA 125 predicts a poor prognosis the patient has no cancer progression in the next 12 months (Fayers et al 1993). However, as an indicator of response or progression, CA 125 is more reliable.

Recently, definitions for response and progression based on serial CA 125 estimations have been proposed (Rustin et al 1993).

- *50% Response:* response to a specific treatment has occurred if after two samples there has been a 50% fall of serum CA 125 levels, confirmed by a 4th sample
  or
  75% Response: response has occurred if there has been a serial fall of serum CA 125 over three samples of more than 75%.

(In each the final sample has to be at least 28 days after the previous sample.)

These definitions are particularly useful for clinical trials where they indicate which new treatments are active more easily and cheaper than by the use of standard response criteria.

Detection of progression or relapse

Using the definitions below it is possible accurately to predict progression during initial therapy by serial CA 125 measurements. Ineffective, toxic and expensive therapy can thus be withheld.

- Progression is predicted if after two samples there is a 25% rise confirmed by a fourth sample, or a serial rise of 50% over three samples, or elevation over 100 U ml^{-1} for over 2 months without a 50% fall.

A simpler definition can be used in patients on follow-up after their initial therapy. A doubling from the upper limit of normal has been shown in several studies to predict progression when off treatment with almost 100% specificity. However, although the use of CA 125 estimation to define progression may reduce the number of radiological investigations performed, there is no evidence at present that early reintroduction of chemotherapy or searching for a resectable site of relapse produces any survival benefit. Therefore, serial CA 125 measurements during follow-up when off therapy cannot be recommended as a routine investigation. However, once there is any clinical suspicion of relapse, serial CA 125 levels at that point are likely to be the most effective investigation to confirm the presence of recurrent tumour.

Prostate cancer

Prostate specific antigen (PSA) is now widely accepted as the most useful tumour marker in patients with prostate cancer. PSA is a serine protease produced by prostate epithelium with the function of liquefying the gel which surrounds spermatazoa to enable them to become fully mobile. In serum, PSA is found either free or complexed to proteins. PSA is elevated in a higher proportion of men with prostate cancer than is prostatic acid phosphatase.

Diagnosis and screening

Elevated levels of PSA (>4 ng ml^{-1}) occur in about 65% of men with localized stage A prostatic cancer, but can also occur in 30–50% of men with benign prostatic hypertrophy (BPH), a condition common in men of similar age group to those who develop prostate cancer (Beastall et al 1991). Clearly, therefore, measurement of PSA alone is not sufficiently sensitive to be used in population screening for prostate cancer. The combination of PSA and rectal examination, followed by prostatic ultrasound in patients with abnormal findings, has been proposed for detecting early prostate cancer. Unfortunately, many screen-detected cancers will already have spread outside the prostate. In a study where healthy men with a PSA of >4 ng ml^{-1} underwent rectal examination and ultrasonography, only 59% of patients with PSA levels of 4.0–9.9 ng ml^{-1} and 13% with levels of >10 ng ml^{-1} with screen-detected cancers had localized tumours at surgical staging (Catalona et al 1991). Recent advances in assay methods give quantitative measurement of the free PSA. It appears that the ratio of free to total PSA is low (about 10%) in prostate cancer compared to >16% in BPH and prostatitis. Using this ratio should increase the specificity, as 93% of patients with a PSA of >4 ng ml^{-1} and a ratio of >15.4% had BPH and not prostatic cancer (Prestigiacomo & Stamey 1995). Until the results of large-scale studies are available, it remains unclear whether screening can reduce the mortality from prostate cancer and it cannot be recommended outside clinical trials.

Staging

PSA measurement may help to reduce the number of staging investigations in patients with prostate cancer. Patients with PSA levels of <20 ng ml^{-1} can be assumed to have no bone metastases and do not necessarily need bone scans. However, as a PSA of >20 ng ml^{-1} can occur in a patient with a bulky, poorly differentiated tumour without distant metastases, bone scanning is still necessary for patients with a PSA of >20 ng ml^{-1}. PSA is inferior to transurethral ultrasound in the detection of capsular invasion, with 30% of patients over-staged and 25% understaged by PSA. Lymph node metastases are usually associated with elevated PSA, and a PSA value of 20 ng ml^{-1} appears to have a positive and negative predictive value similar to CT scanning in the detection of nodal disease.

Prognosis/monitoring response/detection of recurrence

As the PSA level correlates with prostatic volume and tumour differentiation, it is not surprising that a high pretreatment PSA is associated with a poor prognosis. PSA levels fall rapidly to normal after complete removal of tumour by radical prostatectomy, although the rate of fall is slower after successful radiotherapy or endocrine therapy. There is evidence that a serial rise in PSA can precede other evidence of disease progression in the patient with a past history of prostate cancer who develops back pain, the presence of an elevated PSA level suggests the development of bone metastases.

Hepatocellular carcinoma

Serum AFP is elevated at presentation in 50–80% of UK patients with hepatocellular carcinoma (HCC). Although HCC is one of the most common malignant tumours in the world today, the relatively low incidence in the UK does not justify general population screening, although such screening may be justified in areas such as China with high-incidence populations. In the UK, serial AFP estimation and ultrasound examination can be justified, however, for selective screening of high-risk populations (i.e. patients with cirrhosis, chronic hepatitis B or haemochromatosis) because patients who have successful resection of a solitary, screen-detected tumour have a higher chance of long-term survival. Elevated AFP is not specific for the diagnosis of HCC, and histological confirmation is essential. Patients with HCC may have a normal AFP, especially if the tumour arises in a non-cirrhotic liver. In addition, modest elevations of AFP occur in about 20% of patients with hepatitis, cirrhosis, biliary tract obstruction and alcoholic liver disease and in up to 10% of patients with hepatic metastases. Despite these caveats, a massively elevated AFP in a patient with known cirrhosis is virtually diagnostic of HCC.

Breast cancer

A variety of tumour markers have been studied in patients with breast cancer, including CEA and tissue polypeptide antigen (TPA) and several polymorphic epithelial mucin markers (HMFG1, HMFG2, MSA, MCA, CAM-26, CAM-29 and CA 15-3). The most widely investigated mucin marker in breast cancer is CA 15–3. The commercially available CA 15-3 kit utilizes a sandwich technique which employs two monoclonal antibodies: the 115D8 antibody as the capture antibody and the DF3 antibody as the tracer antibody.

Diagnosis and screening

Although elevated levels of CA 15-3 are found in 55–100% of patients with advanced breast cancer, serum CA 15-3 is raised in only 10–46% of patients with primary breast cancer and in about 10% of patients with early (T1-2 NOMO) operable disease. As 2–20% of patients with benign breast disease have elevated levels, it is clear that mucin assays such as CA 15-3 are lacking in both specificity and sensitivity as a screening tool. No other tumour marker or combination of markers contribute to the diagnosis of breast cancer (Nicolini et al 1991).

Prognosis/monitoring response to treatment

Elevated preoperative levels of CA 15-3 have been shown to be associated with a poorer prognosis (Kallioniemi et al 1988). However, this may well be due to the association between CA 15-3 and tumour burden, and there is no convincing evidence to date that measurement of CA 15-3, or any other tumour marker, provides significant independent prognostic information. Although tumour marker levels can fall with reduction in tumour burden following systemic therapy, there is sufficient variation between patients to preclude the use of tumour marker estimation to define response.

Early detection of relapse

The observation that over 60% of patients who develop recurrent breast cancer have raised levels of CA 15-3 suggests a potential value in early detection of recurrence. The use of a panel of tumour markers might further increase the pick-up of recurrent disease. However, it is questionable whether such early detection of relapse will alter survival and thus whether the patient will benefit.

Other cancers and concluding remarks

Neuron-specific enolase is elevated in many patients with advanced small cell lung cancers and in children with neuroblastoma where it is used for screening.

Paraprotein levels are very important in the management of patients with myeloma where β_2-microglobulin may be of prognostic value.

Carcinoid tumours can be monitored by urine levels of 5-hydroxyindole acetic acid (5HIAA), and polypeptides such as gastrin or glucagon are useful in the management of rare gastrointestinal tumours.

Squamous cell carcinomas are associated with elevated levels of squamous cell carcinoma antigen (SCC) as well as cytokeratin fragments. SCC and CA 125 give valuable prognostic information in patients with cervical carcinoma, and may indicate relapse before scans.

Calcitonin and calcitonin-gene-related peptide are used in the diagnosis and screening for medullary thyroid carcinoma.

There are many other markers not mentioned, either because they are not considered to be of clinical value or because information related to value is inadequate. Many cytokines, growth factors, shed receptors, oncogenes and oncogene products are being investigated as tumour markers, and some may well prove to be useful. Despite many claims there are no markers that are of use as general cancer screens.

REFERENCES

Allen-Mersh T G, Kemeny N, Niedzwiechid et al 1987 Significance of a fall in serum CEA concentration in patients treated with cytotoxic chemotherapy for disseminated colorectal cancer. Gut 12: 1625–1629

Bagshawe K D, Harland S 1976 Immunodiagnosis and monitoring of gonadotrophin producing metastases in the central nervous system. Cancer 38: 112–118

Bagshawe K D, Dent J, Webb J 1986 Hydatidiform mole in England and Wales 1973–1983. Lancet ii: 673–677

Bast R C, Klug T L, St John E et al 1983 A radioimmunoassay using a monoclonal antibody to monitor the course of epithelial ovarian cancer. New England Journal of Medicine 308: 883–887

Beastall G H, Cook B, Rustin G J S, Jennings J 1990 A review of the role of established tumour markers. Annals of Clinical Biochemistry 28: 5–18

Begent R J, Rustin G J S 1989 Tumour markers: from carcinoembryonic antigen to products of hybridoma technology. Cancer Surveys 8: 107–121

Bosl G J, Lange P H, Nochomovitz L E 1981 Tumour markers in advanced non-seminomatous testicular cancer. Cancer 47: 572–576

Catalona W J, Smith D S, Ratliff T L et al 1991 Measurement of prostate specific antigen in serum as a screening test for prostate cancer. New England Journal of Medicine 324: 1156–1161

Coppack S, Newlands E S, Dent J et al 1983 Problems of interpretation of serum concentrations of alphafoetoprotein (AFP) in patients receiving cytotoxic chemotherapy for malignant germ cell tumours. British Journal of Cancer 48: 335–340

Fayers P M, Rustin G J S, Wood R et al 1993 The prognostic value of serum CA 125 in patients with advanced ovarian cancer: An analysis of 573 patients by the Medical Research Council Working Party on Gynaecological Cancer. International Journal of Gynaecological Cancer 3: 285–292

Gold P, Freedman D S 1965 Specific carcinoembryonic antigen of the human digestive system. Journal of Experimental Medicine 122: 468–481

Jacobs I, Prys Davies A, Bridges J et al 1993 Prevalence for screening for ovarian cancer in postmenopausal women by CA 125 measurement and ultrasonography. British Medical Journal 306: 1030–1034

Kallioniemi O P, Oksa H, Aaran R et al 1988 Serum C A 15-3 assay in the diagnosis and follow up of breast cancer. British Journal of Cancer 58: 213–215

Kohn J, Ragavan D 1981 Tumour markers in malignant germ cell tumours. In: Peckham M (ed) The management of testicular tumours. Edward Arnold, London, p 50–69

Lennon T, Houghton J, Northover J on behalf of the CRC/NIH CEA Trial Working Party 1994 Post-operative CEA monitoring and second-look surgery in colorectal cancer: trial results. British Journal of Cancer 70: 16

Mead G M 1995 International consensus prognostic classification for metastatic germ cell tumours treated with platinum based chemotherapy: final report of the international germ cell cancer collaborative group (IGCCG). Proceedings of the American Society of Clinical Oncology 14: 235

Medical Research Council Working Party on Testicular Tumours 1985 Prognostic factors in advanced, non-seminomatous germ cell testicular tumours: result of a multicentre study. Lancet i: 8

Newlands E S 1991 Gestational trophoblastic tumours. In: Blackledge G R P, Jordan J A, Shingleton M (eds) Textbook of gynaecological oncology. Saunders, London, p 454–463

Nicolini A, Colombini C, Luciani L et al 1991 Evaluation of serum CA 15-3 determination with CEA and TPA in the postoperative follow up of breast cancer patients. British Journal of Cancer 64: 154–158

Nielsen O S, Munro A J, Duncan W et al 1990 Is placental alkaline phosphatase (PLAP) a useful marker for seminoma? European Journal of Cancer 26: 1049–1054

Prestigiacomo F, Stamey T A 1995 Clinical usefulness of free and complexed PSA. Scandinavian Journal of Clinical and Laboratory Investigation 55 (suppl 221): 32–34

Rustin G J S, van der Burg M E L, Berek J S 1993 Tumour markers. Annals of Oncology 4 (suppl 4): s71–s77

Seckl M J, Rustin G J S, Bagshawe K D 1990 Frequency of serum tumour marker monitoring in patients with non-seminomatous germ cell tumours. British Journal of Cancer 61: 916–918

SECTION 5

Postoperative

27. Postoperative care

J. J. T. Tate

Postoperative care of the surgical patient has three phases:

- Immediate postoperative care (the recovery phase)
- Care on the ward until discharge from hospital
- Continuing care after discharge (e.g. district nurse visits).

The intensity of postoperative monitoring depends upon the type of surgery performed and the severity of the patient's condition.

THE RECOVERY PHASE

Basic management

Immediately after surgery patients require close monitoring, usually by one nurse per patient, in a dedicated recovery ward or area adjacent to the theatre. Monitoring of airway, breathing and circulation is the main priority, but a smooth recovery can only be achieved if pain and anxiety are relieved; monitoring the patent's overall comfort is essential. The nature of the surgery will determine the intensity of monitoring and any special precautions, but children, the elderly, patients with coexisting medical disease and patients who have had major surgery all require special care.

Management of the general comfort of the patient includes:

- Relief of pain and anxiety
- Administering mouthwashes (a dry mouth is common after general anaesthesia)
- The patient's position, including care of pressure points
- Prophylactic measures against
  (a) atelectasis by encouraging deep breathing, and
  (b) venous stasis by passive leg exercises.

These steps, including the prophylactic measures, all start in the recovery area and will continue on the main ward.

Airway and breathing

Patients may have an oral airway, a nasopharyngeal airway or, occasionally, may still be intubated on arrival in recovery; all secretions must be cleared by suction and the artificial airway left until the patient can maintain their own. Breathing may be depressed and a patient hypoxic due to three factors:

- Airway obstruction
- Residual anaesthetic gases
- The depressant effects of opioids.

Oxygen is given, ideally by mask, and the oxygen saturation monitored by a pulse oximeter. Special care is needed for patients with a new tracheostomy. If there is concern about vomiting and the risk of aspiration, patients can be sat up or nursed head-up rather than supine.

Circulation

Blood pressure is recorded quarter-hourly or, after major surgery, continuously via a radial artery cannula. The pulse rate is recorded regularly and continuously monitored by a pulse oximeter. The wound and any drains are monitored for signs of reactionary bleeding.

Before patients are returned to the ward their calculated fluid losses should be replaced with blood, blood products or crystalloids, and, ideally, fluid balance achieved. Monitoring of central venous pressure (CVP) can assist fluid balance management in severely ill patients or after major surgery. Urine output measurement may also provide useful information.

The patient's temperature is monitored as there may be a significant drop during surgery, which should be corrected before they leave the recovery room (e.g. space blanket). As the temperature rises peripheral vasodilatation may occur and this can lead to hypotension after the patient has returned to the ward, if not anticipated.

Special factors

Specific medical conditions and certain types of surgery will require additional monitoring. Some examples are:

- Diabetes mellitus – blood sugar monitoring
- Cardiac disease – electrocardiogram (ECG) monitor
- Orthopaedic surgery – monitoring of distal perfusion in a treated limb, position of limb, maintenance of fracture reduction, examination for peripheral nerve injury
- Neurosurgery – quarter-hourly neurological observations, intracranial pressure monitoring (intraventricular catheter or a transducer in the subarachnoid space)
- Urology – catheter output (after transurethral prostatectomy bladder irrigation is usually implemented and pulmonary oedema can develop if glycine has been absorbed into the circulation; fluid balance is particularly important)
- Vascular surgery – distal limb perfusion.

Pulse oximeter

The pulse oximeter is an essential piece of equipment for the management of the postoperative patient. It monitors three parameters: pulse rate, pulse volume and oxygen saturation. The fingertip sensor contains two light-emitting diodes (LEDs); one red, measuring the amount of oxygenated haemoglobin, the other infrared, measuring the total amount of haemoglobin. The actual amount of oxygen carried in the blood relative to the maximum possible amount is computed – this is the oxygen saturation (S_aO_2). The delivery of oxygen to the tissues depends on:

- Cardiac output
- Haemoglobin concentration
- Oxygen saturation (S_aO_2).

The relationship between oxygen in the blood and S_aO_2 is linear and thus easy to interpret. A fall in oxygen reaching the tissues can be detected far more rapidly with S_aO_2 monitoring than by clinical observation of the lips, nailbeds or mucous membranes for cyanosis (which may only be apparent when the S_aO_2 is 60–70%) or by measuring arterial blood gases. However, pulse oximetry does not indicate adequate ventilation; the S_aO_2 can be normal due to a high inspired oxygen level. Arterial blood gases measure pH, arterial oxygen and carbon dioxide tensions (P_aO_2, P_aCO_2), bicarbonate and base excess. These measurements are affected by many variables and can be difficult to interpret. The P_aO_2 has a non-linear relationship to the oxygen content of the blood (the oxygen dissociation curve), and hence oxygen saturation is easier to use in practice. P_aCO_2 reflects the rate of excretion of carbon dioxide by the lungs and is inversely proportional to the ventilation (assuming constant production of carbon dioxide by the body). The base excess and bicarbonate reflect acid–base disturbances and may be used in conjunction with the P_aCO_2 to distinguish respiratory from metabolic problems.

CARE ON THE WARD

Patients may be discharged from the recovery area when they are able to maintain their vital functions independently (i.e. full consciousness and stable respiratory and cardiovascular observations). On the ward the aim is to maintain a stable general condition and detect any complications early (Box 27.1). Initially, closer and more frequent observation is necessary and the priorities are the same as in the recovery room. Nursing staff perform routine observations; medical staff must undertake additional, clinical monitoring dictated by the nature of the case, including daily review of drug prescriptions. General care includes those measures described previously and control of pain. Early ambulation can reduce the risk of thrombotic complications. Patients who cannot mobilize require particular attention to skin care and pressure areas. Appropriate explanation of the results of the operation and the expected postoperative course should be given to the patient and relatives. The nature of the surgery or underlying disease will determine additional specific management (e.g. physiotherapy after orthopaedic surgery, stoma care for a new stoma).

Pain control

It is impossible for a patient to make a smooth recovery from surgery without adequate pain control (see Ch. 28). There has been a general shift from intermittent intramuscular analgesia to intravenous analgesia, either by continuous infusion or patient-controlled bolus, or epidural analgesia after major surgery. An epidural is particularly useful after major abdominal surgery, but insertion of an epidural catheter in patients who have received a preoperative dose of heparin for deep vein thrombosis prophylaxis is controversial and contraindicated if the patient has a coagulopathy. For day surgery or minor operations oral analgesia is suitable and narcotics can still be used if required. Non-steroidal anti-inflammatory drugs (NSAIDs) are popular but most be avoided in some patients, including asthmatics and those with a history of peptic ulcer or indigestion. Rectal administration of NSAIDs to a sedated patient should only be given with preoperative consent.

Box 27.1
The postoperative ward round – a daily checklist

A fresh assessment of each patient is required at each ward round, often daily but more frequently for seriously ill patients. Only a few factors may change on each occasion but all should be considered.

*Look at the **patient**, look at the **charts**, look at the **drug chart** and **communicate***

Enquire
- General comfort
- Pain control
- Thirst
- Specific symptoms

Examine
- General condition
- Respiration and chest (oxygen saturation if appropriate)
- Surgical wound
- Peripheral circulation/nerves (vascular/limb surgery)
- Drains and tubes (content, kinks or blockage, loss of vacuum)
- Pressure areas
- Drip sites

Check
- Pulse and blood pressure
- Temperature
- Urine output
- Fluid balance (assess insensible loss, e.g. sweating, diarrhoea)
- Special monitoring (e.g. diabetics – blood sugars)
- Results of blood tests/investigations

Review
- Nutrition/oral fluid and dietary intake
- Analgesia management
- Intravenous fluid prescription (volume, sodium and potassium need)
- Antibiotic prescription
- Other postoperative drugs
- Regular prescription medicines (when to start oral medication)

Inform
- What operation/treatment has been done and result
- Comment on progress over previous 24 hours
- Expected course over next few days
- Results of investigations/histology
- Likely day of discharge (identify any special requirements early)

Communicate
- Receive reports from named nurse, physiotherapist, etc.
- Advise changes of management
- Advise frequency/nature of observations required
- Write in the notes

Fluid balance

Fluid balance is important after major surgery and easier if a urinary catheter is in situ allowing accurate charting of urine output. Visible fluid losses are recorded on a fluid balance chart at regular intervals (e.g. hourly for urine output, 4-hourly for nasogastric aspirations, and 12- or 24-hourly for output into drains) and totalled every 24 hours. Unrecorded fluid losses (e.g. evaporation from skin and lungs, losses into hidden spaces such as the intestine, and diarrhoea) must be estimated and added to the recorded losses to calculate the patient's subsequent fluid requirements (see Ch. 8). For the typical 70-kg patient, intravenous fluid requirement after operation is 2.5 litres per day, of which 0.5 litre is normal saline and the remainder 5% dextrose; potassium being added after the first 24 hours once 1.5 litres of urine have been passed. Typically, the sodium requirement is 1 mmol kg^{-1} (normal saline contains 140 mmol l^{-1} of sodium) and potassium 1 mmol kg^{-1}. If the dissection area at operation has been large there will be a greater loss of plasma into the operation site and this may need to be replaced with colloid (e.g. Haemaccel) in the early postoperative period. In addition to these basic requirements, gastrointestinal losses are replaced volume-for-volume with normal saline with added potassium. Daily plasma urea and electrolyte measurement are advisable while the patient is dependent on intravenous fluids.

Clinical monitoring should include asking the patient about thirst, assessing central and peripheral perfusion, examination of dependent areas for oedema and auscultation of the chest. Tachycardia is an important sign that can indicate fluid overload or dehydration, but is also caused by inadequate analgesia.

Oliguria (defined as a urine output of less than 20 ml h^{-1} in each of two consecutive hours) in postoperative patients is caused by hypovolaemia in the majority of cases, but always consider a blocked catheter or cardiac failure. Hypovolaemia may be due to:

- Unreplaced blood loss
- Loss of fluid into the gastrointestinal tract
- Loss of plasma into the wound or abdomen
- Sequestration of extracellular fluid into the 'third' space.

Patients in whom fluid balance is difficult to manage, or where there is a particular risk of cardiac failure, may require central venous pressure monitoring or even left atrial pressure recording.

Blood transfusion

Haemoglobin measurement will be a guide to the need for blood transfusion unless plasma or extracellular fluid loss causes an artificially high measurement; this is most likely in the first 24 hours after surgery and it is generally not necessary to monitor haemoglobin levels more than 72 hours postoperatively. In a stable patient, a top-up transfusion is indicated if the haemoglobin level is less than 8 g% (determined by studies in Jehovahs Witnesses), while above this level patients should be given oral iron. If blood transfusion is given, frequent, regular monitoring of pulse, blood pressure and temperature are routine to detect a transfusion reaction. A major ABO incompatibility can result in an anaphylactic hypersensitivity reaction (flushing/urticaria, bronchospasm, hypotension). Incompatibility of minor factors is usually less severe and is indicated by tachycardia, pyrexia and possible rash and pruritus. The transfusion should be stopped, some blood sent for culture (both from patient and donor blood) and the remainder of the unit returned to the blood bank for further cross-matching against the patient's serum. However, if the reaction is mild it may be appropriate to give steroids or an antihistamine and to continue the transfusion (see Ch. 7).

Nutrition

Nutrition in postoperative patients is frequently poorly managed and treatment delayed. Dietary intake should be monitored in all patients, but usually only requires specific management in patents undergoing major abdominal surgery or in whom eating or swallowing is impossible. A basic indication for postoperative nutritional support is inability to eat (actual or expected) for more than 5 days. Serum protein is a crude but easily measured index of nutrition, and measurement of weight is useful over a period of time; more specific tests such as skin-fold thickness or estimation of nitrogen balance are used infrequently (see Ch. 9).

If nutritional support is required, enteral feeding is preferable if possible, because it has a lower complication rate than parenteral nutrition. Fluid balance and electrolyte monitoring are required and treatment should be given to reduce diarrhoea, which may be precipitated by high-calorie regimes. Parenteral feeding requires monitoring of the venous access point for sepsis, plasma and urinary electrolytes, blood sugar, plasma trace elements (e.g. magnesium) and liver function. The patient's fluid balance must be carefully managed.

Surgical drains

Nasogastric tubes

Nasogastric tubes drain fluid and swallowed air and should be left on free drainage at all times with intermittent aspiration (4-hourly). There is rarely a need to leave a nasogastric tube spigoted; once drainage has fallen below 100–200 ml per day, the tube can be removed.

Chest drains

Pleural drains are attached to an underwater seal because the pleural space is at subatmospheric pressure. If the lung does not expand fully, then low-pressure, high-volume suction may be added. When a drain is bubbling it should not be clamped because there is a danger of tension pneumothorax if the clamp is forgotten or left too long; however, it is essential that the bottle is never raised above the level of the patent's chest or else there is a risk that fluid will syphon back into the pleural cavity.

The drain is removed when:

- Bubbling has stopped for 24 hours
- There is no bubbling when the patient coughs
- The daily chest X-ray shows that the lung is fully expanded.

Check X-rays should be taken at 24 and 48 hours after removal of the drain.

Drains at the operative site

Drains at the operative site are used for the removal of anticipated fluid collections, not as an alternative to adequate haemostasis, and are usually simple tube drains or suction drains (check daily that the vacuum is maintained). Such drains should be removed early; if left in place they will not reduce the risk of a subsequent abscess and may introduce infection. If there is a chronic collection of fluid (such as an abscess or empyema) the drain may be left for several days to create a track. This type of drain is often removed a few centimetres at a time over several days (shortening) in an attempt to prevent the track closing too quickly; a sinogram may be used to confirm that the abscess cavity is shrinking.

Complications

All drains have similar potential complications:

- Trauma during insertion
- Failure to drain adequately due to

Table 27.1 Maximum doses of local anaesthetic agents

	Plain solution	With adrenalin
Lignocaine	200 mg (20 ml of 1%)	500 mg (50 ml of 1%)
Bupivicaine	150 mg (30 ml of 0.5%)	200 mg (40 ml of 0.5%)
Prilocaine	400 mg (80 ml of 0.5%)	600 mg (120 ml of 0.5%)

(a) incorrect placement
(b) too small size
(c) blocked lumen
- Complications due to disconnection
- Introduction of infection from outside via the drain track
- Erosion by the drain of adjacent tissues
- Fracture of drain during removal (retained foreign body)

DAY-CASE SURGERY

After day-case operations the postoperative period is inevitably short, but management should follow the same basic principles outlined above. Special considerations are that the patient is being discharged to a suitable environment, pain control and possible side-effects of sedation and anaesthesia. Patients who have had a general anaesthetic or sedation must be accompanied home and should not drive for at least 24 hours. Written advice and instructions should be given both to the patient and their accompanying relative or friend.

Local anaesthetic

The main problems with local anaesthesia are systemic toxicity of the anaesthetic agent and reactionary haemorrhage if adrenalin has been employed. All the commonly used local anaesthetics (lignocaine, bupivicaine and prilocaine) are cardiotoxic. Initial symptoms are paraesthesiae around the lips, tinnitus and/or visual disturbance. These are followed by dizziness, which may progress to convulsions and cardiac arrhythmia and collapse. Such complications are prevented by strict adherence to maximum dosage schedules (Table 27.1).

Treatment of systemic toxicity is directed firstly towards maintaining ventilation; hypotension is uncommon in the absence of hypoxia.

- Give 100% oxygen and maintain the airway, by intubation if necessary

- Control convulsions with intravenous diazepam
- Establish an ECG monitor; various arrthymias can occur (bretylium is the drug of choice for ventricular arrhythmia)
- If cardiac arrest occurs, start with high energy (360–400 J) DC shock and continue resuscitation attempts for at least 1 hour.

Sedation

For sedoanalgesia or sedation alone (e.g. endoscopy patients) particular attention is paid to monitoring respiration. During upper gastrointestinal endoscopy, delivery of oxygen by nasal spectacles is mandatory. All sedated patients should have a pulse oximeter attached during the procedure and until they are fully awake. The use of the antagonist flumazenil to reverse the sedative effects of benzodiazepines can be associated with delayed respiratory depression as the reversal agent may have a shorter half-life than the sedative itself. Midazolam, with a shorter half-life, is preferred to diazepam. All patients given sedation should be observed for at least 2 hours before being sent home.

CARE AFTER HOSPITAL DISCHARGE

The key is good communication. The patient should understand what treatment they have had, its effect, the likely time period required to complete their recovery and special restrictions on normal activity. Whenever appropriate, the relatives should also have this information. As many complications (e.g. wound infection) occur in the first week or two after hospital discharge, it is essential that the patient's GP is aware of the diagnosis and treatment given and also what information the patient has received. Ensure arrangements are made to communicate histology results to the patient and plans for additional investigation or treatment have been made and explained to the patient.

PROBLEMS IN THE POSTOPERATIVE PATIENT

The incidence and nature of postoperative complications depends upon the nature and extent of the operative intervention (see Ch. 31). Many are self-evident, but some specific problems are discussed below.

Cyanosis/respiratory inadequacy

The time between onset of respiratory problems and surgery may suggest the cause. In the recovery phase, it may be due to inadequate reversal of anaesthesia or excess opiates and the anaesthetist should be called.

Opiate overdosage usually presents in a drowsy patient with shallow, infrequent breaths, while airway obstruction is associated with obvious efforts to breathe, indrawn intercostal muscles and agitation.

Airway obstruction

If a patient is in respiratory distress give verbal reassurance and 100% oxygen by mask. If cyanosed, check the pulse as the most common cause is cardiac arrest. If breathing appears obstructed, call for anaesthetic help and:

- Inspect the mouth for foreign bodies (e.g. vomit, slipped denture and surgical swab after surgery in the mouth)
- Extend the neck and pull the jaw forward to clear the tongue from the back of the mouth and get an assistant to maintain the position
- Insert an oral airway
- If the patient has had a thyroidectomy, open the wound (skin and deep fascia) at the bedside
- If the patient has had surgery in the mouth, throat or neck, or there is no improvement with an airway in place, perform a cricothyroidotomy without delay
- Check that the patient can exhale
- Monitor the oxygen saturation and obtain blood gases and chest X-ray as soon as possible.

Do not attempt to intubate a patient after surgery in the mouth or neck unless experienced – do a cricothyroidotomy and call an anaesthetist. In an emergency, a large-gauge intravenous cannula can be used for cricothyroidotomy but requires jet ventilation, whether the patient is breathing or not, because of the small lumen (attach rigid oxygen line to cannula via the barrel of a 5 ml syringe). During insertion, check that the needle is in the trachea, which may be displaced, by aspiration of air and be careful not to pass it straight through the back. The cannula can kink or displace and should be replaced as soon as possible with a purpose-made device.

Normal breathing

Cyanosis in a patient who appears to be breathing normally may be due to a problem in the lungs or circulation. Listen to the chest for bronchospasm (wheeze is absent in severe bronchospasm) and for uniform air entry. Is the patient asthmatic? Is this a hypersensitivity reaction? Loss of air entry in the upper chest suggests pneumothorax and in the dependent part of the chest, haemothorax or pleural effusion. Has the patient had attempts at intravenous line insertion in the neck?

Acute circulatory problems which can cause cyanosis are loss of venous return (massive sudden blood loss), pump failure (myocardial infarct) and obstruction (massive pulmonary embolus). Check the blood pressure and get an ECG. Other possible causes include severe adverse drug reaction and severe sepsis (air hunger).

Hypotension

The commonest cause of hypotension in a postoperative patient is hypovolaemia, either due to inadequate fluid replacement or bleeding. Myocardial infarction needs to be considered and excluded. Poor management of pain control, either too much or too little analgesia, may be a factor and hypotension is a side-effect of an epidural (local anesthetic drugs may cause dilation of the main capacitance vessels). It is difficult to confirm that an epidural is responsible without turning it off; however, treatment by volume replacement is the same whether hypotension is caused by hypovolaemia or the epidural.

An assessment of the overall clinical situation may suggest an obvious cause of hypotension in a given patient. If not:

- Increase the rate of intravenous fluids
- Elevate the legs
- Give oxygen up to 50% by mask
- Obtain an ECG (dysrhythmia, acute ischaemia, signs of pulmonary embolus)

If the ECG is normal, place a central venous pressure line whilst giving additional intravenous fluid. Listen to the chest to exclude tension pneumothorax (chest trauma, chest surgery, surgery around the oesophageal hiatus, or failed neck line) and consider pulmonary embolus and septicaemia. If no cause is apparent, and the blood pressure responds to volume, hidden blood loss is likely.

Hypertension

This may be dangerous in patients with ischaemic heart disease, cerebrovascular disease or following vascular surgery. Obtain anaesthetic assistance with the management of such patients if a cause cannot be found; the commonest causes of hypertension are inadequate control of pain and/or anxiety, urinary retention and shivering.

Postoperative infection

The patient's temperature is a basic, but crude, observation for infection. Clinical monitoring includes exam-ination of the chest and inspection of the wound. The upper limit of normal temperature is 37°C, but there is considerable variation and occasionally a patient may be pyrexial despite a temperature below this 'magic' figure. The timing of postoperative pyrexia may suggest a cause (e.g. after a large bowel resection: pyrexia within the first 48 hours – chest infection; fifth or sixth day – an anastomotic leakage or wound infection; tenth day – venous thrombosis).

If a patient develops a pyrexia, a routine 'infection screen' is carried out:

- Examine the chest – chest X-ray; sputum for culture; ECG (if ? pulmonary embolus)
- Examine the wound – wound swab for culture
- Enquire about urinary symptoms – urine culture
- Examine for signs of deep vein thrombosis
- Examine intravenous sites (phlebitis) and other catheter sites (epidural)
- Examine pressure areas
- If a child – look in the ears and mouth
- If cause uncertain – send blood cultures; measure white cell count; consider the underlying disease (e.g. pyrexia of malignancy)
- Consider hidden infection (e.g. subphrenic or pelvic abscess).

Delayed gastric emptying/aspiration

Abdominal surgery is frequently associated with delayed gastric emptying and impaired colonic motility, even though small bowel activity, and hence bowel sounds, may return relatively early. If there is intra-abdominal sepsis, metabolic disturbances, or retroperitoneal haematoma or inflammation there may be prolonged inactivity of the small bowel also (paralytic ileus). Colonic pseudo-obstruction occurs most often in elderly patients confined to bed (e.g. after fracture or orthopaedic surgery) and postpartum. Reintroduction of diet too soon can lead to gastric dilation with vomiting and the risk of aspiration. Monitoring nasogastric aspirates, abdominal distension and the passage of flatus determines the timing of reintroduction of normal diet. However, a restricted intake of oral fluids (30 ml h^{-1}) is permissible almost without exception, and increases patient comfort.

Gastric aspiration can be life-threatening:

- Place the patient head-down in the recovery position
- Suction out the mouth
- Give 100% oxygen by mask
- Pass a nasogastric tube to empty the stomach
- Examine for bronchospasm – if present give nebulized

salbutamol ± intravenous aminophylline and consider intubation and ventilation
- Obtain chest X-ray
- Arrange early chest physiotherapy.

Steroids are not thought to be helpful.

FURTHER READING

In addition to the chapters in this book referred to in the text, several pocket-sized texts aimed at trainee anaesthetists are available and provide useful guidelines on the management of acute postoperative problems:

Eaton J M, Fielden J M, Wilson M E Anaesthesia action plans. Abbott Laboratories Ltd., Abbott House, Norden Road, Maidenhead, Berks SL6 4XE

28. The management of postoperative pain

R. Fernando   P. M. Robbins

Pain relief after surgery is still inadequately managed despite the development of new drugs and more effective techniques to control postoperative pain. The traditional approach to postoperative pain is the use of a fixed dose of intramuscular opioid on an intermittent pro re nata (PRN) schedule (e.g. morphine 10 mg, prn, 3-hourly). This approach is simple, cheap, requires no special equipment and sometimes it may actually work. A standard dose of intramuscular opioid such as morphine (10 mg) can result in a five-fold difference in peak plasma concentrations of morphine among different patients, with the time taken to reach these levels varying by as much as seven-fold. In addition, the plasma concentrations of opioid needed to provide analgesia, the minimum effective analgesic concentration (MEAC), may vary by up to four-fold between patients. Therefore the 'standard' dose prescribed is only optimal for a few patients and the PRN ('as needed') part of the order is often interpreted by nursing staff to mean 'as little as possible'.

Additional problems with postoperative pain are:

- The management of postoperative pain is often delegated to the most junior doctor
- The fear of drug addiction and side-effects such as respiratory depression lead to nursing staff withholding medication
- The time delay between the request for analgesia and the final administration of a drug may increase the amount of a patient's pain.

HOW DOES POSTOPERATIVE PAIN ARISE?

Pain involves four physiological processes: transduction, transmission, modulation and perception. Pain begins when local tissue damage, a noxious stimulus, occurs during surgery which causes the release of inflammatory substances (prostaglandins, histamine, serotonin, bradykinin and substance P). This leads to the generation of electrical impulses (transduction) at peripheral sensory nerve endings, or nociceptors. These electrical impulses are conducted by nerve fibres (A-delta and C fibres) to the spinal cord (transmission). Further relay to the higher brain centres can be modified within the spinal cord (modulation) before an individual perceives a painful stimulus (perception). Therefore pain can, in theory, be *blocked* at various levels in this complex chain. Non-steroidal anti-inflammatory drugs (NSAIDs) can reduce the peripheral inflammatory response by reducing prostaglandin production. Local anaesthetic drugs injected into the epidural space can block impulses to the spinal cord by acting on spinal nerve roots. Opioids can produce analgesia through modulation by binding to opioid receptors in the spinal cord and other higher brain centres such as the periaqueductal grey, the nucleus raphe magnus and the thalamus, whereas binding to opioid receptors in the cerebral cortex can affect the perception of pain.

WHY SHOULD WE TREAT POSTOPERATIVE PAIN?

Apart from the humanitarian aspect, there are several physiological reasons for treating postoperative pain.

Respiratory effects

Surgery involving the upper abdomen or chest reduces vital capacity, functional residual capacity and the ability to cough and deep breathe. This in turn can lead to retention of secretions, atelectasis and pneumonia. Inadequately treated pain aggravates these changes, while analgesia improves respiratory function.

Cardiovascular effects

Pain causes an increase in sympathetic output (tachycardia, hypertension and increasing blood catecholamines) which leads to increasing myocardial oxygen demand, which may in turn increase the risk of

---

Box 28.1

Pain associated with different surgical procedures (decreasing order of severity)

- Thoracic surgery
- Upper abdominal surgery
- Lower abdominal surgery
- Inguinal and femoral hernia repair
- Head/neck/limb surgery

---

postoperative myocardial ischaemia, especially in those patients with pre-existing cardiac disease.

Neuroendocrine effects

The stress response to surgery and pain includes the secretion of catecholamines and catabolic hormones. This increases metabolism and oxygen consumption and promotes sodium and water retention.

HOW SHOULD WE TREAT POSTOPERATIVE PAIN?

The management of postoperative pain does not begin *after* the completion of surgery. Preoperative counselling about the operation, the nature of the pain and the methods available to treat it may help the patient to cope better with postoperative pain. Intraoperative opioids used by the anaesthetist during general anaesthesia or the provision of regional blocks such as lumbar epidurals may further reduce postoperative pain. In the ideal world of postoperative pain relief, each individual patient should be jointly assessed preoperatively by the surgeon, anaesthetist and nursing staff. The site and nature of the surgery (Box 28.1), the type and extent of the surgical incision, the physiological and psychological make-up of the patient may all be relevant in the planning of postoperative analgesia. This sort of work-up rarely occurs in practice.

METHODS AVAILABLE TO TREAT POSTOPERATIVE PAIN

Opioids

Opioids act at opioid receptors in the spinal cord and higher brain centres to produce analgesia. Side-effects include nausea and vomiting, delayed gastric emptying, urinary retention, pruritus, respiratory depression and sedation.

Oral opioids

These include codeine, dihydrocodeine and dextropropoxyphene. For example:

- Codeine phosphate, 30–60 mg, 6-hourly
- Codydramol (= dihydrocodeine 10 mg + paracetamol 500 mg), 1–2 tablets, 6-hourly
- Coproxamol (= dextropropoxyphene 32.5 mg + paracetamol 325 mg) 1–2 tablets, 6-hourly.

The oral route for opioids is not recommended initially after major surgery for the following reasons:

- The use of opioids during general anaesthesia can lead to postoperative nausea and vomiting and delayed gastric emptying
- Intra-abdominal surgery can result in postoperative ileus
- Orally absorbed opioids from the gut reach the liver via the splanchnic blood flow where they are highly metabolized (first-pass metabolism) causing insufficient plasma concentrations of drug.

Despite this, oral opioid combinations with paracetamol (codydramol or coproxamol) are adequate for treating mild pain after day-case surgery or 3–4 days after major surgery when parenteral opioids are no longer needed.

Intramuscular opioids

These include morphine, diamorphine, pethidine and 'omnopon'. For example:

- Morphine, 10 mg, 3-hourly
- Pethidine, 75 mg, 3-hourly.

This is the most common route used today, for the reasons given above. It is convenient and is associated with few side-effects, although the degree of analgesia varies between patients. Up to 40% of patients on a PRN intramuscular opioid regime may have inadequate pain relief. Care needs to be taken when multiple doses of intramuscular opioids are administered to shocked patients with poor peripheral perfusion. In such cases a large depot of opioid can accumulate intramuscularly to be later released into the bloodstream when the peripheral circulation is restored with unpredictable and often dangerous results.

Intravenous opioid continuous infusions

These include morphine and pethidine. For example:

- Morphine, 50 mg in 50 ml saline (1 mg ml^{-1}), infusion rate 1–10 ml h^{-1}

Child Morphine mg = ½ wt in 50ml
0 – 4ml /hr

- Pethidine, 250 mg in 50 ml saline (5 mg ml^{-1}), infusion rate 1–8 ml h^{-1}.

A continuous infusion of opioid through an intravenous cannula can abolish wide swings in plasma drug concentration found with the intramuscular route and allow adjustment of the rate to the individual needs of a patient. An initial intravenous loading dose of opioid is usually needed before an infusion is started, otherwise it may take several hours for the drug to reach the patient's MEAC to achieve pain relief. Unfortunately, plasma drug concentrations may continue to increase with such regimes, leading to sedation and respiratory depression. Therefore regular monitoring is essential, with the infusion rate being changed as necessary. Naloxone should be available to reverse opioid side-effects such as excessive sedation and respiratory depression.

Intravenous opioid patient-controlled analgesia

These include morphine, diamorphine and pethidine. For example:

- Morphine, 50 mg in 50 ml saline (1 mg morphine per ml)
  Bolus = 1 ml (1 mg morphine)
  Lock-out time = 5 min
  4-hour limit = 30 mg morphine
- Pethidine, 250 mg in 50 ml saline (5 mg pethidine per ml)
  Bolus = 2 ml (10 mg pethidine)
  Lock-out time = 5 min
  4-hour limit = 300 mg pethidine

Intravenous opioid patient-controlled analgesia (PCA) is superior to both intramuscular and continuous infusion routes because it allows the patient to self-administer small doses of opioid when pain occurs. PCA is administered using a special microprocessor-controlled pump which is triggered by depressing a button held in the patient's hand. When triggered, a pre-set amount (the bolus dose) is delivered to the patient, usually via a separate intravenous line. A timer prevents the administration of another bolus for a specified period (the lock-out interval). Before a PCA is started, a loading dose of opioid must be given to achieve adequate analgesia. Background infusions of opioid are no longer used with PCA because of increasing side-effects. The theoretical basis of PCA is that, since individual patients require different plasma opioid concentrations to achieve an MEAC, each patient will control the frequency of opioid boluses to achieve good pain relief with minimal side-effects. From a safety aspect, if the patient

becomes oversedated on PCA, they cannot give themselves another bolus. This will lead to a fall in plasma opioid concentration to safer levels. Regardless of this, regular monitoring of patients with PCA is essential. Naloxone should once again be available to treat respiratory depression and excessive sedation.

Miscellaneous routes of opioid administration

Transdermal. Fentanyl, a potent short-acting opioid, has been used in a drug-containing patch which adheres to the skin. The drug diffuses through the skin and into the bloodstream. Unfortunately, the dose cannot be titrated to the patient's needs and it takes several hours to achieve a MEAC.

Sublingual. Since the drug is delivered directly into the bloodstream via the sublingual route, first-pass metabolism is avoided. Sublingual buprenorphine, a partial agonist, is available, but has a 20% incidence of nausea and vomiting and a 50% incidence of sedation or drowsiness.

Epidural. This route is discussed below.

Local anaesthetics

Local anaesthetic (LA) drugs (e.g. bupivacaine, lignocaine and prilocaine) block the conduction of nerve impulses when applied to peripheral nerves or nerve roots. Sensory and sympathetic nerve fibres are blocked by smaller amounts of LA compared to motor nerves. In the treatment of postoperative pain, LA drugs injected close to a peripheral nerve (digital nerves in a ring block) or a plexus of nerves (brachial plexus in an axillary block) will block painful stimuli arising from an area supplied by those nerves. Bupivacaine is the most commonly used LA drug due to its long duration of action (2–3 hours).

All LA drugs can cause toxic effects if given in large doses or if accidental intravascular injection occurs. Central nervous system and cardiovascular toxicity can result in restlessness, convulsions, hypotension and cardiorespiratory arrest. Suggested safe maximum doses of LA are 2 mg kg^{-1} for plain bupivacaine and 3 mg kg^{-1} for plain lignocaine. LA solutions are also available with small amounts of adrenaline (e.g. 1 in 200 000) which, acting as a vasoconstrictor, reduces the absorption of the LA, thereby allowing larger amounts of LA to be given. Injection of adrenaline-containing solutions is absolutely contraindicated in areas supplied by end arteries, such as the fingers, toes and the penis, since prolonged ischaemia may lead to tissue necrosis.

Local infiltration to wound

For example:

- Bupivacaine, 0.25%, 10–20 ml, after inguinal hernia repair.

Catheters can also be used to constantly infuse LA into the wound to provide analgesia.

Nerve blocks

For example:

- Bupivacaine, 0.5%, 1–4 ml, penile block for circumcision
- Bupivacaine 0.25%, 10 ml, ilioinguinal/iliohypogastric nerve block for hernia repair.

These blocks can be performed by the anaesthetist while the patient is anaesthetized.

Epidural block

For example:

- Single-shot caudal epidural for paediatric circumcision using bupivacaine, 0.25%, 0.5 ml kg^{-1}
- Continuous epidural infusions for abdominal or thoracic operations:
  (a) Bupivacaine 0.25%, 30 ml + diamorphine 5 mg + saline 30 ml
      Concentration: bupivacaine 0.125% + diamorphine 0.008%
      Infusion rate = 2–8 ml h^{-1}
  (b) Bupivacaine 0.5%, 10 ml + fentanyl (50 μg ml^{-1}) 2 ml + saline 38 ml
      Concentration: bupivacaine 0.1% + fentanyl 0.0002%
      Infusion rate = 2–12 ml h^{-1}

Plain LA solutions such as bupivacaine 0.25% can be administered into the epidural space intermittently through an epidural catheter or, more usually, continuously via an infusion pump to block nerves within the spinal canal. Excellent analgesia can be obtained with this technique especially for thoracic and major abdominal operations. Side-effects of LA used in epidural blocks include hypotension (sympathetic block), muscle weakness of the legs (motor block) and urinary retention.

Most hospitals in the UK use epidural infusions consisting of combinations of low-dose LA (e.g. bupivacaine 0.1%) and opioid (e.g. fentanyl 0.0002%). Such low-dose combinations are synergistic. Side-effects related to epidural opioids alone include nausea and vomiting, pruritus, sedation and delayed respiratory depression. Low-dose mixtures by reducing the amount of both LA and opioid, actually reduce the side-effects of both drugs. However, monitoring of the patient is still important. Naloxone should once again be available to reverse opioid side-effects such as excessive sedation and respiratory depression. Typically, patients receiving low-dose LA + opioid epidural infusions have superior analgesia, improved cardiovascular stability, and the ability to move about due to a reduction in motor block.

NSAIDs

For example:

- Mefenamic acid, 500 mg, orally, 8-hourly
- Diclofenac sodium, 100 mg, rectally, 12–15 hourly (oral preparation also available)
- Ketorolac trometamol, 10 mg, intravenously/intramuscularly, 4–6 hourly.

NSAIDs block the synthesis of prostaglandins by inhibiting the enzyme cyclo-oxygenase (prostaglandin synthetase). Prostaglandins mediate several components of the inflammatory response, including fever, pain and vasodilation.

NSAIDs are usually only suitable for the treatment of mild to moderate postoperative pain. However, if used in conjunction with opioids, they may also reduce the amount of opioids used to treat postoperative pain. In this way opioid side-effects such as nausea and vomiting can also be reduced. This is the concept of 'balanced analgesia'. Diclofenac sodium (Voltarol) is widely used in the UK, usually in suppository form to provide analgesia after many minor day-case operations including gynaecological laparoscopy. Due to its long duration of action (12 hours) diclofenac can be given preoperatively to provide analgesia into the postoperative period. Diclofenac is also generally safe to administer to patients with stable asthma who have *no* history of allergy or worsening asthma with aspirin or other NSAIDs. Other problems with diclofenac apply to NSAIDs in general:

- Gastric ulceration – avoid NSAIDs in patients with a history of gastric ulceration
- Nephrotoxicity – renal function can be altered by NSAIDs secondary to prostaglandin inhibition, but only usually in patients with pre-existing renal problems
- Impaired haemostasis – due to the inhibition of the prostaglandin thromboxane A$_2$ within platelets, NSAIDs may also increase the risk of bleeding.

Pre-emptive analgesia

A hypothesis exists that surgery, which produces a barrage of pain signals to the spinal cord, is a 'priming' mechanism which sensitizes the central nervous system. This is said to lead to enhanced postoperative pain. The rationale behind several studies is that by providing presurgery, or pre-emptive, analgesia using parenteral opioids, regional blocks or NSAIDs, either individually or in combination, these sensitizing neuroplastic changes can be prevented within the spinal cord leading to diminished postoperative pain requirements. Therefore the concept of pre-emptive analgesia may have implications in reducing not only acute postoperative pain, but also chronic pain states such as post-thoracotomy chest-wall pain and postamputation lower limb stump pain. Taken to an extreme, a single dose of analgesic drug administered before surgery could theoretically abolish postoperative pain. Unfortunately, no current study proves the existence of pre-emptive analgesia in humans.

MONITORING OF POSTOPERATIVE ANALGESIA

The effectiveness of any postoperative analgesic regime as well as any side-effects need to be assessed regularly. Pain scores, sedation scores and respiratory monitoring should be used to optimize any form of analgesia.

Monitoring of pain

This can be done in a variety of ways. For example:

- *Visual analogue score (VAS)* – patients are asked to mark their pain score on a 10-cm scale ranging from 0 = no pain to 10 = worst pain imaginable.
- *Verbal rating score (VRS)* – patients rate their pain as 1 = no pain, 2 = mild pain, 3 = moderate pain, 4 = severe pain.

Pain scores can be difficult to interpret since individual patients vary in their perception of pain. VAS and VRS are the most commonly used methods when adjusting analgesic regimes such as opioid PCA or epidural infusions. Most pain scores only measure pain when the patient is resting. Obviously such a score will change when, for example, a patient after upper abdominal surgery attempts to cough to clear secretions or receives chest physiotherapy. Therefore pain scores on coughing or moving will be just as important as those at rest.

Monitoring of sedation and respiration

For example, a *sedation score* may be:

0 = No sedation (patient alert)
1 = Mild sedation (occasionally drowsy; easy to arouse)
2 = Moderate sedation (often drowsy; easy to arouse)
3 = Severe sedation (difficult to arouse).

The major fear with opioids, administered by any route (intravenously, intramuscularly or epidurally) is that of respiratory depression. Epidural opioids have the added risk of delayed respiratory depression. This risk is extremely small. Highly lipid-soluble opioids such as fentanyl have a lower risk of this complication than does morphine which is less lipid soluble. Of course the general medical condition of the patient must be considered, since elderly patients with cardiorespiratory disease are at a higher risk of this potentially dangerous complication. Traditionally it has been assumed that intermittent observation of a patient's respiratory rate by a ward nurse is adequate to detect respiratory problems. The development of pulse oximetry, which allows a patient's blood oxygen saturation (S_pO_2) to be measured non-invasively using a simple finger probe, has shown that episodes of hypoxaemia may occur despite a normal respiratory rate with any form of opioid analgesia. In fact an increasing level of sedation may precede respiratory depression. Therefore it is important regularly to monitor not only pain scores but also sedation scores and respiratory rate. A sedation score of 3 or a respiratory rate less than 8 breaths per minute should be treated immediately with intravenous naloxone.

If pulse oximetry is used, a S_pO_2 of less than 94% in a patient breathing air should be treated with supplemental oxygen through nasal cannulae or a face mask.

Measurement of S_pO_2 using pulse oximetry is already a minimum monitoring standard during anaesthesia and the immediate recovery period. Several studies which have extended the use of pulse oximetry to the postoperative period on the ward have detected periods of hypoxaemia 3–4 days after major surgery. The relationship of these events to the risk of myocardial ischaemia is a subject of ongoing research. In the future, the gold standard of patient monitoring could well be the pulse oximeter which will be allocated to patients scheduled for surgery when they first arrive in hospital. Continuous monitoring of S_pO_2 will then occur preoperatively (to obtain baseline values) and postoperatively. On this basis the use of postoperative oxygen therapy on the ward could be extended to more patients at risk of hypoxaemia. Note, however, that pulse oximetry alone gives no information about the adequacy of respiration or the

Box 28.2

Intravenous opioid PCA standing orders

1. PCA drug concentration: Morphine 1 mg ml^{-1}
2. Bolus dose: Morphine 1 mg (= 1 ml)
3. Lock-out interval: 5 minutes
4. 4-hour limit: 30 mg Morphine
5. If pain not controlled after 1 hour, *increase* bolus dose to: . . . . . . mg = ... ml of morphine
6. If pain still not controlled after 1 hour, *reduce* lock-out interval to: . . . . . . min
7. If pain still not controlled, call acute pain service (APS) (bleep . . . . . .) for further advice
8. No systemic opioids or other CNS depressants to be given
9. Monitor: heart rate/blood pressure/pain score/respiratory rate/sedation score.
   Monitor hourly for the first 8 hours, then 2–3-hourly
10. SIDE-EFFECTS:
    (a) Sedation score = 3. **Action:** Call APS (Bleep . . . . . .)
    (b) Respiratory rate < 8/min. **Action:** Call APS (Bleep . . . . . .)
    (c) Sedation score = 3 + Respiratory rate < 8/min. **Action: Give intravenous naloxone 0.4 mg STAT and fast bleep APS**
    (d) Nausea and vomiting: **Action:** Metoclopramide, 10 mg, i.v./i.m.
          or Ondansetron, 4 mg, i.v./i.m.
    (e) Pruritus:
        Mild   **Action:** Give chlorpheniramine (Piriton), 10 mg, i.m., 8-hourly
        Severe **Action:** Give naloxone, 40 μg, i.v. bolus (repeat if needed)
    (f) Urinary retention. **Action:** In/out bladder catheter

Box 28.3

Epidural opioid/local anaesthetic infusion standing orders

1. Drugs: **fentanyl** (50 μg ml^{-1}, 2 ml) + **bupivacaine** (0.5%, 10 ml) + **saline** (38 ml)
   Concentration = fentanyl 0.0002% + bupivacaine 0.1%
2. Infusion rate: 2–12 ml h^{-1}
3. If in pain, increase rate by 2 ml h^{-1} each hour, until maximum rate
4. If pain still not controlled, call APS (Bleep . . . . . .) for further advice
5. If epidural bolus given by APS, check blood pressure every 5 minutes for 30 minutes
6. No systemic opioids or other CNS depressants to be given
7. Monitor: heart rate/blood pressure/pain score/respiratory rate/sedation score.
   Monitor hourly for the first 8 hours, then 2–3 hourly
8. SIDE-EFFECTS:
    (a) Sedation score = 3. **Action:** Call APS (Bleep . . . . . .)
    (b) Respiratory rate < 8/min. **Action:** Call APS (Bleep . . . . . .)
    (c) Sedation score = 3 + respiratory rate < 8/min. **Action: Give intravenous naloxone 0.4 mg STAT and fast bleep APS**
    (d) Nausea and vomiting. **Action:** Metoclopramide, 10 mg, i.v./i.m.
          or Ondansetron, 4 mg, i.v./i.m.
    (e) Pruritus:
        Mild   **Action:** Give chlorpheniramine (Piriton), 10 mg, i.m., 8-hourly
        Severe **Action:** Give naloxone, 40 μg, i.v. bolus (repeat if needed)
    (f) Urinary retention. **Action:** In/out bladder catheter

level of sedation. As such it can only be useful if used in combination with regular nursing observations.

ACUTE PAIN SERVICE (APS)

Each hospital should have an APS team as recommended in 1990 by the Royal College of Surgeons of England and the Royal College of Anaesthetists. This team should be responsible for the day-to-day management of patients with postoperative pain. The establishment of an APS requires a multidisciplinary approach using medical, nursing and pharmaceutical expertise. Anaesthetists have a major role to play, since they not only initiate postoperative analgesic regimes such as PCA and epidural infusions, but also are familiar with the drugs and equipment used in such cases. Many hospitals have an acute pain nurse coordinating an APS. Problems which require more medical input can be referred to a designated doctor, using the anaesthetist on-call. Protocols or standing orders for PCA and epidural regimes for the ward staff are invaluable (Boxes 28.1 and 28.2).

CONCLUSION

Currently, in the treatment of postoperative pain there is no single analgesic therapy which can treat all aspects of pain without causing side-effects. The emphasis should be on a 'balanced analgesic' technique, especially after major surgical procedures, using NSAIDs in combination with other drugs such as opioids or local anaesthetics. Using such principles, we may be able not only to improve analgesic efficacy, but also to reduce analgesic-induced side-effects.

FURTHER READING

Commission on the Provision of Surgical Services 1990 Report of the Working Party on Pain after Surgery. Royal College of Surgeons of England and the College of Anaesthetists, London

Ferrante F M, Vade Boncouer T R 1993 Postoperative pain management. Churchill Livingstone, Edinburgh

Liu S, Carpenter R L, Neal J M 1995 Epidural anesthesia and analgesia, their role in postoperative outcome. Anesthesiology 82: 1474–1506

McQuay H J 1992 Pre-emptive analgesia. British Journal of Anaesthesia 69: 1–3

Ready L B 1990 Acute postoperative pain. In: Anesthesia, 3rd edn. Churchill Livingstone, Edinburgh, p 2135–2145

Sabanathan S 1995 Has postoperative pain been eradicated? Annals of the Royal College of Surgeons 77 (3): 202–209

Souter A J, Fredman B, White P F 1994 Controversies in the perioperative use of nonsteroidal antiinflammatory drugs. Anesthesia and Analgesia 79: 1178–1190

29. The body's response to surgery

J. P. S. Cochrane

The body responds to trauma with local and systemic reactions that attempt to contain and heal the tissue damage, and to protect the body while it is injured. The response is remarkably similar whether the trauma is a fracture, burn, sepsis or a planned surgical operation, and the extent of the response is usually proportional to the severity of the trauma.

The systemic response, produced by many different mediators, increases the metabolic rate, mobilizes carbohydrate, protein and fat stores, conserves salt and water, and diverts blood preferentially to vital organs. It also stimulates important protective mechanisms such as the immunological and blood clotting systems.

The response aids survival if no other help is available, but some of its features are not ideal in a hospital setting. Moreover, severe trauma can lead to a harmful overreaction of the response in which systemic changes cause progressive organ dysfunction, with lethal consequences.

INITIATION OF THE RESPONSE

Various noxious stimuli produce the response but they rarely occur alone, and multiple stimuli often produce greater effects than the sum of single responses. The response is modified by the severity of the stimulus, the patient's age, nutritional status, coexisting medical conditions, medication and whether or not the trauma or operation has affected the function of any particular organ. Recent trauma or sepsis will also modify the response to a subsequent surgical operation.

Pain. Stimuli from the skin, musculoskeletal system, visceral stretch receptors, especially those pulling on the mesentery stimulate the sympathetic nervous system, ACTH and vasopressin (AVP).

Tissue injury. Cell death leads to cytokine release. If sufficient cytokines are produced in the wound they will enter the systemic circulation and the acute-phase response occurs.

Infection. Endotoxin from the cell walls of Gram-negative bacteria is the most powerful stimulus for release of one of the cytokines, tumour necrosis factor (TNF), from macrophages. Infection can also enter the circulation from the bowel if the mucosal barrier is impaired.

Hypovolaemia. Most injuries lead to hypovolaemia, either from haemorrhage, plasma loss in burns or third-space losses. This stimulates baroreceptors, releasing AVP, catecholamines, renin–angiotensin and aldosterone, and leads to impaired excretion of sodium and water. If there is hypoperfusion, toxins and metabolites may be released into the circulation.

Starvation. If starvation accompanies trauma it causes the body to use muscle bulk as a source of protein and the immune response is impaired.

Hypoxia, hypercarbia or pH changes. Chemoreceptors in the carotid and aortic bodies react to these changes and stimulate the sympathetic nervous systems, ACTH and AVP.

Energy substrates. Hypoglycaemia stimulates ACTH, growth hormone, β-endorphin, AVP and catecholamines. Certain amino acids also have particular effects.

Fear and emotion. These stimulate the sympathetic nervous system, AVP and ACTH.

Temperature. Hypothermia, whether due to decreased heat production in prolonged hypovolaemia or starvation, increased heat loss in burns, or induced for cardiac surgery, stimulates the hypothalamus and leads to increased secretion of AVP, ACTH, growth hormone, thyroxine and catecholamines.

SYSTEMS CONTROLLING THE RESPONSE

Four principal systems produce the response:

Sympathetic nervous system. The immediate fight and flight reaction may help the injured person avoid further injury, but it has short-lasting effects on metabolism.

Acute-phase response. The wound becomes a 'cytokine organ' whose metabolism and local healing responses are controlled by cytokines and other mediators that are produced by different cells in the wound. In severe trauma, cytokines produce a systemic 'acute-phase' response, with profound changes in protein metabolism, and immunological stimulation, effects that are mostly beneficial but in severe trauma can be lethal.

Endocrine response. This includes not only the hypothalamic–pituitary–adrenal (HPA) axis, but also growth hormone, AVP, thyroxine, insulin and glucagon, causing some metabolic effects, particularly changes in carbohydrate and fat metabolism. This response appears to protect not so much against the stress, but more against the body's acute-phase response from overreacting.

Vascular endothelial cell system response. This affects vasomotor tone and vessel permeability, so it affects perfusion, circulating volume and blood pressure and can lead to septic shock.

Sympathetic nervous system

The central and peripheral sympathetic systems are stimulated particularly by pain and hypovolaemia, and this has direct actions and indirect effects by releasing adrenaline from the adrenal medulla and noradrenaline predominately from peripheral ganglia. These catecholamines have both α and β effects on sympathetic receptors that prepare the body rapidly for fight and flight by cardiovascular, visceral and metabolic actions.

Cardiovascular effects. Blood is redistributed from the viscera and skin (α effects) to the heart, brain, and skeletal muscles (β_2 effects) and there is an increase in heart rate and contractility (β_1 effects).

Visceral effects. Non-essential visceral functions such as intestinal motility are inhibited and bladder sphincter tone is increased. Other actions are: bronchodilatation (β_2); mydriasis (α_1); uterine contraction (α_1) and relaxation (β_2); and visual field increases.

Metabolic and hormonal effects. Blood glucose rises due to increased breakdown of liver and muscle glycogen and by gluconeogenesis (α_1), and indirectly by suppression of insulin secretion (α_2) and stimulation of glucagon secretion (β). Other hormonal actions are stimulation of growth hormone (α) and renin (β_1). Lipolysis is stimulated in adipose cells, and ketogenesis is stimulated in the liver.

Acute-phase response

Local effects

Noxious stimuli such as infection, trauma, toxins, haemorrhage or malignancy, attract granulocytes and mononuclear cells to the site of injury, and these cells together with local fibroblasts and endothelial cells release cytokines. *Cytokines* are peptides produced by a variety of cells (unlike true hormones) and produce mainly paracrine (direct cell-to-cell) effects. Interleukins (IL) 1, 2 and 6, tumour necrosis factor (TNF) and the interferons are the main cytokines. Their actions help to contain tissue damage by contributing to the inflammatory reaction through vasodilatation, increased permeability of vessels, migration of neutrophils and monocytes to the wound, activation of the coagulation and complement cascades, and proliferation of endothelial cells and fibroblasts.

Systemic effects

If cytokine production is large enough, systemic effects that encourage energy conservation occur (e.g. fever, malaise, headache and musculoskeletal pains). They may also produce a leukocytosis, activation of immune function, release of ACTH and glucocorticoids, activation of clotting cascades, an increase in ESR, and a decrease in circulating levels of zinc and iron (inhibiting the growth of microorganisms requiring iron). They also affect the serum levels of *acute-phase reactants* (APRs) which are host-defence proteins synthesized in the liver; most increase (e.g. C-reactive protein, fibrinogen, complement C3, α-antichymotrypsin, caeruloplasmin and haptoglobin), but the levels of albumin and transferrin decrease.

IL-6. This is the main mediator of this altered hepatic protein synthesis.

TNF. TNF (Cachetin), released primarily from macrophages by bacterial endotoxin, causes anorexia, tachypnoea, fever and tachycardia, with proliferation of fibroblasts and widespread effects on neutrophils; it stimulates production of other cytokines, ACTH, APRs, and amino acids from skeletal muscle, hepatic amino acid uptake, and elevation of plasma triglycerides and free fatty acids. High concentrations cause multiple organ dysfunction syndrome (MODS).

IL-2. This enhances immune function by T-lymphocyte proliferation and by enhancing the activity of natural killer cells.

IL-1. In low dosage IL-1 causes fever, neutrophilia, low serum zinc levels, increased APR synthesis, anorexia, malaise, and release of ACTH, glucocorticoid and insulin; in high dose the features of MODS.

Interferons. Interferons such as γ-interferon, are glycoproteins produced by T lymphocytes which activate macrophages, enhancing both antigen presenting and processing as well as cytocidal activity. γ-Interferon is synergistic with TNF, inhibits viral replication and inhibits prostaglandin release.

Prostaglandins. These are important components of the inflammatory response. They can be produced by all nucleated cells except lymphocytes. They increase vascular permeability and cause vasodilatation and leukocyte migration.

Leucotrienes. These are 1000 times as effective as histamine at increasing postcapillary leakage, and they cause increased leukocyte adhesion, vasoconstriction and bronchoconstriction.

Kallikreins and kinins. Bradykinin release is stimulated by hypoxia and it is a potent vasodilator which increases capillary permeability, producing oedema, pain and bronchoconstriction and affects glucose metabolism.

Interactions between APRs and the endocrine response. IL-1 and IL-6 can activate the HPA axis by increasing ACTH secretion and also directly stimulates glucocorticoid release from the adrenal gland. Glucocorticoids initially help cytokines to regulate APRs, but if glucocorticoid levels remain elevated they inhibit cytokine production.

Endocrine response

The HPA axis is stimulated mainly by the injury itself, but probably its most important function is to control the effects of systemically released cytokines.

ACTH. This is released from the anterior pituitary by neurological stimuli reaching the hypothalamus, or by hormones such as AVP, angiotensin II or catecholamines. The ACTH response to stress is not inhibited by administered steroids. ACTH stimulates the adrenal cortex to release glucocorticoids and also potentiates the action of catecholamines on cardiac contractility.

Glucocorticoids. These usually have only a 'permissive' action (allowing other hormones to function), but the increased levels after trauma have important metabolic, cardiovascular and immunological actions proportional to the severity of the trauma.

Cortisol is the main glucocorticoid. Its serum level usually returns to normal 24 hours after uncomplicated major surgery, but it may remain elevated for many days in extensive burns or if infection supervenes. It stimulates the conversion of protein to glucose (catabolic action); it stimulates the storage of glucose as glycogen; it is an antagonist of insulin, and this assists gluconeogenesis to increase plasma glucose (diabetogenic action); it helps to maintain blood volume by decreasing the permeability of the vascular endothelium, enhancing vasoconstriction by catecholamines and suppressing synthesis of prostaglandins and leucotrienes (anti-inflammatory action); and it inhibits secretion of IL-1 and IL-2, antibody production and mobilization of lymphocytes (immunosuppressant action).

If the glucocorticoid response is absent (due to previous long administration of steroids or adrenalectomy) the injured person may die from hypoglycaemia, hyponatraemia or circulatory failure.

Aldosterone. The inevitable release of ACTH after trauma stimulates a short-term release of aldosterone from the adrenal cortex, but the rise may be prolonged if other stimuli such as hypovolaemia or vasomotor changes (which activates the renin–angiotensin system in the kidney) occur. A rise in plasma potassium concentration can also stimulate aldosterone release. Aldosterone causes increased reabsorption of sodium and potassium secretion in the distal convoluted tubules and collecting ducts, and hence a reduced urine volume.

Arginine vasopressin (AVP). This is released from the posterior pituitary by pain, a rise in plasma osmolality (via osmoreceptors in the hypothalamus), hypovolaemia (via baroreceptors and left atrial stretch receptors), anaesthetic agents or a rise in plasma glucose. Its actions on the distal tubules and collecting ducts in the kidney lead to increased reabsorption of solute-free water; it causes peripheral vasoconstriction, especially in the splanchnic bed; and it stimulates hepatic glycogenolysis and gluconeogenesis. Its secretion increases for about 24 hours after operation, and during this time the kidney cannot excrete 'free' water (water that is not solute led), so the urine osmolality remains higher than that of plasma. After head injury, burns or prolonged hypoxia there may be continued secretion of AVP, resulting in oliguria and hyponatraemia.

Insulin. In the ebb phase after injury, plasma insulin concentration falls because catecholamines and cortisol make the β-islet cells of the pancreas less sensitive to glucose. Glucagon also inhibits insulin release, and cortisol reduces the peripheral action of insulin; less carbohydrate is transported into cells and blood sugar rises. In the flow phase, plasma insulin rises but blood sugar remains elevated because various intracellular changes make the tissues resistant to insulin.

Glucagon. Secretion of glucagon from the α-islet cells of the pancreas increases after injury and this plays a small part in increasing blood sugar by stimulating hepatic glycogenolysis and gluconeogenesis. It also stimulates hepatic ketogenesis and lipolysis in adipose tissue. Cortisol prolongs its actions.

Thyroxine. Total T4 (but not usually free T4) and total and free T3 (the more active hormone) decrease after injury, because cortisol impairs conversion of T4 to T3.

Heat shock proteins (HSPs). These are produced

by virtually all cells in response to many stresses (not just heat), mainly via the stimulus of the HPA axis, and they are also elevated in certain tissues in chronic diseases. The ability to produce them declines with age and they appear to protect cells from the deleterious effects of stress and to inhibit synthesis of APRs.

5-Hydroxytryptamine. This is a neurotransmitter produced from tryptophan. It is found in entero-chromaffin cells of the intestine and platelets. It is released when tissue is injured. It causes vaso-constriction and bronchoconstriction, increases platelet aggregation and increases heart rate and contractility.

Histamine. This is released from mast cells, platelets, neurons and the epidermis by trauma, sepsis and hypotension. Its main action is to cause local vasodilatation and increased vascular permeability, so large concentrations may lead to hypotension. It acts on H_1 cell surface receptors to increase histamine precursor uptake and cause bronchoconstriction, and increased intestinal motility and cardiac contractility; it also acts on H_2 receptors, which inhibit histamine release and produce changes in gastric secretion, heart rate and immunological function.

Growth hormone. This is released from the anterior pituitary as a result of neurological stimulation of the hypothalamus or by a rise in circulating levels of catecholamines, ACTH, AVP, thyroxine or glucagon. Its plasma levels increase after trauma, hypovolaemia, hypoglycaemia, or a decrease in plasma fatty acids or increase in serum arginine. Its main effects are to promote protein synthesis and enhance breakdown of lipid and carbohydrate stores. It increases plasma fatty acids and ketone bodies through direct stimulation of lipolysis and potentiation of catecholamine effects on adipose tissue and by stimulation of hepatic ketogenesis. It is also associated with a fall in insulin levels, which allows plasma glucose to rise.

Endogenous opioids. Endogenous opioids such as β-endorphin increase after trauma. They produce analgesia, a rise in blood sugar, a lowering of blood pressure and effects on immune function.

Vascular endothelial cell system response

The scattered 'endothelial organ' weighs about 1.5 kg and after trauma produces short-lived substances that have primarily local actions, affecting local vasomotor tone and coagulation, but it can also produce systemic effects on the immune function by affecting platelet and lymphocyte binding. Endothelial cells such as granulocytes can produce oxygen-free radicals (OFRs) in response to ischaemia and shock. These lead to cell damage by peroxidation of cell membrane unsaturated fatty acids.

Nitric oxide (NO). This is a powerful vasodilator which is produced mainly by endothelial cells but also by macrophages, neutrophils, Kuppfer cells and renal cells. It is inactivated by haemoglobin and opposed by endothelins. Its other action is to increase the production of APRs.

Endothelins (ETs). These are a family of potent vasoconstricting peptides with mainly paracrine actions. They are released by thrombin, catecholamines, hypoxia, cytokines and endotoxins. They counteract NO and prostacyclins to maintain vasomotor tone.

Platelet-activating factor (PAF). This is released from endothelial cells by the action of TNF, IL-1, AVP and angiotensin II. When platelets come into contact with PAF they release thromboxane that causes platelet aggregation and vasoconstriction. PAF also reduces the permeability of endothelial cells to albumin and may also affect glucose metabolism.

Prostaglandins. These cause vasodilatation and reduce platelet aggregation.

Atrial natriuretic peptides (ANPs). These are potent inhibitors of aldosterone secretion and are released by atrial tissue (a specialized endothelium) in response to changes in chamber distension. They can also be released by the CNS. It is not yet clear what role they play in the response to injury.

CLINICALLY APPARENT SYSTEMIC EFFECTS OF THE RESPONSE

Hypovolaemia

Most severe injuries cause hypovolaemia, particularly if they are accompanied by blood, gastrointestinal fluid or plasma losses. The acute phase response of vasomotor changes and increased vessel permeability causes fluid loss into the 'third space', the name for a sequestered part of the extracellular fluid (ECF), which includes oedema fluid in the wound, the peritoneal cavity or the lungs. ECF may also shift into cells.

Impaired excretion of water and sodium

Trauma is rapidly followed by a rise in plasma AVP and aldosterone which cannot be suppressed by fluid replacement. During this time there is no free water clearance (so urine osmolality stays higher than plasma osmolality), with impaired excretion of water and sodium. After about 24 hours (depending on the severity of the trauma) these hormones come under normal control mechanisms, so they may stay elevated if there is continuing hypovolaemia. Therefore, a major but uncomplicated surgical operation with adequate fluid replacement is usually followed by 24 hours of impaired free water clearance and about 5 days of impaired sodium excretion. Thus the oliguria which occurs can be increased by increased fluid intake, but only at the expense of an increasing positive balance (i.e. only a proportion of the fluid given will be excreted because part of that fluid passes to the 'third space'). Retention of sodium and bicarbonate may produce a metabolic alkalosis, which impairs the delivery of oxygen to the tissues. The diuresis that occurs when this 'third-space' fluid mobilizes is a welcome sign of recovery.

Pyrexia

There is usually a 1–2°C increase in body temperature after injury, even in the absence of infection, because the increased metabolic rate is accompanied by an upward shift in the thermoregulatory set-point of the hypothalamus. Fever has some detrimental effects, but more are beneficial.

Metabolism after injury

There is an initial 'ebb' phase (Fig. 29.1) of reduced energy expenditure after injury for up to 24 hours. This changes to a catabolic 'flow' phase with increased metab-olism, negative nitrogen balance, hyperglycaemia, increased heart production, increased oxygen consumption and weight loss. The increase in metabolic rate ranges from about 10% in elective surgical operations to 50% in multiple trauma and 200% in major burns. This may last for days or weeks depending on the severity of the injury, previous health of the individual and medical intervention; it is less marked at the extremes of age or in previously malnourished individuals. Once started it cannot be stopped rapidly by controlling infection, correcting hypovolaemia or blocking pain. If recovery occurs it is followed by an anabolic phase in which weight gain is accompanied by restoration of protein and fat stores.

Lipids

Lipids are the principal source of energy following trauma. Lipolysis is produced mainly by catecholamines and increased sympathetic nervous system activity, and also by lower plasma insulin, a rise in ACTH, cortisol, glucagon, growth hormone and, probably, cytokines. Ketones are released into the circulation and are oxidized by all tissue except the blood cells and the CNS. Free fatty acids provide energy for all tissues and for hepatic gluconeogenesis.

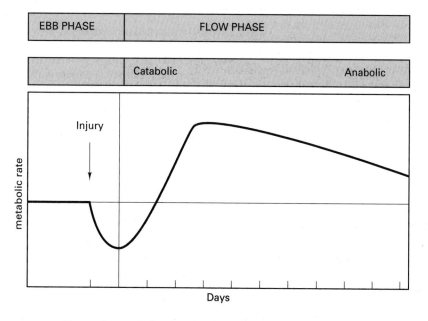

Change in metabolic rate related to preoperative level

Fig. 29.1 Change in metabolic rate relative to preoperative level.

Carbohydrates

Hyperglycaemia occurs immediately after injury, because glucose is mobilized from stored glycogen in the liver by catecholamines and glucocorticoids, and because insulin resistance of peripheral tissues impairs their uptake of glucose (the 'diabetes of injury'). This helps to maintain the volume of ECF, and therefore the circulating volume, by shifting water out of cells, and it provides energy for obligate tissues such as the CNS, leukocytes in the wound and red cells (cells not requiring insulin for glucose transport). In major injuries the inflammatory cell infiltrate can account for 70% of glucose uptake.

Body glycogen stores can only maintain blood glucose for about 24 hours. Subsequently it is maintained by gluconeogenesis, stimulated by corticosteroids and glucagon, and this is helped by the initially suppressed insulin levels encouraging the release of amino acids from muscle. Even when insulin levels rise they do not suppress this increased hepatic gluconeogenesis because it is required for the clearance of lactate and amino acids, which are not used for protein synthesis.

Amino acids

Shortly after injury, skeletal muscle protein breakdown supplies the three- to four-fold increased demand for amino acids (unless there is an exogenous protein source); this reaches a peak after 1 week, and may continue for several weeks. The nitrogen loss is proportional to the severity of the trauma, the extent of sepsis and to the muscle bulk (so it is greatest in fit young males). A loss of 40% of body protein is usually fatal because it causes the intestinal mucosa to atrophy resulting in failure of the mucosal barrier to infection; this is probably the main cause of MODS. The mobilized amino acids are used for gluconeogenesis, oxidation in the liver and other tissues, and for synthesis of APRs. Glutamine is a major energy source for the gastrointestinal tract, for lymphocytes and for fibroblasts during catabolism, and may become an 'essential' amino acid at this time. The catabolic phase is followed by an anabolic phase produced by growth hormone, androgens and 17-keto-steroids.

Albumin

Serum albumin falls after trauma because its production by the liver decreases, and its loss into damaged tissue increases due to the action of cytokines and prostaglandins on vessel permeability. The accompanying shift of fluid out of the intravascular compartment is a contributing cause of dysfunction in various organs.

Changes in plasma electrolytes

Hyponatraemia is a common occurrence after injury, partly because of the dilutional effect of retained water (due to AVP), and partly because sodium drifts into cells (impaired sodium pump). It does not indicate sodium deficiency as it occurs at a time when the total body sodium is usually elevated. Serum potassium may rise due to cell death, liberation of potassium by protein catabolism and from impaired potassium excretion.

Acid–base disturbances

The commonest change is a metabolic alkalosis because intense reabsorption of sodium in the distal tubules of the kidney is accompanied by excretion of potassium and hydrogen ions. This impairs oxygen delivery to the tissues because it affects the oxygen–haemoglobin dissociation curve. In more severe injuries, a metabolic acidosis is common due to poor tissue perfusion and anaerobic metabolism. This may decrease myocardial contractility and produce arrhythmias as well as decrease the effect of catecholamines on the myocardium and peripheral vessels.

Other blood changes

A leukocytosis occurs which appears to be due mainly to cytokine-stimulated release of neutrophils from bone marrow. An increase in C-reactive protein and fall in serum albumin are the most easily measured evidence of altered hepatic APR synthesis. Serum iron levels fall.

Wound healing

The systemic responses give 'biological priority' to wound healing, but a wound will still heal more slowly if there are other major injuries.

Immunological responses

Trauma leads to impairment of the immune system, with defects in cell-mediated immunity, antigen presentation, neutrophil and macrophage function, complement activation and bacterial opsonization. This occurs at a time when the initial injury has usually breached mechanical defences, when catabolism impairs the mucosal barrier in the bowel and when many factors contribute to produce pneumonia and other infections.

Cardiac effects

The cardiac index may rise to more than $3.5\,l\,min^{-1}\,m^{-2}$ after severe trauma, unless there is inadequate preload, previous cardiac disease or acquired cardiac dysfunction.

Pulmonary effects

Areas of lung may be underventilated if secretions obstruct bronchioles and this may lead to shunting of blood and a decreasing P_aO_2 and increasing P_aCO_2. Increased respiratory drive will lead to a respiratory alkalosis and a fall in P_aCO_2. Acute lung injury occurs when there is an increasing pulmonary vascular reaction with microemboli, endothelial changes and interstitial oedema.

Coagulation changes

Stimulation of the coagulation cascade and platelets leads to a state of hypercoagulability that may be beneficial at the site of injury but increases the risk of venous thrombi forming. If coagulation is triggered away from the wound, for example by Gram-negative bacteria or hypoxic damage to endothelial cells, then disseminated intravascular coagulation can result.

Systemic inflammatory response syndrome (SIRS)

Severe trauma can lead to this harmful overreaction of the acute-phase response that is defined by set criteria of fever, heart rate, respiration rate, arterial oxygen saturation and white cell count. Bacterial translocation through the bowel is believed to be an important event in this progression. The central problem is impaired extraction of oxygen in the tissues, and this may be due to vasoconstriction and microthrombi impairing the microcirculation, or to a metabolic blockade within individual cells.

Septic shock is a less useful term because the hypotension and perfusion abnormalities with lactic acidosis and oliguria that occur in this condition due to sepsis can also occur in conditions that are not primarily septic.

SIRS may progress to the *multiple organ dysfunction syndrome (MODS)* in which the acutely ill patient has dysfunction of one or more organs, such that intervention is needed to maintain homeostasis. Although the organ dysfunction may be primary and caused directly by the injury, it is usually secondary to progressive SIRS. Pulmonary dysfunction is pivotal in SIRS and particularly in MODS, and the shunting of blood, reduced compliance and diffuse infiltrates on X-ray are described in milder form as being 'acute lung injury' or in more severe form as 'adult respiratory distress syndrome' (ARDS), which has a 50% mortality. Liver and kidney dysfunction are the next commonest occurrences, and if three organs dysfunction the mortality reaches 90%. The majority of patients who die from burns, trauma or sepsis develop this syndrome.

WAYS OF AFFECTING THE RESPONSE

Although the local response to trauma is beneficial, the systemic response becomes less helpful as the degree of trauma increases, and in a hospital setting it is an advantage to suppress and control the response. In trauma and emergency surgery, pain, bleeding, hypoxia and anxiety have often been present for some hours before surgery starts, whereas in elective surgery it is usually possible to control these stimuli and thereby reduce the systemic response.

Reduce the stimuli that cause the response:

- Less trauma – care in handling tissues; minimally invasive surgery
- Control of infection – antibiotics; enteral feeding maintains the mucosal barrier to infection (selective gut decontamination with antibiotic combinations is still being investigated)
- Remove source of toxins – debride wounds and drain pus
- Control of pain – analgesics, local and regional blockade, given if feasible before the noxious stimuli occur
- Correct hypovolaemia – prompt replacement of fluids and electrolytes lost; transfusion for haemorrhage and colloid for plasma losses
- Correct metabolic alkalosis or metabolic acidosis
- Correct hypoxia – attention to airway, breathing; administration of oxygen
- Remove fear and stress – explanation; administer analgesics or anxiolytics.

Metabolic manipulation

Protein administration to malnourished patients improves their immune function but has no immediate benefit on wound healing. *Enteral feeding* has particular benefits over the parenteral route because it helps to maintain the gut mucosal defence barrier. Increased intake of arginine (which improves weight gain, nitrogen balance, wound healing and immune function) and glutamine (which improves nitrogen balance and prevents the redistribution of body water) can be helpful.

Maintaining ambient *body temperature* at 32°C,

especially in burns patients, may improve nitrogen balance by reducing the need for increased metabolism to replace heat losses.

Drug administration

Ways of manipulating the body's response to trauma are being sought but are still experimental. Many agents are only effective if given before the injury or sepsis occurs, and it is difficult to block deleterious responses and still preserve beneficial ones.

Steroids, antiendotoxin antibodies, anti-TNF antibodies, IL-1 receptor antagonists and specific platelet activating factor (PAF) receptor antagonists have increased survival in septic animals but have not yet shown clear advantages in humans, although some are effective if given before the injury. Other agents that have been used are adrenergic blockers (decrease the metabolic rate), aspirin (attenuates cytokine actions), growth hormone (stimulates protein synthesis), mannitol (hydroxyl radical scavenger), propanolol (improves postoperative nitrogen balance), allopurinol (inhibits free radical formation) and atrial natriuretic factor (natriuretic).

30. Wound healing

N. Woolf

The biological objectives of wound healing are two-fold:

1. To restore the integrity of epithelial surfaces should this have been lost. In this way, the underlying tissues are protected against
   (a) an abnormal environmental milieu (e.g. abnormal drying or wetting of the exposed surface)
   (b) infection
   (c) the ingress of non-living foreign material.
2. To restore the tensile strength of the subepithelial tissue.

Healing by primary and secondary 'intention'

Whatever the type of wound, the basic mechanisms involved in healing are the same, and the differences described are largely those of degree rather than of kind. However, almost by convention, the healing of cleanly incised wounds, where the edges are in close apposition, tends to be considered separately from those in which there is extensive loss of epithelium, a large subepithelial tissue defect which has to be filled in by scar tissue and where the edges cannot be brought together with sutures. These two circumstances are described in archaic terminology as being 'healing by first intention' or 'healing by second intention', these terms first appearing in a surgical treatise published in 1543, though Thomson (1813) in 'Lectures on Inflammation' gives the credit for introducing these terms to Galen.

The healing of an incised wound

Incision involves the division of:

- Epidermis
- Dermal connective tissue fibres and matrix
- Subcutaneous tissue
- Blood vessels.

Severing of blood vessels obviously leads to haemorrhage with the resulting accumulation within the tissue defect of platelets and pre-eminently among the plasma proteins, *fibrinogen* and *fibronectin*. Clotting mechanisms are activated and the former becomes converted to a clot consisting of polymerized fibrin, which is stabilized by fibronectin binding to it by means of a glutaminase bridge. 'Fibronectin' is the term used for a set of large, extracellular matrix glycoproteins, and the gel formed by fibrin and fibronectin acts in the early stages of healing as a 'glue' which helps to keep the severed edges of the tissue apposed. It has a number of other possible roles in wound healing, and indeed is one of the key substances involved in healing, but these can be best considered after the morphological events which make up the healing process have been described.

Purely as a matter of convenience, these events can be considered under two headings: those which concern the *epidermis*; and those taking place within the *dermis*.

EPIDERMAL EVENTS

Within a few hours of wounding, a single layer of epidermal cells starts to migrate from the wound edges to form a delicate covering over the raw area exposed by the loss of epidermis. This migratory process can be studied in vitro by observing the behaviour of epidermal cells when small cubes of excised skin are cultured at 37°C in appropriate nutrient media. Under these circumstances, the epidermal cells begin to spread over the five raw dermal faces, and eventually the whole cube of dermal tissue is enclosed by epidermis like a small parcel. The jargon term applied to this spreading process is *epiboly*. The idea that cell movement plays a significant part in this is supported by the fact that substances such as cytochalasin B, which are known to interfere with cell migration, inhibit epiboly.

Mechanisms involved in cell migration

Epidermal cell migration across the area of epithelial loss depends on interaction between the keratinocytes at or near the wound edges and the extracellular matrix glycoprotein fibronectin. The fibronectins are large two-chained glycoproteins which are present both within plasma and within tissues. Originally they were thought to be cell surface proteins but it is now realized that they constitute part of the extracellular matrix and exert much of their effect by providing sites which act as ligands for receptors on a wide variety of cell types. This ligand–receptor binding mediates cell-matrix adhesion. The binding sites often include the tripeptide arginine-glycine-aspartate (colloquially known as RGD sites). The receptors on cells, which serve as ligands for the RGD sequence, belong to what is known as the *integrin family* of receptors; this includes those surface molecules on phagocytic cells which mediate adhesion to the endothelial cells in the microcirculation. Differences between plasma and tissue fibronectins appear to be mediated by post-translational modifications, differences in splicing being particularly important. In relation to the epidermis in wounds, the type of splicing of fibronectin mRNA resembles that which is found in early embryogenesis. Keratinocytes from normal, *unwounded skin* do *not* possess receptors which bind to fibronectin, being tightly attached to basement membrane which contains laminin and collagen type IV. Those derived from wounds, however, express a fibronectin receptor which is very similar to a fibronectin receptor expressed on fibroblasts. As already stated, the wound is infiltrated by a gel rich in fibronectin and the activated keratinocytes preferentially adhere to the RGD sequences on the fibronectin and thus migrate across and, indeed, through this matrix.

Epithelial cell proliferation

Epidermal cell movement can provide an initial covering for very small wounds, but in most instances epithelial re-covering cannot be accomplished without proliferation of epidermal cells, the new cells being derived from the stem-cell compartment of the epidermal cell population which is made up of the basal cells just above the dermal–epidermal junction. From about 12 hours after wounding, there is a marked increase in mitotic activity in the basal cells about three to five cells from the cut edges. This is preceded by an increase in DNA synthesis of about 30% over normal, and similar cycles of increased DNA synthesis and mitosis follow. The new epidermal cells grow under the surface fibrin/fibronectin clot and for a little distance down the gap between the cut edges to form a small 'spur' of epithelium, which afterwards regresses. If the wound has been sutured, a similar downgrowth of new epidermis occurs in relation to the suture tracks and, on occasion, these may form

the basis of keratin-forming cysts within the dermis – so-called 'implantation dermoid cysts'.

DERMAL EVENTS

Within the first few hours after wounding a mild acute inflammatory reaction takes place with the usual influx of neutrophils into and around the wound (up to day 1 after wounding). This is followed by migration of macrophages into this area (1–2 days after wounding) – a key event since it is these cells that orchestrate the complex interplay of chemical signs which now takes place.

Viewed in an operational sense the objectives of this phase of the healing process are:

1. Demolition and removal of any inflammatory exudate and tissue debris.
2. Restoration of the tensile strength of the sub-epithelial connective tissue. This involves:
   (a) chemoattraction of cells which synthesize and secrete collagen and other connective tissue proteins, i.e. fibroblasts;
   (b) expansion of the existing small fibroblast population by stimulating the cells to proliferate; and
   (c) stimulation of these new fibroblasts to secrete extracellular connective tissue proteins.
3. Causing the ingrowth of new small blood vessels into the area undergoing repair; this is particularly important where there has been a substantial degree of tissue loss, leaving a large defect to be filled in with scar tissue. This involves:
   (a) budding of new endothelial cells from small intact blood vessels at the edges of the wound; and
   (b) chemoattraction of these new endothelial cells into the fibrin/fibronectin gel within the wounded area.

In a surgical wound, fibroblasts and myofibroblasts appear in the wound between 2 and 4 days after wounding, and endothelial cells follow about 1 day later. The infiltration of macrophages and fibroblast proliferation are followed, as stated above, by the ingrowth of new capillary buds which are derived from intact dermal vessels at the margins of the wound. Initially these buds consist of solid ingrowths of endothelial cells, but these soon acquire a lumen. An essential starting step for the ingrowth of new vessels is local degradation of the basement membrane of the existing capillary, this local defect permitting the budding of new endothelial cells. At this stage newly formed capillaries have little basement membrane substance and, compared with a normal capillary, are extremely leaky. This combination of a richly vascularized gel in which both inflammatory cells and collagen-producing fibroblasts are present is known as *granulation tissue*.

This name, which in biological terms is meaningless, derives from the fact that when the raw surface of a large wound is inspected it shows a granular appearance rather like that seen on the surface of a strawberry. Each of these granules contains a loop of capillaries and hence bleeds easily if traumatized.

Collagen production

The ultimate development of tensile strength in a wound depends on the production of adequate amounts of collagen and on the final orientation of that collagen. Collagen is the only protein which contains large amounts of the amino acids hydroxyproline and hyroxy-lysine. Within 24 hours of wounding, protein-bound hydroxyproline appears within the damaged area and within 2–3 days some fibrillar material may be seen, though at this time it lacks the dimensions and the typical 64 nm banding of polymerized collagen. Within a few weeks of the infliction of a surgical wound the amount of collagen in the wounded area is normal, though preoperative tensile strength is not regained for some months. This suggests that replacement and remodelling of the collagen formed early in wound healing is an important part of the whole process.

Each type of collagen (there are about ten, of which types I, II and III are the chief fibrillar collagens) consists of three peptide α chains which are wound round each other in a helical pattern. These chains are synthesized in the rough endoplasmic reticulum of the fibroblast following translation of the mRNA for each chain. They then undergo post-translational hydroxylation of their proline and lysine moieties and the hydroxylysine is then glycosylated. Linkage of the three chains is accomplished through the medium of disulphide bonds. The three chains then become twisted into a helix and the molecule passes to the Golgi zone. Assisted by the microtubules, the soluble procollagen molecules are secreted into the extracellular environment. Solubility is conferred by the presence of an extra peptide. This is removed by a peptidase, and the cleaved molecules then assemble into fibres which gain tensile strength by cross-linking. The typical periodicity of the collagen fibres is due to the assembled molecules having a staggered arrangement. On some occasions, the control mechanisms which determine an appropriate amount of new collagen for healing a given wound are faulty and excess collagen may be formed, leading to the formation of a bulky scar which stands proud of the surrounding surface. This is known as a *keloid*.

Healing of wounds associated with a large tissue defect

A large volume of tissue loss can occur in cases of severe trauma or extensive burns, or, much less frequently, in relation to certain surgical procedures. Qualitatively there are few differences between the healing of such a wound and that of an incised wound, though of course there are quantitative differences, since the formation of granulation tissue, and ultimately of scar tissue, must be on a far larger scale. One feature of the healing process in large tissue defects which is not seen in relation to healing of incised wounds is wound contraction.

Wound contraction

Two or three days after the formation of large open wounds, the area of raw tissue starts to decrease. This is the expression of a real movement of the wound margins and is quite independent of the rate at which covering by a new epithelial layer can take place. In some fur-bearing animals the raw area may decrease in size by as much as 80% in 2 weeks, and, sometimes, the degree of contraction may be so great as virtually to close the wound.

The wound contraction occurs at a time when relatively little new collagen is being formed in the dermis and subcutaneous tissue, and it therefore seems unlikely that shortening of collagen fibres at the wound margins is responsible for the contraction. Indeed, inhibition of collagen formation does not interfere with the process of wound contraction.

A currently favoured hypothesis is that the contraction is brought about by the action of cells which appear at the margins of the wound in the first few days and which, on electron microscopy, show features suggesting both fibroblast and smooth muscle differentiation. This has led to the term *myofibroblast* being applied to them. Use of appropriation antibodies shows that these cells contain actin, but no smooth-muscle-type myosin has been found within their cytoplasm. In any circumstances, for a pulling force to be exerted there must be a connection between the object being pulled and whatever is applying the force. In wound contraction the connection is provided by fibronectin molecules which form bridges between collagen fibres on the one hand and receptors on the myofibroblasts on the other. Thus strips of granulation tissue from healing wounds can be made to shorten in vitro by any pharmacological agents which cause actin fibrils to contract. It has been postulated that a similar mechanism is responsible for the contracture of dermal connective tissue seen in such conditions as Dupuytren's contracture.

GROWTH FACTORS AND CYTOKINES IN WOUND HEALING

It is clear from what has been said in the previous sections that the cellular events in wound healing must depend on a series of 'instructions' which:

- Cause the cells concerned in repair, (e.g. fibroblasts and endothelial cells, to *migrate* into the wound)
- Cause these cells, and also the epithelial cells which must cover the raw surface, to *proliferate*.

These instructions consist of a set of chemical signals derived from a number of sources. Some, which have as their principal function a mitogenic effect on the cells to which they bind, are known as growth factors. The other, chiefly derived from inflammatory cells, are known as cytokines.

Growth factors

Growth factors are peptides which may reach their specific targets via one or more of three pathways:

- The *endocrine pathway*, where the growth factors are synthesized at some considerable distance from their targets and are delivered to them via the bloodstream
- The *paracrine pathway*, where the growth factors are synthesized and released by cells which are in the close neighbourhood of their targets
- The *autocrine pathway*, in which the same cells both synthesize and use the growth factor.

Growth factors can be divided into two groups depending on the phase in the life of a stem cell during which they operate.

A *competence* growth factor is capable of moving a cell out of the G_0 phase back into cycle, while a *progression* growth factor has a mitogenic effect only on cells which are not in the G_0 phase.

Typical competence growth factors, which are likely to be involved in the healing process as well as in a number of other pathological situations such as atherogenesis, interstitial fibrosis within the lung and the formation of fibrous tissue stroma in relation to tumours, are platelet-derived growth factor and fibroblast growth factor, while the progression growth factors are represented by such molecules as insulin-like growth factors 1 and 2 (the somatomedins) and epidermal growth factor.

Platelet-derived growth factor

Platelet-derived growth factor (PDGF) is a basic protein which has a molecular weight of about 30 000. It consists of two peptides (an A chain and a B chain) which are bound by disulphide bridges. Reduction of the disulphide bridges causes the mitogenic activity of the growth factor to be lost. The B chain is the gene product of the cellular proto-oncogene c-*sis*.

The name 'platelet-derived growth factor' is somewhat misleading in two senses. Firstly, while it is certainly stored in the α granules of platelets and released from them when the platelets are activated, the growth factor is synthesized and secreted from other cells as well. These include:

- Endothelial cells
- Macrophages
- Arterial smooth muscle cells
- Cells from certain tumours.

Secondly, PDGF has a number of functions apart from its undoubted powerful, mitogenic effect. These include:

- It is chemotactic for the same cells for which it is a mitogen
- It increases intracellular synthesis of cholesterol and also increases binding of low-density lipoprotein (LDL) by increasing the number of LDL receptors expressed on the plasma membrane of the target cell
- It increases prostaglandin secretion, initially by making more of the starting material (arachidonic acid) available, and later by stimulating the synthesis of cyclo-oxygenase
- It induces changes in cell shape accompanied by a reorganization of actin filaments within the cells
- It induces increased synthesis of RNA and protein
- It is a potent vasoconstrictor.

Thus PDGF can carry out both tasks which were outlined at the beginning of this section. It can attract mesenchymal cells into the wound (with the exception of endothelial cells which do not possess the PDGF receptor) and it acts as a mitogen and stimulator of protein production.

PDGF and other growth factors bind to receptors which, after ligand–receptor interaction, act as tyrosine kinases.

The binding of PDGF to its receptor produces a conformational change in the latter which induces it to act as tyrosine kinase. The phosphorylation of tyrosine residues which follows affects at least two proteins which may have an important part to play in the signal transduction pathway triggered by tyrosine kinases.

The first of these is a novel lipid kinase which phosphorylates phosphatidylinositol at the 3-position to yield metabolites such as 1,3-phosphatidylinositol 4-phosphate and 1,3,4-phosphatidylinositol 4,5-biphosphate which have been found in cultured cells transformed by oncogenes.

The second is a cytoplasmic serine–threonine kinase which is believed to be involved in the transmission of signals from cell plasma membranes to the cytoplasm and possibly to the nucleus. This kinase is the gene product of the protooncogene c-*raf*. The c-*raf* kinase can also be activated via protein kinase-C in cells which have been rated with phorbol ester.

The transduction of the mitogenic signal from the cell membrane is followed within a few minutes by activation of the protooncogenes c-*fos* and c-*myc* and also by the activation of the genes which code for the production of the contractile protein actin and for the production of β-interferon.

Epidermal growth factor and transforming a growth factor α

Epidermal growth factor (EGF) is a 53-amino-acid polypeptide which is cleaved from a larger precursor protein. It was discovered by the Nobel laureate Cohen in the course of experiments in which he was engaged in a search for a nerve growth stimulating factor in the salivary glands of baby mice, such a factor having been discovered previously in the salivary glands of snakes. However, extracts of these glands when injected into baby mice caused their eyes to open prematurely and their incisor teeth to grow faster, these effects being due to a stimulation of epidermally derived tissues. The factor was purified and is now known as *epidermal growth factor*, though it stimulates mitogenesis in connective tissue as well as in epithelial cells. The salivary glands and, as shown recently, the lacrimal glands also, are storage sites for EGF which can be released in saliva and tears. Thus, licking one's wounds in the literal rather than in the metaphorical sense may be of definite biological advantage, as may be the irrigation of the cornea by tears in corneal abrasion or ulceration. EGF, or a molecule with considerable homology, is also produced in the Brunner's glands in the duodenum and its metabolite, urogastrone, may be measured in the urine. In rodents EGF may be found in the plasma but in humans blood-borne EGF is concentrated within platelets, for the most part in the α granules. Since EGF protein can also be found in the bone marrow in the cytoplasm of megakaryocytes, it seems almost certain that platelet EGF is derived from synthesis within the megakaryocytes rather than by uptake from the plasma.

In experimental wounds the application of EGF has been found to accelerate significantly the rate of epidermal regeneration. EGF has also been shown to have a beneficial effect on the dermal component of healing in experimental wounds, causing an increase in proliferation of dermal connective tissue and an increase in the tensile strength of incised wounds. In humans, also, topical application of EGF accelerates the healing of donor sites for skin grafts.

There is no evidence that EGF is produced by any of the cells taking part in the healing process, though, as already stated, platelets store EGF. However, there is another factor, known as *transforming growth factor α* (TGF$_a$), which shows a considerable degree of homology with EGF and which can be produced by both epidermal cells and by macrophages in healing wounds. TGF$_a$ binds to the same receptor on target cells as does EGF and has the same mitogenic effect. In this way TGF$_a$ may be a direct mediator of wound healing.

Transforming growth factor β

Transforming growth factor β (TGF$_\beta$) is a polypeptide, first discovered in culture media conditioned by transformed cells, but is produced by almost all cell lines in culture. In the presence of EGF it acts as a mitogen, but in some assays has also been found to inhibit growth. It is possible that these contradictory actions may be a reflection of the different types of assay used and may not tell us much about what is happening in vivo. There is, however, good evidence that macrophages in healing wounds express mRNA for TGF$_\beta$ as well as for TGF$_a$. TGF$_\beta$ has also been shown to be a powerful chemoattractant for monocytes and its release from the first wave of inflammatory cells migrating into the wound may act as a mechanism for recruiting additional monocytes/macrophages.

Summary

The pattern of expression of growth factors in healing wounds supports the idea that the macrophage plays a leading role in the healing process, as does some other evidence such as the observations that:

- Wound fluid stimulates cell division and promotes the ingrowth of new vessels
- Ablation of macrophages in animals slows the process of wound healing
- Macrophages in wounds also express other growth factors such as insulin-like growth factor 1.

CYTOKINES

'Cytokine' is the term used for a group of protein cell regulators which includes such members as:

- Lymphokines
- Monokines
- Interleukins
- Interferons.

Growth factors could also, with some justification, be called cytokines, and treating them as a separate class of regulator, as has been done here, is somewhat artificial, if convenient.

The four classes referred to above are low-molecular-weight proteins (usually less than 80 kDa). They tend to be produced rapidly and locally and can act in either an autocrine or a paracrine fashion. They are produced by a wide range of cells and have many overlapping actions which are mediated by their binding to high-affinity receptors on their target cells. The response of an individual cell to a given cytokine is dependent on the cell type, what other chemical signals are being received at the same time, and the local concentration of the cytokine. Two cytokines which play a significant role in wound healing are interleukin-1 (IL-1) and tumour necrosis factor α (TNF$_a$) (syn. cachectin).

IL-1 (formerly known as endogenous pyrogen) is a small (17 kDa) protein which is produced by a wide variety of cell types, those having relevance for healing being macrophages and epidermal cells. IL-1 has many biological actions, which in relation to healing include a proliferative effect on dermal fibroblasts and up-regulation of collagen synthesis by the fibroblasts. It also increases collagenase production and this may be one of the ways in which the collagen in wounds is remodelled so as to achieve maximal tensile strength.

TNF$_a$ is another monocyte/macrophage product which is released following tissue injury or infection. It is the main factor responsible for macrophage-mediated tumour cell killing and is also responsible for the wasting (cachexia) which is seen in certain chronic bacterial and parasitic infections. Its biological activity has a remarkable overlap with that of IL-1, though it does not appear to have the immunoregulatory functions of that molecule. Its receptors, however, are quite distinct from those of IL-1 and presumably the similarities in their actions indicate that they stimulate the same 'second messenger' systems. The expression of TNF$_a$ by monocytes and macrophages requires activation of these cells. This may be brought about in a number of ways, such as:

- Interacting with fibrin (which is always present in wounds)
- Binding of TGF$_\beta$
- The action of α-interferon
- The action of endotoxin.

TNF$_a$ is a potent stimulus for the ingrowth of new blood vessels in healing wounds, being not only chemotactic for endothelial cells but also being the agent responsible for the focal degradation of capillary basement membranes which precedes the migration of endothelial cells into a healing wound.

Can cell proliferation in healing occur because of *loss* of some factor which restrains cell division? – The chalone theory

The foregoing sections dealing with growth factors and cytokines presupposes a model of epithelial proliferation in which cell division is *driven* by binding of mitogenic signals to their specific receptors on fibroblasts, endothelium and epidermal cells. Another model put forward before the discovery of growth factors, suggests that the cell proliferation occurring in healing is due to the loss of some normal restraint that controls the rate of cells turnover in labile cells and, for most of the time, represses cell division in stable cells during postnatal life. The hypothesis in this model is that repression of mitosis is mediated by a group of substances which have been extracted, but never purified, from a number of cells types, of which the epidermis is one. These substances, which appear to be glycoproteins, have been called *chalones* (from the Greek: *chalinoeion* = to bridle or restrain). It is postulated that normal numbers of a given cell population are maintained as a result of the secretion of chalones from fully differentiated cells, the result being a 'damping down' of cell division in the stem cell compartment of the cell population. When, for example, epidermal cells reach the end of their natural term, become keratinized and are shed, the chalone level would fall slightly and new epidermal cells would be recruited as a result of decreased repression of stem cell division. If cell loss on a large scale were to occur (as in wounding), there would be a sudden marked drop in chalone concentration locally and a corresponding wave of mitotic activity which would persist until the original cell mass had been restored. The model is a neat and attractive one but is lacking in hard evidence. Until this is forthcoming it deserves the Scottish verdict: 'not proven'.

FACTORS WHICH MAY INTERFERE WITH WOUND HEALING

Failure to heal satisfactorily can be the result of either systemic or local factors.

Systemic factors

Nutrition

Protein. The state of nutrition of the patient is a potent factor in determining the success or failure of the healing process. There may be at least two explanations for this. Firstly, the undernourished patient shows evidence of depression of the immune system and wound infection, and the inflammatory response to this may delay healing. Secondly, a deficient protein intake may inhibit collagen formation and so inhibit the regaining of tensile strength. In this regard, sulphur-containing amino acids such as methionine seem to be particularly important, and increasing the intake of this amino acid alone can partially offset the effects of a low protein intake on wound healing.

The role of vitamin C. Vitamin C holds the most prominent place among the individual dietary factors which can affect healing. It has been known since the seventeenth century that scurvy is associated with poor healing of wounds and fractures. Indeed, there are colourful descriptions of old wounds, acquired honourably or otherwise in combat, breaking down after the onset of scurvy. While we owe our knowledge of how to avoid scurvy to the maritime founders of our once far-flung Empire, it was not until well into this century that vitamin C was discovered by Szent-Gyorgy. Once this was done it was possible to examine the effects of vitamin C deficiency on experimental wounds. Vitamin C lack was found to inhibit the secretion of collagen fibres by fibroblasts and this was due to a failure of hydroxylation of proline in the endoplasmic reticulum of the fibroblast. In addition Vitamin C concentrations in biological fluids appear to affect the production of galactosamine and hence the deposition of chondroitin sulphate in the extracellular matrix of granulation tissue.

Vitamin A. Vitamin A has important functions in relation to morphogenesis, epithelial proliferation and epithelial differentiation. Data relating to its effect in the context of wound healing are scanty but it is believed to promote the epithelial component of the process.

Zinc. A role for zinc in wound healing was discovered more or less by accident. In the course of a study on the effects of certain amino acids on wound healing, a phenylalanine analogue which had expected to impair healing instead accelerated it. Careful study of this analogue revealed that the sample used had been contaminated by zinc. Further studies showed that zinc does indeed accelerate the healing of experimental wounds. Zinc deficiency, such as is found in patients who have been on parenteral nutrition for long periods and in patients with severe burns, is associated with poor healing and this is reversed by the administration of zinc.

Steroid hormones

Many studies show that glucocorticoids have an inhibitory effect on the healing process and on the production of fibrous tissue. Indeed advantage is taken of this by administering steroids in situations where inappropriate scarring is taking place, such as in interstitial fibrosis in the lung. It is still not clear whether steroids exert their effect indirectly by damping down the inflammatory process or whether they directly affect one or more of the mechanisms which have been outlined in the foregoing sections.

Local factors

The presence of foreign bodies or infection

The presence of infection or of a foreign body will increase the intensity and prolong the duration of the inflammatory response to injury and will inhibit a satisfactory conclusion to the healing process. It is worth remembering that fragments of dead tissue, such as bone, and other elements of the patient's own tissues which have become misplaced, such as hair or keratin, act as foreign bodies.

Excess mobility

Even the least observant will have noticed that a cut across a joint, such as an interphalangeal joint, will take longer to heal than one which is not subjected to frequent movement. Excess mobility in a wound will, inevitably, increase the time taken for a wound to heal. This is of particular significance in relation to fracture healing (which is why the severed ends of the bone are immobilized) but applies in other tissues as well.

Perfusion and venous drainage

The degree of arterial perfusion and the efficacy of venous drainage play key roles in the healing of injured tissues. Where the arterial perfusion is compromised by stenosis or occlusion of the supplying vessel, a quite trivial injury may give rise to a disproportionate degree of tissue damage and healing may be delayed or even completely inhibited. Adequate venous drainage is also important, and impairment of this may play a part in the genesis of chronic ulcers, which often occur on the anterior surface of the legs in elderly patients. Histological examination of the margins of these lesions suggests that drainage is compromised by the presence of cuffs of polymerized fibrin round the venules. This can, in part, be prevented by administration of the synthetic steroid stanazolol. Suboxygenation of normally perfused tissue such as may occur in the presence of severe anaemia will also lead to defective healing.

The presence of diabetes mellitus, especially if this

is of long standing, will also impair healing. This is particularly noticeable on the soles of the feet, where quite trivial injuries may develop into very chronic, non-healing ulcers. Blood vessel disease affecting both the large muscular arteries of the lower limb (atherosclerosis and its complications) and changes in the walls of arterioles and capillaries probably makes the major contribution to failures of healing in diabetics, but these patients show increased susceptibility to infection (particularly if their diabetes is badly controlled) and may have a sensory neuropathy as well which makes them more liable to sustain injuries to their extremities.

REPAIR IN SOME SPECIALIZED TISSUES

Bone

The processes involved in the early stages of fracture healing are basically the same as those which have been described in the foregoing sections. Thus the tissue defect created by the fracture is, in the first instance, made good by well-vascularized connective tissue in a manner similar to what occurs in the healing of large open wounds.

Once this stage has passed, important new features are imposed on the basic model of healing. These are necessary because bone, unlike soft tissues, requires mechanical and weight-bearing efficiency of a high order. These needs are met through the operation of two types of specialized cell:

- The *osteoblast*, which lays down seams of uncalcified new bone (osteoid)
- The *osteoclast*, a multinucleated cell probably of macrophage lineage which resorbs bone and which, therefore, plays a key part in the remodelling of the new bone formed in the course of fracture healing.

Stages of fracture healing

1. When a bone is fractured, tearing of blood vessels takes place, *haemorrhage* results and the defect between the fractured ends of the bone becomes filled with blood clot and other plasma-derived proteins.

2. As in any other tissue, the injury elicits an *acute inflammatory reaction*, though the degree of neutrophil infiltration is mild. The combined effect of the haemorrhage and the inflammatory oedema causes loosening of the periosteum from the underlying bone ends and this results in a fusiform swelling at the fracture site.

3. Some degree of bone necrosis is almost inevitable and is due to cutting off the blood supply to some areas as a result of damage to blood vessels. It takes 24–48 hours for the first morphological evidence of bone necrosis to become apparent, the marrow being the site of the first changes. Fat necrosis is seen, and if haemopoietic marrow is involved the cells lose their nuclear staining. So far as the bony tissue itself is concerned, the extent of necrosis depends on the anatomy of the local blood supply, and some sites such as the talus, the carpal scaphoid and the head of the femur are particularly likely to show significant ischaemic necrosis after fracture. Empty lacunae, the dead osteocytes having disappeared, are a reliable indication of bone necrosis.

4. *Macrophages* now invade the fracture site and commence the process of demolition. This is followed by the formation of granulation tissue, and about four days after fracturing the bone the mass of blood clot has been replaced by granulation tissue which also extends upwards and downwards within the marrow cavity for a considerable distance from the fracture site. Within the granulation tissue small groups of cartilage cells are beginning to differentiate from connective tissue stem cells.

5. *The formation of provisional callus.* 'Provisional callus' is the term used to describe a cuff of woven bone admixed with islands of cartilage which serves to unite the severed portions of bone on their external aspect but not across the gap between the bone ends. The origin of the callus is from two sources, and the relative proportions of these vary depending on a number of factors. The first and more important is the periosteum. The cells on its inner aspects proliferate and begin to lay down woven bone (i.e. bone in which the collagenous osteoid tissue is not deposited in a lamellar or 'onion skin' fashion but in series of short bundles of parallel fibres, each bundle having a different orientation). Where the periosteum has been raised from the external surface of the bone (see above) the new woven bone fills the gap so that there are two cuffs of new bone around the periosteal aspect of the separated fragments. These cuffs then extend upwards and downwards until they meet, though there is, as yet *no* direct union across the gap between the separated bone ends. The degree of efficiency with which its external callus formation occurs depends on the adequacy or otherwise of the blood supply around the fracture site. Some of the new blood vessels are derived from the periosteum itself, while others come from the muscle and other soft tissues which abut on the fractured bone. The amount of cartilage admixed with this periosteal new bone is small in human fractures which are healing well, but tends to be greater in cases where the local blood supply is poor or where the fractured bone ends have not been properly immobilized. The second source of provisional callus is the medullary cavity where, following on the formation

of granulation tissue, fibroblasts and osteoblasts start to proliferate and lay down bone matrix. Some of this is deposited on trabeculae of dead bone while the remainder forms new trabeculae.

6. *Healing across the fracture gap.* The provisional callus, as stated above, extends round the separated ends of the fractured bone but does not bridge the actual gap *between* the separated portions of bone. Well after the provisional callus has been formed the clot which fills the gap between the fragments is invaded, first by granulation tissue capillaries and then by osteoblasts. Ossification within this gap may occur as a primary event, the osteoblasts being derived from the provisional callus. In some cases the bone ends are united by fibrous tissue and over a period of time this is replaced by woven bone. This takes far longer than direct ossification and is more likely to occur if the fracture has not been properly immobilized or if there is any other factor present which is likely to inhibit healing (i.e. infection or extensive and severe periosteal damage). Occasionally the fibrous tissue filling the gap is not replaced by bone (non-union) and weight bearing by the affected limb is not possible. In cases of delayed or non-union, some improvement may be brought about by electrical stimulation, which appears to accelerate ossification at fracture sites.

7. *Remodelling.* Once union has occurred and the patient is bearing weight, the lumpy new cortical bone gradually becomes resorbed and smoothed out and the excess medullary new bone is similarly removed, with restoration of a normal medullary cavity. Woven bone, which is quite rapidly formed and which is much less efficient at weight bearing, is resorbed completely and is replaced by lamellar bone. This is a lengthy process and restoration to normal may take up to a year.

Nervous tissue

The central nervous system

Most neurons cannot be replaced once they have been lost, though there is some evidence to suggest that a limited degree of regeneration can take place in the hypothalamic–neorohypophyseal system. In contrast to the peripheral nerves where injury is not associated with any marked tendency towards scarring, necrosis within the central nervous system elicits the proliferation of glial cells and the formation of new glial fibres which, together with the ingrowth of capillaries, may constitute a physical barrier to the regeneration of new neuronal fibres.

Peripheral nerves

When an axon is severed, the nerve cell shows chromatolysis (i.e. it swells and the Nissl granules which represent zones of the endoplasmic reticulum studded with many ribosomes disappear). The axon swells and becomes irregular, and its lipid-rich myelin sheath splits and later breaks up. The surrounding Schwann cells proliferate and accumulate some of the lipid released from the damaged myelin.

Soon new neurofibrils start to sprout from the proximal end of the severed axon and these invaginate the Schwann cells, which act as a guide or template for the new fibrils. The neurofibrils push their way down through the Schwann cells at a rate of about 1 mm per day. Eventually they may reach the appropriate end organ and their myelin sheaths are reformed as a result of the secretory activity of the Schwann cells and, in this way, a degree of functional recovery is attained. In some instances neurofibril sprouting takes place but the fibrils do not grow down existing endoneurial channels, and grow instead in a haphazard fashion. The end result may thus be a tangle of new nerve fibres embedded in a mass of scar tissue, the whole being called a traumatic or 'stump' neuroma.

Complications

31. Complications – prevention and management

J. A. R. Smith

In surgical practice no procedure is without risk. Any decision on management must balance the benefits of surgery and the risks of offering treatment against the risks and side-effects of the regimen under discussion. However, recognizing what the likely complications are allows an accurate assessment of the risk factors involved and the use of selective appropriate prophylaxis, allowing both early diagnosis and treatment of the established problem.

RISK FACTORS

Risk factors may be general, applicable to all surgical procedures or more specific to the operation and complication concerned.

Age

Any procedure at the extremes of age is more likely to be hazardous. In older age this relates more to those conditions which are found more commonly in the elderly, such as neoplastic, peripheral vascular and respiratory diseases, rather than to older age per se. The incidence of cardiovascular disease rises with age (Table 31.1). This is associated with an increased risk of postoperative myocardial infarction over the age of 50 years, the risk being 6% with a 70% mortality. In the elderly, there is an increased risk of atrial fibrillation and hypertension with a consequent risk of serious dysrhythmia and death.

Table 31.1 Risk of cardiovascular disease with age

Age (years)	Incidence of cardiovascular disease (%)
40–50	6
60–70	41
70–80	100

With increasing age there is a reduction in arterial oxygen tension, especially over 80 years. This is compounded by the increase in physiological dead space and by the decrease of lung capacity, vital capacity, maximal breathing capacity, forced expiratory volume and peak expiratory flow rate.

Renal function deteriorates with age, partly because of vascular disease, partly because of loss of nephrons and partly secondary to impaired cell function. Therefore fluid overload and acid–base and electrolyte disturbance are more common in the elderly.

The older patient is more likely to be on medication for various disorders, so that the risk of drug interaction is higher.

At the other end of the spectrum, surgery in the neonatal period is also hazardous. The margins of safety in tolerance of fluid infusion are much less, but diarrhoea is common and accurate replacement of fluid and electrolytes is difficult. There is an increased susceptibility to acid–base disturbance.

Thermoregulation is poor, so that the risk of hypothermia is considerable. Congenital abnormalities are often multiple and major. Enzyme systems are immature, so that jaundice may occur, and general and drug metabolism may be affected adversely.

The physical size of the child and the delicacy of the tissues make surgery more difficult.

Obesity

It is important to distinguish between patients who are overweight (up to 10% over their ideal body weight), those who are obese and those who are morbidly obese (greater than 40% over their ideal). Operating on any fat patient is difficult. Exposure can be limited, and the view obscured by adipose tissue. This makes accidental trauma a greater risk. Vessels are less well supported and therefore more likely to bleed and to retract, making wound haematoma more common.

Fat patients are less mobile and, by sheer weight, exert

direct pressure on calf veins while lying on the operating table, increasing the risk of venous thromboembolism.

There is an association in some obese patients with atherosclerosis and the consequences of peripheral vascular disease.

In orthopaedic practice, obesity may be associated with an increased risk of arthritis and such patients are poor candidates for joint replacement because of the extra strain placed on the artificial joint. A number of such patients are referred for dietary advice and even for vertical gastric stapling in preparation for joint replacement. However, it must be recognized that there is very little evidence that weight reduction is associated with a reduced incidence of postoperative complications.

Cardiovascular disease

The presence of any cardiovascular disorder increases the risk of serious morbidity and mortality in the postoperative period.

Myocardial infarction

Recent myocardial infarct is the most serious predisposing factor (Table 31.2). The risk is highest if surgery is performed in the first 6 months after infarction, but even after 3 years the risk is higher than in a patient of similar age without history of infarct. Furthermore, the risk of mortality from infarction is high (25–70%).

Angina

The more severe the symptoms of angina the higher the risk of cardiovascular complications in general, and infarction in particular.

Dysrhythmias

Atrial fibrillation and heart block carry the worst prognosis. The risk is reduced, but not abolished, when medical control of the dysrhythmia is achieved.

Table 31.2   Risk of myocardial infarction with time

Time since infarct	Incidence of further infarction after surgery (%)
0–6 months	55
1–2 years	22
2–3 years	6
>3 years	1
No infarct	0.66

Cardiac valve disease

Any valve disease or artificial valve is at risk of colonization with bacteria after surgery, so that even for clean surgery prophylactic antibiotics are indicated. In addition to the risk of fibrillation or atrial thrombosis, the presence of valvular disease impairs cardiovascular responses to surgery and to infused fluids.

Cardiac pacemaker

The patient with a fixed-rate pacemaker cannot produce a tachycardia and is therefore particularly vulnerable to hypovolaemia. Care is required if diathermy is used.

Arteriosclerosis

The incidence of atheroma increases with age and is associated with a similar increase in cardiovascular complications. The patient aged 50 years has a 23% incidence of atheroma and a 0.66% incidence of infarction. Over age 70 years the incidence of atheroma approaches 100%.

Hypertension

There is no clear relationship between hypertension and cardiovascular complication after abdominal surgery. In cardiac surgery there is an increased risk of myocardial infarction in the hypertensive patient. It is important to remember that in removing a phaeochromoctyoma the blood pressure can fluctuate widely, with consequent risk of a cerebrovascular accident.

Other factors

The combination of respiratory and cardiovascular disease is very serious because of the resulting arterial hypoxia. This is more likely to be found in older patients.

If renal function is impaired the risk of fluid overload is increased greatly.

Down to a haemoglobin level of 10 dl^{-1} a normal myocardium can compensate well. Below this level, or in the presence of myocardial disease, peripheral hypoxia is more likely. Subendocardial ischaemia and fibrosis may also result.

Respiratory disease

Smokers and patients with bronchiectasis and emphysema are at increased risk of respiratory complications. More common problems such as tonsillitis, bronchitis and even coryza make respiratory infection more common in the postoperative period and indicate the need to postpone elective surgery.

With advancing age there is a greater reduction in arterial oxygen tensions, the decrease being greater over age 80 years. Age also produces reductions in total lung and vital capacities, and in peak expiratory flow rate and forced expiratory volume. The physiological dead space is increased and the alveolar–arterial oxygen difference is greater. Thus any respiratory complication produces more severe hypoxaemia. In addition, it is estimated that the combination of cor pulmonale and ischaemic heart disease produces a mortality of about 50%.

Diabetes mellitus

Insulin-dependent diabetics are high-risk patients for a number of different reasons.

Metabolic factors

Maintenance of blood sugar can be difficult in the perioperative period, and even non-insulin-dependent diabetics may require insulin for a short time. The metabolic response to surgery results in hyperglycaemia, and if complications such as infection arise both hyperinsulinaemia and hyperglycaemia may coexist – so-called insulin 'resistance'.

The major danger is the development of severe ketoacidosis; this is most commonly seen in undiagnosed or poorly controlled diabetic patients.

Infection

In diabetes, polymorphonuclear phagocyte function is impaired. The incidence of peripheral vascular disease affecting both medium and small vessels is increased. Diabetic neuropathy reduces sensation to touch and pain, so that skin ulceration is more common. It is also suggested that a higher sugar level in blood and tissues encourages bacterial growth.

For all these reasons, infective complications are more common and are more likely to give rise to serious morbidity.

Wound healing

The reduced blood supply and impaired polymorph function, combined with the increased risk of infection, all contribute to impaired wound healing.

Peripheral vascular disease

There is an increased risk of atheroma affecting both medium and small arteries. If gangrene does result, infection is more common for the reasons given above, and because of the ulceration. Thus wet gangrene is more common in diabetic patients.

Renal disease

In diabetes mellitus of 20 years' duration there is a 15% incidence of glomerulosclerosis. Impaired renal function makes fluid and electrolyte balance more complex. Furthermore, diabetic patients are more sensitive to protein depletion, and are at risk of severe ketoacidosis during a surgical illness.

DRUG THERAPY

Corticosteroids

The longer the patient is on steroid therapy and the higher the dose, the greater the risk of complications.

Glucocorticoids interfere with the mobility and phagocytic activity of polymorphonuclear leukocytes, so that acute inflammation and the handling of bacteria are impaired. Thus deficient wound healing and wound infection are more common.

Ground substance is reduced and capillary fragility greater, so that wound haematoma is more common, contributing both to impaired wound healing and to infection. However, experimentally, the short-term use of methylprednisolone has not been associated with impaired healing of colonic anastomoses.

Intake of steroids in the 6 months before surgery may be associated with impaired stress response. The output of endogenous glucocorticoid is an essential part of the response to surgery and anaesthesia, and is depressed by exogenous steroid therapy. In order to avoid this complication the patient should receive 100 mg hydrocortisone intravenously at induction of anaesthesia, continued 6-hourly for 48 hours, and then reduced gradually either to zero or to the preoperative intake over the next 5–7 days.

Remember that steroid therapy may delay the diagnosis of postoperative complications or make them more likely to occur. Exacerbation of peptic ulcer disease is one example – and ulcer perforation may be masked by the anti-inflammatory effect of glucocorticoids. More contentious is the role of immunosuppressive dosage of steroids in the pathogenesis of neoplasia. There is some evidence that the incidence of head and neck tumours and the virally induced tumours may be increased in transplant patients, but this does not apply to the more common tumours of lung, breast or gastrointestinal tract.

In orthopaedic practice the patients may well be on steroids for rheumatoid arthritis. These patients have an increased risk of osteoporosis and therefore of pathological fractures. Furthermore, joint replacement in these patients is more hazardous, both because of the bone thinning and because of the general complications mentioned above.

Antibiotic therapy

The most serious complication of antibiotic therapy is anaphylaxis, closely followed by hypersensitivity. There remains a significant problem of the development of resistant strain, such as methicillin-resistant *Staphylococcus aureus* (MRSA). Therefore, use antibiotics for specific indications and for a clearly defined duration.

From the surgical point of view, pseudomembranous colitis, caused by *Clostridium difficile*, is a more urgent problem. It seems likely that exposure to antibiotics, combined with hypovolaemia or hypotension, is required for colitis to develop. Treatment with vancomycin or metronidazole intravenously is usually effective. Occasionally, total colectomy is required for resistant cases.

The aminoglycosides have potential for ototoxicity and nephrotoxicity, such that peak and trough blood levels must be monitored. Gentamicin causes ototoxicity in 3% of patients, more commonly in the elderly and in those with impaired renal function. Nephrotoxicity occurs in 2% of patients.

Cytotoxic agents

In addition to general problems such as gastrointestinal upset and hair loss, patients on cytotoxic chemotherapy who undergo surgery risk several complications.

Depression of the white cell count and function interfere with acute inflammation, increasing the incidence of wound infection and of impaired wound healing.

Reduction in cell-mediated immunity increases the risk of the development of a second neoplasm, as exemplified by a 3% incidence in patients successfully treated for primary lymphoma.

Bone marrow depression is common and, in addition to the problems of infection, especially with opportunistic organisms, there is a risk of purpuric eruption and frank bleeding.

Cyclosporin

Cyclosporin A carries the risk of depressing immune responses, but more specifically it can result in depression of renal function. Often this is a barrier to continued therapy with this agent.

BLOOD TRANSFUSION

Incompatibility

Major incompatibility reactions are now rare, even with emergency cross-matching. In patients who have had repeated transfusions, minor group incompatibility is more common. This involves, in order of importance, Kell Duffy or Kidd systems. Do not attribute all febrile reactions to incompatibility. Transfusion of pyrogens, or antibodies to white cells, are alternative explanations for a febrile reaction.

Consequences of storage

Because of the finite lifespan of red cells, lysis is an inevitable consequence of storage. Transient jaundice after massive transfusion is not of dire consequence, but the potential for hyperkalaemia is significant.

Acid citrate dextrose is the most commonly used anticoagulant. Transfused citrate may bind free calcium and result in hypocalcaemia. On storage, both platelets and clotting factors are consumed within some hours. Thus transfused stored blood cannot be relied upon to correct haemorrhagic tendencies.

The level of 2,3-diphosphoglycerate falls in stored red cells. The resulting shift of the oxyhaemoglobin dissociation curve to the left increases the affinity of haemoglobin for oxygen. Delivery of oxygen at tissue level is thereby reduced.

Stored red cells become more rigid, thus impairing capillary circulation and encouraging sludging.

Transmission of disease

In the past, both syphilis and hepatitis B were transmitted by transfusion, but this has been virtually abolished by more stringent screening. More recently, the human immunodeficiency virus (HIV) has been transfused, mainly to haemophilic patients, with disastrous consequences.

Alteration in immunity

There is clear evidence that transplantation of a kidney is less likely to result in rejection after blood transfusion. The reduction in efficacy of cell-mediated immunity has deleterious effects in the surgical management of cancer patients. It is suggested that in colon cancer perioperative transfusion results in a poorer prognosis, even when groups are matched for stage of disease, degree of operative trauma, age, sex and other factors.

Other neoplastic processes, and the relevance of blood transfusion to prognosis, are under investigation.

There is clear evidence that in colorectal surgery the use of blood transfusion is associated with an increased risk of infective complications in the postoperative period. However, more recent evidence would suggest that this risk is not identified in patients undergoing joint replacement in orthopaedic practice.

TYPE OF PATHOLOGY

Obstructive jaundice

Effect on coagulation

The coagulation factors are manufactured in the liver. Interference with liver function by back-pressure and hepatocellular damage limits the production process. In addition, fat-soluble vitamin K is not absorbed in the absence of bile salts, further interfering with the production of prothrombin.

All patients with obstructive jaundice have an increased risk of haemorrhage, which can be corrected by the systemic administration of vitamin K_1, and by the infusion of fresh frozen plasma, depending on the results of the clotting screen. The intravenous route for vitamin K_1 reduces the risk of intramuscular haematoma, but does of course require the presence of the medical practitioner or a specially trained nurse. In practice this may limit the value of this route of administration.

Effect on wound healing

Disturbance of protein metabolism is also caused by the back-pressure causing hepatocellular disruption. Standard teaching has it that this results in impaired healing of wounds and anastomoses, with a consequent increase in the incidence of wound dihiscence and incisional herniae. More recent evidence suggests that only in obstructive jaundice due to a neoplastic cause is the problem of wound failure significant. However, sufficient doubt remains for all such patients to be considered at high risk.

Effect on infective complications

It is well established that opening the common bile duct produces a three-fold increase in the incidence of wound infection relative to cholecystectomy alone. This effect is compounded by the presence of obstructive jaundice, especially when the obstruction is secondary to stones or postoperative stricture. The incidence of infected bile is at least 75%, and even with malignant obstructions incidences of 25% have been reported. The more often the bile duct is operated upon, the more likely is there to be infection secondary to infective bile in the postoperative period.

Wound infection and wound haematoma also contribute to the incidence of impaired wound healing. Infections play a significant role in the hepatorenal syndrome (see below). Because of reduced efficacy of the reticuloendothelial (Kupfer) cells in the liver, the incidence of septicaemia and endotoxinaemia is increased. Increased mortality and morbidity result from ascending cholangitis.

Effects on renal function

Following surgery for obstructive jaundice, patients are at risk from acute renal failure – 'the hepatorenal syndrome'. There are a number of theories as to aetiology.

Acute renal failure is also a complication of Gram-negative septic shock, believed to be caused by the effects of endotoxin. These include activation of complement by the alternative pathway, and inappropriate disseminated intravascular coagulation. Microthrombi in the renal parenchyma interfere with renal function, but it is likely that other toxic substances, released by the activation of complement, also interfere with renal function. It is said that at least some part of renal failure occurs because the tubules are blocked by excess bilirubin. Histological evidence of this is variable, and at best it is only a contributing factor.

The hormones responsible for maintaining fluid and electrolyte balance are metabolized in the liver, so that disturbance of hepatic function may interfere with such hormonal activity.

Because of the difficulties with haemostasis, these patients are at greater risk of hypovolaemia. Protect them by ensuring that they receive adequate fluid infusion, and a good diuresis in the perioperative period.

Effects in drug metabolism

It is generally assumed that drug metabolism is altered in the presence of obstructive jaundice. The evidence for this belief is not strong. A particular problem applies to drugs which are oxidized in the liver. In surgical practice great caution is recommended with analgesic and sedative therapy with, for example morphine-like agents. A number of cytokines have been implicated, including tumour necrosis factor, interleukin, etc.

Neoplastic diseases

Venous thromboembolism

Gynaecological patients undergoing major resection for pelvic carcinoma are at particular risk of this complication.

The association between superficial thrombophlebitis migrans and pancreatic carcinoma is well established. The incidence of deep vein thrombosis (DVT) is also higher in patients with carcinomatous disease, probably because of factors released by tumours affecting the thrombotic cascade. Furthermore, oncological procedures tend to be prolonged, with greater operative trauma, often requiring blood transfusion.

Wound healing

It is generally stated that patients with carcinoma are at higher risk of both primary wound failure (dehiscence) and later incisional herniation. This relationship has been most clearly confirmed in malignant obstructive jaundice, where malnutrition together with impaired protein metabolism in the liver combine to cause impaired healing. The whole concept of cancer cachexia is complex, but the resulting protein malnutrition is of greatest significance with regards to wound healing.

Patients with ovarian carcinoma have a high incidence of ascites with omental and peritoneal deposits. Surgery on such patients not only involves relatively rapid loss of protein-rich fluid but also the accumulation of fluid in the postoperative period is associated with abdominal distension and impaired wound healing.

MINIMALLY INVASIVE SURGERY

No field of surgical practice has escaped the introduction of minimally invasive procedures. Although most such procedures require a general anaesthetic there is evidence of more rapid recovery from surgery, earlier discharge and earlier return to normal activities. The fact that the wounds are much shorter and that tissue manipulation is less are probably important.

On the down side, the learning curve for this new form of operation can be quite long. Hand–eye coordination and the handling of tissues at a distance means that tactile sensitivity is not as great as in conventional surgery. Visual fields are limited, which is of particular importance when laser, diathermy or intracorporeal suturing are being applied. A particular problem exists when diathermy is being used and capacitance coupling may occur resulting in burn injuries at the trocar site. If laser-assisted dissection techniques are used, not only do all normal precautions for the use of lasers have to be taken but also great care must be exercised to avoid inadvertent tissue damage. Clear understanding of the characteristics of the different forms of laser used is essential.

TYPE OF SURGERY

Orthopaedic

Operations on the hips and pelvis have an increased risk of DVT. Both with extensive elective procedures and after major trauma, DVT is also more common, especially if blood transfusion is required.

Although the incidence of infection following most types of orthopaedic surgery is low, the consequence of infection (e.g. after joint replacement) is catastrophic. The combination of infection and the presence of a foreign body (i.e. a joint prosthesis) means that the chances of eradicating infection by antibiotics is minimal. Removal of the prosthesis is likely to be required.

The problem with steroid therapy in patients with rheumatoid disease has been mentioned above. In orthopaedic surgery the problem of the use of tourniquets is well established, and tourniquet time must be kept to a minimum. Of even greater importance is assessment of the vascular supply, especially to the lower limbs. Unless this is done, then the potential hazard of, for example, knee replacement, are greatly increased, and significant skin ischaemia may complicate badly planned incisions.

Gynaecology

Trauma to the pelvic veins increases the risk of iliofemoral thrombosis. Extensive oncological eradication carries all the risks relevant to cancer surgery (see above).

Thoracic/upper abdominal

Wound pain in these procedures increases the risk of respiratory complications, especially in the elderly (see above).

Prolonged operations

It has always been stated that long operations increase the risk of respiratory problems, fluid and electrolyte imbalance and DVT. However, prolonged 'keyhole' operations by the laparoscopic route have proved relatively free of complications, and it seems likely that such factors as intraoperative trauma, blood transfusion, loss of fluid and heat from exposed cavities and tissues are more important than the duration per se. The fact that minimal access surgery has been performed does not mean that complications such as DVT, wound infection and wound herniae will not occur, and it is important that these common complications are not overlooked when problems arise in patients who have been treated in this way.

COMPLICATIONS AND THEIR MANAGEMENT

Venous thromboembolism

Risk factors

- Obesity
- Age
- Malignant disease
- Length of operation
- Pelvic and hip surgery
- Past history of DVT or pulmonary embolism
- Varicose veins
- Pregnancy
- Oral contraceptive pill.

Incidence

The incidence varies with the type of operation and the risk factors mentioned. Overall it is estimated that for every 1000 operations there will be 100 DVTs, ten pulmonary emboli and one death. Pelvic and hip surgery, prolonged procedures and operations for neoplasia carry the highest risk of venous thrombosis.

Diagnosis

Early diagnosis is difficult and clinical diagnosis inaccurate. Experimentally [^{125}I]fibrinogen scanning is sensitive in detecting developing thrombi, but is of no value for established thrombosis.

Doppler ultrasound scans are increasingly valuable, but only for peripheral sites. For iliofemoral thrombosis and more proximal lesions, venography is the definitive method of diagnosis. Two-criteria isotope venography shows great promise for the future.

Prophylaxis

Because of the difficulties of diagnosis, prophylaxis is the cornerstone of management. Such risk factors as obesity, contraceptive pill, etc., should be corrected if clinically possible.

The time of maximum risk of a thrombosis developing in surgical practice is during the operation when the three factors of stasis, endothelial trauma and increased coagulability are most prevalent.

Mechanical and electrical methods of stimulating muscle function, thereby maintaining blood flow, are of value, but have been superseded by pharmacological methods.

Subcutaneous calcium heparin (5000 units), injected 2 hours before surgery and continued postoperatively 12-hourly for 5 days or until the patient is fully mobile, is effective for all but high-risk patients. Up to now, orthopaedic surgeons have used full anticoagulation with warfarin to minimize the risk of DVT in major joint replacement. The new low-molecular-fragment heparin may well replace this method and reduce the risk of perioperative haemorrhage.

Treatment

If the thrombosis can be shown to be confined to the calf and is less than 5 cm long, no anticoagulation is indicated. Analgesics and support stockings may well be helpful.

Take care when actively treating patients with a dyspeptic history or with a history of cerebrovascular accident.

Most patients require:

- Intravenous heparin, a loading dose of 10 000 units being followed by continuous intravenous infusion to prolong the activated partial thromboplastin time (APTT) by twice the control level
- Anticoagulation with warfarin for at least 3 months.

Complications

Pulmonary embolism may be fatal or multiple, producing pulmonary hypertension. Diagnosis is on the basis of a radioisotope perfusion lung scan. If surgery is contemplated, as for a major embolism in a specialist centre, pulmonary angiography should be performed if time allows. Alternatively, thrombolysis with streptokinase or urokinase may be used. The alternative is full anticoagulation, as described for DVT.

Postphlebitic limb is more likely to follow an occlusive iliofemoral thrombosis. Treatment is symptomatic with support stockings and analgesics or aimed at treating the venous ulcers which can complicate this condition, probably secondary to liposclerosis.

Respiratory complications

Respiratory complications are the most common following surgery, but because of the various risk factors involved a true incidence is difficult to establish.

Risk factors

Arterial oxygen tension falls gradually with age, especially over 80 years. Cardiovascular disease is more common. There is a reduction in vital capacity, lung capacity, peak expiratory flow rate and forced expiratory volume.

Smoking increases the risks, as do obesity, excessive sedation, immobility, pre-existing lung disease and myocardial disease; the combination of heart and lung disease is particularly dangerous.

The type of operation is important. Cardiothoracic, upper abdominal and vertical wounds all reduce expiratory movement and increase the risk of respiratory complications.

Pathology

The commonest problem after surgery is atelectasis. Small plugs of mucus block minor air passages and cause localized collapse. The plugs can usually be coughed clear by physiotherapy, but if not superinfection may result. Pulmonary embolus (see above) may also predispose to infection. Pleural effusion often complicates pulmonary pathology such as infection, infarct or metastatic disease, or may result from a subdiaphragmatic abscess or pancreatitis. It may also follow general causes such as congestive cardiac failure and hypoalbuminaemia. Pneumothorax can arise during ventilation, and may be caused by cannulation of central veins for monitoring central venous pressure or for parenteral nutrition.

Adult respiratory distress syndrome (ARDS) is the most serious pulmonary complication in surgical practice. It may complicate severe sepsis, fluid overload, chest trauma, fat emboli and inhalation pneumonitis. The cause is unclear, but contributing factors are: changes in type I and II alveolar cells, with loss of surfactant and alveolar collapse; impaired capillary to alveolar diffusion; arteriovenous shunts; the effects of endotoxin, resulting in complement activation by the alternate pathway and disseminated intravascular coagulation; and the effects of hyperoxide radicals.

It is now quite clear that a number of agents are important in producing the 'sepsis syndrome', such as tumour necrosis factor, interleukin-6 that is a V1, etc., and the identification of such agents has therapeutic implications with the development of antibodies to them.

Management

Wherever possible, correct risk factors such as weight and smoking habit before surgery. In all patients at risk,

ensure adequate analgesia without excessive sedation, and regular physiotherapy, administered not only by the therapist but also by the nursing and medical staff and indeed the patient.

Carefully monitor the pulse, respiratory rate and temperature, which all rise in patients with atelectasis and infection. Give appropriate antibiotics to patients who are pyrexial despite conservative measures, are ill, are at high risk (as in combined myocardial and pulmonary disease), or who have features of ARDS. Administer supplementary oxygen by mask. Give ventilatory support if the P_aO_2 falls below 75 mmHg.

Infective complications

Risk factors

Alimentary surgery not only has a higher incidence of infection but this is often associated with endogenous organisms. In 'clean' surgery, infection is usually secondary to exogenous agents.

The risk is increased in the presence of obesity, haematoma formation, diabetes mellitus, glucocorticoid therapy, immunosuppression, malnutrition and obstructive jaundice. Wounds may be classified as: *clean*, such as thyroid or hernia surgery; *potentially contaminated*, as in elective gastrointestinal surgery; *contaminated*, as following bowel perforation; and *dirty*, where there is faecal contamination. The incidence of infection, morbidity and mortality increases from clean to dirty, and is greater in all categories if surgery is performed as an emergency. However, it cannot be emphasized too strongly that, although the incidence of wound infection after clean procedures is low, the consequences of such infection may be catastrophic (e.g. in a joint replacement or after valvular heart replacement).

Prophylaxis

Identify the patients at risk. This refers both to those patients in whom the incidence of infection is higher and those for whom infection is particularly hazardous, such as those having joint or valve replacement, or those with cardiac valve disease. Reduce or control risk factors if possible. Ensure that your surgical technique is as perfect and as meticulous as possible. Select the appropriate antibiotic to give the greatest protection and tissue penetration, but take into account possible patient allergies and the cost involved. Give one dose intramuscularly with the premedication, or intravenously at the time of induction. Give more than one dose only if the operation is longer than 4 hours, or if there has been contamination. In this case, treatment rather than prophylaxis is indicated. Remember the value of mechanical bowel preparation.

Controversy persists about the need for and timing of shaving the operative area, the agent used for skin preparation, the value of intracavity antibiotics or antiseptics and the use of plastic drapes for wound protection. However, the use of 'danger' towels, separate knives for incising skin and deeper tissues and changing gloves after anastomoses, are now of historical interest only.

It is difficult to overemphasize that antibiotics are no substitute for gentle handling of tissues, careful haemostasis, judicious use of diathermy, and avoiding strangling tissues with ligatures and sutures.

Treatment

Wound infection. Open the wound to allow adequate drainage. Obtain pus for culture, to establish the infecting organism(s) and antibiotic sensitivity. Irrigate the wound for adequate drainage and debridement. Formally reopen and surgically debride dirty wounds. If clean wounds become infected, consider cross-infections and investigate the likely sources.

Use antibiotics only if specifically indicated (for cellulitis or septicaemia) or if the consequences of infection would be disastrous (see above).

If the wound infection is chronic, consider the possibility of specific organisms such as *Actinomyces*, a foreign body in the wound such as a suture, an associated fistula as may occur in Crohn's disease, or associated factors such as irradiation and perineal wounds. Remember the danger of synergistic infections and dermal gangrene.

Postoperative abscess. These are usually intraperitoneal but can be found deep in the wound. Localize the abscess and attempt drainage, if necessary under ultrasound or computed tomography (CT) control. Monitor resolution of the cavity radiologically if necessary. Exclude anastomotic leakage as a cause (see below).

If the patient remains toxic or the cavity fails to resolve, proceed to operative drainage and definitive treatment of any underlying cause.

Septicaemia and septic shock. The septic complications mentioned above may progress to septicaemia and septic shock in patients who are debilitated by disease or drug therapy, such as steroids or cytotoxic chemotherapy. However, some organisms may be particularly virulent from the outset.

After surgery it is vital to remain alert for all septic problems. In terms of recognizing the more serious conditions remember the danger signs, which are:

- Persistent, often swinging pyrexia with tachycardia
- Signs of toxicity – flushed warm skin, glazed eyes, tachypnoea
- Falling urinary output – less than 40 ml h^{-1}
- Hypoxaemia.

Once the condition is suspected urgent effective therapy is essential to avoid low-output septic shock with its associated high mortality (>50%). The nature of death in such patients is multiple organ failure, and while a patient may survive failure of a single organ system such as the kidneys, the more organs which fail the higher the mortality. This problem is most likely to be encountered when diagnosis and localization of a septic focus is delayed, and when inadequate initial treatment is instituted.

Principles of treatment are:

- Ensure adequate circulating blood volume using a mixture of crystalloid and colloid fluids, aiming for a central venous pressure of 10–15 cmH$_2$O in a ventilated patient
- Oxygen supplementation
- Versatile intravenous antibiotic
- Ventilatory support if the P_aO$_2$ is less than 75 mmHg
- Cardiac support with such drugs as dopamine, dobutamine, digitalis and catecholamines, as indicated
- Attention to renal function with dialysis for established renal failure
- Early recognition and treatment of any evidence of multiple organ failure.

More controversial are the methods used in some centres to ensure gastrointestinal decontamination. This involves a combination of enteral antibiotic and antiseptic agents, combined with a parenteral antibiotic, and this is gaining popularity. The value of enteral glutamine and/or α-ketoglutarate is considered vital in several intensive care units.

Anastomotic leakage

Anastomotic leakage may complicate any anastomosis, but is seen most commonly following oesophageal and colorectal surgery. In the latter group, leakage results in a three-fold increase in operative mortality.

Anastomoses below the pelvic peritoneal reflection are associated with an increased risk of leakage, both clinical and radiological. The clinical rate always underestimates the true incidence of leakage, as detected by

Table 31.3 Rates of clinially evident and radiologically detected leaks following colonic anastomoses performed above and below the pelvic peritoneal reflection

Location of anastomoses	Detected leaks (%)	
	Clinical	Radiological
Above pelvic peritoneum	1.2	18.3
Below pelvic peritoneum	16	33

gastrografin or barium enema (Table 31.3).

Predisposing factors

The general factors are similar to those which apply to wound healing in general, such as nutritional deficiencies (particularly protein, vitamin C and zinc), old age and impaired local blood flow from general conditions such as arteriosclerosis and cardiac disease.

Local factors include tension at the anastomosis and poor surgical technique with regard to preparing the bowel ends, handling of tissues, excessive use of diathermy and the insertion and ligation of sutures. Contamination of the anastomosis with liquid faeces prejudices healing, as does an inadequate vascular supply to one or both sides of the anastomosis. Less important factors are the suture materials, the number of layers employed, and whether a stapling or suturing technique is used. However, there is preliminary evidence that tumour recurrence is lower in experimental studies when stainless wire is used for the anastomosis and, in clinical work, if the anastomosis is stapled.

Presentation

Gastrointestinal contents may be identified in the wound or at a drain site. An intra-abdominal abscess or more serious septic complication may develop. There may be prolonged ileus, unexplained pyrexia or tachycardia, sudden collapse postoperatively or development of an internal fistula.

Where there is any doubt, confirmation can often be obtained from a gently performed X-ray using a contrast medium. In this regard, gastrograffin is preferable to barium since leakage of barium has much more serious contents if present free in the peritoneal cavity.

Management

Management depends on the state of the patient and the volume draining. When the volume is small (i.e. less than 500 ml per 24 hours) and the patient is well, the initial treatment should be conservative:

- Restricted oral intake
- Intravenous fluids
- Correct fluid, protein, electrolyte, acid–base and vitamin deficiencies
- Treat associated sepsis
- Institute nutritional support.

If such treatment fails to produce resolution, so that the output is high, or the patient is adversely affected by peritonitis, shock or infection, more interventional treatment is indicated:

- Adequate resuscitation
- Antibiotic cover
- Surgery.

The surgical procedure depends on the operative findings, but the principles are:

- Thorough peritoneal lavage with tetracycline and warmed saline (1 gl l^{-1})
- Identification of the leak and any associated pathology such as Crohn's disease
- Resection of the affected area (never try to insert a few extra sutures)
- Be prepared to establish a proximal stoma and a distal mucous fistula or carry out a Hartmann's type procedure of closing the distal stump
- Very occasionally, if contamination is slight, and conditions are satisfactory, an expert surgeon may elect to excise the margins and re-form the anastomosis
- As a rule, after restoring the patient's health and nutritional status, the bowel ends are trimmed and rejoined.

Problems with the wound

Failure of wound healing may result (in descending order of importance) in wound dehiscence, incisional hernia or superficial wound disruption. Wound dehiscence should now be less than 0.1%. Incisional hernia is more common but should occur in less than 10% of abdominal wounds.

Risk factors

General risk factors include:

- Respiratory disease
- Smoking
- Obesity
- Obstructive jaundice, especially secondary to malignant disease

- Nutritional deficiencies of protein, zinc and vitamin C
- Malignant disease
- Steroid therapy
- Emergency procedures.

Local risk factors include:

- Wound infections
- Impaired blood supply
- Foreign body in wound
- Irradiation to the area
- Type of wound (clean incised wounds heal better than ragged traumatic wounds)
- Site of wound (the anterior tibial area is notorious for wound breakdown and inappropriate length-to-width flap wounds heal less well)
- Poor surgical technique.

The best results are obtained by closing the abdominal wall en masse with a non-absorbable suture such as Nylon or an absorbable suture with prolonged tensile strength such as polydioxanone.

Prevention

As in all complications the cornerstone of success is to recognize risk factors, correct those which can be corrected and use an appropriate surgical technique for all wounds.

Management of superficial disruption

- Evacuate haematoma and/or pus
- Excise and remove slough
- Remove any foreign body
- Irrigate with, for example, hydrogen peroxide and povidone–iodine
- Pack gently to avoid too rapid healing over of the skin, but avoid trauma to granulation tissue
- Carefully monitor healing by secondary intention
- Use newer materials such as Kaltosler or Sorbisan.

Management of wound dehiscence

The mortality reported following abdominal wound rupture varies from 24% to 46%.

- Recognize the problem early
- Do not overlook premonitory serous discharge from the wound, a prolonged ileus or low-grade pyrexia
- Resuscitate the patient
- Re-explore the abdomen and perform adequate peritoneal lavage
- Proceed to resuture the abdomen under general anaesthetic, using an adequate length of non-absorbable suture without tension
- Use 1 cm bites about 1 cm apart
- Avoid pulling suture tightly in the tissues
- It may be helpful to decompress the small bowel in retrograde fashion to reduce intra-abdominal tension.

Recurrence is uncommon, but incisional herniation complicates approximately 25% of cases.

Management of incisional hernia

The indications for surgical intervention are obstruction, pain or increasing size. However, first spend time reducing such risk factors as obesity, smoking, constipation and prostatism, and in assessing overall prognosis. Not all patients require or want surgical repair. In elderly and high-risk patients, an abdominal support controls symptoms in the majority of cases.

If you decide to proceed to herniorrhaphy, a number of options are available. The one selected depends on the site and size of the defect, the quality of the tissues, and your preferences.

Following repair, the mortality should be less than 1% and the recurrence rate 5–10%. However, if a patient is greater than 50% over ideal body weight at the time of repair, a satisfactory result is less likely.

Hypertrophic and keloid scarring

Hypertrophic scars are limited to the wound area and do not advance after 6 months. Keloid scars are more extensive and continue to expand beyond 6 months, but fortunately are much less common.

Predisposing factors are pigmented skin, burn trauma wounds on posterior aspects, younger age groups, and a past history of keloid scarring.

Pathology. There is excessive production and contraction of fibrous tissue. The synthesis of collagen is increased but the scar contains embryonic or fetal collagen. Only in hypertrophic scars is there an increased lysis of collagen.

The main complication is joint deformity, but the cosmetic problems can be considerable in exposed sites and with younger patients.

Management. Successful treatment is difficult, and should not be contemplated until 6 months from injury. There is no treatment for hypertrophic scars, and keloid scars should not be approached until they are mature.

Re-excision with and without pressure or plastic procedures is as disappointing as radiotherapy. Greater success has been claimed for injection of steroid into the wound. The mode of action appears to be increased collagen lysis, with depression of the proliferation of fibroblasts. Injection of triamcinolone can be repeated at intervals of 1 or 2 weeks, depending on the result achieved.

Haemorrhage

Incidence

The incidence and severity of haemorrhage complications are not easy to quantify. Re-exploration of a wound to evacuate haematoma and to secure haemostasis is uncommon. Wound haematoma and local bruising are sufficiently common to make it difficult to differentiate a complication from a normal sequel of surgery.

Predisposing factors

- Obesity
- Long-term steroid therapy
- Jaundice
- Recent transfusions of stored blood
- Coagulation diseases
- Platelet deficiencies
- Anticoagulant therapy
- Older age (secondary to increased capillary fragility)
- Severe sepsis with disseminated intravascular coagulation.

Pathology

It is conventional to consider primary haemorrhage within 24 hours of surgery, which is usually a technical problem of haemostasis, and secondary haemorrhage. This usually occurs 5–10 days after operation and is due to local infection, sloughing of a clot or erosion of a ligature.

Prevention

It is vital to recognize patients at risk and to reverse risk factors whenever possible. Even patients on long-term warfarin can be 'covered' by subcutaneous or intra-venous heparin, on the basis that the latter agent can be reversed more rapidly than the warfarin.

Cooperation with a haematologist is essential in managing patients with coagulation disorders to infuse specific factors as required. Timing is vital (e.g. fresh platelets after splenectomy). Vitamin K is used to reverse the problems associated with the obstructive element of jaundice.

Control of infection is essential. Above all, make sure your surgical technique is meticulous.

Management

The need for intervention is dictated by the patient's symptoms and vital signs. Where haemorrhage is overt it is usually easier to decide whether exploration of the wound and cavity is indicated or not. When bleeding is internal reliance cannot be placed on any intracavity drain.

Check a clotting screen to assess any established and to identify any new problem. Correct any deficit appropriately with vitamin K by injection for problems with the clotting mechanism, expressed as the international normalized ratio (INR). Use specific factors for deficiencies, fresh frozen plasma, and fresh platelets as indicated by the results of the coagulation study. Do not undertake surgical exploration until any deficit has been corrected at least in part. It is unusual to identify a specific bleeding point.

The principles are:

- Evacuate the blood and clot
- Identify any bleeding point or points, and control them appropriately
- If a troublesome ooze persists, try the effect of a haemostatic agent such as Spongistan, or a collagen derivative
- If control remains difficult, pack the raw surface for 24–48 hours
- Consider leaving the superficial wound open, and give thought to the benefits of laparostomy (leaving the main wound open, packed with sterile packs) when a deeper source is suspected and recurrent bleeding is feared, as after pancreatic surgery – this facilitates re-exploration.

32. Intensive care

J. Jones

An intensive care unit (ICU) (also sometimes called an intensive therapy unit (ITU)) provides a safe environment for treating the critically ill. It is reasonable to believe (though it has never been proved), that a hospital's sickest patients, whatever the nature of their disease, will benefit from being managed in a separate area, specially equipped for their needs. It must also be cost-effective to concentrate the resources necessary for the care of the very sick into a single space. The Department of Health recommends that 1–2% of the acute beds in a hospital should be allocated to intensive care, a figure increasingly regarded by people who work in ICUs as too low.

Of all the resources an ICU must be able to command, the most important is staff. The best bedside monitor is a competent nurse, and every ICU worthy of the name should have a nurse at each bedside for all the time that the bed is occupied. There should, in addition, be a senior nurse in charge of the unit. Shortages of suitably qualified nurses, and of the money with which to pay them, limit the availability of intensive care.

There must be a doctor always on duty within the ICU and free from commitments elsewhere. He or she does not have to be an anaesthetist, but must be able to intubate patients. A consultant should be immediately available. Although 75% of ICUs in the UK are run by anaesthetists, successful intensive care requires the cooperation of specialists of many disciplines (see Intensive Care Society 1990). It is vital to the successful management of very sick patients that specialist colleagues be called in whenever necessary. Microbiologists can give immensely helpful advice on antibiotic therapy and infection control. Involve a renal physician early in the care of a patient with suspected real failure. 'Does the patient have renal failure?' is a better question than, 'How soon can you dialyse the patient?'.

The Intercollegiate Committee on Intensive Care proposes that Senior House Officers (SHOs) in medicine, surgery and anaesthetics should all spend 3 months of their training in intensive care. Some years are likely to pass before suitable training programmes can be set up and recognized. Until they are, surgical SHOs should involve themselves as heavily as possible in the management of their firm's patients when they pass through the ICU.

INDICATIONS FOR ADMISSION

It should be clear from the above that intensive care is expensive, and should be offered only to patients who really need it, and who may be expected to benefit from it. Such patients fall, in descending order of priority, into three categories, those who need:

1. *Mechanical support of a vital function.* In practice, the mechanical support most frequently employed is a ventilator. It may also be an intra-aortic balloon pump to augment cardiac output, a machine for haemofiltration or haemodialysis, or even an extracorporeal oxygenator. None of these can safely be used anywhere but in an ICU.

2. *Close monitoring.* Patients who need intensive monitoring always require the continuous attention of a specially trained nurse, and often need frequent medical interventions such as blood transfusions or infusions of drugs that improve myocardial contractility (inotropic drugs).

3. *'Heavy' nursing.* Under this heading fall patients (nearly always surgical) who need scrupulous care of skin, wounds and drains, and whose fluid balance and nutrition call for careful attention. Such patients need a great deal of nursing time, but a less sophisticated level of nursing skill than patients in the first two categories.

It is now fashionable to point out that patients in the second two categories may, perhaps, be effectively, and more cheaply, managed in a High Dependency Unit (HDU) leaving the scarce and expensive facilities of the ICU more readily available to patients with organ failure, i.e. those in the first category.

It is not reasonable to refuse admission to the ICU to

a patient simply on the grounds that he or she is old. Old people can be very resilient, and have been shown to respond to intensive care just as well as younger ones with similar disorders. Equally, it is not good practice to make the ICU a final common pathway to the mortuary. For example, patients with respiratory failure due to diffuse metastatic infiltration of the lungs should not, as a rule, be supported with artificial respiration in the hope that chemotherapy will grant them a few more months of life.

Scoring systems in intensive care

Numerous systems have been devised to try to quantify the severity of a patient's illness, of which the Acute Physiology and Chronic Health Evaluation (APACHE II) system is the the most widely used in this country. A patient's score is calculated by computer from data on a dozen physiological parameters (such as blood pressure and haemoglobin concentration) plus the Glasgow Coma Score (see p. 41), weighted by the patient's age, general health and diagnosis. The more severe the patient's illness, the higher the APACHE II score will be. Higher APACHE II scores are associated with higher mortality rates, but the APACHE II score is not an established reliable predictor of outcome in the individual case.

If consistently performed, APACHE II scores together with data on hospital mortality could be a useful tool for audit purposes. Unfortunately, there is great variation in the way ICUs collect their APACHE II data. The Intensive Care National Audit Centre (ICNARC) hopes to collect data from large numbers of (and eventually from all) ICUs in the UK in a standardized way. ICUs will then be able to compare their performance with others.

OXYGEN DELIVERY AND OXYGEN CONSUMPTION

The amount of oxygen available to the tissues is given by the equation:

$$\begin{array}{ccc} \text{Oxygen} & \text{Cardiac} & \text{Arterial} \\ \text{delivery} = & \text{output} & \times \quad \text{oxygen content} \\ Do_2 & CO & C_aO_2 \end{array}$$

Normal values (Nunn & Freeman 1964):
$$1000 \text{ ml min}^{-1} = 5000 \text{ ml min}^{-1} \times 20 \text{ ml dl}^{-1}$$

Also:
$$\begin{array}{cccc} \text{Arterial} = & \text{Hb conc.} & \times & O_2 \\ \text{oxygen} & & & \text{carried} \\ \text{content} & & & \\ C_aO_2 & Hb & & \text{ml/g Hb} \end{array}$$

Normal values at full saturation:
$$20 \text{ ml dl}^{-1} = 15 \text{ g dl}^{-1} \times 1.34 \text{ ml/g Hb}$$

An adequate supply of oxygen to the tissues thus depends on:

- Cardiac output (CO)
- Hb concentration
- percentage saturation of Hb (S_aO_2).

The volume of oxygen consumed by the tissues at rest is given by:

$$\begin{array}{ll} \text{Oxygen} & = CO \times \text{(Arterial oxygen content} \\ \text{consumption} & \quad - \text{ Mixed venous oxygen} \\ & \quad \quad \text{content)} \\ Vo_2 & = CO \times (C_aO_2 - C_vO_2) \end{array}$$

Normal values:
$$250 \text{ ml min}^{-1} = 5000 \text{ ml min}^{-1} (20 \text{ ml dl}^{-1} - 15 \text{ ml dl}^{-1})$$

In normal circumstances, therefore, oxygen delivery exceeds consumption by a comfortable margin (Table 32.1). In very sick patients, however, oxygen delivery may fall because of:

- A low cardiac output
- Anaemia
- Respiratory disorders causing the S_aO_2 to fall.

Unfortunately, especially if they have sepsis, such patients may also have a higher than normal oxygen consumption. If oxygen delivery is inadequate to supply the tissues' needs, the consequences will be:

- Lactic acidosis
- A low C_vO_2
- Organ failure.

Direct estimations of the adequacy of tissue oxygen supply are not easy to make. It is possible to measure both serum lactate and mixed venous oxygen saturation levels, but both are difficult to interpret. It has been suggested that the intracellular pH of the mucosa lining the gastrointestinal tract is a good indicator of the adequacy of the oxygen supply to the bowel. The pH of saline sampled from an intragastric balloon may mirror the pH within gastric mucosal cells, but doubt has also

Table 32.1   Blood gas analysis: normal values

pH	7.35–7.45
PaO$_2$	75–100 mmHg, 10–13.3 kPa (see text)
PaCO$_2$	36–44 mmHg, 4.8–6.0 kPa
SaO$_2$	95–100%
Base deficit	± 2.5
HCO$_3^-$	22–26 mM l^{-1}

Table 32.2

	HR	BP	CO	Extremities	CVP
Hypovolaemic		↓	↓	Cold	↓
Cardiogenic	↑	↓	↓	Cold	↑
Anaphylactic	↑	↓	↓	Rash sometimes warm at first	↓
Septic	↑	↓	↑ at first Then ↓	Warm at first Cold later	↓

been expressed as to the usefulness of such measurements.

It is, therefore, crucial in intensive care:

- To monitor and support the cardiovascular and respiratory systems in order to maintain a satisfactory, or even supranormal, tissue oxygen supply
- To monitor and support the function of the vital organs which demand adequate perfusion with oxygenated blood.

SHOCK

Shock can be defined as inadequate tissue perfusion due to acute circulatory failure. It may be classified as hypovolaemic, cardiogenic, anaphylactic or septic (see Table 32.2). Oxygen delivery to the tissues is always reduced, sometimes critically.

1. *Hypovolaemic shock.* Hypovolaemic shock is due to a reduction in the circulating volume, after haemorrhage, plasma loss (as in burns) or loss of water and electrolytes (e.g. intestinal obstruction, diabetic ketoacidosis and Addisonian crisis). The venous return to the heart is reduced, and the cardiac output and blood pressure fall. Tachycardia and peripheral vasoconstriction, reflexly mediated by the baroceptors, partially compensate for the hypotension. Splanchnic vasoconstriction, and underperfusion of the gut, may be associated with an increased permeability of the intestinal mucosa to bacteria or endotoxin. Hypovolaemia may thus be a precursor of sepsis.

2. *Cardiogenic shock.* In cardiogenic shock, the primary defect is a fall in cardiac output. Causes include myocardial infarction and cardiac compression (tamponade. In the elderly, impaired myocardial perfusion secondary to hypovolaemia may cause acute cardiac failure. Hypotension, tachycardia and vasoconstriction are again seen, but the cardiac filling pressure (central venous pressure (CVP)) will be raised because the heart is unable to eject all the blood that is returned to it.

3. *Anaphylactic shock.* The clinical features of anaphylactic shock are those of acute histamine release. This is often secondary to the administration of drugs to which the patient is sensitive, of plasma substitutes or of contrast medium. Profound vasodilatation causes hypotension with a fall in venous return and cardiac output. Urticarial rashes, bronchospasm and spasm of the gut also occur. There is an increase in capillary permeability, which may add an element of hypovolaemia.

4. *Septic shock.* Septic shock is due to overwhelming infection. The clinical features, which may be caused by the release of a variety of vasoactive substances such as bacterial endotoxin, are at first vasodilatation, opening of arteriovenous shunts and increased capillary permeability. The extremities are initially warm, and the cardiac output high. Later, loss of fluid from the circulation brings about the signs of hypovolaemia. Impaired organ function due to inadequate perfusion and oxygen delivery may occur in all forms of shock, but multiple organ failure, with the development of coagulopathy and the adult respiratory distress syndrome (ARDS), is a particular feature of continued sepsis.

The treatment of all forms of shock is, in part, supportive, and careful monitoring of the patient (see below) is essential if support is to be appropriate. Support must be promptly given if organ failure is not to supervene. However, support is not all-important. Prompt treatment of the cause of shock may be crucial to the patient's survival. There is no point in relying simply on massive blood transfusion, attentively monitored, in a patient whose hypovolaemia is due to a ruptured ectopic pregnancy or to a leaking aortic aneurysm. Similarly, supportive treatment will not cure a patient with septic shock due to a ruptured bowel or to an empyema. Early surgery, after initial resuscitation, is the best treatment for patients of this sort.

CARDIAC SUPPORT

Monitoring the cardiovascular system

The measurement of cardiac output (CO) is an invasive procedure and, fortunately, is not essential in every patient in the ICU. Estimates of the adequacy of cardiac output can be made by monitoring other variables which are easier to measure. These include:

- The electrocardiogram (ECG)
- The blood pressure (BP)
- The core–peripheral temperature gradient
- The central venous pressure (CVP).

In addition, estimates of the adequacy of tissue perfusion can be made from simple clinical observations. A patient who is alert and passing urine must be supplying his brain and kidneys with enough oxygenated blood for them to function.

ECG

Since:

$$CO = Heart\ rate \times Stroke\ volume$$

continuous monitoring of the ECG provides reliable information of one determinant of the CO. The ECG will also demonstrate any arrhythmias; depression or elevation of the ST segments may be a warning of inadequate myocardial oxygenation.

Blood pressure

The blood pressure may be measured intermittently using a cuff or displayed continuously on a monitor after arterial (usually radial) cannulation. Since:

$$BP = \frac{CO}{Systemic\ vascular\ resistance\ (SVR)}$$

the blood pressure is often a reliable guide to the adequacy of the cardiac output. However, in the presence of vasoconstriction, which may be secondary to inadequate filling of the circulation or to primary cardiac failure, a normal blood pressure can be associated with a low cardiac output. Further information on the state of the circulation can be obtained from the peripheral temperature.

Peripheral temperature

The core (rectal or oesophageal)–peripheral temperature gradient has been shown to be a reliable guide to the cardiac output (Joly & Weil 1969). Clearly, a patient with warm, pink feet cannot be vasoconstricted.

Central venous pressure

Clinical estimation of the jugular venous pressure is made by observing the level of the external jugular veins above the angle of Louis in a patient propped up to 45°. Can-

nulation of a central vein (usually the subclavian or internal jugular) enables the CVP to be measured, either intermittently using a water manometer or continuously using a transducer. Zero is taken from the level at which the right atrium is presumed to be (the midaxillary line if the patient is lying flat). Because the zero level is somewhat arbitrary, and, in any event, alters when the patient moves to a different position, single measurements of the CVP are not very helpful. However, a low CVP (normal range 5–10 mmHg) which rises only transiently on the rapid administration of 200 ml intravenous fluid is strongly suggestive of an empty circulation. A persistently elevated CVP with a normal venous waveform (i.e. the high value is not due to a blocked cannula) in the presence of peripheral vasoconstriction suggests myocardial failure (Sykes 1963) (Fig. 32.1).

Measurement of CVP is an invasive procedure. The complications are:

- Pneumothorax
- Accidental arterial puncture causing haematoma or haemothorax
- Misplacement (check the position of the catheter with a chest X-ray)
- Air embolism if the catheter is opened to the atmosphere with the patient sitting up
- Infection – especially if the catheter is handled frequently or left in for too long.

If we monitor all the variables above, then in many patients we will be able to infer:

- Whether or not the cardiac output is adequate.
- Whether a low cardiac output is due to
  (a) insufficient filling of the circulation, or
  (b) impaired myocardial function.

Furthermore, we will be guided as to whether matters may be improved by infusing intravenous fluids, or using drugs to improve cardiac performance. Finally, we will be able to follow the results of whatever therapy we institute. In only a few patients will it be necessary to monitor any further variables.

Pulmonary artery catheterization

The CVP is a reliable indicator of cardiac filling (or preload) if both right and left ventricles are functioning similarly. Although the right and left ventricles function similarly in most patients, there are circumstances in which the performance of one may be impaired while the other continues to work normally.

The left ventricle is usually the one afflicted by ischaemic heart disease, with or without myocardial infarction. Left ventricular ischaemia, especially in the elderly, may

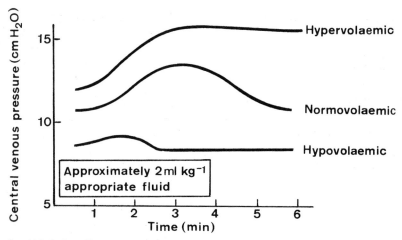

Fig. 32.1 Effect of rapid infusion of intravenous fluid on central venous pressure (Sykes 1963).

follow hypovolaemic or septic shock. Some cardiac valvular lesions and cardiomyopathies affect solely or predominantly the left ventricle. Right ventricular performance may be impaired in the presence of normal left ventricular function in pulmonary hypertension of any cause. In all these circumstances, it is desirable to measure the left atrial pressure as well as the right. It is also useful, in some patients with hypoxaemia and diffuse pulmonary shadowing, to monitor the left atrial pressure to ascertain whether the underlying cause is left ventricular failure or primary pulmonary disease, such as ARDS.

The least invasive way to measure left atrial pressure is to float a balloon-tipped catheter (often known as a Swan–Ganz catheter) into the pulmonary artery through an introducer placed in a central vein. The catheter is advanced until, with the balloon inflated, it 'wedges' in a branch of the pulmonary artery. The pressure at this point, the pulmonary capillary wedge pressure (PCWP), corresponds in most circumstances to the left atrial pressure. Deflation of the balloon reveals a pulmonary artery pressure tracing.

Pulmonary artery catheterization carries the risks of central venous catheterization, as listed above, and, in addition, those of:

- Dysrhythmia during passage
- Knotting and misplacement
- Trauma to cardiac valves
- Pulmonary infarction if the balloon is kept inflated all the time
- Pulmonary artery rupture
- Problems with the balloon:
  (a) rupture,
  (b) leakage,

  (c) embolism
- Thrombosis and embolism of the catheter.

The septic complications of pulmonary artery catheterization include bacterial endocarditis, and it is recommended that, to minimize this risk, the catheter should be withdrawn after 72 hours.

Measurement of the cardiac output

Once a pulmonary artery catheter is correctly placed, it is possible to measure the cardiac output. If the catheter incorporates a thermistor, the method of thermal dilution may be employed. This is the method most commonly employed in ICUs. (Other methods employ the Fick principle or indicator dilution.)

Cardiac output computers are often programmed to calculate additional physiological variables. For example, if the cardiac output and blood pressure are measured, the systemic vascular resistance (SVR) can be calculated. Such more sophisticated information is extremely useful in patients with complicated disorders. For instance, the circulatory derangements in patients with trauma and sepsis may combine hypovolaemia with cardiac dysfunction; these patients may also have respiratory problems which further reduce oxygen delivery. The more information we have about cardiac performance, the better we shall be able to choose drugs which may improve it.

Improving cardiac performance

General measures

1. Ensure that an optimal degree of cardiac filling has been achieved.

2. Correct any coexisiting abnormalities such as hypoxaemia (see respiratory support), acidosis (lactic acidosis occurs if oxygen delivery is impaired), hyper- or hypokalaemia and hypocalcaemia.

3. Correct any dysrhythmias. (Apart from specific antidysrhythmic drugs, atropine raises the cardiac output in sinus brachycardia.)

Drugs which increase cardiac output

Sympathomimetic drugs. These agents act on α- or β-adrenergic receptors or both (see Table 32.3). Dopamine in low doses improves renal perfusion through a direct effect on dopaminergic receptors (see section on Renal support). All these agents can increase cardiac output at the cost of increased myocardial oxygen consumption. The α-agonists cause vaso-constriction, which may be of benefit in septic shock when SVR may be very low, but which increases cardiac work.

Vasodilators. (Examples, nitroglycerine, sodium nitroprusside.) These drugs bring about a fall in SVR, and reduce the work and oxygen consumption of the heart. Some of them act predominantly on the capacitance vessels and reduce CVP (or preload), which may improve the performance of the failing heart. Because the use of vasodilators is associated with a fall in BP, patients receiving these drugs must be closely monitored.

Phosphodiesterase inhibitors. (Examples: enoximone, milrinone.) Drugs in this recently introduced category increase cardiac output and reduce SVR. Unlike β-adrenergic agonists, they do not cause tachycardia or a rise in myocardial oxygen consumption. They would appear to be most useful in cardiac dysfunction associated with peripheral vasoconstriction.

RESPIRATORY SUPPORT

Arterial oxygen saturation (S_aO_2)

To recapitulate the equations given earlier (p. 316), oxygen delivery to the tissues depends on:

- Cardiac output (discussed in cardiac support)
- Haemoglobin concentration
- S_aO_2.

S_aO_2 is related to arterial oxygen tension (P_aO_2), as shown by the oxygen dissociation curve (Fig. 32.2).
Note that:

- The normal P_aO_2 in a healthy young person at sea level is 100 mmHg (13.3 kPa), and corresponds to an S_aO_2 of almost 100%.
- The pO_2 of mixed venous blood (p_vO_2) is 40 mmHg (5.3 kPa), which is associated with an S_aO_2 of 70%.
- The normal P_aO_2 falls with advancing age. The normal P_aO_2 for an 80-year-old is 60 mmHg.
- At a P_aO_2 of 60 mmHg, Hb is 90% saturated.

Measurement of arterial oxygen saturation

S_aO_2 may be continually and non-invasively monitored using a pulse oximeter. A sensing probe is attached to a finger or earlobe and the pulse rate and S_aO_2 are digitally displayed. The device is generally reliable, although it may fail in the presence of intensive peripheral vasoconstriction, and can give inaccurate figures for S_aO_2 if the patient has methaemoglobinaemia or jaundice. The pulse oximeter is an excellent simple guide to the adequacy of tissue oxygenation. If a patient has a peripheral pulse which can be sensed and an S_aO_2 of 90% or more, he must be perfusing at least his finger or earlobe with oxygenated blood.

Table 32.3   Properties of some sympathetic amines

	α-Receptors (agonists $\rightarrow$ vasoconstriction rise in B P)	β-Receptors (agonists $\rightarrow$ tachycardia, improved contractility, vasodilatation)	Other receptors
Adrenaline	α-agonist at high doses	β-effects predominate at low doses	
Noradrenaline	α-agonist	Some β_1 effects	
Isoprenaline		β-Agonist	
Salbutamol		β_2-Agonist	
Dopamine	Resembles noradrenaline at high doses		Agonist at dopaminergic receptors $\rightarrow$ enhanced renal perfusion at low doses
Dobutamine	Closely resembles dopamine; believed by some to cause less tachycardia and to be a more effective inotrope		

Table 32.4 Causes of respiratory failure

Ventilatory failure (PaCO$_2$ ↑ ; PaO$_2$ ↓)
  Deranged mechanics
    Obstructive airways disease
    Chest wall lesions
      Kyphocoliosis
      Chest trauma—flail chest
  Deranged control
    Depression of the respiratory centre
      Drugs
      Trauma
      Increased intracranial pressure
    Spinal cord lesions
      Trauma above C3.4
      Motor neurone disease; poliomyelitis
  Peripheral neuropathy
  Neuromuscular lesions
    Myasthenia gravis
    Botulism
    Relaxants
Hypoxaemic failure (PaO$_2$ ↓ ; PaCO$_2$ ↓ or normal)
  Collapse
  Consolidation
  Contusion
  Oedema
    LVF
    ARDS
  Pulmonary emboli

Arterial blood gas analysis

Most machines measure the pH, pO_2 and pCO_2 of a sample of blood directly, and will derive values for variables such as bicarbonate and base excess. It is essential to obtain a sample of arterial blood if P_aO_2 is to be estimated, but an 'arterialized' capillary specimen from the back of the hand will give a reasonable idea of the arterial pH and P_aCO_2. Normal values are shown in Table 32.1.

Blood gas analysis thus yields information on:

- Whether or not the patient is hypoxaemic
- Whether the patient is underventilating (P_aCO_2 elevated) or overventilating (P_aCO_2 low) their alveoli
- Whether the patient is acidotic or alkalotic, and whether the acid–base disturbance is respiratory or metabolic.

End-tidal carbon dioxide analysis

At the beginning of expiration, gas from the respiratory dead space leaves the airways first, with alveolar gas emerging at the end. Continuous monitoring of the expired carbon dioxide concentration (using infrared absorption) will therefore display a peak concentration of carbon dioxide at the end of each expiration. Since alveolar and arterial carbon dioxide tensions are closely matched, measurement of end-tidal carbon dioxide tension provides a guide to P_aCO_2. Like pulse oximetry, end-tidal carbon dioxide analysis is a continuous and (in a patient connected to a breathing system) non-invasive method of assessment of respiratory function. An end-tidal carbon dioxide analyser is also a good warning of disconnection from a ventilator.

Hypoxaemia (low P_aO_2)

General causes

- Low inspired oxygen tension:
  - (a) high altitude
  - (b) negligent anaesthesia
- Hypoventilation – (see Ventilatory failure, Table 32.4)
- 'Shunting' of venous blood into the arterial system:
  - (a) pulmonary disease causing venous admixture (see Hypoxaemic failure, Table 32.4)
  - (b) low cardiac output
  - (c) congenital cyanotic heart disease with right-to-left shunts.

In most patients, hypoxaemia has a respiratory cause.

Hypoxaemia in the postoperative period

Immediately after surgery, a patient is liable to underventilate because of pain, or because of the residual effects of drugs used in anaesthesia (especially opiates and muscle relaxants). For reasons not fully understood, general anaesthesia causes a degree of venous admixture (ventilation/perfusion mismatch). If the patient's temperature has been allowed to fall during the operation, he will start shivering as he wakes up and will consume an excess of oxygen.

If satisfactory pain relief is not achieved the patient will not breathe or cough properly, nor will he cooperate with physiotherapy. Retained respiratory secretions, pulmonary collapse and infection may follow. Obviously, the patient's prospects are worse if surgery has been major or if he has pre-existing chest disease, usually due to smoking. It has been explained elsewhere that poisoning the patient with large doses of opiates in the hope of providing pain relief will, in its turn, produce respiratory depression. More sophisticated analgesic techniques have complications of their own.

It may be helpful to admit a patient who is at high risk of chest complications to the ICU for a night or two after his operation. The ICU staff can provide the close supervision that a patient with, say, an epidural infusion requires. They can also monitor his S_aO_2 and P_aO_2, and maintain his oxygenation with controlled oxygen

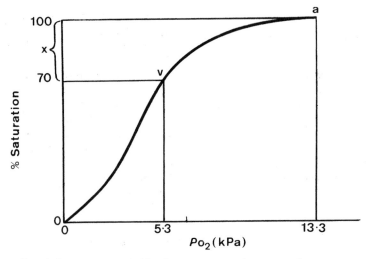

Fig. 32.2   The oxygen dissociation curve: a = arterial point; v = venous point; x = arteriovenous oxygen content difference.

therapy. Chest physiotherapy always seems to be better performed in the ICU, possibly because the nursing staff here have a good understanding of it. It must be more economical to keep a patient for a short, elective period in the ICU than to admit him as an emergency with respiratory failure due to pneumonia a few days later and to ventilate him artificially for (perhaps) weeks.

Artificial ventilation (intermittent positive pressure respiration (IPPR))

Indications

- Respiratory failure, which may be ventilatory or hypoxaemic
- Cerebral oedema
- Prophylaxis.

Respiratory failure. A detailed list of the causes of both types of respiratory failure is given in Table 32.4.

Ventilatory failure is the consequence of inadequate movement of gas in and out of the lungs. Failure to excrete carbon dioxide causes the P_aCO_2 to rise (hypercarbia), and the P_aO_2 falls proportionately. The physical signs of hypercarbia are tachycardia, hypertension and vasodilatation in the cutaneous and cerebral circulations. The resultant rise in intracranial pressure may cause headache, confusion and papilloedema. Ventilatory failure is usually due to deranged respiratory mechanics or to disordered respiratory control (see Table 32.4). Excessive carbon dioxide production due to intravenous feeding has also been incriminated (Ashkenazi et al 1982).

Hypoxaemic failure occurs when large quantities of venous blood pass through the pulmonary circulation without participating in gas exchange, i.e. when non-ventilated or underventilated alveoli remain perfused. Ventilation/perfusion mismatch of a minor degree is normal; severe derangements occur if large numbers of alveoli are collapsed, or are filled with blood, pus or fluid instead of gas (see Table 32.4). The P_aCO_2 does not rise in hypoxaemic failure; overventilation of the remaining functional alveoli keeps it at a normal level. If the P_aO_2 falls below 60 mmHg, hypoxaemia reflexly stimulates the respiratory centre, and the P_aCO_2 will fall below 40 mmHg. The physical signs of hypoxaemia are cyanosis and confusion.

Cerebral oedema. If the intracranial pressure is raised, hyperventilation can bring about a temporary fall in cerebral blood flow and in intracranial pressure. Artificial ventilation is also indicated in patients with cerebral oedema to prevent hypoxaemia or hypercarbia, both of which may cause the intracranial pressure to rise even further.

Prophylaxis. In a number of patients, respiratory failure may fairly confidently be predicted, and elective ventilation will prevent the development of dangerous hypoxaemia and/or hypercarbia. It has already been mentioned that some postoperative patients may benefit from a period of respiratory monitoring in the ICU. In others, usually those in whom the cardiac output, haemoglobin concentration and S_aO_2 may all be erratic, artificial ventilation may be continued after surgery until the patient's condition has stabilized. Cardiac and major vascular surgery almost invariably demand a period of elective postoperative artificial ventilation.

Benefits of artificial ventilation

In all the circumstances mentioned above, artificial ventilation will ensure:

- The elimination of carbon dioxide
- Improved oxygenation by:
  (a) reducing respiratory work and oxygen consumption by the respiratory muscles
  (b) enabling very high inspired concentrations of oxygen to be administered
  (c) recruiting collapsed or oedematous alveoli (especially if positive end-expiratory pressure is employed) in hypoxaemic respiratory failure.

Management of artificial ventilation

1. Establish an artificial airway with

- Endotrachial tube (oral or nasal)
- Tracheostomy.

This must subsequently be properly cared for. The inspired gases must be humidified to prevent drying of respiratory secretions, and great care must be taken not to introduce infection.

2. Suppress the patient's drive to spontaneous respiration:
(a) Unless the patient is comatose or weak, it will probably be necessary to use drugs for the purpose, initially at least:

  Opiates – provide analgesia as well as depression of the respiratory centre, and are the first choice for most surgical patients
  Benzodiazepines – reduce anxiety and cause amnesia
  Muscle relaxants – are inhumane in the conscious patient, and particularly hazardous if the patient is accidentally detached from the ventilator. Their place is extremely limited.
(b) Once artificial ventilation is established, a moderate degree of hypocarbia or the choice of a mode of artificial ventilation which permits some spontaneous respiratory effects (e.g. synchronized intermittent mandatory ventilation (SIMV) may keep the patient 'settled' on the ventilator with minimal sedation).

3. Monitor the patient and the machine.

Hazards of artificial ventilation

- Complications of the artificial airway:
  (a) trauma from the endotracheal or tracheostomy tube
  (b) obstruction due to inspissated secretions
  (c) misplacement
- Accidental disconnection of the patient from the ventilator
- Barotrauma from positive pressure to the respiratory tract:
  (a) pneumothorax
  (b) surgical emphysema
- Circulatory embarrassment – positive intrathoracic pressure may impede venous return to the heart
- Acute gastric dilatation
- Sodium and water retention
- Introduction of microorganisms into the respiratory tract.

Weaning from artificial ventilation

It may not be possible to wean a patient from his ventilator until he has recovered from the condition which brought him to it. This is a very simple point, but is constantly forgotten or ignored. For example, a patient with hypoxaemic respiratory failure due to a chest infection should be apyrexial, with clear sputum, resolution of the physical signs in the chest, a falling white cell count and some radiological improvement. It is not enough to demonstrate that the blood gases conform more closely to the ideal since IPPR was instituted. The longer the patient has been artificially ventilated, the more protracted the weaning process will be. Malnutrition, especially if associated with hypophosphataemia (Aubier et al 1985) can make weaning difficult.

A patient may be weaned by separating him from his ventilator for short periods of spontaneous respiration, which are gradually extended. Alternatively, the gradual and progressive reduction of support using a technique such as SIMV may be tried.

Extubation can be considered when the patient has demonstrated:

- A capacity to breathe spontaneously for an indefinite period.
- An ability to cough effectively.

The longer the time of weaning has been, the longer the tube will have to be left in place after weaning is over.

RENAL SUPPORT

Renal failure is a frequent occurrence in ICUs. An episode of hypotension, of any cause, may result in renal hypoperfusion and failure. Patients with sepsis may develop multiple organ failure, coagulopathy and ARDS, and in this group renal failure is often a terminal event. Generally, however, acute renal failure (acute tubular necrosis) is reversible, and the patient will recover if he is supported through his illness.

A patient who develops acute tubular necrosis will come to no immediate harm if his renal failure is diagnosed and promptly treated. Acute renal failure usually presents as oliguria, and it is crucial not to confuse it with oliguria due to some other cause. In a surgical patient in the ICU, the other causes of oliguria are:

- Obstruction to the flow of urine, most commonly due to a partially blocked catheter (N.B.: there are only two causes of anuria: renal cortical necrosis, which is irreversible, and a completely blocked catheter, which can be changed at once)
- Sodium and water retention occurring:
    (a) as part of the 'stress response' to surgery
    (b) in response to an episode of renal hypoperfusion, past or present
    (c) in response to an inadequate fluid intake.

Figure 32.3 outlines the immediate management of a surgical patient with oliguria. Having once excluded obstruction and hypovolaemia, the urine osmolality should be measured. An osmolality close to that of plasma (280–320 mOsm l^{-1}) is suggestive of renal failure, and the patient should, until the skilled advice of a specialist in renal medicine has been obtained, be treated as if the diagnosis were certain. There is little to do except:

- Infuse dopamine at 3 $\mu g\,kg^{-1}\,min^{-1}$ to improve renal perfusion.
- Restrict the basic fluid intake to 20 ml h^{-1} plus the previous hour's output
- Watch the serum potassium, checking the level 4-hourly. If it is above 6 mm l^{-1} it may be controlled, for some hours at least, with 50% glucose (50 ml boluses or 20 ml h^{-1}) with soluble insulin (1 unit for each 2–4 g glucose)
- Check blood gas measurements 4–6 hourly, to see if metabolic acidosis develops
- Measure and keep all the urine which is passed for 24 hours. Send 24-hourly aliquots for electrolyte and creatinine estimations. The serum creatinine level must be measured daily.

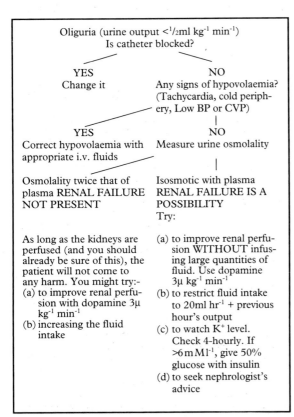

Oliguria (urine output $<\frac{1}{2}$ml kg^{-1} min^{-1})
Is catheter blocked?

YES — Change it

NO — Any signs of hypovolaemia? (Tachycardia, cold periphery, Low BP or CVP)

YES — Correct hypovolaemia with appropriate i.v. fluids

NO — Measure urine osmolality

Osmolality twice that of plasma RENAL FAILURE NOT PRESENT

Isosmotic with plasma RENAL FAILURE IS A POSSIBILITY
Try:

As long as the kidneys are perfused (and you should already be sure of this), the patient will not come to any harm. You might try:-
(a) to improve renal perfusion with dopamine 3μ kg^{-1} min^{-1}
(b) increasing the fluid intake

(a) to improve renal perfusion WITHOUT infusing large quantities of fluid. Use dopamine 3μ kg^{-1} min^{-1}
(b) to restrict fluid intake to 20ml hr^{-1} + previous hour's output
(c) to watch K$^+$ level. Check 4-hourly. If >6 m Ml^{-1}, give 50% glucose with insulin
(d) to seek nephrologist's advice

Fig 32.3 First-aid management of oliguria in the surgical patient

The other causes of oliguria are associated with a concentrated urine of high osmolality. As long as adequate renal perfusion is ensured, the patient will not develop renal failure. Attempts may be made to increase the urine volume by giving more fluid. They will not necessarily be successful in the presence of the stress response, but a good flow of urine is comforting to the doctor.

It is absolutely essential *not* to treat the patient who is passing isosmotic urine – i.e. a patient who may have renal failure – with repeated 'fluid challenges' amounting to several litres over a few hours. Remember the words of a wise nephrologist: 'No patient with renal failure ever died of dehydration, but, every day, one dies of pulmonary oedema'.

Of course, it is also essential to obtain expert advice as soon as possible. It is usual to persist with conservative treatment unless:

- It is difficult to control the serum potassium
- The serum creatinine is rising steeply
- Fluid restriction is undesirable because of the need to feed the patient intravenously.

Active treatment, haemofiltration, or haemodialysis, is indicated in the above circumstances. Peritoneal dialysis is an alternative if the patient has not had recent abdominal surgery.

ALIMENTARY SUPPORT

The importance of feeding

It has been pointed out elsewhere in this book that patients who are starved break down their own tissues to meet their energy requirements. The catabolic response to surgery, trauma and sepsis promotes the breakdown of protein as well as of fat, so that many patients in the ICU are liable to sustain substantial nitrogen losses. Loss of muscle bulk in patients on ventilators may make weaning more difficult (Larca & Greenbaum 1982).

Enteral feeding is preferable to intravenous because it is:

● Cheaper
● Less fraught with complications
● Protective against stress ulceration of the stomach (Pingleton & Hadzima 1983).

Unfortunately, many surgical patients in the ICU are unable to absorb enteral feeds, and intravenous feeding must be resorted to. In some ICU patients, nutritional requirements are so large that only intravenous feeding can meet them. It has already been mentioned that intravenous feeding, especially if glucose is the main source of calories, increases carbon dioxide production, which can be a respiratory embarrassment.

Prevention of stress ulceration

Very sick patients are liable to acute peptic ulceration, with consequent gastrointestinal haemorrhage. Routine prophylaxis is recommended, but it is uncertain which method is the best. The choices are as follows:

1. Enteral feeding, when it is feasible, is simple, safe and reliable.
2. Elevation of the gastric pH using one of the following:

● Antacids, which may be instilled through a nasogastric tube, are effective, although large doses are required to raise the gastric pH above 4. Antacids containing magnesium may cause hypermagnesaemia in patients with renal failure.
● H_2-receptor blockers (cimetidine or ranitidine) can be administered parenterally. These drugs are, however, expensive and have side-effects which include interference with the metabolism of other drugs, notably benzodiazepines, thrombocytopenia and arrhythmias.

The neutralization of gastric acidity, unfortunately, permits the colonization of the stomach by Gram-negative microorganisms, which may go on to infect the lungs.

3. Sucralfate, which has to be enterally administered, appears to have a protective effect on the gastric mucosa with very little effect on the pH of gastric juice. It has yet to be shown conclusively that its use in the prophylaxis of stress ulcers is associated with a lower incidence of hospital-acquired (nosocomial) pneumonia than is the use of H_2-receptor blockers. It is certainly cheaper.

Selective decontamination of the digestive tract

Because the Gram-negative organisms which normally colonize the digestive tract have such deadly effects if they migrate, attempts have been made to decontaminate the bowel itself by the prophylactic administration of non-absorbable antibiotics. Routine selective decontamination has been claimed to reduce the incidence of infection in patients with trauma (Stroutenbeek et al 1984). The universal pursuit of the practice would certainly add to the cost of intensive care and might promote the emergence of resistant bacterial strains.

FURTHER READING

Hinds C J 1987 Intensive care: a concise textbook. Baillière Tindall, London

REFERENCES

Ashkenazi J, Weissman C, Rosenbaum S H et al 1982 Nutrition and the respiratory system. Critical Care Medicine 10: 163–172

Aubier M, Murciano D, Legogguic Y et al 1985 Effect of hypophosphataemia on diaphragmatic contractility in patients with acute respiratory failure. New England Journal of Medicine 313: 420–424

Intensive Care Audit 1990 Intensive Care Society, London

Intensive Care Society 1984 Standards for intensive care unit. Biomedica, London

Intensive Care Society 1990 Intensive Care Service in the UK. ICS, London

Joly H R, Weil M H 1969 Temperature of the great toe as an indication of the severity of shock. Circulation 39: 131–138

Larca L, Greenbaum D M 1982 Effectiveness of intensive nutritional regimes in patients who fail to wean from mechanical ventilations. Critical Care Medicine 10: 297–300

Nunn J F, Freeman J 1964 Problems of oxygenation and oxygen transport during haemorrhage. Anaesthesia 19: 206–216

Pingleton S K, Hadzima S K 1983 Enteral alimentation and gastro-intestinal bleeding in mechanically ventilated patients. Critical Care Medicine 11: 13–16

Stroutenbeck C P, van Saene H K F, Miranda D R et al 1984 The effect of selective decontamination of the digestive tract on colonisation and infection rate in multiple trauma patients. Critical Care Medicine 10: 185–192

Sykes M K 1963 Venous pressure as a clinical indication of adequacy of transfusion. Annals of the Royal College of Surgeons 33: 185–197

33. Dialysis

J. E. Scoble   J. F. Moorhead

INDICATIONS

Dialysis therapy replaces the excretory functions of failed kidneys in patients with acute or chronic renal failure. As with all illnesses prevention is vital, encompassing optimal fluid, drug and infection management in acute renal failure and treatment of exacerbating factors, especially hypertension, in chronic renal failure. It is important to realize that with most renal replacement therapies, excretory function equivalent to only 10% of normal renal function, and of course no endocrine functions are provided by the artificial kidney. Dialysis therapy uses two principles to imitate the kidney and provide effective renal therapy.

PRINCIPLES

Diffusion

The first principle is diffusion of a solute from a region of high concentration to a region of low concentration, as shown in Figure 33.1. In renal failure, waste products such as urea or creatinine are present in high concentrations in the blood. Dialysis fluid (either peritoneal or haemo) contains neither and, provided the membrane between the two is permeable to these solutes, net movement will occur from the blood to the dialysis fluid. In peritoneal dialysis the membrane is the peritoneum and in haemodialysis it is an artificial membrane. It is important to note that some substances such as calcium and bicarbonate are present in low concentrations in the blood but in high concentrations in the dialysis fluid. Provided the membrane is permeable to these, net movement will occur from the dialysis fluid to the blood.

Ultrafiltration

The second principle is ultrafiltration in which solvent moves through a membrane driven either by a hydrostatic or osmotic pressure difference as shown in Figure 33.2. The glomerulus in the kidney uses the hydrostatic

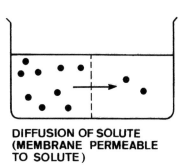

DIFFUSION OF SOLUTE (MEMBRANE PERMEABLE TO SOLUTE)

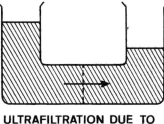

ULTRAFILTRATION DUE TO HYDROSTATIC GRADIENT

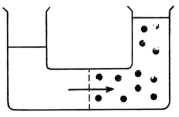

ULTRAFILTRATION DUE TO OSMOTIC GRADIENT (MEMBRANE IMPERMEABLE TO SOLUTE)

Fig. 33.1 Diffusion of a solute from a region of high concentration to one of low concentration.

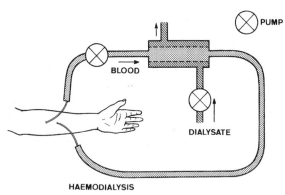

Fig. 33.2 Ultrafiltration.

pressure difference between the glomerular arteriole and the renal tubule to ultrafiltrate 180 litres per day under normal circumstances. Similarly, in haemodialysis a pressure difference which can be varied at will can be exerted between the blood and the dialysis fluid by a blood pump. This results in net fluid movement. In fact under certain circumstances the dialysis fluid can be disconnected and pure ultrafiltration occurs from the blood to the perimembrane space in the artificial kidney. In peritoneal dialysis where the 'blood pump' is the heart, ultrafiltration would be extremely slow if it were not for the fact that increased osmotic pressure is exerted on the dialysis-fluid side of the peritoneal membrane by increasing the concentration of glucose in the dialysis fluid. Thus both haemodialysis and peritoneal dialysis as conventionally used rely on both diffusion and ultrafiltration.

DEVELOPMENT OF METHODS

Although the principles of dialysis appear relatively simple, the practical problems are very large. Kolff in Holland was the first to devise a practical haemodialysis machine and use it to dialyse a woman with acute renal failure. It is interesting to note that the patient was 69 years old, underlining the fact that since the beginning of dialysis the majority of patients have been in the older age group. The major problems with the early dialyses were the large extracorporeal volume of blood and poor access to the vasculature. Scribner transformed haemodialysis by inventing a semipermanent arteriovenous external shunt which could be regularly disconnected and attached to a machine. This enabled regular dialysis for patients with chronic renal failure rather than, as previously, once or twice on patients with acute renal failure. An arteriovenous shunt can be placed in the leg or arm, providing immediate vascular access for dialysis,

but since it involves the placement of foreign material in the body, infections are not uncommon. There is also a danger of accidental disconnection and patients with shunts are limited in their ability to swim or bathe. The arteriovenous shunt still remains a useful form of access for acute renal failure.

The next step forward was the introduction of the Cimino–Brescia arteriovenous fistula formed either in the fore or midarm by side-to-side anastomosis of an artery and vein. The vein is then exposed to arterial blood pressure, enlarges, and arterializes over a period of 4–6 weeks. The advantages are that repeated punctures by large-bore needles are relatively simple and the veins do not clot. Very high dialysis blood flows can usually be achieved, increasing the efficiency of dialysis and shortening time on the machine. Once the needles are removed after dialysis there is no foreign material present and the patient can easily bathe or swim. The disadvantages are that steal syndromes can occur in the hand, aneurysms can form on the fistula and, if the arteriovenous flow through a more proximal fistula is very large, heart failure may be precipitated. The arteriovenous fistula is now the preferred form of vascular access in haemodialysis patients. There are, however, patients in whom it is impossible to form fistulae, perhaps because previous venous access has caused clotting of forearm veins, or the veins are thin walled and of very small diameter.

Urgent access may be achieved by a tunnelled subclavian catheter or, more temporarily, by direct subclavian access. When required, catheters may be placed in the internal jugular, subclavian or femoral veins. When suitable arteries and veins are not available or have already been used, some centres use a Gortex graft to link an artery and vein. The graft itself can be needled, but if infection occurs it may prove impossible to eradicate.

Peritoneal dialysis has been used for the management of acute renal failure using a hard catheter inserted percutaneously midway between the umbilicus and pubic symphysis, care being taken to avoid the aorta by directing the point of the obturator towards the pelvis. This has the advantage of easy and rapid placement in a unit not having access to haemodialysis. The disadvantages are that after 48 hours infection may occur and in many patients previous abdominal surgery makes placement of the catheter impossible. Although initially used on a weekly basis for chronic renal failure it came to be used only for acute renal failure until the late 1970s. Tenkhoff developed a soft catheter which needs to be placed surgically; it has one to three cuffs on it which stimulates a local fibrous reaction. This seals the catheter track and stops both leakage and passage of

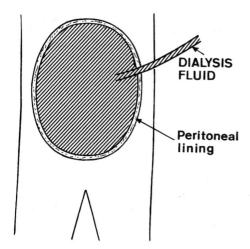

Fig. 33.3 Peritoneal dialysis.

infection around the catheter. The advantage of this system is that it can be used long term as chronic ambulatory peritoneal dialysis (CAPD). In this system the peritoneal fluid is changed four times a day. The advantages are that the patient is independent of any machine and is permanently undergoing dialysis, making fluid balance easier. The disadvantage is that it is relatively inefficient and peritonitis may occur, necessitating stopping treatment.

AVAILABLE DIALYSIS TREATMENTS

The dialysis treatments on offer seem confusing, with a large number of different names. The principles though are those already outlined. A glossary of what is available follows.

Haemodialysis

In haemodialysis, blood is pumped through the centre of the fibres of an artificial kidney and dialysate is pumped around the fibres in a countercurrent direction (Fig. 33.2). The dialysate may contain either bicarbonate or acetate as a pH buffer. High-flux dialysers use a very permeable membrane, but this requires specialized monitoring equipment because of potential large fluid fluxes. This method may enable shorter dialysis periods and may prevent dialysis amyloid by depletion of circulating β_2-microglobulin. Some units may still use intermittent haemodialysis in the management of acute renal failure, but management of fluid balance is more difficult using this method than the haemodiafiltration described below.

Peritoneal dialysis

This may be acute with a hard catheter or chronic with a Tenkhoff catheter (Fig. 33.3). Chronic ambulatory dialysis requires peritoneal dialysis solution to be changed four times a day with the fluid dwelling in the abdomen between changes. Intermittent peritoneal dialysis is usually controlled by a machine and the patient is attached for a period of 6–8 hours and the cycle of fluid-in/dwell/fluid-out takes approximately 30 minutes.

Haemofiltration

This is used mainly in the intensive care unit (ICU) and depends on an ultrafiltrate being produced from blood driven through a filter usually by the patient's arteriovenous pressure difference; it does not require the complicated air detectors required in a pumped system (Fig. 33.4). The filters used have very low resistance to the passage of fluid from the blood through the membrane. If, in addition to this, a dialysate solution is passed around the filter, both dialysis and ultrafiltration can occur. With this method a clearance of approximately 20–30 ml min^{-1} can be achieved. It is in essence a slow haemodialysis, but does not require a haemodialysis machine and can continue for many hours or even days at a time, facilitating intravenous drug and nutrition administration in the ICU setting.

PROBLEMS WITH DIALYSIS

Compared with a well-functioning transplant dialysis, therapy with an artificial kidney of any kind is always second best. There are many patients, however, either awaiting transplantation or who have rejected a number of transplants, who need long-term dialysis therapy. The aim of dialysis is to maximize the well-being of the patient on the therapy. The quality of life on dialysis has been dramatically improved by erythropoietin. This treats the severe anaemia seen in many patients on dialysis and improves their exercise tolerance. Renoprival erythropoeitin deficient anaemia, however, is only one

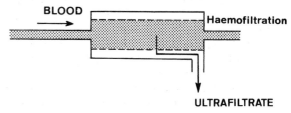

Fig. 33.4 Haemofiltration.

of a number of long-term complications of dialysis, of which the first recognized was renal osteodystrophy, a combination of osteoporosis, hyperparathyroidism and osteomalacia. Early use of phosphate binders, vitamin D administration of 1,25-dihydroxycholecalciferol (or an analogue) and, later, total parathyroidectomy has meant that severe bone disease is seen much less often. The second major complication is a specific form of amyloid caused by the non-excretion of β-microglobulin. This eventually may cause severe arthropathy and may affect other organs. It is thought that some of the modern high-flux artificial kidneys for haemodialysis may decrease this problem. The third major problem is cystic changes which occur in the kidneys of patients on long-term dialysis. This may lead to haemorrhage or, occasionally, malignancy. This condition has been termed 'acquired multicystic kidney disease', to differentiate it from the inherited polycystic kidney disease which predates dialysis.

CONCLUSION

Dialysis therapy replaces sufficient renal function to avoid death but it does not in any way provide normal renal function. The aims of dialysis treatment are to maximize the well-being of the patient until recovery occurs in acute renal failure, or transplantation in chronic renal failure.

FURTHER READING

Bellomo R, Boyce N 1993 Acute continuous hemofiltration: a prospective study of 110 patients, with a review of the literature. American Journal of Kidney Disease 21: 508–518

Davenport A, Will E J, Davidson A M 1993 Improved cardiovascular stability during continuous modes of renal replacement therapy in critically ill patients with acute hepatic and renal failure. Critical Care Medicine 21: 328–338

Golper T A 1992 Indications, technical considerations and strategies for renal replacement therapy in the intensive care unit. Journal of Intensive Care Medicine 7: 310

34. Chronic illness, rehabilitation and terminal care

A. C. Kurowska   A. Tookman

In patients with chronic and terminal illness effective symptom control forms the basis of management. For such patients the primary aim of treatment is not necessarily to prolong life but to make life as comfortable and meaningful as possible. A significant number of patients experience functional limitations because of their disease or its treatment. Many of these can be treated by rehabilitation techniques which enable them to develop to their maximum potential.

A *terminally ill* patient is one in whom an accurate diagnosis has been made and cure is impossible. Usually prognosis is of the order of months or less. Treatment is aimed at relief of symptoms. The majority of such patients have far advanced cancer, but patients with non-malignant disease also fall under this definition, e.g. the end-stage of diseases such as renal failure, chronic obstructive airways disease, multiple sclerosis, acquired immune deficiency syndrome (AIDS) and motor neurone disease.

A *chronically ill* patient has a longer and less predictable prognosis. Many of these patients are likely to have non-malignant disease, e.g. inflammatory bowel disease, peripheral vascular disease and post-trauma. However, some malignant conditions have a protracted course, e.g. breast and prostatic cancer.

Patients with malignancy will form a large proportion of the case-load of patients with chronic and terminal illness who are seen by general surgeons.

OBJECTIVES

Since patients with incurable illness present with complex problems, an approach which focuses on the whole patient, rather than simply on the disease, is needed. It should:

- Address the psychological, social, spiritual and financial needs of the patient as well as their physical symptoms
- Provide effective symptom control

- Offer control, independence and choice. This will enable the patient to participate in decisions about the management of his problems. For the terminally ill patient this would include negotiating the most appropriate place for the patient to die (home, hospice or hospital)
- Support 'the family' (i.e. all those who are important to the patient) as well as the patient
- Provide bereavement counselling for the terminally ill patient's 'family'.

To achieve these aims an interdisciplinary team approach is essential. The team includes the patient and their 'family'.

The proportion of all deaths occurring in hospital has increased over the last 15 years. Figures show that 65% of cancer deaths occur in hospital. The recent development of palliative care support teams, based in the hospital and/or the community, has led to marked changes in this trend in certain area. Effective use of these teams will enable patients to choose the most appropriate place to spend their terminal illness. For example, one team has reported that of patients under their care 50% of deaths occur in the patient's own home and 34% in a hospice.

Such teams exist to provide support and expert advice to the professionals and other carers involved in the patient's management. It is therefore important that the surgeon be familiar with the local teams both within the hospital and in the community.

COMMUNICATION

Communication with patients who have advanced incurable illness is always difficult. Chronic and terminal illness can be seen as a failure and can generate feelings of inadequacy, fear and despair in the doctors. These fears lead to the use of certain tactics in order to keep patients at a safe emotional distance.

Such tactics include prematurely reassuring patients

of one's ability to control physical symptoms when the real issue is their underlying emotional fears. For example, when a patient complains of pain a quick reassurance is given that it can be got rid of rather than exploring the significance of the pain to the patient. Another tactic is the use of selective attention to physical symptoms – a patient may complain of losing weight and constipation and say 'I am worried'; the doctor ignores the worry expressed and proceeds to discuss the constipation! Other tactics include changing the topic when emotional issues are raised, asking closed questions and even physical avoidance by walking past the end of the patient's bed.

As well as avoiding the use of distancing tactics, clear explanations of the physical and functional outcome of surgery should be given. Understanding of the rationale for treatment helps patients handle side-effects better and enhances trust in the physician. Studies of psychological reactions to cancer have shown that patients who are given accurate facts about their diagnosis and treatment adapt better to radical surgery. The opportunity to prepare psychologically for the major physical changes associated with procedures such as radical mastectomy, colostomy and head and neck surgery facilitates postoperative adaptation.

When patients have radical surgery, especially when associated with cosmetic deformity, issues surrounding 'loss' need to be explored. Such issues include altered body image, sexuality, social role and anxieties related to death and dying. The professionals involved must be sensitive to the psychological needs of patients and educate these patients in order to ease their acceptance of their new image and readjust their goals. Often these issues are not discussed at all. The rehabilitation process should start as soon as the diagnosis is made. Nurse specialists (e.g. breast, stoma, incontinence advisors) can be very useful.

There are some fundamental principles of good communication:

- The patient's concerns should be dealt with before professional concerns
- Each topic should be fully covered before proceeding to the next
- All the problems should be elicited before giving advice or attempting any solution
- Non-verbal cues are very important
- It is helpful to clarify and summarize what the patient reports

Remember it is not always a question of 'What should the patient know?' but rather 'What does the patient want to know?'

COMMON EMOTIONAL REACTIONS TO LIFE-THREATENING ILLNESS

Anxiety

This is a normal reaction to a serious illness. One of the commonest emotional reactions to a life-threatening illness is fear. It is important to find out precisely what the patient fears since many anxieties are based on fears that can be resolved (see below). Normal levels of anxiety should be acknowledged and accepted; however, the patient must be assessed for signs of clinical anxiety.

Such signs include a persistently anxious mood which is subjectively different from normal worrying; difficulty in distracting the patient from his worries; feelings of tension and restlessness, insomnia, autonomic hyperactivity (e.g. palpitations, sensation of choking) and panic attacks. Anxiolytics may be helpful in this group of patients.

Denial

It is important to assess whether the denial is causing harm (e.g. refusal of necessary medication, psychological turmoil). In many patients it represents a successful coping strategy, in which case breaking down the denial may cause unnecessary distress.

Anger

This can be displaced onto staff and/or onto the relatives. It is important not to react with anger but to try to accept and understand. It needs to be explained to the relatives that the patient is not really angry with them, but is displacing the anger he feels towards the disease onto them.

Despair/depression

Despair is a normal reaction to a life-threatening illness which should be recognized and acknowledged. However, it is important to look for signs of clinical depression.

The classical somatic symptoms of depression, e.g. weight loss, anorexia and lethargy, carry less importance in the assessment of patients with terminal illness as they are often a manifestation of the cancer. Important clues are a persistently depressed mood which is subjectively different from normal sadness; difficulty in distracting the patient; a lowering of interest in and enjoyment of social activities; crying, irritability, poor sleep and feelings of guilt. Suicidal ideas may be present. These patients should be treated with antidepressants.

Common fears in patients with life-threatening illness

- Fear of unrelieved symptoms especially pain
- Fear of death and the process of dying
- Fear of dying alone
- Fear of incompleted tasks (e.g. will has not been made)
- Fear of loss and separation (family, job, income, etc.)
- Fear of loss of dignity (confusion, incontinence, loss of control)
- Fear of altered body image
- Fear of retribution in the afterlife.

UNDERLYING PRINCIPLES OF SYMPTOM CONTROL

A positive but realistic attitude should be encouraged and assurance given that a considerable amount can be achieved. A problem-oriented individualized approach is the key to effective symptom control. For each symptom:

1. *Diagnose the cause and treat appropriately.* An accurate diagnosis is important for good symptom control. A careful history and examination can be more revealing than extensive investigations, which can be impractical and distressing. Investigations may be important but should only be carried out if they alter subsequent management.

The treatment of a symptom varies considerably depending on the underlying pathology. For example, in a patient with cancer, vomiting may be due to:

- Raised intracranial pressure
- Drugs
- Hepatomegaly
- Intestinal obstruction, etc.

Each of the above requires specific management.

Since many symptoms are multifactorial in origin it is important to recognize the contributory factors and address each as far as possible. Other intercurrent illnesses are common in debilitated patients, hence it is vital to consider non-malignant as well as malignant causes.

If the diagnosis is tentative but it is not appropriate to investigate further, symptomatic relief must be given. Very often a therapeutic trial will indicate the cause; for example, a trial of steroids in a confused patient with suspected cerebral metastases who is too unwell to undergo a computed tomography (CT) scan.

2. *Explain symptom to patient.* Fear is an important contributory factor in the patient's interpretation of any symptom. The fact that the doctor understands the

---

Box 34.1	
Approximate incidence of common symptoms in patients with far advanced cancer	
Physical	
Weakness	80%
Pain	70%
Anorexia	70%
Dyspnoea	50%
Cough	50%
Constipation	50%
Nausea and vomiting	40%
Psychological	
Depression	30%
Anxiety	30%

---

symptom, can explain its cause and can offer treatment is reassuring.

3. *Discuss the treatment options.* Patients should be given adequate and accurate information on treatment options in order to make informed choices. This enhances the patient's sense of control. Therapy need not be limited to drugs. Other measures may be appropriate such as radiotherapy, nerve blocks, physiotherapy, psychological therapies (counselling, hypnotherapy), etc.

4. *Set objectives that are realistic.* It is frustrating for both patient and staff alike if expectations are set that will never be achieved.

5. *Anticipate.* In patients with advanced illness symptoms (Box 34.1) may change rapidly, if such changes are anticipated much distress may be avoided. For example, deterioration in a patient's condition may make it impossible for them to continue with oral medication. Such deterioration should be anticipated and injectable preparations should be available. This particularly applies in the home care setting and can avert an unnecessary crisis.

6. *Ensure relatives remain informed and supported.* It is important to treat the 'whole family'.

PAIN

Pain is a common symptom in chronic and terminal illness and one that is particularly feared by cancer patients. Pain can be alleviated or modified in all patients. Proper pain assessment leads to effective management. The principles outlined here have been developed in the context of management of patients with advanced cancer, but are applicable to patients who have non-malignant pain secondary to chronic disease.

Diagnose the cause of the pain

The majority of patients with far advanced disease have pain at more than one site. Each pain should be evaluated individually.

In order to establish the cause of any pain it is essential to take a careful history, particularly noting:

- The site of pain and any radiation
- The type and severity of pain
- When the pain started and any subsequent changes
- Exacerbating and alleviating factors
- Analgesic agents already used.

Physical examination often confirms the diagnosis. On occasion it may be appropriate to investigate the patient with X-rays, isotope bone scans, CT scans, etc.

Pain may be due to a malignant or non-maligant cause. In one third of patients with advanced cancer who complain of pain the underlying pathology is non-malignant.

It is always important to assess how significant the pain is for the individual patient – how does it affect him and alter his lifestyle?

Common causes of pain in cancer patients

Bone pain

This is due to metastatic disease or local infiltration by adjacent tumour. It is characteristically a deep gnawing pain made worse by movement. The bone is often tender on percussion.

Visceral pain

Due to tumour mass in the lung or internal organs of the abdomen and pelvis. The tumour causes pain by a variety of mechanisms:

1. *Soft tissue infiltration.* Deep-seated pain which is due to complex pathology. The tumour invades and/or stretches pain-sensitive structures (e.g. parietal and visceral pleura, peritoneum, nerve plexuses, and local bony structures).

2. *Stretching of a capsule.* The capsule of an organ is sensitive when stretched. The most common example of this is right hypochondrial pain due to stretching of the liver capsule. The pain can be very severe, and a sudden exacerbation of liver pain may be due to a bleed into a local deposit.

3. *Stretching of a hollow organ.* Distension of hollow viscera (small and large intestines, bladder, ureters, etc.) can cause severe spasmodic colicky pain.

Nerve pain

Nerves can be infiltrated or compressed. Nerve destruction pain may be burning, lancinating, and associated with abnormal sensations (e.g. hyperaesthesia). Nerve compression pain is more often a deep ache. Destruction of nerve plexuses, nerve roots or peripheral nerves may result in deafferentation pain (dermatomal pain associated with sensory changes in the painful area). Pain of central origin (brain or spinal cord) is often unilateral and manifests itself as spontaneous pain and hypersensitivity, including dysaesthesiae of a disagreeable kind. Nerve compression and nerve destruction may, of course, coexist.

Myofascial pain

Musculoskeletal pains are common in chronically ill patients. They radiate in a non-dermatomal pattern. Typically there are localized hypersensitive areas of muscle known as trigger points, which are tender to pressure.

Superficial pain

In weak, debilitated patients bedsores may be unavoidable and give rise to distressing pain.

Realistic objectives

In nearly all patients pain can be significantly modified and in many patients total freedom from pain can be achieved. In a few patients pain can prove to be an intractable symptom, unresponsive to most treatments. It is these patients that provide the greatest challenge and in whom all avenues of achieving pain relief must be explored.

Realistic goals

- Freedom from pain at night – should always be achievable
- Freedom from pain at rest – usually achievable
- Freedom from pain on mobility – may not be achievable.

Treat appropriately

This clearly depends on the cause – not all pain requires analgesia; e.g. the pain of constipation is best treated with laxatives, not analgesics! However, when indicated, analgesics must be prescribed correctly.

Analgesic treatment of pain

The variety of analgesics available for use in the treatment of pain can be daunting. It is better to use a few drugs really well than many badly. The following 'three-step' regimen is effective in the majority of situations:

Step 1: *Non-opioids for mild pain*
      Paracetamol

If pain not relieved with two paracetamol 6-hourly move on to

Step 2: *Weak opioids for mild/moderate pain*
      Coproxamol – dextropropoxyphene (central action) + paracetamol (peripheral action)

If pain not relieved with two coproxamol 4–6 hourly move on to

Step 3: *Strong opioids for moderate/severe pain*
      Diamorphine/morphine (tabs/solution) or MST (morphine slow-release tablets).

Principles of prescribing opioids

Opioids should be given so that pain is suppressed and, if possible, not allowed to break through: pain due to advanced disease is unlikely to remit. Therefore *regular prescribing* is essential.

Analgesia should be given in an adequate dose and the dose titrated upwards until the pain is controlled. Therefore there is *no maximum dose* of morphine/diamorphine.

Diamorphine/morphine *should not be prescribed* p.r.n. for pain unless it is for pain that breaks through the *regular* analgesia.

Strong opioids of choice

Diamorphine or morphine (tablets or solution). Quick-acting preparations. Prescribe 4-hourly (day and night). The short duration of action means there is rapid response to alterations of dose. They are therefore used when the patient first starts on opioids in order to estimate the overall opioid requirement of that individual.

Morphine sulphate slow release. Long-acting preparation. Prescribe 12-hourly. When the patient's pain is stable on 4-hourly diamorphine/morphine they should be converted to the equivalent dose of morphine sulphate slow release in order to simplify their regime.

In certain circumstances it is possible to start patients

Table 34.1 Approximate opioid equivalents

Drug	Dose	Diamorphine equivalent (mg)	Duration of action (h)
Dextropropoxyphene (Coproxamol)	32.5 mg	3	5–6
Dihydrocodeine (DF118)	30 mg	3	3–5
Pethidine	50 mg	6	2–3
Diconal (dipipanone 10 mg + cyclizine 30 mg)	1 tablet	5	3–5
Methadone	5 mg	5	6–8
Dextromoramide (Palfium)	5 mg	10	2–3
Buprenorphine (Temgesic)	200 μg	10	6–8
Phenazocine	5 mg	15	5–6

on morphine sulphate slow release straight away (e.g. outpatients with moderate pain where urgent control of pain is not necessary).

These two strong opioids will be suitable for virtually all needs. There are other strong opioids that may have a role in pain management (e.g. methadone, fentanyl). However, their precise role is yet to be determined.

Choosing the dose

The dose depends on previous analgesic requirements.

If not on any previous analgesic, start with 5 mg diamorphine/morphine 4-hourly or 10 mg morphine sulphate slow release 12-hourly.

If on weak opioid (e.g. coproxamol) start with 5–10 mg diamorphine/morphine 4 hourly or 30 mg morphine sulphate slow release 12-hourly.

If on other strong opiod use Table 34.1 to convert to equivalent dose of diamorphine/morphine 4-hourly. Titrate the dose as indicated by the level of pain control achieved.

For all practical purposes conversion of diamorphine to morphine sulphate slow release can be done on a milligram for milligram basis, e.g. diamorphine 10 mg 4-hourly = diamorphine 60 mg in 24 hours = morphine sulphate slow release 30 mg 12-hourly.

Summary

If a patient has significant pain then adequate, effective analgesics should be started early.

Valuable time can be wasted using an array of ineffective moderate analgesics. In particular this can mean that the terminally ill patient may spend a substantial portion of his remaining life with uncontrolled pain. Opioids are the most effective strong analgesics.

Routes of administration

If the patient is able to swallow use the oral route. However, at times it may be necessary to give opioids rectally, transdermally or parenterally.

Indications for rectal/parenteral opioids

- In the last few hours/days of life when the patient is unable to swallow
- Dysphagia
- Nausea and vomiting
- Gut obstruction
- Unable to tolerate taste/number of tablets.

Small-volume injections are more acceptable. Diamorphine hydrochloride is highly soluble (1 g in 1.6 ml) and is therefore the drug of choice for parenteral use. *Subcutaneous* injections are effective and this is the route of choice. Diamorphine undergoes first-pass metabolism in the liver and therefore the subcutaneous dose should be half the oral dose.

If the patient is going to require more than two or three injections a subcutaneous infusion pump should be considered. This is a small battery-driven device that will inject the contents of a syringe over a 24-hour period. It can be used in the home as well as in the in-patient setting.

Examples of doses that are equipotent:

- Oral diamorphine 20 mg 4-hourly
- Subcutaneous diamorphine 10 mg 4-hourly
- Subcutaneous diamorphine 60 mg per 24 hours in syringe pump.

Fears of prescribing opioids

Fears about prescribing opioids are common and generally without foundation. They may lead to patients having effective analgesia withheld.

Fear of addiction

It has been shown in many studies that psychological addiction does not occur. Patients reduce and/or stop their opioid if their pain is controlled by another method (e.g. nerve block, surgical fixation). Since chemical dependence occurs (as is the case with many drugs) morphine should be gradually reduced. It must never be stopped abruptly.

Fear of tolerance

Tolerance occurs only to a minor degree and for practical purposes is not relevant. If the dose of opioid needs to be increased it is as a result of an increase in pain secondary to further advance of the tumour.

Fear of respiratory depression

With careful attention to dosage this does not occur. In fact opioids are used in the palliative care setting to alleviate dyspnoea by reducing ventilatory demand and hence the sensation of breathlessness.

Fear of hastening death

Opioids do not hasten death when correctly prescribed. The exhaustion caused by unrelieved pain may do so.

Predictable side-effects of morphine/diamorphine

- *Constipation occurs in >95% of patients.* Regular prophylactic laxative should always be prescribed.
- *Nausea and vomiting occur in approximately 30% of patients.* An antiemetic should be prescribed if nausea or vomiting occurs but it is not necessary to prescribe antiemetics prophylactically unless the patient is primed to vomit (e.g. gastrointestinal tumour, already nauseated). The antiemetic of choice for opioid-induced nausea is haloperidol. Nausea due to opioids is usually self-limiting so the antiemetic can be withdrawn after 10–14 days.
- *Drowsiness occurs in about 20% of patients.* This side-effect wears off after approximately 5 days on a stable dose.
- *Other side-effects.* These include: dry mouth, which is very common and should be treated with simple local measures; confusion and hallucinations are extremely rare (<1% of patients) and other causes should be excluded; twitching can occur on high doses.

Opioid-resistant pain

Some pains are either partially sensitive or insensitive to opioids. These pains will need to be managed with an additional or alternative drug or some other technique.

Bone pain. Although partially sensitive to opioids this pain frequently requires the addition of a non-steroidal anti-inflammatory drug. Localized bone pain can often be treated with radiotherapy. Surgical fixation may be indicated if there is a pathological fracture. Prophylactic fixation should be considered (if >75% of the cortex is eroded spontaneous fracture is highly likely).

Nerve pain. This is very often opioid insensitive. Steroids are useful in nerve compression. Nerve infiltration/irritation may respond to drugs which alter neurotransmission (e.g. low-dose tricyclic anti-depressants, anticonvulsants). Radiotherapy and nerve blocks may also be indicated.

Liver capsule. This pain is partially opioid sensitive. Steroids are very useful in this context as they may reduce the liver swelling and relieve capsular stretching.

Colic. If due to constipation treat with laxatives! If due to tumour obstruction antispasmodics may be required.

Meningeal pain/raised intracranial pressure. Steroids are the drug of choice. Radiotherapy should be considered.

Lymphoedema. Non-steroidal anti-inflammatory drugs and steroids can be helpful. Physical treatment plays an important role (massage, compression hosiery and intermittent pneumatic compression).

Muscle spasm. Benzodiazepines or baclofen can be used.

Infection. It may be appropriate to treat infections in order to relieve pain.

Joint/myofascial pain. Non-steroidal anti-inflammatories should be used in conjunction with opioids. Local injections of steroid into joints and trigger points may be of value. Physiotherapy can also be helpful.

Superficial pain. Patients with bedsores need to be kept off the pressure areas with regular turning. An effective patient support system (e.g. sheepskin, low-loss airbed) is helpful.

Remember pain may be aggravated by psychological factors

If management is solely directed at physical factors, one may fail to control pain adequately in some patients. It is important to treat coexistent depression or anxiety, and if appropriate offer counselling, diversionary activities, etc.

Complementary therapies

Although scientifically unproven, these seem to benefit some groups of patients. If the patient perceives these therapies as adding to their overall well-being then one should support the patient, provided the treatment does not harm the patient or interfere with their conventional management.

Injection techniques in cancer pain

Nerve blocks have a place in palliative care. They are highly effective when used in a selected group of patients (approximately 4% of patients with pain will benefit). Various 'injection techniques' can be used. Although some of these techniques need expertise and specialized equipment to perform, simple techniques can be performed at the bedside.

Nerve blocks

Nerve blocks can be considered when there is:

- Unilateral pain
- Localized pain
- Pain due to involvement of one or two nerve roots
- Abdominal pain arising from 'upper' gut
- Rib pain.

The patient needs careful assessment as to the cause of the pain before a block is carried out. This assessment will determine the exact site at which the pain pathways should be interrupted.

Many procedures can be performed using local anaesthetics and steroids. These blocks can give good pain relief outlasting the effect of the anaesthetic and are safe procedures. The pain relief from a nerve block may be transient and repeated blocks may be necessary. Careful patient selection is vital. A nerve block should not be offered as a 'last resort' but only if there is a reasonable chance of success.

Major neurolytic procedures may carry the risk of serious side-effects. For example:

- Intraspinal neurolysis for nerve root pain can produce urinary and faecal incontinence
- Coeliac plexus block for upper abdominal pain can cause postural hypotension.

Once again careful patient assessment is vital.

WEAKNESS AND IMMOBILITY

Weakness is a common and distressing symptom in patients with advanced illness. When due to general debility it is very difficult to treat. Reversible causes such as cord compression and cerebral metastases must be excluded.

It is important to acknowledge the problem and explain to the patient that it is a result of the illness. This allows realistic goals to be set, which in itself can reduce the patient's distress. Even very sick patients need to feel a sense of control. Simple measures such as a wheelchair can help them achieve this.

Steroids improve weakness in a proportion of patients. The response, however, is often short lived and side-effects, such as proximal myopathy and poor wound healing, must be taken into consideration. Therefore patients must be carefully selected and the time at which steroids are introduced has to be carefully assessed.

A patient who is immobile and confined to bed will lose muscle strength. A normal person loses 10–15% of his muscle strength when completely rested for one week and it takes 60 days to restore that strength. It is therefore not surprising that muscle weakness quickly develops in the immobile cancer patient, especially in the common situation where protein catabolism is increased. If immobility continues contractures can develop, leading to impaired ability to self-care. Contractures are more likely when soft tissue damage is present and with improper positioning in bed. Good nursing care and regular physiotherapy are essential for these patients.

When patients are debilitated and immobile, pressure sores can rapidly develop. This is aggravated by increased protein catabolism and negative nitrogen balance as well as other factors (e.g. diabetes, steroids). Damage can be minimized if pressure on the skin is intermittent. Early prophylaxis with scrupulous nursing attention and the use of effective patient support systems (e.g. special mattresses, low-loss airbeds) will limit damage and help prevent distressing pain.

Autonomic dysfunction and impaired peripheral circulation are the cardiovascular consequences of immobility. There is an increased likelihood of deep venous thrombosis and pulmonary embolism.

Atelectasis as a result of reduced aeration of the posterior lungs predisposes patients to chest infection.

Urinary retention and urinary infection are more common in immobile patients.

Immobility, anorexia and weakness lead to reduced peristalsis and constipation.

Loss of proprioceptors in skin of feet will lead to an inability to balance which can take many weeks to recover.

ANOREXIA

This symptom is common. It occurs in approximately 70% of patients with advanced cancer. It is important to decide whose problem it is – the patient's or the carers'. The family need to understand that as death approaches it is normal to lose interest in food. At this stage the goal of eating is enjoyment, not optimal nutrition.

Causes

- Tumour bulk and associated biochemical abnormalities (hypercalcaemia, uraemia, etc.)
- Oral problems (e.g. thrush, oral tumour)
- Constipation
- Drugs, radiotherapy
- Depression or anxiety.

It must be remembered that fear of vomiting may lead to avoidance of food (as opposed to true anorexia). Psychological factors such as anxiety and depression can manifest as lack of appetite. Presentation of food is important – it should be in small portions and well presented.

If the above factors have been attended to and it is still felt to be a problem for the patient, steroids can be tried as an appetite stimulant.

DYSPHAGIA

Site of dysphagia

The site of dysphagia can be predicted from the symptom complex. Drooling, leaking of food and retention of food in the mouth indicate a buccal cause; nasal regurgitation, gagging, choking and coughing suggest pharyngeal pathology; a sensation of food sticking behind the sternum and pain between the shoulder blades imply oesophageal obstruction.

Table 34.2 Common causes of dysphagia in patients with advanced disease.

Problem	Implication	Example of cause
Solids then liquids	Obstruction	Tumour mass. External compression
Solids and liquids simultaneously	Neuromuscular cause	Terminal dysfunction in very weak patients. Perineural tumour infiltration with head and neck tumours which damage cranial nerves (V, IX, X). Bulbar palsy
Painful	Mucosal causes	*Candida* (N.B.: only 50% of patients with oesophageal *Candida* have clinically apparent oral *Candida*). Post-radiotherapy

Management

It is important to explain the cause (Table 34.2) to the patient so that any dietary adjustments are understood. Restriction to liquids or soft foods may be necessary.

Any associated pain should be treated. Mucaine is useful for the local pain of *Candida* or radiotherapy, but many patients require opioids for satisfactory pain relief. *Candida* should be actively treated with topical or systemic antifungals. If patients are unable to swallow even liquids, drugs should be given by another route. A subcutaneous infusion of drugs (analgesics, etc.) is both effective and well tolerated.

If it is appropriate to attempt to relieve the obstruction, then possibilities include radiotherapy, endo-oesophageal tubes, dilatation and laser therapy. Steroids by reducing oedema may palliate dysphagia for a significant period. They can be particularly useful in the management of dysphagia syndrome associated with head and neck tumour.

Endo-oesophageal tubes should be considered in patients who are relatively independent and active, but are not appropriate for the moribund. Gastrostomy is rarely indicated in patients with incurable malignant obstruction. It does not solve the problem of saliva aspiration. In patients with carcinoma of the stomach or oesophagus, by the time severe obstruction occurs the prognosis is very short. Gastrostomy itself and its postoperative complications have a significant morbidity and mortality and can even contribute to terminal discomfort. However, with the advent of percutaneous techniques gastrostomy now has a role in selected patients.

Nasogastric tubes and gastrostomies may be appropriate for patients with a longer prognosis (e.g. those with neurological problems, certain malignancies of the head and neck and cerebral tumours).

A belief that adequate nutrition is essential and the pressure to act may lead to overtreatment of dysphagic patients.

In irreversible total obstruction or terminal neuromuscular dysfunction secretions must be reduced to a minimum using hyoscine.

Dehydration should be looked on as a natural process in the last few days of life. It helps relieve a number of symptoms and intravenous fluids tend to exacerbate discomfort by increasing bronchial secretions, gastrointestinal fluid (thereby increased likelihood of vomiting), urine flow (leading to need for catheter), etc.

NAUSEA AND VOMITING

Nausea and/or vomiting occur in approximately 40% of patients with far-advanced cancer. The cause must be

Table 34.3 Common causes of nausea and vomiting in advanced disease

Cause	Symptomatic treatment
Drugs	If possible withdraw the drug
Metabolic (hypercalcaemia, uraemia, etc.)	Treat with centrally acting antiemetics
Bowel obstruction	(e.g. cyclizine/haloperidol)
Gastric statis Squashed stomach syndrome*	Treat with prokinetic antiemetic and/or asilone
Gastric irritation (e.g. NSAIDs, gastric ulceration)	H$_2$ antagonist
Constipation	Laxatives
Raised intracranial pressure	Steroids

NSAID, non-steroidal anti-inflammatory drug.
*Squashed/small stomach syndrome is a constellation of alimentary symptoms seen in patients with large epigastric mass/gross hepatomegaly. It is manifested as early satiation, epigastric fullness, epigastric pain, flatulence, hiccoughs, nausea, vomiting and heartburn.

found in order that rational treatment can be offered (Table 34.3).

If an antiemetic is needed, most nausea and vomiting in patients with advanced illness can be controlled using just three antiemetic drugs. Most antiemetics act at one of the three sites shown in Table 34.4.

Sometimes more than one antiemetic will be necessary. If this is the case it is common sense to combine drugs which act at different sites, i.e. a neuroleptic with an antihistamine. The antiemetic must be delivered by a suitable route. There is little point giving a drug orally if the patient is vomiting! Rectal or parenteral routes should be chosen in these situations. A 24-hour subcutaneous infusion by means of a syringe driver is a simple and effective method of drug delivery. (Syringe drivers are discussed in more detail later.)

BOWEL OBSTRUCTION

Gastrointestinal obstruction occurs in approximately 4% of patients with advanced cancer. It occurs more

Table 34.4 Main sites of action of antiemetic drugs

Main site of action	Class of drug	Example
Central		
Chemoreceptor trigger zone	Neuroleptic	Haloperidol
Vomiting centre	Antihistamine	Cyclizine
Peripheral	Prokinetic	Domperidone

commonly in those with colonic primary (10%) and ovarian primary (25%).

Surgical management in patients with known malignancy is indicated if the patient's general condition is good, they have low-bulk disease and an easily reversible cause seems likely. Previous laparotomy findings must be taken into consideration. Surgery remains the primary treatment because 10% of obstructions in such patients prove to be non-malignant, 10% represent a new primary and approximately 60% will not reobstruct.

With conservative treatment (drip and suck) 30% of obstructions resolve spontaneously. Therefore this management should be considered prior to proceeding to surgery.

Neither of these strategies should form part of the management of irreversible obstruction in patients with far-advanced cancer. The majority of such patients have obstruction at multiple sites. The aim is symptom control with drugs. Intravenous fluids and nasogastric tubes are rarely needed.

Medical management of bowel obstruction

Obstruction may be proximal, in which case the predominant symptom is vomiting, or distal, when the predominant symptom is colicky pain. Nausea is often more distressing than vomiting. The aim is to eliminate nausea, reduce vomiting to a maximum of once or twice a day and treat associated pain.

Baines et al (1985) reported on this form of management in 38 patients with advanced malignant disease. They found that nausea and vomiting was well controlled in 90% of patients, colic in 100% and pain relief was total in 90% with only mild residual pain in 10%. The median survival was 3 months and 24% survived >6 months.

CONSTIPATION

The need to treat constipation is usually a consequence of failing to use prophylactic laxatives (virtually all patients on opioids should have a regular laxative). A rectal examination is essential on any patient complaining of constipation or diarrhoea to assess for impaction. Use a laxative that combines a softener and stimulant (e.g. Codanthramer).

SYRINGE DRIVERS IN SYMPTOM CONTROL

Syringe drivers delivering subcutaneous infusions of analgesics, antiemetics, anticholinergics and tranquillizers are commonly used in patients who would require regular parenteral medication (Table 34.5). The

---

Box 34.2
Medical management of bowel obstruction

Diet	No restrictions but small meals appropriate
Nausea and vomiting	Cyclizine 150 mg per day via syringe pump. If partial/no success combine with haloperidol 5–10 mg per day via syringe pump
Reverse obstruction	If constipated attempt to clear with softeners. Docusate 100–200 mg three times daily, tablets/syrup (Consider dexamethasone 16 mg per day by subcutaneous infusion to reduce oedema)
Pain	Diamorphine in appropriate dose in pump according to previous analgesic requirement and level of pain. Halve the oral dose to get equivalent subcutaneous dose, i.e. subcutaneous/oral potency = 2 : 1
Colic	If colic persists despite the above, add hyoscine hydrobromide 1.2 mg per day to pump

Gastrokinetic antiemetics such as metoclopramide or domperidone are contraindicated – they will exacerbate vomiting

---

subcutaneous route is simple, safe, effective and acceptable to most patients. Indications for the use of such syringe drivers have already been discussed above in the context of pain control.

THE MANAGEMENT OF THE TERMINAL PHASE OF THE ILLNESS

When a patient who has advanced illness enters into the terminal phase (normally a day or so prior to death) *all*

Table 34.5 Drugs commonly used in the syringe driver

Drug class	Drug	Dose
Analgesics	Diamorphine	According to need
Antiemetics	Haloperidol	5–10 mg per 24 hours
	Cyclizine	150 mg per 24 hours
	Methotrimeprazine	100–200 mg per 24 hours
For bronchial secretions	Hyoscine hydrobromide	1.2–1.8 mg per 24 hours
Terminal agitation	Midazolam	20–60 mg per 24 hours

medication should be reviewed. All drugs should be stopped apart from those aimed at symptom control. Communication is vital and explanation should be given to the patient and their carers about anticipated changes in the patient's condition. Reassurance should be given that symptoms will remain controlled and the patient kept comfortable. Often it is appropriate to use a syringe driver to administer medications.

Analgesia. This should be continued even if a patient becomes unconscious. The patient may still perceive pain and in addition abrupt withdrawal of opioids can result in an unpleasant withdrawal reaction. If a patient is on regular opioids they will need to be continued at an equivalent dose subcutaneously. If the patient will require more than a few injections a syringe driver should be started.

Agitation. This can be a problem and causes must be looked for and treated appropriately, e.g. retention of urine requires catheterization. However, it is not uncommon for patients to become agitated and confused shortly before death. If a tranquillizer is indicated, use subcutaneous midazolam (5–10 mg, 4–6-hourly). Midazolam (20–60 mg per 24 hours) can be combined with diamorphine in a syringe driver.

Bronchial secretion. This can be controlled using subcutaneous hyoscine hydrobromide (600 μg, 4-hourly) as required. It can also be added into the syringe driver together with the diamorphine and midazolam. If this symptom does not respond to repeated doses of hyoscine, try bumetanide 2 mg intramuscularly.

Crises. In some circumstances it may be appropriate to prescribe drugs for a crisis. For example, if it is likely that the patient may have a major bleed (haemoptysis, haematemesis, etc.) prescribe diamorphine and midazolam as a 'crisis pack' to be given in the event of such an emergency. Such crises can be of great distress to the patient and the family and need to be handled with speed and sensitivity.

The rules of symptom control should always be followed, even at this stage of the illness. Symptoms should be evaluated and appropriate treatment instituted. It is important to anticipate problems and to communicate well with all concerned. It has been shown that 'peaceful' death leads to far fewer bereavement problems in the family.

BEREAVEMENT

Support offered to the family both during the patient's illness and at the time of the patient's death not only helps them to cope better but reduces the likelihood of future complications. Evidence suggests there is higher physical and psychiatric morbidity and possibly increased mortality in those recently bereaved.

People avoid grieving individuals because they feel helpless, awkward, embarrassed, they do not wish to feel sad themselves and they fear releasing strong emotions.

Normal stages in the process of grief

Denial

Death represents an enormous threat to the individual. Even if the death is anticipated the reaction of the bereaved person is often one of shock and disbelief. They feel numb and immobilized. The response of the individual depends very much on the circumstances of the death. Religious beliefs and cultural background will influence their reactions.

Developing awareness

Gradually an awareness of the reality of the loss develops and various emotional reactions can emerge such as depression/sadness, anger, guilt, loneliness. In addition, outbursts of grief, with episodes of anxiety and anguish associated with crying, restlessness and preoccupation with the dead person are common. A strong sense of the physical presence of the deceased, at times amounting to a visual awareness, should not be misinterpreted as abnormal. It is during this phase that the bereaved often present to their GP with physical and psychological symptoms. Stress, irrational behaviour, lethargy and physical illness which mimics the symptoms of the deceased are common complaints.

Resolution

Ultimately the individual gains a new sense of self-identity and adjusts to their new role in society. Gradually there develops a resolve that they will cope, and a feeling that it is now appropriate to develop new social contacts.

Bereavement counselling

It is important to interpret normal reactions to loss. Many people who are undergoing a normal grief reaction interpret their symptoms as evidence of psychiatric illness. For example, they may feel the dead person is present or actually see the dead person. Reassurance can be given that such reactions are expected and will resolve with time.

The survivor will need to accept the reality of the loss in order to deal with its emotional impact. It is vital that they have time to talk about the dead person so that they can identify and express their feelings. Anger and guilt are common emotions. Anger may be directed at the deceased, other family members, professionals involved in the patient's care, God, etc. Such anger needs ventilating. Depression may result from self-directed anger (guilt), thus it is important to check for clinical depression and suicidal ideas. Feelings of anxiety and helplessness may make the survivor feel unable to cope. Exploring the resources the bereaved person utilized before the loss will enable them to see that they can indeed cope. When sadness occurs the bereaved person needs to be given permission to cry.

The recently bereaved person needs to adjust to their new role. Major life-changing decisions in the immediate bereavement period should be actively discouraged. As time passes a degree of emotional withdrawal from the deceased and the formation of new social contacts should be encouraged.

It is important to identify those who are likely to have a difficult bereavement since they are at risk of developing psychiatric illness in the bereavement period (e.g. psychosis, clinical depression, extreme anxiety states). Some individuals may resort to alcohol, drugs, denial, idealization, etc., as a way of coping with loss. They should be referred early to the appropriate agency (psychiatrist, bereavement counsellor, etc.).

Important risk factors for abnormal bereavement reaction

Those at increased risk of difficult bereavement include those:

- With a close, dependent of ambivalent relationship
- Undergoing concurrent stress at the time of bereavement
- With memories of a 'bad' death (e.g. uncontrolled symptoms)
- Who have a perceived low level of support (the carer's perception is more important than the actual support in determining outcome)
- Experiencing strong feelings of guilt/reproach
- Unable to say goodbye, who feel there are things left unsaid (e.g. sudden or traumatic deaths or absence at the time of death).

FURTHER READING

Baines M, Oliver D J, Carter R L 1985 Medical management of intestinal obstruction in patients with advanced malignant disease: a clinical and pathological study. Lancet ii: 990–993

Directory of Hospice and Palliative Care Services in the United Kingdom and Republic of Ireland. 1995 Hospice Information Service, St Christopher's Hospice, London

Doyle D, Hanks W C, Macdonald N 1993 Oxford textbook of palliative medicine. Oxford University Press, Oxford

Maguire P, Faulkner A 1988a Communication with cancer patients: 1. Handling bad news and difficult questions. British Medical Journal 297: 907–909

Maguire P, Faulkner A 1988b Communication with cancer patients: 2 Handling uncertainty, collusion and denial. British Medical Journal 297: 972–974

Parkes C M 1972 Bereavement: studies of grief in adult life. Tavistock and Pelican, London; International Universities Press, New York

Regnard C, Davies A 1986 A guide to symptom relief in advanced cancer. Haigh & Hochland, Manchester

Stedeford A 1985 Facing death. Heinemann, London

Twycross R G 1994 Pain relief in advanced cancer. Churchill Livingstone, Edinburgh

Twycross R G, Lack S A 1986 Control of alimentary symptoms in far advanced cancer. Churchill Livingstone, Edinburgh

Twycross R G, Lack S A 1990 Therapeutics in terminal cancer, 2nd edn. Churchill Livingstone, Edinburgh

General considerations

35. Critical reading of the literature

R. M. Kirk

Even as late as the turn of the twentieth century many surgeons could learn from their masters and thereafter add to their knowledge only as a result of experience.

The rate of change of surgical practice has gradually increased so that now it would be considered negligent for a surgeon to fail to keep up to date with the literature.

Textbooks are in part out of date before they are published, since the time from writing to being put on sale is often 2 years. Some annuals contain reviews of the literature contributed by experts in the field. They offer a digest of many papers, interpreted by a single, albeit authoritative, author.

In each subject there are a few 'core' journals which publish important papers that have been refereed by at least two experts. Competition to publish in these prestigious journals is severe, so the editors are able to select only the best articles. As a rule the research or investigation that has led to the publication has been well authenticated. Many of us accept without question the findings and conclusions of the articles we read in these journals. This is sometimes a dangerous assumption.

LOGIC OF SCIENCE

Advances in science are made in many ways and by many different people. There are no identifiable characteristics of successful originators of discoveries. Very often advances result from attempts to solve a problem. Sometimes, in a blinding flash, an idea strikes out of the blue. Ideas bounced between people working in the same or different fields may be productive. Louis Pasteur stated, '*Dans les champs, le hasard ne favorise que les espris préparé*' ('In the field of observation, chance favours only the prepared minds'). This emphasized the fact that many of us have the opportunity to make discoveries but may fail to recognize them unless we are receptive. Those of us engaged in any form of medical practice meet unusual circumstances, but only a few pick up those that give fresh insights.

Chance observations, juxtaposition of circumstances that suggest an association, and attempts to solve problems may throw up questions. These may stimulate provisional solutions or possible methods of achieving them. Such suppositions are termed *hypotheses*. These need to be tested.

The great scientific philosopher, Sir Karl Popper, pointed out that it is not possible to prove a statement, but it is possible to disprove it. He used as an example a possible statement about the colour of swans. Most of the swans we see are white, and one might deduce that all swans are white. It is impossible to *prove* that all swans are white because it is impossible to be sure one has seen every swan. However, it is possible to disprove the hypothesis by merely seeing a single swan that is not white. And, of course, there are famous black swans on the Freemantle River in Western Australia.

Popper stated that an investigator who constructs a hypothesis should try to falsify it, not to prove it. If the hypothesis cannot be disproved, then it is reasonable to adopt it for use until a better hypothesis emerges or the present one proves to be fallacious.

Unfortunately, although we pay lip service to Popper's views, in practice they are rarely applied. Pick up any scientific journal and you will find the authors marshal their evidence to prove their hypothesis. It becomes the duty of readers to identify the defects in the evidence presented.

CONSTRUCTION OF SCIENTIFIC PAPERS

Scientific reports can be expressed in many ways. The famous Nobel prize winning discovery by Crick and Watson, that DNA exists as a double helix, was reported in a short letter to *Nature*.

However, when an investigation has been carried out, it is conventional to construct the report in a standardized way for easy reference. The article is traditionally now published in a journal that will be read by others interested in the subject. We scan the Contents list looking for articles of particular interest, read the summary of perhaps one or two, read excerpts of perhaps one, and from time to time avidly read every word of an article of particular interest.

Titles. This states as succinctly as possible what the paper is about. It is chosen so that key words can be included in the great American contribution to science, the *Index Medicus*. In this way, the work can be easily traced.

Summary. This should, as briefly as possible state what was done, what was found and the conclusion that was reached. In this way a reader scanning the journal, seeing the title, can quickly decide whether the work is sufficiently relevant to be worth reading further.

Introduction. This states why the work was done. It gives the background facts that define the question that the authors wish to answer.

Methods. This tells what was done, giving all the relevant information.

Results. These state what was found.

Discussion. What do the results mean? The discussion places the results in the context of previous work.

Conclusion. This is not essential if the summary is well expressed, but in some cases there is a need for an expansion or rearrangement of the end statement of the discussion, perhaps pointing the way to future work.

References. References to published work gives corroboration to statements made in the text that were not specifically investigated in the reported work.

CRITICAL READING

There is insufficient time to read every paper on any subject of interest and check the authenticity of the references. It is of great educational value to critically read an article on a topic of personal interest to you.

Introduction. This may start with the wrong premise, or one with which you do not agree. Read at least some of the papers referred to by the authors in constructing their hypothesis.

Method. The design of experiments and investigations may be poorly described. It is important that the authors give full information so that you can judge whether it is logical and well conducted.

Results. Do they provide full, reliable information on which you can base a judgement?

Discussion. Do the authors read more into their results than is justified by the findings?

WHAT DO YOU LEARN?

1. Most importantly you practice making up your own mind about the 'facts' that are presented to you on the basis of the evidence placed before you. You are not just a passive accepter of the opinions of others. This gives you the confidence to reject evidence you consider unreliable, and confidence in your own good sense rather than relying unthinkingly on 'experts'.

2. You may not know the fine points of statistics (see Ch. 36, but you can decide whether they have been properly applied. Too often, when reading statistical comparisons of like groups that we are told differ in one respect only, this is not so. Biological variation is so great that not too much can be read into small differences. Sometimes you can identify these. Ignoring differences between compared populations is often said to be, 'comparing apples with pears'. You may also detect imperfections in the way in which two populations have been compared. The clear demonstration of claimed 'prospective, double-blind', clinical trials is sometimes fudged. 'Follow-up' is used without making clear who carried it out and how it was performed. Sometimes the 'raw' data are not given but are displayed in an indirect manner in derived data or graphs, so you cannot see individual results.

3. When comparing diagnostic methods or treatments, authors may make erroneous claims that one is better than another. For example, earlier diagnosis and treatment of a malignant tumour may appear to improve life expectancy when compared with diagnosis and treatment at a later stage. In fact the progress of the disease may be unchanged and the apparent life-expectancy improvement following early treatment may represent the 'lead time' that it would take for an early tumour to develop to the stage it has reached when detected later.

4. Because it is usual for authors to provide only the evidence in support of their hypothesis (and contradictory evidence they can demolish), we rely upon independent investigations to support or challenge the findings and conclusions. Therefore do not accept uncritically a single paper, especially if it runs counter to the accepted view.

5. If you read the literature you will discover that the results of investigations do not always agree. By selectively quoting the literature, support for the authors' views can be corroborated. Always look for other articles on the subject that are not quoted by the authors.

6. During your career you will see patients with unusual, perhaps unique, conditions. If you have kept up with your reading you may recognize those that should be investigated or reported to your colleagues. Your familiarity with the surgical literature will have prepared you for creating a logically argued and acceptable publication.

36. Numeracy in surgical biology and surgical practice

H. Dudley   J. Ludbrook

This chapter was said by one of the editors to be 'hard going', particularly for those whose first language is not English. We consider this not so much to be a matter of vocabulary and comprehension but of *attitude*: surgeons, for the most part, have not been brought up to think in numerical terms. It is time that they were and we are fairly unrepentant because all the content is at elementary level and is, we think, essential knowledge for what James Calnan has called the contemporary 'alert' surgeon. By this we take him to mean someone who brings a critical intellect to what goes on in the surgical world and wishes to have some knowledge of how to handle numbers so as to:

- Understand what is meant by such terms as *probable* or *likely*
- Assess data quoted in articles or textbooks for their veracity and relevance
- Follow the process of diagnosis
- Participate intelligently in clinical experiments – including clinical trials.

We consider that it is inappropriate in modern clinical practice for any clinician to leave the above matters, and especially the analysis of raw data derived from experiment, entirely to a statistician to produce descriptions and interpretations out of a hat (more usually a computer these days, but the magical element tends to persist). Nor is it safe to use computer packages for calculation or to reach a diagnosis without having some understanding of their basis. It is not necessary for the surgeon to have detailed knowledge of a wide range of statistical tests, but some quite simple principles are as much a part of clinical education as are learning to use a knife or dissecting forceps with skill.

We have to admit that making the contents of this chapter into *examinable* material is not easy. In consequence we must frankly admit that, though we believe it to be of great importance, the candidate for any examination which tests *surgery in general* is fairly unlikely to be questioned on these matters in the immediate future.

We have to appeal to the student of surgery to read, learn and inwardly digest what follows as part of their duty to modern surgical practice rather than because it will be essential to surmount the next assessment hurdle.

CLINICAL STATISTICS

Our definition is the knowledge required to take a reasoned approach to *data* derived either by merely collecting information in the field or by designing an experiment to study a defined area. There are two components of this process.

Description pools a varying number of observations into what might be called a 'statistical shorthand'. We look in the data that we have in order to find some measure of the *central tendency* (e.g. an average) of a group or series of observations such as height or metabolic rate. In addition, we calculate a measure of the *dispersion* of the individual values around the central figure (e.g. standard deviation (see p. 352) or range). Descriptions of these kinds may allow us to make some simple inferences, say about the usual or average height in the British, weight in Australians or metabolic rate in Bantus, depending where our measurements have come from. As we shall see, measures of dispersion also allow us to say how often an observed difference from the average might occur; this is often the first step in analysis.

Analysis takes three main forms. Firstly, *comparison* which is the principle behind most simple statistical testing when, for example, we compare two groups of patients undergoing colonic surgery one of whom has had antibiotic M and the other antibiotic N to try to prevent wound infection. If valid inferences are to be drawn, strict rules govern such comparisons. Secondly, analysis can *break down the variability* between observations into its components – such as that which may be the result of measurement errors and that which is truly a consequence of different treatments or different conditions to which patients are exposed. Third, the fate of a group or groups of individuals with a specific condition can be followed over time to assess the effects of different treatments or circumstances – generally known as *life table analysis*.

STATISTICAL INFERENCE

To draw conclusions from numerical observations involves two things. Firstly, it is very uncommon that, in making a numerical assessment, we can study all those *subjects* (the word is used in a general sense for patients, rats or laboratory measurements) which create the 'population' about which we want to make an inference. It is not easy to measure the height of every Briton, or the weight of every Australian. In consequence, we must take a *sample* from what we believe to be the population about which we want to draw conclusions. Obviously, any such sample must represent (that is have the same characteristics) as the population. Here is a circular argument: unless we know the characteristics of the population we cannot take a representative sample. But we do not know about it – that is why we are studying it. So the only hope is take what we believe is a *random sample*, that is one in which any individual in the population has an equal chance of being selected and, consequently, in which there is no bias towards, say, sex, age or any other characteristic. The detailed techniques for this are largely beyond this introductory account, but we will give some guidelines later (see p. 350).

Secondly, if we have to sample, then any inference we make about the population must be hedged around with a statement of uncertainty or probability of how our sample reflects the population. If we could have studied the whole population we would be certain about inferences – they would be 100% valid. The smaller the sample the less the chance that it necessarily predicts the behaviour of the population because, in spite of our intention of taking a random sample, we may perchance have more women than men in a proportion that is not found in the population, more old than young and so on. This leads on to a consideration of *probability*.

Probability

For our purpose, a definition is necessary, though if one gets too involved in the underlying theory this can be difficult to achieve. We use the term in day-to-day speech, yet it remains a somewhat elusive concept.

We can first of all define *mathematical or prior probability* which is a prediction based on what we know about a system. An example would be the toss of an unbiased coin: if we concede that it will never land on its edge, then it is right to say that, in a *long run* of tosses, it will come down on half the occasions heads and

the other half tails. This leads to a statement that the probability is 0.5 for a head and 0.5 for a tail. However, even with our prior understanding of the system, we cannot tell from that statement whether the next toss will be a tail or a head, and therefore when we talk about probability in practice we usually mean the quantifying of the occurrence of events over a long run of experiences. This is sometimes called *numerical or frequentist probability* and in our coin tossing example implies that if we toss a coin 100 times we would expect to get *roughly* 50 heads and 50 tails, though we might observe some slight imbalance unless we carried on our experiment to many thousand tosses. So when we say that the probability of an occurrence of a serum bilirubin concentration of 2.5 mg l^{-1} is 0.02, we are indicating that in a long series of observations this value will turn up 2 times in 100 samples taken from what we believe to be a healthy population. This has a bearing on the interpretation of laboratory results (see also Diagnosis, p. 359).

Such an approach to probability also applies to the interpretation of statistical analysis. The precise definition of probability used in this context is somewhat complicated, but an approximate one is that if we were to repeat an experiment 100 times we would not expect to get results the same as or more extreme than those observed to alter our interpretation on, say, more than five ($P = 0.05$) or more than one ($P = 0.01$) occasions. We will discuss later how we can transfer such a statistical statement into a biological one (see p. 358). (We should emphasize that this is an account under what is called the *population* model which can be challenged, but in this elementary introduction we disregard that problem.)

There are some simple rules about probability which we need to assume not only for statistical purposes but also when we consider diagnosis (see p. 359). Their logico-mathematical basis need not concern us. They are:

1. *The sum of independent probabilities must always equal 1.* Thus if we are thinking about three horses in a race one may have a probability of 0.5 of winning, one of 0.3 and one of 0.2 (always assuming that all three do not fall at the first fence, which in this calculation is given a probability of zero). Similarly for diseases. Given that there are three diagnostic possibilities only, then each will have a probability based on the evidence available, but their sum cannot equal more or less than one.

2. *The probability of the simultaneous occurrence of two or more independent events is the multiplicand of their separate probabilities.* The probability, on the basis of symptoms and clinical findings of my having an acute torsion of the testis (say 0.005) and acute appendicitis (say 0.2)

together as the cause of my right iliac fossa pain would be $0.005 \times 0.2 = 0.001$.

From the foregoing it is apparent that a major task of statistics is to quantify uncertainty in terms of probability values and that this is done against the framework of what will happen if we try out or experience over and over again.

HYPOTHESES AND THEIR EVALUATION

When we use statistical description of analysis we most usually have some expectation of what we are going to find – what sort of central tendency and dispersion or what degree, if any, of difference in a comparison. Statisticians and surgical biologists have a problem of communication because of the different ways they tend to set up their expectations or, to use the technical word, hypotheses. A biologist is usually interested in a comparison that is expected to yield a difference and *designs the experiment* accordingly, though in fairly rare circumstances disproval of a difference, say between the outcome of two operations, may be important. The statistician by contrast, *undertakes the analysis* using the concept of the *null hypothesis* – that is to say that the starting point is the assumption that a difference does *not* exist. There is of course nothing incompatible about the two approaches, but it does sometimes cause confusion in writings about statistical analysis.

If the null hypothesis is rendered unlikely by the results produced in an experiment and their analysis, then an *alternative hypothesis* must exist. In clinical work there is an advantage in distinguishing between a *specific* and a *non-specific hypothesis* as a challenge to the null one. To explain more precisely what is meant, let us take as our starting point the null hypothesis that there is no difference in final outcome in patients with breast cancer between those who, on the one hand, have a local excision and a 'watch' policy with later axillary dissection if indicated, and on the other hand those who have a routine axillary clearance. Our results might suggest that the null hypothesis is wrong and the non-specific alternative is then that one or other treatment is better (or worse). Before the study is done we could, if we wish, set up a more specific alternative that in practical terms we would only be interested in a difference of a given magnitude and/or direction because we would only alter treatment if there were clear indications that this would effect the lives of many women, and also perhaps alter the way resources are allocated. The non-specific alternative aims at an explanation in a biological sense; the specific alternative addresses the practical side of how we are going to proceed. Choosing between the two

objectives may be important in defining the size of the samples we have to take (see p. 350) as well as in the non-statistical sense of deciding what is really important for our patients and the health system in which we work. A decision on whether we are out to establish or refute a non-specific or a specific hypothesis is thus an important part of the design of any comparison.

PROBING THE TRUTH OF HYPOTHESES NUMBERS NEEDED

Because, as we have seen, a sample is almost always necessary, there is an element of uncertainty about our inferences in relation to the population from which we believe the sample has been taken. What we must now explore is how prepared we are to:

- Accept that the null hypothesis is true (a real difference does not exist) when our results suggest that it is false (a real difference does exist) and
- Fail to reject the null hypothesis when a difference does exist in nature but our experimental design has been unable to detect it.

We have already, in considering probability, implied the answer to the first. When we say our results can be interpreted that there are less than 5 chances in 100 repetitions of the experiment which will give us an answer we would interpret differently (though of course this does not mean exactly the same numerical answer), we are effectively rejecting the null hypothesis. Statisticians call this the α *probability* or the *probability of a type I error*. The conventional level is 0.05, but the stringency is determined by context. For example, it would not be satisfactory for interpretation of comparative data from two channels of data in an aircraft's blind landing system to accept that there would be 5 chances in 100 that they could safely disagree. Similarly, if we are going to base our clinical behaviour in a life-threatening problem or one with considerable morbidity on the outcome of some statistical comparison, then we might want to set our level of falsely rejecting conventional practice (the null hypothesis) at 1 chance in 100 or even 1 in 1000. To achieve this goal requires in many circumstances a larger sample, and so it is important in designing the experiment to decide what α probability we feel is necessary.

Our second statement is what Feinstein has termed 'the other side of statistical significance', i.e. failing to reject the null hypothesis when there is a difference really present. This is a *type II error* and the chance that we might commit it is known as the β *probability*. The bigger our samples, the more precisely they tend to define the underlying population and its variability and the more sensitive should be comparisons to detect a difference between subsamples. We can set (by mathematical techniques that do not need to concern us here) a β probability based on the importance of the difference we think may be there and of the need to detect it.

The ultimate thing needed to determine sample size is, if desired, to define a specific alternative hypothesis in terms of the size of the difference in which we are interested. If we want to reject the null hypothesis in favour only of a big difference, we may not need very large numbers to find out that we cannot achieve this. However, if we are interested in a very small difference, we may have to take large samples so as not to miss it.

POWER

We can conclude the foregoing discussion, and particularly that related to type II errors, by referring to what is currently an 'in word' – power. The power of an *investigation*, by which we mean the overall study, is its ability to avoid failing to find a difference which exists in nature. The power of a statistical *test* is its ability, given the size of the difference expected and the size of the required sample, to detect such a difference. Ideally, for both we would like the power to be 100%, but usually we have to settle for less. When statistical comparisons are designed, we need to make an estimate of power in both senses. Because power is a fairly intricate concept (and also so as to retain statistical respectability) we need also to obtain statistical advice. Though we must heed the latter, we must also recognize that it is not always enlightened by a clear understanding of the clinical problem, particularly in terms of the alternative hypothesis.

Given that we have followed the pathway outlined above and defined the size of a difference we are interested in (i.e. the alternative hypothesis) and the level of α and β that we will accept, then there are statistical techniques and tables which will give us the appropriate sample size. A 'guesstimate' of this kind is an essential preliminary to undertaking a comparison, especially in that it may show that the sample size is much larger than it is possible to achieve either from the pool of patients available or with the time and resources at your disposal.

In practice, the best way of not becoming too involved in statistical subtleties is to choose a problem for which a large difference is likely to be found on biological grounds, to make sure that it is possible to recruit a large sample, and to refine measurement so that it is as precise as possible. Then statistical analysis will either not be needed or will be simple to carry out and should provide an unequivocal answer.

SAMPLING

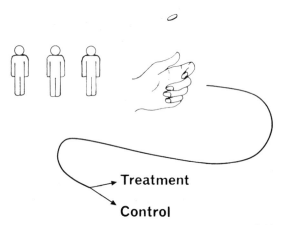

Fig. 36.1   Allocating to random treatment from an available queue of patients.

MORE ABOUT SAMPLING

We have defined 'random sampling' as taking a number of individuals from a population using some technique to ensure that each member of it has an equal chance of being chosen. We have also said that this is difficult if we do not know about the population. In clinical practice we often have to deal with an 'available' sample such as all Mr W's outpatients or Miss M's inpatients operated upon for a particular condition. Because of this we must be careful not to make inferences which draw the same conclusion about, say, Professor N's patients unless it can be shown that the last group is comparable in a large number of ways (such as age, sex and stage of disease) to the first group. Even then, it is wise to be cautious both in inference and in pooling Professor N's patients with those already studied (see Meta-analysis p. 357).

In clinical work we are more often interested in making what might be called an *internal comparison*. We have two antibiotic regimens proposed for the prophylaxis of wound infection. Which is the better? For this purpose we take all the patients at our disposal and randomize them to receive one or other agent (Fig. 36.1). We are then creating two random *subsamples* in which we expect all characteristics of the series of patients that we have at our disposal to occur with approximately equal frequency so that we do not introduce extraneous factors which might alter outcome in one way or another. Two such subsamples is the simplest, but in theory we could have any number. The process of random allocation into subsamples can be done using a table of random numbers (e.g. an odd number assigns to one subsample and an even to the other) a computer random-number generator, envelopes drawn from a prepared pack or odd–even birth dates. Alternate allocation is *not* random.

Finally, we must note that an internal comparison of the kind we have described means that we can only make *direct* and *valid* inferences about the study subsamples. The same restraints apply to generalizing the information to all patients treated in the same way. We consider this matter in more detail below (p. 358).

SCALES OF MEASUREMENT AND THE CHOICE OF STATISTICAL DESCRIPTIONS AND COMPARISONS

Measurement is essential to our understanding of the physical–scientific world. We can, somewhat arbitrarily, distinguish three scales (Fig. 36.2): *nominal* or *categorical*, such as male/female (Fig. 36.2a); *ordinal*, where we can state a difference but not its precise magnitude, such as taller/shorter or lighter/heavier (Fig. 36.2b); and *interval*, when we refer what we measure to an established scale, such as a metre stick or a weighing machine usually with equal intervals specifying its points but, in its ideal form, continuous (Fig. 36.2c). It is obvious that our arbitrary scales shade into one another. Male may be male and female may be female, but intermediate forms exist; black is black and white is white, but we all recognize grey. Continuing the analogy, we recognize spectral colours in a rainbow but we can define light more precisely in terms of wavelength, although, even here, as with all interval measures, how precisely we do so is determined by the instruments we have available. The scale against which a measurement is made has a considerable effect on both statistical description and analysis.

Categorical scales lead to descriptions which are usually expressed as proportions or ratios. Proportions can lose a lot of their meaning if they are carried to absurdity – for example when we say that for every female on the waiting list for hernia surgery there are 3.35 males. What we may ask is: 0.35 of a male?

For statistical comparison of proportions, the tests used are usually based mathematically on the binomial theorem. The two commonest are the χ^2 *(chi-squared statistic)* and *Fisher's exact test* (see Box 36.1). The latter is only called 'exact' because it gives a precise value for *P*, not because it yields more penetrating analysis of the data.

Ordinal scales tell us the position of individual values in the rank of all the measurements made – any value (except those at the two extremes) is greater than, less than or equal to some other. For description we can use the rank order to determine the central value, which is known as the *median*. In an odd-numbered series

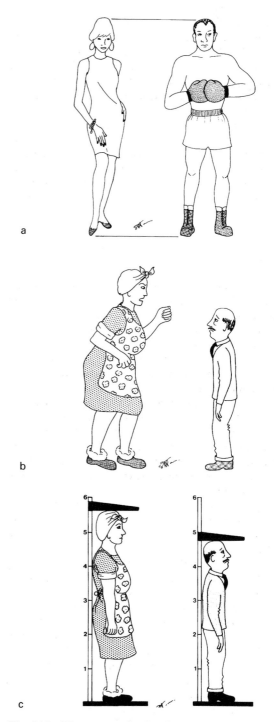

Fig. 36.2 The concept of scales of measurement: (a) categorical – male and female; (b) ordinal – I am bigger than you; (c) interval – I am 5 ft 9 in., you are 4 ft 10 in.

Box 36.1

A 2 × 2 table for two different methods of managing a condition (often called a *contingency table*) reads as follows:

Treatment	Outcome		
	Death	Survival	Total
A	41	216	257
B	64	180	244
	105	396	501

What is the probability that A (mortality 41 out of 257 = 16%) is better than B (mortality 64 out of 244 = 26%)?

The statistic to calculate for this compares the *observed* values (O) with those *expected* (E) if there was no difference between A and B. For example, the expected value for deaths under treatment A is:

$$\frac{\text{Total deaths (105)}}{\text{Total patients (501)}} \times \text{Total treated by A (257)}$$

This is 54 so we have a difference of (41 − 54) = − 13 between the observed and expected values. To be able to manipulate negative values we square them to get rid of the negative sign. Then we express the difference as a ratio between observed and expected:

$$\frac{(O - E)^2}{E}$$

or

$$\frac{(41 - 54)^2}{54} = 0.313$$

It is clear that the bigger the discrepancy between the observed and expected values, the bigger the statistic is going to be.

We make this calculation for each cell in the table and add the results together. Statisticians have calculated the chance (probability) of values for this statistic (χ^2) occurring by chance and we can read these off from a table. For example, (χ^2) for the table given above is 7.37 (using a slightly more sophisticated method of calculation which includes a correction factor), for which $P < 0.0066$. On statistical grounds, it is probable that treatment A will be associated with fewer deaths than Treatment B.

(Fisher's exact test gives $P = 0.0059$ for the same data. The choice between χ^2 or the Fisher test is somewhat subtle. Anyone interested can consult Ludbrook & Dudley (1994.)

the median is truly the middle number; for an even-numbered series it is defined as the average of the two central values. Dispersion of the values should strictly only be given by the range of the values from lowest to highest, but we can refine that by looking at the range which encloses a given proportion of the values observed (quartiles for example). Comparative analysis of ordinal data is best done with a method which compares rank order (see Box 36.2). Such tests (also often referred to as *non-parametric*) have the additional advantage that they do not make any assumptions about how the measurements are *distributed* in some underlying population from which the samples have been drawn, i.e. whether it is a normal distribution, a log–normal one or some other (rarer) form. In consequence, these tests are also often appropriate for comparisons of samples in which the measurements have been made on interval scales, but we cannot infer from this the way in which they are distributed in the population. However, it is important to remember that similar dispersions (scatter) of the values in the subsamples which are being compared *must* be present.

Interval scales permit the relatively precise assignment of a number to a measurement, and thus the use of arithmetic. The central value is the *average or mean* obtained by summing all the values and dividing by their number. Dispersion is obtained by squaring the deviations of the values from the mean (which gets rid of any negative signs), adding them together and again dividing by the number of observations (or, more precisely, in the case of a sample, by one less than this). This gives an 'average' value for the squared deviations about the mean in both directions and is known technically as the *variance*. The square root of the variance is the *standard deviation* (SD). If the dispersion of values around the mean is symmetrical we can draw either an approximate (for a sample) or an ideal curve (for a population) which is the familiar bell-shaped one for which one standard deviation from the mean embraces about 66% and two standard deviations about 95% of the values (see Box 36.3). The mathematics of this *normal curve* are well understood by statisticians, but not commonly (or necessarily) by surgeons. What we must note is that the word 'normal' has not quite the same sense as it does in biology (see p. 358).

A further descriptive measure of variation is the *standard error of the mean* (SEM) which is an estimate of the likely variation that would be found in the mean if the experiment was repeated many, many, times. Its value is found by taking the square root of the standard deviation divided by the number of observations in the sample. It is *not* a good measure for a description of the sample as a whole, and when investigators show SEMs in diagrams

Box 36.2

If we have two sets of data we can order them by rank using the convention: Low value = Lowest rank. We assign ranks to both sets in ascending order.

There are four possibilities (shown in the figure below):

1. All *x*s have a lower rank than all *y*s.
2. All *y*s have a lower rank than all *x*s.
3. The ranks of *x*s and *y*s alternate.
4. There is a 'mix' of ranks between the *x*s and the *y*s.

It is intuitively obvious that for (1) and (2) the *x* and the *y* samples are not likely to have come from the same population, whereas in (3) there is no way of denying on simple inspection that they might have done. In (4) there is some probability that they might be either from the same or from different populations and this can be determined mathematically from a knowledge of the sample size and the rank sum for one sample (which automatically determines the rank sum for the other). The values are read off against probability tables.

(For more detail see Siegel & Castellan (1988). For simplicity, in this explanation paired values in the *x* and *y* samples have been ignored.)

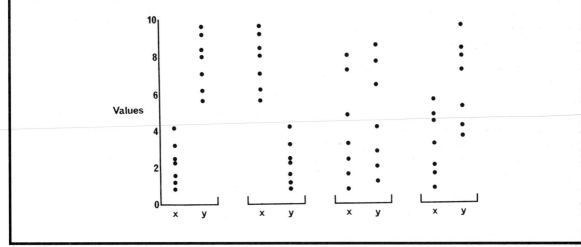

it usually means that they are trying to minimize what is in fact a wide dispersion of their results. However, the SEM has important uses in statistical tests and in relation to confidence intervals (see p. 352).

The analysis of data on an interval scale is often known as *parametric*, because the assumed population distribution is mathematically defined (*parametrized*). The normal distribution is the most common, but there are others, such as the binomial distribution. The normal distribution can be redrawn as one of 'probability density'. The maximum frequency of values in such a symmetrical distribution is at the mean, and therefore the mean is the 'most probable' value. Moving away from the mean the values get less frequent, so that by the time we reach 2 SDs the probability is down to 5 times in 100 (0.05) that this value will be found (see Box 36.3 for further details).

We are less often interested in determining the prob-

ability of a single value with respect to a mean than we are in comparing two sets (samples) of values to see if they are probably or improbably drawn from the same population (this is a precise statistical statement, but what we are really doing is seeing if they are different in some respect which would make it unlikely that, if that population existed, both would plausibly represent it). The principle is the same as that outlined in Box 36.3: a ratio is calculated which relates differences between the means of the samples and their dispersion (standard errors). The ratio will be large if there is a large difference between the means and/or a small standard error, and small if the reverse holds true. This is one form of the familiar *Student's 't'* statistic that crops up in so much biological work.

Analysis of variance (ANOVA), which gives a partition of the variability within and between samples, is based on a similar argument, but we will not go into this here.

Box 36.3

Two normal curves are shown. In the first is a set of values for the concentration of serum sodium in a large sample which we assume is biologically normal. The vertical lines are placed at one and two standard deviations from the mean (most frequent) value which in this instance is 135 mmol l^{-1}. Because of a mathematical relationship (which need not concern us here), one standard deviation on either side of the mean encloses approximately 66% of the values and two standard deviations enclose 95%. The two 'tails' shown as hatched areas thus each represent 2.5% of the population. The second figure shows this in graphical terms. Given a value of serum sodium concentration greater or less than the mean, we can compare it with the curve and say that it lies either within one, or two, or more standard deviations from the mean. We can then translate this into a probability statement to say that it has a probability of 0.33, 0.25, or less of being representative of the normal population.

Statisticians generalize this argument by transforming the curve so that it has a mean of zero and, as in the second figure, is charted in terms of an x axis expressed as standard deviations. It is then possible to calculate a *standardized deviate*, which is the ratio of the distance a value is from the mean to the standard deviation (the measure of the dispersion of all values). When the curve is expressed in this way we can assign a probability to the values of the standardized deviate obtained. For example, a value of 145 mmol l^{-1} would have a standardized deviate of 1.194, the probability of occurrence of which would be $P = 0.05$.

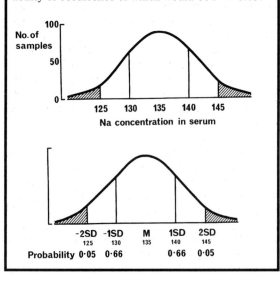

Na concentration in serum

Probability 0·05　0·66　　0·66　0·05

Note. The statistical expert will point out that nothing has been said about either 'estimates' or 'degrees of freedom'. These are technical statistical terms which govern probability calculations. Degrees of freedom are equivalent to the number of independent comparisons that can be made between items in a sample, which in turn is usually one less than the number of observations. Any deeper consideration is beyond the immediate needs of the surgical biologist.

OTHER FORMS OF ANALYSIS

Regression

It is sad that the general mathematics of statistics are beyond the comprehension of most of us because it is possible to derive nearly all the common analytical techniques which are used in clinical work by starting with regression. To be able to do so would simplify the whole matter of trying to understand statistical reasoning, because it would show that there is such a common and unified background. Anyone who is serious about more advanced statistical applications to clinical and biological work should attempt to grasp some of the theory of regression analysis, but most surgeons will probably be content with a nodding acquaintance.

Everyone is familiar with Cartesian coordinates (Fig. 36.3), and indeed they have already appeared in this account. A straight line drawn with reference to these can be described algebraically as a simple linear equation with three terms:

$$y = ax + b$$

which simply means that when $x = 0$, $y = $ b; and as x changes value so will y. In this sense the values of x and y are *co-related* and it is usual to say that y is the *dependent* variable. Of course a lot of biological relationships are

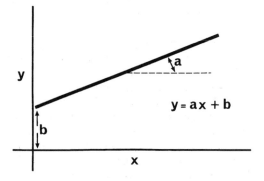

Fig. 36.3 Two-dimensional Cartesian coordinates: a, slope of the curve; b, intercept.

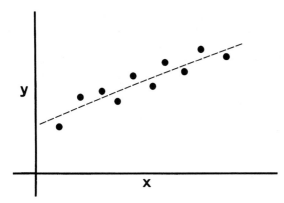

Fig. 36.4 A 'real-life' curve with the values to one or other side of the perfect line.

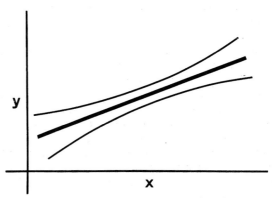

Fig. 36.5 Confidence limits for the data shown in Fig. 36.4. Values within the confidence limits have a given probability (usually 95% or 0.95 is the level chosen) of being part of the population described by the curve.

much more complicated than this, but the linear model is the one most important for statistical work.

The relationship described by the equation is an ideal one – the sort we might hope to get, for example, when we calibrate a measuring instrument; if it is a 'good' instrument, we get a series of values for y which correspond to known values of x so that a straight line can be drawn directly through them. However, in real life it is more usual to find (either because of the inaccuracies of the observations we make or because there are other 'disturbing' factors which affect the value of y) a plot which looks more like the one in Figure 36.4. There is still indubitably a relationship present – as x gets bigger so does y, but the relationship is now less precise. We can do four things with the data in Figure 36.4:

1. 'Fit' a straight line to it, which is done by finding the linear equation of a line that passes as close as possible to all the points. The mathematical way of doing this is to minimize the sums of the squares of deviations from the line, and for this reason the method is known as *least squares*. We will not give the details of the calculation – they can be found in any text on statistics, and computer programs are available to do the work for you.

2. Derive a statistic which gives some idea of how far from the line the individual values of y are and thus how much of the value of y can be ascribed to (or correlated with) the value of x. The usual statistic for this is the *correlation coefficient* (r) which, for mathematical reasons that do not concern us, ranges from $+1$ through 0 to -1. The correlation in Figure 36.3 is 1, and in figure 36.4 it is somewhat less than 1; if there is no relationship of the values of y to x then the coefficient is 0: and if it is -1 then the relationship is again perfect, but in this case as x gets bigger, y gets smaller.

Though the correlation coefficient has a distinguished statistical history, it is not a very good measure to apply except in carefully chosen circumstances, and for the statistically unsophisticated it may be frankly misleading. It does not give a *direct* estimate of the amount of variability of y that is related to change in x, though this can be obtained by squaring the coefficient. Thus a correlation coefficient of 0.5 means that a quarter of the variability of y is associated with x. Furthermore, it does not tell us anything about the *slope* of the regression line. Very precisely measured values of x and y may give us a coefficient which is highly significant (that is highly significantly different from 0) but in which there is only a very small change in y for a given change in x, and the result may therefore not be of much interest.

3. Predict a value of y from a value of x. How precisely this can be done depends on how tightly the observed values of y relate to the regression line, which also means how close to 1 is the correlation coefficient. We can get a numerical idea of this by calculating a confidence interval (usually that which encloses 95% of the possible values of y), shown as the curved lines in Figure 36.5. At the extremes of the range for measured xs these confidence lines get further away from the fitted line. The reason for this need not concern us – we need only consider the fact that the prediction of y from x becomes less and less precise.

4. If we have two different sets of data which purport to relate x and y, two regression lines can be drawn to see if either their slope or intercept are the same or different and calculate how likely this is the outcome of a real difference or could have arisen by chance. The difference can take two forms: differences in intercept and difference in slope. (The techniques can be found in Gardner & Altman (1989).)

So far this discussion has concentrated on the simplest

case of two-dimensional Cartesian coordinates. However, we do not need to stop there. We can easily envisage a three-dimensional system where the value of y is related to the value of two variables x and z; the point shown in Figure 36.6 is in the three-dimensional 'space' defined by the x, y and z coordinates. Going beyond this into four- or higher-dimensional spaces is not easy to visualize but is mathematically possible, and is the basis for forms of analysis which, for example, indicate how well the presence or absence of a disease or some measure of its severity is predicted by independent variables such as age, sex, smoking or life-styles. Such analysis can be done either with categorical or continuous variables.

CLINICAL TRIALS

Prospective randomized controlled clinical trials (PRCCTs)

These are a special case of statistical comparison. There is an established treatment (this can be either an operation or a drug) and a new way of managing a clinical situation. How do we decide whether to adopt the new or persist with the old? We set up an experiment so that by sampling as described on page 350 we create two random subsamples, one of which receives the standard treatment and the other the new one. The following factors must be considered carefully before such a study can be successful.

- A precisely defined outcome measure. Life or death, wound infection or no wound infection?
- How big a difference (alternative hypothesis) are we interested in? That is, how big a difference has there to be to alter our clinical behaviour?
- In consequence of the size of the difference we estimate may exist or in which we are interested, how

many patients will we have to study in order to minimize the risk of type I and type II errors? We regard it as both statistically and ethically improper to start a trial until this matter has been explored.

- Can we find and randomize that number of patients for our study?
- How 'blind' (by which is meant neither the patient, the investigator nor any assessor of outcome knows who has had what treatment) can we make the study? It is easy to blind both patient and investigator to a pill by having a dummy version to act as a placebo; it is much more difficult to blind a surgeon to which operation he does or the patient to whether or not an operation has been done.

Another important factor in surgical prospective randomized trials is what might be called 'technical efficiency'. Every surgeon knows that he/she is comfortable with a procedure which has been learnt well and done frequently, but less so with a new but potentially better technique. Initially the new procedure may be associated with difficulties and complications or may simply be unsuccessful (as with some surgeons' initial attempts to do various refined types of vagotomy or the radical resections recommended by some for gastric cancer). If a comparison is begun during the learning period, then the new procedure is very likely to be shown to be less satisfactory than the old. In consequence, comparative trials should not be set up until the 'learning curve' has been climbed. However, the difficulty is that if the start-up period makes both the patient and the surgeon feel that there are *perceived* advantages from the new, then mounting a randomized trial may prove impossible, because either the patient is reluctant to be recruited or the surgeon is hesitant to request permission. Recent examples are simple mastectomy versus local excision for breast cancer and laparoscopic versus open cholecystectomy. In such circumstances we may have to admit that the full rigour of a PRCCT is impossible and instead try to make careful, continuous assessment of results to see if they conform to our expectations and ideals (see Ch. 37).

A final point about PRCCTs is that they become progressively more difficult to mount as results improve and the end-point for comparison (e.g. wound infection, hernia recurrence or even death) gets less and less common. When wound infection rates are less than about 5% then it takes about 1000 patients to make a comparison between two techniques which might result in a further 3% reduction. This is often beyond available resources or alternatively it is impossible to keep all the other factors that might influence the outcome stable over the period required. Multicentre studies can help

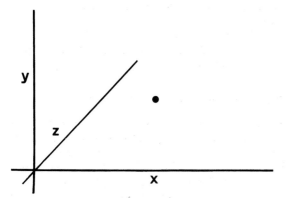

Fig. 36.6 Three dimensional Cartesian coordinates. A y value for a given value of x and z will be found somewhere in the space enclosed by the coordinates.

here, but they introduce their own problems. For all the above reasons, although they are powerful tools, PRCCTs have such limitations that they cannot be the only way that new knowledge comes to be applied to surgical management. They are often recommended or started without realizing their difficulties and drawbacks, and in consequence *some* reliance has still to be placed on careful objective observation and interpretation.

Survival analysis

Quite frequently in clinical practice we want to find out after something has been done to a patient what happens over the years – the influence, for example, of a treatment or a method of presentation on the outcome of patients with colorectal cancer. Ideally, we would like to operate on a very large number of patients all at the same time and then follow them up to see how many die on each day over the next 5 or 10 years. Usually this is impossible and patient numbers have to accumulate over time. We also, in that we all die sometime, have to compare the deaths that occur in our group with those that would occur anyway from other causes. We may further be interested in subsampling to compare two methods of management. All these give rise to statistical difficulties, though they can all be allowed for. Detailed accounts of life table analysis and follow-up are beyond this simple introduction and advice should *always* be taken before embarking on such a study, though the rules given for controlled clinical trials do apply. An example of a life table analysis is shown in Figure 36.7.

Meta-analysis

In recent years techniques have been developed in statistics which permit the pooling of results from individual studies and their reanalysis by statistical means. As we pointed out on page 350, there must be good grounds for feeling that the studies are biologically comparable – for example, the operations done for varicose veins by one group are technically the same as those done by another – there being no statistical way one can compare chalk with cheese. In addition, certain statistical rules must be observed and the new calculations must be done with methods which guard against overinterpretation. Finally, it is doubly important to express results in terms of 'confidence' which we discuss in more detail below. Though undoubtedly useful in trying to reach an overview or consensus on a new treatment, caution should be exercised in regarding meta-analysis as giving authoritative guidance to the clinician.

ALTERNATIVES TO PRCCTs

The controlled trial, as described on the previous pages, has become something of a central dogma of clinical comparison. This is in some ways a good thing because its widespread adoption has got rid of a great deal of cant, opinion and rigid adherence to out-moded practices. Nevertheless, though in many respects it remains the ideal, it is not always feasible, for the reasons we have already given. Are there any alternatives?

Historical controls

The use of past experience to compare with what is currently being done is always criticized because the 'background' may have changed from the past to the present: surgeons have become more skilled; the severity of the disease process under study may have changed; the population from which we draw samples has developed or lost some biological property such as immunity; and ancillary treatment (e.g. antibiotics, intensive care, nutrition) may more effectively support a new surgical procedure which is inherently no better or different from the old. All this is true, but even so it can be possible to draw some useful conclusions from comparison of the past with the present. Some rules which govern the use of historical controls are:

1. Stability of the population (its nature and the outcome of treatment) from which the samples have been taken over several periods of previous study. The data for this are often lacking.

2. Caution in drawing conclusions from the outcome of a comparison. A formal statistical comparison is *not* usually justified on technical grounds (though it is often undertaken), so that differences to which importance is ascribed must be large. There should be some collateral support from other studies or from scientific understanding of mechanisms for the inferences that are drawn.

3. Historically controlled studies which indicate a particular course of action should be confirmed by prospective analysis.

Prospective studies

The last observation serves as an introduction to the *controlled prospective study*. This is a potential intermediate stage between a retrospective analysis and a PRCCT. It is no good starting out on the latter until a 'baseline' has been established, that is until we really know what is happening *now*. For example, there is no point looking for an improvement in survival in the surgical treatment of colon cancer unless we know how

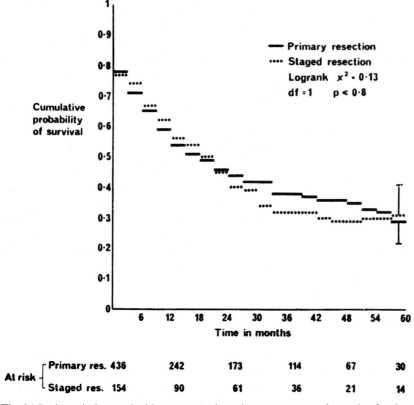

Fig. 36.7   A survival curve, in this case comparing primary versus staged resection for obstructing colon cancer. The curve has been constructed using what is known as the log-rank method. The horizontal bars at each probability level give the 95% confidence intervals. All these overlap.

good, or bad, the results are at the moment. Such studies in the real world can often direct us to critical points where improvements in surgical practice can be made without recourse to elaborate controlled comparisons. They can also have a valuable 'halo' effect (sometimes known as the 'Hawthorn effect' after the town in which it was first demonstrated) in improving clinical practice, because it is well known that concentrating attention on a particular area nearly always improves results. In the often confused, multivariable, circumstances of clinical practice, prospective studies with a recognition of their limitations still have an important place.

Scenarios

There is a new proposal for diagnosis or management – for example ultrasound or laparoscopy for the investigation of acute lower abdominal pain. In the scenario method, conventional management is taken to the point where the new technique would be used – in acute abdominal pain for example, after a full history and

clinical examination and perhaps a white cell count, a decision is made on how to proceed were the technique (say laparoscopy) not available (a scenario rather than what really happens). The technique is then applied and the extent to which it alters decision-making assessed. The scenario and real outcomes are compared both with each other and with the final outcome. Clearly this approach has a considerable subjective element, but it is an effective and economical way of first testing new ideas.

STATISTICAL AND BIOLOGICAL INFERENCE

The foregoing account has been based almost entirely on the idea that we use statistics to analyse date in order to prove or disprove a hypothesis at a predetermined level of probability. In a way this does not make very good sense in clinical practice, because we are then faced with a second decision: given that we have established that repetitions of our experiment or trial will come out differently only 5 times in 100, what in fact do we do with our next patient? Do we or do we not give the new treatment? The answer is that we usually do, but sometimes we can have more confidence in making a dichotomized decision of this kind if we look at the confidence intervals which surround the difference which we have shown. We are not in fact using any new statistical information in doing this, just altering our attitude towards how we study the results.

Confidence intervals give us the values on either side of a mean or median within which we can find a given proportion of the results of the population about which we have drawn a conclusion. (For their calculation see Gardner & Altman (1989).) It is usual to calculate the 95% intervals. If we take a simple example of the effect of two acid-reducing agents on maximal acid output, we might find the effects shown in Figure 36.8. In Figure 36.8a the mean of acid output with one agent is greater than that with the other and the difference is significant at the $P < 0.05$ level using a t-test. However, the 95% confidence levels overlap, and so we might find quite a number of subjects who got as good a result with either agent. If the confidence limits do not overlap, as in Figure 36.8b, then we would have greater confidence that the one agent was the better for us to use. In a sense, what confidence intervals tell us is the size of the mean difference and how widely the individual values are likely to be distributed around these means. Figure 36.7 shows how this method of display can also be applied to a life table.

Similar calculations can be done on ordinal and categorical data, so when, for example, we are comparing outcomes in terms of life and death, we can compare two survival curves and see if their 95% confidence intervals overlap or not.

STATISTICAL AND BIOLOGICAL SIGNIFICANCE

Statistics is full of pitfalls about meaning. One of them involves the use of the word 'significance'. The previous pages have given its *statistical* meaning – it is the probability value assigned to the occurrence of events in a long run of 'trials' such as coin tossing, or the outcomes

of a repeatedly performed surgical operation, or 'comparisons' such as the relative efficacy of two antibiotics. It tells us about *chance* or *likelihood* (though the latter word is sometimes used with a more specialized meaning we need not consider here). It does *not* tell us anything about the nature or magnitude of any difference we may observe. So when we say a difference is 'highly significant' or 'very highly significant' this just means that the outcome is less and less likely to have arisen by chance and not that it is bigger or more important. As we have seen, the same is true for the correlation coefficient (see p. 355). Of course a highly significant result may be important when our prime interest is not to do something which may turn out to be wrong – we have already given the example of a blind landing system (p. 349) – but this is not usually our objective in clinical practice. So in studying results we should be more interested in the size of the difference we observe and in the confidence which surrounds our measures.

DIAGNOSIS

Much of the interest in this matter has been the result of pioneer work by surgeons and is especially relevant to their work. By diagnosis we mean either the definition of a pathological entity such as acute appendicitis or the choice of a management option such as how to proceed in further investigation of acute lower abdominal pain – should it be by another investigation or by opening the abdomen? Clinical surgery and medicine have tended to concentrate on the former, in spite of the recognition in some areas that the latter can be more important for the welfare of the patient. 'Better to look and see rather than wait and see' is an example of taking a management decision without having a clinicopathological diagnosis and, until recently, was rightly given priority over reaching a precise diagnosis in the management of the acute abdomen.

We can distinguish three interrelated methods by which diagnoses are made.

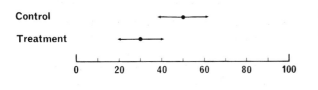

a

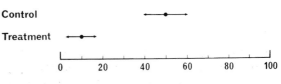

b

Fig. 36.8 Confidence intervals. Hypothetical values for a difference in mean between two methods of acid reduction. In (a) there is overlap of the 95% confidence intervals; in (b) there is not.

Pattern recognition

This is probably the commonest way of both teaching diagnostic technique and of proceeding in clinical practice. It is the basis on which virtually all textbooks have been written since the Aphorisms of Hippocrates which, in effect, are largely descriptions of patterns. If we have the 'running together' (the literal meaning of *syndrome*) of central abdominal pain, followed by pain, tenderness and guarding in the right iliac fossa, we say that this is the 'pattern' of acute appendicitis, just as a flat surface supported by four legs is the pattern of a table. The pattern does not need to be complete for us to make the inference that it is there; for example, no central pain, which is not uncommon in the elderly if the appendix infarcts early in the course of the episode, or no tenderness and guarding if the organ is in the pelvis. Similarly, if we see a drawing of a table with a leg missing, we would still be likely to infer that a table is what is meant to be depicted. However, the more items that are absent from the pattern the less confidence that can be put in our statement that *this* is appendicitis or *that* is a table. As we have seen in the section on probability, confidence and probability are closely related, and in recognition of an incomplete pattern we are saying: 'given such and such items of history and clinical examination (perhaps supplemented by certain tests) appendicitis is *probably* present'.

Bayesian reasoning

What we have just discussed (the probable presence of a pattern) leads to the second method of making a diagnosis, which is based on a further term in probability: *conditional probability*. If there is a population of N patients, n of whom have appendicitis at any one time, then if we were to draw a patient from that population the probability that he or she has appendicitis is

$$P_A = \frac{n}{N}$$

However, if instead of just drawing a patient at random we looked only at patients with acute abdominal pain, we should expect to find a different and somewhat higher probability which is the *conditional probability* of the patient having acute appendicitis given that he or she also has acute abdominal pain. There are a variety of ways that this can be written, but the usual one is $P_{A|S}$, where we have used S to indicate the symptom of acute abdominal pain.

Can we make use of this? The answer is 'yes', given that we have studied the population in the past for this symptom and its relation to the disease processes in which we are interested. A prior study of the population tells us how often acute abdominal pain occurs in acute appendicitis and how often it is found in the same population without acute appendicitis being present or, what amounts to the same thing when other disorders are present. Then we can write the equation:

$$P_{A|S} = \frac{P_{S|A} \times P_A}{P_S}$$

The more often acute abdominal pain without appendicitis is found in the population the smaller will be the probability of acute appendicitis given acute abdominal pain, in accordance with the probability axioms given on page 348.

On its own this does not appear to add very much, but do not forget that we can add probabilities; we can easily sum the probability of acute appendicitis given acute abdominal pain, to the probability of appendicitis given pain in the right iliac fossa, the probability of acute appendicitis given tenderness in the right iliac fossa, and so on. Therefore, for an individual patient we can develop a probability value given any combination of symptoms and signs.

Calculations of this kind, which are known as 'Bayesian' after the English divine who first tentatively described them, are mathematically trivial but arithmetically tedious so that they are usually done on a computer. They have been tested extensively in such conditions as acute abdominal pain, back pain and dyspepsia. In the first they give an order of probabilities that is more precise than unaided clinical evaluation, particularly by the inexperienced.

Bayesian techniques are most useful in:

- Ensuring that data about the patient are properly gathered, because the computer forces the clinician to be precise
- Providing assistance to the clinician rather than taking over the diagnostic role; such assistance can also help *teach*.

Sequential reasoning

The third diagnostic technique that has achieved a good deal of prominence is *sequential reasoning*. Psychologists have established that we can only consider a small number of items at a time (unlike the computer using Bayesian methods) – not more than five or six. In such circumstances it is necessary to make a decision having considered these items and then to go on to consider more information or, what amounts to the same thing, take some course of action. For example, having put abdominal pain and tenderness and guarding in the right

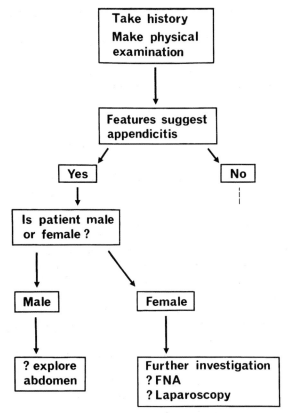

Fig. 36.9 A sequential decision chart (see text for full explanation). FNA = fine needle aspiration

iliac fossa together to arrive at the conclusion that there is lower right quadrant peritoneal irritation, we might then say: 'Is the patient male or female?' If the answer is 'male' we might be prepared to explore the right iliac fossa; if it is 'female', and because of the more frequent occurrence of other causes, we might seek further evidence from an ultrasound examination or laparoscopy. This is an example of *binary decision-making* (yes/no, go/no go) and can be built up into quite complex trees or algorithms (see Fig. 36.9). Algorithms are useful for sorting out how to make decisions in complicated circumstances and also for teaching purposes; they prove less satisfactory at the bedside. However, in the future they may form one basis for *expert systems*, in which knowledge is incorporated into a computer program to give an output which advises the clinician what should, on the basis of the evidence, be done next. A number of such systems have already been developed to deal with specific circumstances such as the prescription of antibiotics and, more recently, for the diagnosis of acute abdominal pain.

It should be clear from the foregoing that the three main methods by which we reach a diagnosis are interrelated. Pattern recognition can sometimes, when the pattern is incomplete, be based on probabilities of association. Bayes' theorem is a numerical way of creating a pattern of probabilities. Sequential reasoning takes a few items of a pattern, works on these and arrives at a binary decision (do this or do that) which, though it appears exact, is more often than not probabilistic (probably better to do this than to do that).

ANALYSING DIAGNOSTIC TESTS

It is now common to analyse tests made to determine the presence or absence of a given condition (or, more accurately, for their ability to predict the presence or absence of a condition) in terms of their *sensitivity* and *specificity*. Many surgeons (including the writers) find this fairly confusing, so an example is given in Box 36.4. For simplicity, the example considers only a categorical variable (one in which the outcome is yes/no or positive/negative). In reality, we can set 'cut-off' points for most tests which are on interval scales.

If a test is to be of clinical value it should have high values (see Box 36.4) for sensitivity (few false-negative outcomes) and specificity (few false-positive outcomes). In our example with a cut-off at $50\,000$ RBC ml^{-1} we are not going to have many false-positive outcomes but we may well have some false-negative ones because of lightly bleeding, but nevertheless serious, lesions about which something should be done. If we change the cut-off to $25\,000$ RBC ml then there are more false-positive but fewer false-negative outcomes.

CATEGORIZING DISEASE

On page 351 *et seq.* we considered the various forms of scales. For many years, clinicians and others have used either categorical or ordinal scales to classify disease. Early attempts to stage breast cancer are an example of what amounts to a categorical scale (the axilla is involved or it is not). However, ordinal scales with 'more' meaning 'worse' or 'more advanced' soon superseded these, so that we have, for example, Duke's classification of colon cancer in which there were initially three stages based on histologically detectable tumour burden: confined to the mucosa (A); penetrating the bowel wall (B); and with lymph node metastases (C, sometimes subdivided further into C(I) and C(II) according to the extent of involvement).

The utility of such classifications relates to how they can predict the behaviour of the disease process, and this is reflected in the way in which they are derived.

Box 36.4
Sensitivity and specificity

100 patients with suspected abdominal trauma undergo peritoneal lavage. A cut-off point of positive is selected at 50 000 red blood cells (RBC) per ml. All patients have an end-point confirmation by laparotomy, autopsy or a benign course without intervention. The results are:

	No. RBC/ml lavage	
	>50 000	<50 000
Laparotomy truly needed	90	10
Laparotomy truly *not* needed	20	80

False negatives = 10 out of 100, so that

Sensitivity = 90%

False positives = 20 out of 100, so that

Specificity = 80%

We can 'move the goal posts' by lowering the cut-off point to 25 000 RBC/ml.

	No. RBC/ml of lavage	
	>25 000	<25 000
Laparotomy truly needed	95	5
Laparotomy truly *not* needed	40	60

False negatives = 5 out of a 100, so that

Sensitivity = 95%

False positives = 40 out of a 100, so that

Specificity = 60%

On general grounds these figures show that the more sensitive the test the less its specificity.

There may be at the outset enough knowledge of the disease and its features that we can compare these with outcome; alternatively, we may take what is initially an arbitrary but rational fact or set of facts which are then tested on a series of patients against some end-point such as death. These processes form part of a circle (Fig.

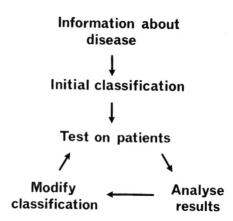

Fig. 36.10   How disease is categorized.

36.10) so that an initially fairly rough classification is refined to improve its predictive value. Thus, though Duke's staging works quite well to predict outcome, adding histological evidence of lymphatic permeation improves its predictive value, as does grading the tumour. However, the factors that go to make up the classification may not be wholly independent – for example undifferentiated tumours are more likely to have lymph node metastases. Some of the techniques of regression analysis (see p. 354) can be used to find out if factors included in a staging of a disease are independent or not, and this technique is now widely applied to establish what it is useful to measure as independent predictors.

As with other uses of measurement in clinical medicine, it is always conceivable that being able to base a classification or staging on an *interval* rather than a categorical or ordinal scale might increase its precision. One of the first successful attempts to do this was when the Birmingham Accident Hospital surgeons used their records to construct a table (more accurately a matrix) which related age and the extent of a burn to the probability of survival. This, at the time it was constructed, clearly told the clinician that, below and above certain ages, burns of a given percentage were not survivable (had a probability of death of 1) and, therefore, that treatment should be directed to palliation only. More recently, a similar approach has been used to develop *scores* for individual situations (trauma, sepsis, severe illness; e.g. the APACHE II score, see Ch. 2). A number of items of data are pooled with or without being given some weighting factor to give them more or less relative importance, and a total score is produced by adding the values for the items together. What weight is given to an individual item is derived from a study of the predictive value of each alone or in combination. This is best undertaken by using regression analysis on a sample of patients with the condition under consideration and an outcome such as death or complications being the dependent variable. As more information becomes available and the size of the sample increases, these values can be modified and the score updated for its predictive capability.

Classifications and scores are very useful in giving us an overview of complex processes, but it must be emphasized very firmly that they have some limitations. Firstly, the score is only as good as the data that go into it and an ill-defined condition studied by analysing only a small or heterogeneous sample will yield values for the score which have wide confidence intervals. Secondly, the figures produced give outcomes which are applicable to *groups* of patients. Thus if, using the old Birmingham burns figures, a 45-year-old male with a 50% burn had a probability of surviving of 0.5 this meant only that if 100 patients of this kind were studied in the future, 50 of them would die. It could not tell you *which* 50. Effort is usually directed to finding in numerical scores a 'cut-off' that will discriminate accurately between a favourable or unfavourable outcome, but the problem is the same as balancing the sensitivity and specificity of a test (see p. 362).

The third point is that a grade or score predicts what has been achieved in management *so far*. It does not necessarily imply that a measurement which predicts a high mortality should lead us to abandon our efforts. New techniques and their application by an enthusiastic team can shift outcome so that a previously bad prognostic score is no longer so. The Birmingham burns probabilities have had to be updated several times as treatment at all stages of severe burns has improved. It is for this reason that socio-economic decisions about *individuals* based on their classification or score should be made with great caution – if at all.

Quality-of-life (QOL) scores {often expressed as quality-of-life years (QLYs)} are a recent example of assigning a value to the outcome of a procedure based on a scoring technique which can then be used to decide which patients should have priority for treatment. For example, hip replacements produce a high value for a large number of QLYs and are therefore good value, while oesophagectomies for cancer are the reverse. Again, such techniques are of analytic value for groups but do not necessarily provide the way to base decisions on individuals in practice. (For those who would like to explore the basis of QOL measurement and its uncertainties a reference is given in the Further Reading section).

Though these are legitimate criticisms of classifications and scores, there is no doubt that they are useful in terms of giving us yardsticks by which we can compare treatment and attempt to single out groups of patients who will or will not benefit from our use of particular techniques. In complex circumstances where outcome is determined by the interplay of many factors, they supply an important 'handle' for more precise study.

SCREENING

Considerations of sensitivity and specificity for a diagnostic test relate directly to the subject of screening. It is widely assumed that if we can detect a disease process before it has led the patient to consult a doctor then the disease is likely to be at a pathologically earlier stage in its evolution and its effects on the patient thus less; it is, we can believe, more susceptible to cure. Though this assumption is probably too simple, it is the basis for screening, either to elicit symptoms which have not alerted the patient to the fact that there is something wrong (e.g. minor intermenstrual bleeding or a change in bowel habit) or to apply a test to a truly asymptomatic group (e.g. undertaking a cervical smear or looking for occult blood in the stool). Fundamental requirements for a screening programme are:

1. The condition for which screening is undertaken is treatable or, in the case of a possible genetic defect, can be pre-empted by some action such as a termination of pregnancy.

2. A *target* population is identifiable which contains the great majority, if not necessarily all, of those at risk. It is not likely to be valuable to screen patients under 45 years of age for occult blood in the stool, and it is a waste of time (and can possibly be dangerous) to undertake mammography to look for breast cancer in women under the age of 40 years. In neither instance is the disease which is being sought completely absent outside these age brackets, but in both it is so rare that it does not justify the work involved.

3. Resources are available to apply the screening technique. It is usual to distinguish between *programmed* and *opportunistic* screening. In the first, the target population which has been identified from prior epidemiological studies is approached and either invited or cajoled into taking part (e.g. cervical smears, stool occult blood, mammography). In the second, if patients present either for a routine examination/procedure or because they have a condition associated with screenable risk factors, the opportunity is taken to screen them (e.g. hypertension in patients undergoing hernia repair, hyperlipidaemia in patients with vascular disease).

4. Given that the condition can be identified by

screening, are the resources and techniques required to manage it also available? It is not very useful to find a possible carcinoma of the breast at mammography and then not to have the facilities for targeted biopsy freely available.

5. There must be a test (or a battery of tests) which have a reasonably high sensitivity and specificity for the condition. Low sensitivity will mean too many false negative results, thus negating the purpose of the screening programme. Low specificity (which as we have seen (p. 362) usually means high sensitivity) will result in a large number of patients being unnecessarily alarmed by the possibility that they have the disease; considerable resources may need to be expended to show that most of them are in the 'false-positive' zone.

Quite often, screening programmes are started without due consideration of the above points. Nevertheless, successful screening programmes for surgical disease are in progress (e.g. mammography for breast cancer and the search for positive occult blood in the stools to detect early colon cancer).

ASSESSING PUBLISHED WORK

Only practice and living in a critical professional atmosphere will enable the surgeon to acquire and sustain the ability to assess published work. However, there are some ground rules which can help make it easier to tell the adequate from the bad. In theory, bad work should not get published because of 'peer review' (the process by which papers submitted to journals are assessed by those who are supposed to know about their content and to possess rigorous standards of judgment about scientific worth). However, this system can let a lot of papers through which, when they are perused, require a critical eye from the reader. This section describes ways of looking at what is called the 'literature' which are applicable to the exit examination for a speciality, but are included here in that establishing good habits is part of training in surgery in general.

Hypothesis

Though straightforward, undirected observations (what social scientists have called 'abstract empiricism') still have a part to play in clinical science, most work that achieves publication is based on some sort of hypothesis; some of the rules that govern hypotheses have already been discussed. In addition, the reader of a paper should ask the following questions:

1. Is there a hypothesis at all? If not, are the observations of interest without one?

2. Is the hypothesis well formulated? By this is meant: Does it have a basis in science or in past experience, or is it just a wild speculation?

3. Is the work and the analysis based on a prospective (a priori) as distinct from a retrospective (a posteriori) hypothesis? The exploitation of a hypothesis is likely to lead to more meaningful conclusions if it is set up before any studies are made, simply because the collection of data or the conduct of an experiment will then be structured more adequately to test it. Thus the comparison of two methods of closure of the abdominal wall should, *before* the study begins, state the hypothesis (e.g. layered closure is better than mass), lay down criteria for the selection of patients, the difference which it is desired to detect and which is clinically important, and the process of randomization. The hypothesis is then a priori and the study is prospective. The alternative, which is frequently encountered in clinical practice, is to have used (perhaps at random, but usually not) different methods of closure in a surgical unit over a period of time and then come up with the hypothesis such as the one above and try to test it by looking back at outcome. Such an a posteriori hypothesis requires retrospective collection and analysis of information, and usually lacks the same rigour as a prospective study simply because the data have not been collected with the hypothesis in mind.

The same problems arise when data which have been collected to test one hypothesis are then reanalysed to test another one that was not originally part of the protocol or was perhaps even thought about when the study began. Neither of these circumstances is fatal to the possibility of getting some useful information out of a study (and statisticians have techniques for dealing with subsidiary or a posteriori analysis), but both should be looked upon with caution, particularly in terms of the inferences drawn by the authors. Though audit is a useful method of quality control (see Ch. 37), it can suffer from the same problem in that a priori decisions are not necessarily taken on the hypothesis of what special quality it is wished to control for.

Design and conduct of the experiment

1. Has the sample been adequately constructed and taken, and is it of sufficient size (see Sampling, p. 350)? Do the authors give any calculations of power?

2. Have the observations/experiments that follow from the hypothesis been adequately made? In these days of high-technology measurement, the investigative tools have to be taken largely on trust (though the referees who peer reviewed the paper should be able to assess

these), but some assessment of the sensitivity of the measurements for the desired purpose is always welcome, although often missing.

Results

Are the differences claimed by the authors of biological, as distinct from statistical, significance (see p. 358)

Introduction and discussion

Do these adequately review the past information? This question begs to a certain extent that of whether the reader is already familiar with the other work done in the field, but some clues can sometimes be gained from: the number of personal comments such as 'it is the author's personal conviction', 'our experience is' and 'we believe', all of which are evidence of special pleading; and if the reference list includes a large amount of self-quotation, this usually implies a selective and therefore biased approach to the analysis of other publications. The discussion should be firmly based on the work reported and correlated with similar work (if any) of others. It should state, either explicitly or implicitly, whether the expectations announced in the introduction (such as the confirmation or refutation of a hypothesis) were fulfilled. A long rambling discussion which includes an extended chain of inference such as 'we have shown *this* and if this means *that* and if at the same time we assume *something additional* then it is worthwhile *speculating* that *maybe* yet *another thing* follows'.

Such tenuous chains of reasoning are not usually quite so blatant as this, but they do tend to exist (often in an attempt to gain priority for new speculative ideas). They call into doubt the scientific clarity of the authors (as well, of course, as the critical faculties of peer reviewers and the editor of the journal in which it appears).

FURTHER READING

Explicable foundations of clinical statistics
Altman D G 1991 Practical statistics for medical research. Chapman & Hall, London [Easier than Berry & Armitage (see below) and excellent for the practising clinician]
Armitage P, Berry G 1994 Statistical methods in medical research, 3rd edn. Blackwell, Oxford. [Hard going but authoritative]
Campbell M J, Machin D 1990 Medical statistics. A commonsense approach. Wiley, Chichester
Gardner M J, Altman D G 1989 Statistics with confidence. British Medical Journal, London

Non-parametric methods
Siegel S, Castellan N J 1988 Non-parametric statistics for the behavioral sciences, 2nd edn. McGraw Hill, New York

Choice of tests for analysing contingency tables (see Box 36.1)
Ludbrook J, Dudley H 1994 Issues in biomedical statistics. Analysing 2 × 2 tables of frequencies. Australian and New Zealand Journal of Surgery 64: 780–787

Clinical trials
Friedman L M, Furberg C D, DeMets D L 1985 Fundamentals of clinical trials. John Wright, Boston

Diagnosis
Bradley G W 1993 Disease, diagnosis and decisions, Wiley, Chichester
de Dombal F T 1991 Diagnosis of acute abdominal pain. Churchill Livingstone, Edinburgh

Assessment of quality of life
Editorial 1995 Quality of life and clinical trials. Lancet **346**: 1–2

37. Audit

B. W. Ellis   J. Simpson

DEFINITIONS

Clinical audit is defined by the Department of Health (DoH) as: 'The systematic, critical analysis of the quality of medical care, including the procedures used for diagnosis and treatment, the use of resources, and the resulting outcome and quality of life for the patient', and states that 'an effective programme of medical audit will also help to· provide reassurance to doctors, their patients, and managers that the best quality of service is being achieved, having regard to the resources available' (DoH 1989). the efficient and effective use of resources is important (Ellis et al 1990), but it is not the first priority of clinical audit.

Clinical audit is the responsibility of clinicians and must be led by them (Standing Committee on Postgraduate Medical Education 1989). The terms 'clinical audit' and 'medical audit' are sometimes used interchangeably, but a consensus has developed whereby *medical audit* refers to the assessment by peer review of the medical care provided by the medical profession to the patient, and *clinical audit* refers to an assessment of the total care of the patient by nurses, professions allied to medicine (such as physiotherapists) as well as doctors. The multiprofessional team has an essential role in patient care and the quality of health care cannot be determined by doctors alone. Most hospitals have now focused their audit activity around clinical rather than medical audit.

A policy document setting out a strategy for moving towards multiprofessional clinical audit (Clinical Audit: Meeting and Improving Standards in Healthcare) was published by the DoH in 1993. A further booklet was issued outlining the practical measures needed to support this move (The Evolution of Clinical Audit) (DoH 1994). These two documents together provide a concise overview of the development of audit and its place in the organization and delivery of health care in England.

HISTORY AND BACKGROUND

While modern-day concepts of audit may be new to many, a critical appraisal of the care dispensed by clinicians is by no means new. There have been many examples of audit activity in a number of guises over the last few centuries. Our forefathers in surgery very often had no option but to learn by trial and error. The openness of their writing, especially in their descriptions of surgical disasters, makes fascinating reading when we can look back with the benefit of hindsight and with our current state of knowledge:

The patient had complete retention. I was induced at length to try forcible catheterization with a straight instrument – an operation which has been recommended by excellent surgeons, especially Dupytren. My attempt was unsuccessful; the instrument bent and did not penetrate the prostrate gland. Retroperitoneal infiltration of urine followed and the patient died. I do not advise anyone to follow my example. In such a case puncture of the bladder by the rectum would have been the proper proceeding [sic]. (Bilroth 1881)

Nor were these expositions confined to the anecdotal. In the same book, T. H. Bilroth, who was then Professor of Surgery in Vienna, noted:

Of 118 operations on the breast alone, eight were fatal; the cause of death in all cases being erysipelas. Of 187 operations on the breast and axillary glands, ... forty patients died from various causes; three deaths occurred from severe secondary haemorrhage, but many of the other cases, who were attacked with septicaemia, pyaemia or erysipelas had also haemorrhage from the axilla.

There then follows a critical appraisal of the various techniques of ligature of veins and the use of antiseptics and caustics.

The improvement in standards of care in surgery as a whole and in the practices of individual surgeons has, until recently, relied on the apprenticeship of the training years, and the dissemination of new learning and good practice through the medium of the book, the journal and the lecture by the 'expert'. Those who were prepared to listen and read were able to change practice where appropriate. Even now many surgeons rely on the annual meetings of the various 'craft' associations for education in current surgical practice.

The roots of modern audit lie in the regular morbidity and mortality meetings held in many hospitals in the UK and the USA in the 1950s and 1960s. The value of these meetings as a means of learning was recognized and formed the basis of broader audit activities.

In the early 1980s, microcomputers made their first appearance on the audit scene and this made it possible to collect and analyse large amounts of information very swiftly. This then gave the clinician a powerful tool to assist in the interpretation of types of work done, throughput and complications. Audit systems are now very powerful, and can rapidly highlight areas of high risk of complication, death, cost, etc. However, there is the danger that some surgeons believe ownership of an 'audit' system to be synonymous with the successful practice of audit. They must appreciate that such systems are merely tools with which we can get a grasp and some understanding of the activity for which we are responsible.

Every hospital in England is responsible for ensuring the development of clinical audit in which every doctor participates (DoH 1989). Whereas before, audit was practised on a voluntary basis, and thus predominantly by enthusiasts, it has now become compulsory and the requirement for audit is written into the job descriptions of all new medical staff. Managers must also be given clear evidence that effective audit is being practised.

From 1989 to 1994, central funding to support audit activity (for instance to employ audit support staff), was allocated directly to hospitals and other healthcare providers via Regional Health Authorities. However, audit is now seen as an integral part of clinical activity and is included as part of the contracting process, with the resources for audit included in purchasers general funding allocations.

ATTITUDES TO AUDIT

The clinician

Some will argue that medical audit is practised already; that ward rounds, clinical presentations, research and morbidity and mortality meetings fulfill this function. However, there are differences between these and medical audit. Medical audit must be seen as a systematic approach to the review of clinical care to highlight opportunities for improvement and to provide a mechanism for bringing them about. As such it endeavours to get away from the 'single interesting case' and look for patterns of care. There should also be a difference in emphasis in the type of case examined. Audit

should initiate investigation into those areas of clinical care that are considered as high risk, high cost, or very common. Audit investigation is also suitable for resolving issues of contention or local interest. The rare and clinically interesting case should be left for the clinical conference.

There remains a view held by many clinicians that the time spent on audit could be much better spent on other activities, such as treating more patients. This is not a wholly spurious argument; a recent evaluation of the audit programme by CASPE Research, while noting the significant achievement of the establishment of organized audit involving medical staff in virtually all healthcare providers, queried the extent to which *meaningful* change in practice had resulted (Buttery et al 1994). There is, nonetheless, general agreement that a regular review of his or her own practice by a clinician in the light of constructive criticism by one's peers can lead to improved delivery of care for the patient. It is important that we do not lose sight of the concept that the principal beneficiary of the process should be the patient.

The manager

With the implementation of purchaser/provider contracts from April 1991 there is now a need to specify the quality of the service provided and to link quality of care with quantity and cost. More explicit quality standards and outcome measures will be specified in contracts between health authorities (the purchasers) and their hospital (the providers). As part of their responsibility for the quality of care, managers will need to have confidence in the local audit programme and to share medical and clinical audit information with doctors and other professionals within agreed rules of confidentiality. Many deficiencies revealed by audit relate to the organization of care and managers' involvement, and commitment is essential to ensure the necessary changes.

The purchaser

Clinical audit should be a major part of the overall quality assurance that purchasers require of the hospitals with which they place contracts. Purchasers wish to know the arrangements for clinical audit, the level of participation by doctors and other professional staff, the topics examined and improvements generated. Clinicians should be directly involved in discussions with purchasers on issues of clinical quality, the content of the audit programme and the development of robust outcome measures.

Clinical decisions should be made, as far as possible, on research evidence of effectiveness. Clinicians are increasingly being asked to develop evidence-based guidelines for the delivery of care and to monitor their use through audit (see Criterion audit, p. 371). However, it is acknowledged that the freedom of clinicians to determine the treatment of individual patients must be preserved (DoH 1993b).

THE IMPLEMENTATION OF CHANGE

If audit is to be effective it must lead to change. Audit may be considered as a cycle, the first component of which is the observation of existing practice to establish what is actually happening. Then, standards of practice are set to define what ought to happen and a comparison made between observed practice with the standard. Finally, change is implemented. Clinical practice is observed again to see whether what has been planned has been achieved. A decision can then be made as to whether practice needs to change further, or whether the standards were unrealistic or unobtainable. This process has become known as the 'cycle of audit' (Royal College of Physicians 1989) and the achievement of change has been termed 'closing the audit loop'.

The provision of information on clinical activity, without any evaluation or suggestions for improvement, has been judged to have almost no effect on clinical practice (Mitchell et al 1985), unless it is targeted at decision-makers who had already agreed to review their practice (Mugford et al 1991). It was also judged to be most effective if presented close to the time of decision-making (Mugford et al 1991). The most commonly used approach, and one of the most effective, involves the publication of guidelines, in the form of notes to junior staff, the display of posters or notices and the redesign of forms or charts. Changes in behaviour may occur. However, these are much less effective when developed by external 'experts'. Involvement in the development of guidelines seems to enhance compliance (Anderson et al 1988). Guidelines need to be reviewed regularly to establish 'ownership' and to incorporate the latest research findings. If they are not valued, they will not be used. Finally, it has been noted that the act of investigating clinical decisions has itself brought about improvements in clinical practice (Gabbay et al 1990).

THE EDUCATIONAL COMPONENT

The educational benefits of clinical audit have been considered in depth by Batstone (1990). It is now seen as vital that doctors in training are taught the basic principles of audit. Equally, conclusions drawn from the audit process should be seen as an important feeder into education.

There can be little doubt that the critical review of current practice and comparisons against predefined standards encourages and acquisition and updating of knowledge. The audit process also enables the identification of key features of clinical practice which should help to make teaching more explicit. However, the evidence for the effectiveness of educational strategies on clinical practice is unclear (Mugford et al 1991).

Through audit, it is possible to identify particular areas where knowledge could be improved or is deficient, suggesting the need for research. Self-evaluation and peer review (common activities in audit) are important components of postgraduate education. In order fully to realize the educational potential of audit, it is essential that the lessons arising from previous audit meetings are reviewed, and the conclusions acted upon.

STAFF FOR AUDIT

Most hospitals in England now have an audit officer and/or audit coordinator. It is their task to enable the implementation of audit and to assist where possible in the execution of the audit process.

While much still rests on the clinical staff to prepare for audit exercises, the audit staff should be able to provide support in:

- Suggesting audit activities
- Helping to prepare audit programmes
- Helping to plan audit studies
- Literature searching
- Screening case records against clinically determined criteria
- Computer assistance with databases/graphics and forms
- Preparing audit reports.

COMMITTEES FOR AUDIT

Shortly after the introduction of the White Paper (DoH 1989), health districts set up district medical audit committees to oversee the implementation of audit and report to management. Now that health districts are in effect the 'purchasers' and the hospitals (either as trusts or directly managed units) 'providers', hospitals now have their own clinical audit committees reporting to their unit management.

An audit committee should draw members from a range of clinical backgrounds so that a wide perspective can be used in the planning of audit at a local level. The chairman needs to be well motivated and prepared to devote time on a regular basis to the task. There should be representation from the nursing profession, primary health care (general practice), education (usually the clinical tutor) and the doctors in the training grades, plus other clinical staff such as pharmacists and physiotherapists. The audit staff should also sit on the committee.

Hospital audit committees have the following functions. They must:

- Coordinate and foster clinical audit for everyone involved in patient care
- Attempt to minimize the perception that audit is a threat
- Highlight the benefits of the audit process for patients and the clinical staff
- Determine existing practice of audit
- Assist clinicians in the implementation of audit methods
- Monitor the results and conclusions of the audit process and check the validity of data and reporting
- Ensure that changes, where indicated by the outcome of audit, are implemented
- Ensure that the outcome of audit is perceived as educational and that doctors are educated in the practice and process of audit
- Train and direct audit officers
- Ensure effective liaison with GPs and management
- Maintain confidentiality
- Estimate funding required for audit
- Prepare annual report and forward programme.

ROYAL COLLEGE OF SURGEONS OF ENGLAND

The College has published guidance on audit: Clinical Audit in Surgical Practice (revised, 1995).

TECHNIQUES IN AUDIT

Donabedian (1966) identified three main elements in the delivery of health care: structure, process and outcome.

Structure. This includes the quantity and type of resources available and is generally easy to measure. It is not a good indicator of the quality of care but should be taken into account in the assessment of process and outcome.

Process. This is what is done to the patient. It includes consideration of the way an operation was performed, what medications were prescribed, the adequacy of notes, and compliance with consensus policies. There is an underlying assumption that the activities under review have been previously shown to produce an optimal medical outcome. This is the area of patient care that can be changed by education.

Outcome. This is the result of clinical intervention and may represent the success or failure of process. For example, outcome could be measured by studies of surgical fatality rates, incidence of complications, or patient satisfaction. It can be considered to be the most relevant indicator of patient care, but it is the most difficult to define and quantify. Mortality and length of stay in hospital are very easily measured outcome indicators, but variations in these outcomes are rarely related directly to the quality of the service being delivered. It may be more important to consider whether patients perceive that their problems have been solved, their quality of life improved and, where appropriate, the duration of their survival.

It is essential when planning an audit exercise to consider which of the above elements of care are being examined and how the changes in each might bring about improved patient care.

A number of audit techniques have evolved and found a place in the regular assessment of clinical practice. These are as follows.

Basic clinical audit. This entails an analysis of throughput, a broad analysis of case type, complications and morbidity and mortality. It is suggested that review of such data is undertaken by each clinical firm at intervals of approximately 3 months. Where possible, figures derived from the data should be contrasted with previous periods of time, other clinical firms, other hospitals or information derived from global audit (see below). There is a danger that this exercise can become a boring repetition of figures. The essential ingredient is to distil out of the data any notable deviations from an accepted 'norm' and then to investigate the reason for this observation. Hence the need for a comparative 'yardstick'.

Incident review. This involves the discussion of strategies to be adopted under certain clinical scenarios. An incident may be taken to be anything from a patient suffering from a leaking aortic aneurysm to the use of a department for an investigation (e.g. emergency intravenous urography). It is expected that such discussions would lead to clear policies for future use, and may result in the production of local guidelines. This audit method is particularly suitable for multidisciplinary or interdisciplinary audit.

Clinical record review. A member of another firm of the same or similar specialty is invited to review a random selection of case notes. Where possible, criteria should be established for this review purpose. Clinical record audit has the advantage of simplicity and requires relatively little additional time or other resources. However, there is a potential disadvantage in that discussion might concentrate too much on the quality of record keeping and not enough on patient care – these two are distinct facets of the clinical process, although related. In practice, a balance between these two components of audit might be encouraged by having the audit meetings chaired by a third clinician who is neither 'auditing' nor 'being audited'.

Criterion audit. This is an approach that can be considered as a more advanced and structured form of incident audit. Retrospective analysis of clinical records is made and judged against a number of carefully chosen criteria. These criteria should encapsulate the key elements in management of a particular topic which should be capable of unambiguous interpretation from the medical record by a non-medical audit assistant. All cases falling within the scope of the topic in question are screened and those that fail to meet any of the criteria are brought forward for further clinical review. The criteria may relate to administrative elements (e.g. waiting time), investigations ordered, treatments considered, outcome, follow-up strategies, etc. Criteria for adequate management of a particular condition can be easily derived from clinical guidelines, if these have been developed. Clinical time is necessary in the preliminary discussion, but the majority of the work can be done by audit assistants. It is applicable to a variety of circumstances and allows the comparison of data between different hospitals (Shaw 1989).

Adverse occurrence screening. A clinical firm decides on a shortlist of events that are worthy of avoidance (e.g. wound infections, unplanned readmissions, delay or error in diagnosis). Details of occurrences are recorded and complex or serious occurrences are reviewed by clinicians. A database is built up which can then be interrogated to identify trends, perform comparative analyses, etc. Cases can be selected by considering all admissions or a sample of them. This technique can also be used for risk management (Bennett & Walshe 1990).

Focused audit studies. Outcome from any other area of audit may dictate the need for a more closely focused area of research. Such a study comes close to an academic research exercise. However, it must always be kept in mind that audit, unlike research, will not lead to new clinical knowledge. Research aims to identify 'the right thing to do' while audit assesses whether 'the right thing has been done' and whether further improvement is required.

Global audit. In any one hospital the number of departments undertaking similar work is often very small. Even between two firms of general surgeons the case mix may be sufficiently different to negate the value of comparative audit. In other specialties there may not be anyone else in the hospital with whom to compare results. Global audit implies the collection of data and its comparison across units, health authorities and even through a whole region (Gruer et al 1986, Black 1991). In 1991, the Royal College of Surgeons set up a comparative audit service in which all surgeons are requested to supply information under a confidential number for comparison with their peers at regular meetings (Royal College of Surgeons 1991). Techniques in data presentation allow such sensitive information to be widely disseminated and discussed, while maintaining an individual clinician's confidentiality (Emberton et al 1991).

Outcome audit. Outcome will depend on the whole of the process of health-care delivery during a patient's episode in hospital and, as such, is a measure of the spectrum of the skills of the medical and nursing staff, the hospital administration and indeed, every person or department with whom the patient comes into contact. There will inevitably be a contrast between the perspectives on outcome between the patient, the GP and the clinician, and much work remains to be done to evolve satisfactory measures. Studies on outcome, especially in the surgical specialties, are likely to be seen as an important measure of the quality of care. The DoH has set up an 'Outcomes Clearing House', based at York University, to enable the dissemination of good practice in this area.

National studies. These were first used over a decade ago to address the question of perinatal mortality in obstetric units. The report of the first confidential enquiry into perioperative deaths (CEPOD) (Buck et al 1987) considered the factors involved in the deaths of patients who died within 30 days of surgery in three regional health authorities. Much was learnt from that exercise, especially the need for doctors in the training grades to be given adequate support and supervision. It was clear that disaster frequently arose when surgeons attempted procedures for which they possessed insufficient skill or training. The enquiry has since developed into a national review (NCEPOD), which publishes annual reports (Campling et al 1993).

ETHICS AND CONFIDENTIALITY

Information used in audit about patients must protect the confidentiality of individual patients and also that of the professionals involved. The audit committee must have clear guidelines on confidentiality. It is vital that there is a consistent policy on confidentiality, particularly where audit activities cross boundaries between specialties or professional disciplines.

With regard to patient confidentiality, the same principles are involved as in the clinical conferences which form part of any academic programme. The matter becomes more complex if professionals other than doctors are involved in audit. It is important to secure an undertaking from all those involved not to talk about what was discussed in an audit meeting outside that meeting. Unless an explicit and convincing case can be made for inclusion of identifying details of a patient in verbal or written presentations, such details should be excluded.

The confidentiality of the professionals involved also requires protection. This is likely to prove difficult in some types of audit, for example where one consultant reviews the clinical records of another consultant's patient. Nevertheless, this type of audit can be successful, provided that the necessary atmosphere of trust and collaboration is fostered. It is always necessary to obtain permission from all consultants involved before starting an audit exercise.

It is important to consider what should happen if audit reveals problems of deficiencies in a given individual's clinical practice. Such a situation is likely to occur infrequently, if at all, but this makes it the more important to anticipate such an eventuality and to make explicit provision for it (Ellis & Sensky 1991).

Ethical committee permission before interviewing patients is occasionally required, but this is usually a local requirement which needs to be checked. In general, audit projects need not involve ethical committees.

COMPUTERS

The past decade has seen a staggering evolution in computing. In the mid-1970s computers were rarely seen outside large corporations and research centres. They were large and difficult for all but the expert to use. Now, in the 1990s we have small, very portable 'notebook' machines the power of which easily matches a computer of two decades ago that would have filled a room. Current desktop and deskside machines are now more powerful than almost any computer of the early 1970s.

The surgical trainee should have a good working knowledge of the basics of computing. He or she should be capable of installing application programs onto a personal computer and have a working knowledge of a word processor, the principles of a spreadsheet and database and be familiar with the use of a graphics program and the graphical user interface found in today's multitasking environments such as Windows (Microsoft Ltd).

Many postgraduate medical centres now offer the use of a microcomputer for the production of graphics and for word processing. Some centres have also installed CD-ROM drives to enable enquiry on databases pub-lished in CD format. The best known, and most useful, medical publication in this format is MEDLINE. With regular update discs access to such a system will replace the need to search Index Medicus; furthermore computer-based searching is not only a great deal faster but it is also more comprehensive and permits searching in many different ways. For those trainees with access to a CD-ROM, a 'download' facility allows the export of selected papers with or without abstracts into a database on a personal computer. The Internet is also finding a place as a reference source including access to systematic reviews of the effectiveness of health-care interventions.

Computing skills are best acquired by practice on the computer itself. Books and manuals tend to get used only to solve problems. A number of programs are available as clinical information systems, which usually have outputs configured to help in the process of audit. Despite some pioneering ventures into the realms of clinical decision-making systems and artificial intelligence, there is still a great deal to be learnt about the clinical as opposed to the administrative capabilities of computing in medicine.

Hospital information systems

As personal computers have grown in power, so have the larger mini and mainframe computers. The role of large computers in hospitals in the UK is currently under review. The DoH has never been keen to prescribe solutions, and the result is that every hospital has the potential to find a different configuration of computer.

A few hospitals have a completely integrated 'hospital information system' covering every function from the recording of clinical data, the scheduling of clinics, to the provision of financial and manpower reports, etc. Such systems are very costly and, at present, not well developed in the UK.

At the other end of this computing spectrum are those hospitals which have a mainframe-type computer running a patient administration system (PAS), including the 'master index' (patients' demographic details) and records of admissions and diagnostic codes. This represents the minimum upon which a hospital manager can rely for information. PAS systems regularly pass aggregated information to a district information system (DIS); it is from the DIS that reports are usually generated.

In those hospitals with the latter configuration there are bound to be many departments which have implemented their own information systems. Surgeons may rely on proprietary clinical information systems, while the accident and emergency department is likely to have its own variant. Operating theatres and maternity departments frequently have departmental systems to help provide the reports necessary for management.

There may also be separate systems installed for manpower, finance, personnel, estates, etc. All of these departmental systems may be required to pass information onto other departments, and, in the context of integrated computer systems, are known as 'feeder systems'.

Current trends seem to favour the introduction of so-called case-mix systems. These pull together information from the clinically orientated feeder systems (or provide their own input modules) and allow interrogation of the common pool of data for resource management, general management and audit. As yet these case-mix systems have yet to prove themselves in the realms of audit; the clinical information may not be derived with sufficient detail.

Only one thing is certain: that the surgical trainee will be involved in the collection of data for the common use of:

- The production of a discharge summary to the GP
- Clinical information for audit
- Information for resource management.

The better systems will provide the trainee with feedback and give him or her the ability to get useful information out of the system.

FURTHER READING

Royal College of Surgeons of England 1994 Guidelines for clinicians on medical records and notes (revised) London
Royal Society of Medicine 1990 Computers in medical audit: a guide for hospital consultants to personal computer based medical audit systems. Royal Society of Medicine Services, London
Shaw C D, Costain D W 1989 Guidelines for medical audit: seven principles. British Medical Journal 299: 498–499
Trent Regional Health Authority 1993 Guidelines on confidentiality and medical audit. Sheffield

REFERENCES

Anderson C M, Chambers S, Clamp M 1988 Can audit improve patient care? Effects of studying use of digoxin in general practice. British Medical Journal 297: 113–114

Batstone G F 1990 Educational aspects of medical audit. British Medical Journal 301: 326–328
Bennett J, Walshe K 1990 Occurrence screening as a method of audit. British Medical Journal 300: 1248–1251
Bilroth T H 1881 Clinical surgery: reports of surgical practice 1860–1876. The New Sydenham Society, London
Black N 1991 A regional computerised surgical audit project. Quality Assurance in Health Care 2: 263–270
Buck N, Devlin H B, Lunn J N 1987 report of a confidential enquiry into perioperative deaths. Nuffield Provincial Hospitals Trust and Kings Fund, London
Buttery Y, Walshe K, Coles J, Bennett, J 1994 The development of audit findings of a national survey of healthcare provider units in England. CASPE Research, London
Campling E A, Devlin H B, Hoile R W, Lunn J N 1993 Report of the national confidential enquiry into perioperative deaths. London
Department of Health 1989 Working for patients (paper No. 6). HMSO, London
Department of Health 1993a Clinical audit: meeting and improving standards in healthcare. Leeds
Department of Health 1993b EL (93) 115 Improving clinical effectiveness. Leeds
Department of Health 1994 The evolution of clinical audit. Leeds
Donabedian A 1966 Evaluating the quality of medical care. Millbank Memorial Federation of Quality 3 (2): 166–203
Ellis B W, Sensky T 1991 A clinician's guide to setting up audit. British Medical Journal 302: 704–707
Ellis B W, Rivett R C, Dudley H A F 1990 Extending the use of clinical audit data. British Medical Journal 301: 159–162
Emberton M, Rivett R C, Ellis B W 1991 Comparative audit: a new method of delivering audit. Bulletin of the Annals of the Royal College of Surgeons 73: 117–120
Gabbay J, McNichol M C, Spiby J, Davies S C, Layton A J 1990 What did audit achieve? Lessons from preliminary evaluation of a year's medical audit. British Medical Journal 301: 526–529
Gruer R, Gordon D S, Gunn A A, Ruckley C V 1986 Audit of surgical audit. Lancet i: 23–26
Mugford M, Banfield P, O'Hanlon M 1991 Effects of feedback of information on clinical practice: a review. British Medical Journal 303: 398–402
Royal College of Physicians 1989 Medical audit. A first report – what, why and how? Royal College of Physicians, London
Royal College of Surgeons 1991 The Royal College of Surgeons Confidential Comparative Audit Service. Bulletin of the Annals of the Royal College of Surgeons 73: 96
Shaw C D 1989 Medical audit: a hospital hand book. King's Fund Centre, London
Standing Committee on Postgraduate Medical Education 1989 Medical audit: the educational implications. SCOPME, London

38. Screening for surgical disease

T. Bates

At first sight, screening the population for the common forms of surgical disease seems a good idea, since it should then be possible to cure the condition before it becomes symptomatic. Cancer of the lung, which is still the commonest malignancy (22 700 male, 11 000 female deaths in England and Wales per year) (Office of Population Censuses & Surveys 1992) has such a poor prognosis that prevention offers the only real hope of a significant impact on death rates but screening programmes have been tried for carcinoma of the colon, stomach, breast, cervix and, more recently, the prostate and ovary. It is possible that screening for non-malignant conditions such as abdominal aortic aneurysm may reduce the number of deaths in elderly men from leaking aneurysm. To be effective, early detection and treatment must lead to fewer deaths from the disease in the screened population, but there are still remaining doubts that this has been achieved. An increased survival time from diagnosis to death could well be due to earlier and therefore more prolonged observation of the natural history of the disease which might be unaffected by the treatment. This situation is known as *lead-time bias*.

The acid test for a screening programme is to compare a screened population with an identical non-screened population and this should ideally be set up as a randomized controlled trial to avoid unrecognized biases (Shapiro 1981, Hardcastle et al 1989). If the disease carries a relatively good prognosis when adequately treated at an early stage, it may take many years of observation to show a difference in the number of deaths between the screened and non-screened groups and this will require considerable resources.

There are many questions which should be answered before very considerable amounts of time, money and effort are committed to a screening programme. These questions must be addressed by several disciplines – clinical scientists in the relevant specialty, epidemiologists with expertise in screening, social scientists and economists.

Is the burden of the disease in the population sufficient to warrant an intervention? Is the screening test accurate in detecting cases in the population to be screened and is the subsequent treatment effective in curing the disease? In trying to answer these three critical questions the following specific issues must be considered.

THE REQUIREMENTS FOR A SCREENING TEST

1. Is the screening test sensitive: i.e. does it detect most of the cases, with few false-negative results?
2. Is the test specific: i.e. does it only detect cancer cases, with few false-positive results?
3. The test must be safe, relatively inexpensive and capable of achieving adequate compliance in the population to be screened.

There are many examples of screening where these criteria have not been met: *o*-tolidine based dyes for detecting occult blood increased the risk of bladder cancer in laboratory staff, and the dose of irradiation used for the first breast screening mammograms is no longer regarded as safe. Investigation and treatment of false-positive cases may lead to psychological or physical morbidity.

THE POPULATION TO BE SCREENED

To screen young people for cancer does not make sense, but cancer of the cervix has become more common in younger women which has led to a reduction in the age at which screening is offered. It is essential to have an accurate register of the population to be screened and in city areas this must be updated frequently if the client is to receive the invitation for screening. Screening the very elderly is likely to show poor compliance and the cost-benefit ratio will therefore be less favourable. Screening high risk-groups (e.g. those with a strong family history) poses special problems and different criteria must be used.

COLORECTAL CANCER (8750 male, 8650 female deaths per year)

Colonoscopy is the gold-standard test for detecting colonic cancer or polyps with both specificity and a sensitivity nearing 100%, but its high cost and low compliance rule this out as a screening test unless a very high-risk population such as a family with familial adenomatous polyposis is being examined.

Colorectal cancer should be an ideal candidate for screening since it seems that many cancers are preceded by benign adenomatous polyps and, furthermore, early cancer (Dukes' A) has a 5-year survival of 90% with conventional operative treatment. However, the best available test is poor. The Haemoccult test is probably the best of several tests for faecal occult blood but it has a relatively low sensitivity (especially for right sided and rectal tumours) and, although the specificity is over 90%, this does give rise to false-positive cases which require expensive and unnecessary investigation.

Hardcastle et al (1989) set up a massive randomized controlled trial of Haemoccult screening which has shown a favourable downgrading of tumours in the screened group, and recent meta-analysis of the three trials which have so far reported mortality data do now show a reduced number of deaths from colorectal cancer in the screened group (Towler et al 1995).

CANCER OF THE BREAST (13 700 deaths per year)

There have been four randomly allocated trials of population screening for breast cancer by mammography and of these only the Swedish Two-Counties study has shown a significant reduction in mortality (Tabar et al 1989). However, a recent overview of these trials and other non-randomized studies shows that all report fewer deaths in the screened versus the non-screened population (Wald et al 1991). There are unconfirmed reports of an initial increase in mortality in the screened group and our understanding of cause and effect is clearly incomplete. Most authorities are confident that the UK National Breast Screening Programme will reduce the number of deaths from breast cancer (Blamey et al 1994), but an unexpectedly high number of cancers presenting between 3-yearly screens (interval cancers) has led to the adoption of two-view instead of single-view mammography for the first screen. There is pressure to increase the upper age limit from 64 to 69 years, since compliance in this age group seems better than was expected.

CARCINOMA OF THE CERVIX (1650 deaths per year)

Unfortunately, no randomized trial of cytological screening for carcinoma of the cervix has been carried out and, although death rates for this disease have fallen in many countries, this fall has often preceded the introduction of screening (Williams 1992).

Up to 60% of women who have developed cervical cancer in the UK had never been screened and the false-negative rate for examination of the smears is about 10%. Not all smears are adequate and cytoscreening is very labour intensive. This situation has been unsatisfactory since the outcome of adequate treatment in cervical intraepithelial neoplasia (CIN) is highly successful. However, there is now an efficient mechanism for the recall and treatment of patients with positive smears based on general practice, and compliance has reached 83% (Austoker 1994a).

CARCINOMA OF THE STOMACH (5000 male, 3300 female deaths per year)

The incidence of cancer of the stomach seems to be falling as colon cancer rises, but these changes may be confounded by the vagaries of death certification.

Cancer of the stomach is much more common in Japan and there is considerable small-area variation in parts of the Middle East. Screening for early gastric cancer seems to be effective in Japan (Hisamichi & Sugawara 1984), but in the UK the search has been less successful and screening by gastroscopy should perhaps be confined to symptomatic patients over 55 (Hallissey et al 1990).

CARCINOMA OF THE PROSTATE (8700 deaths per year)

Screening for carcinoma of the prostate is controversial since the disease mainly affects an elderly population and 30% of men over 50 years have histological evidence of prostatic cancer at necropsy but in only 1% of these is there clinically active disease (Austoker 1994b). The available screening tests, apart from rectal examination, are prostatic specific antigen and transrectal ultrasound. Neither the sensitivity nor the specificity of these tests is high, either alone or in combination, and the treatment of localized prostatic cancer is also controversial. Radical prostatectomy, radiotherapy, hormonal manipulation and a watch-policy are all used in this situation, but there is no randomized trial to indicate survival benefit and it must be important not to cause unnecessary morbidity in elderly men with asymptomatic disease.

CANCER OF THE OVARY (3900 deaths per year)

Evidence for survival benefit from screening is lacking, but a large randomized controlled trial has been set up. The main screening tests are antigen marker CA 125 and transvaginal ultrasound, but other tumour markers and colour Doppler are being evaluated. The sensitivity of CA 125 for early ovarian cancer may be as low as 50%. There must, however, be a strong case for screening a high-risk group with family ovarian cancer syndrome (Austoker 1994c).

SCREENING FOR NON-MALIGNANT SURGICAL DISEASE

Neonatal screening

Congenital disease is increasingly diagnosed as a result of routine antenatal ultrasound screening, but postnatal clinical examination should be carried out for evidence of congenital cardiac and renal abnormalities as well as orthopaedic, sexual and anorectal malformations. Most congenital abnormalities will normally present as a clinical problem in the first few days of life, but it is important to recognize silent conditions such as congenital dislocation of the hip when delay in diagnosis may worsen the outcome.

Abdominal aortic aneurysm (2900 male, 1040 female deaths per year)

There are several population screening studies from the UK and the USA and in men over 65 years ultrasound screening of the aorta shows a prevalence of aneurysm of about 5%, depending on size criteria. This rate may be twice as high in men with hypertension or vascular disease, and the lifetime prevalence in first-degree male relatives may be as high as 50% (Collin 1994). It seems likely that deaths from leaking abdominal aortic aneurysm could be reduced by screening men at age 65 years, with a policy of elective surgery for fit patients with an aortic diameter of say 5.0 cm or more. This has yet to be confirmed by a randomized controlled trial.

WHAT COMPLIANCE IS TO BE EXPECTED?

Compliance varies with the social acceptability and public awareness of the disease, the screening test and the perceived treatment. Screening for breast cancer by mammography will achieve 80% in areas with a stable population, but this may be less than 50% in inner city areas. It is possible that compliance may be affected by fear of mastectomy, and discomfort at the initial screen may reduce attendence for rescreening. There is also some evidence that compliance may change due to media exposure in the short term.

In screening for colorectal cancer, the population's enthusiasm for faecal occult blood test is very low, which leads to poor compliance unless considerable efforts are made to increase public awareness at the time that screening is offered. There are many reasons why people decline screening invitations, but failure to receive the letter is a common cause.

The true refusers are an unusual group of people who have a poor outlook from both a health and a social standpoint. It seems that they neglect or abuse their health in many respects, and it is therefore important not to use them as a control group for comparison with the accepters of screening since whatever comparison is made the refusers will be disadvantaged. Compliance in screening for carcinoma of the cervix by cytology was worst in the socioeconomic group most at risk from the disease, but this seems to be improving.

THE INTERVENTION TO BE USED

It has already been noted that an operation for early bowel cancer has a high cure rate, but we cannot be sure this is the case for breast cancer. In the latter disease the evidence so far fails to show survival benefit in screening women under 50 years and it is therefore logical that screening on a national basis should be confined to older women until there is information to the contrary. Screen-detected breast cancer has many features known to indicate a good prognosis (Klemi et al 1992), but ductal carcinoma in situ is diagnosed in up to 20% of screened cases and the best treatment for this condition is still in doubt. It is possible that fear of overtreatment by mastectomy may lead to a sacrifice of survival advantage by inadequate surgery. Severe dysplasia of the cervix (CIN III) has an extremely good outlook with local treatment and close surveillance. Node-positive carcinoma of the stomach has a 5-year survival rate of less than 10%, but in situ tumours carry a good prognosis if treated with adequate surgery. The Japanese have pioneered more radical surgery for gastric cancer than has been the norm in the West and clinical trials are currently in hand to try and repeat their excellent results in the UK.

WHAT SHOULD BE THE INTERVAL BETWEEN SCREENS?

In the National Breast Screening Programme the current interval between screens is 3 years and in a few trial centres this has been reduced to 2. However, the interval cancer rate is 31% in the first year, 52% in the second and 82% in the third year (Woodman et al 1995). This suggests that the 3-year interval between screens is too long, but it is possible that many interval cancers will be rapidly growing tumours with a poor prognosis. The most appropriate interval for cervical screening is still controversial, and the case for screening in carcinoma of the colon or stomach is not sufficiently secure for the interval between screens to be a major issue.

WHAT IS THE COST?

The economist will want to know the cost per case detected, the cost per case treated and per life saved. The sociologist will want to know the psychosocial cost to those false-positive cases investigated unnecessarily (Ellman et al 1989) and the quality of life in those patients who have cancer detected sooner than it otherwise would have been.

SUMMARY

A screening test for cancer must be able to detect the disease at a stage when earlier treatment will lead to fewer deaths. To achieve this the test must be sensitive, specific and acceptable: the treatment must be effective. The overall cost of a life saved may be difficult to quantify, but this should be taken into account.

REFERENCES

Austoker J 1994a Screening and self examination for breast cancer. British Medical Journal 309: 168–174

Austoker J 1994b Screening for cervical cancer. British Medical Journal 309: 241–248

Austoker J 1994c Screening for ovarian, prostatic and testicular cancers. British Medical Journal 309: 315–320

Blamey R W, Wilson A R M, Patnick J, Dixon J M 1994 Screening for breast cancer. British Medical Journal 309: 1076–1079

Collin R 1994 Abdominal aorta: epidemiology. In Morris P J, Malt R A (eds) Oxford textbook for surgery. Oxford University Press, New York, p 377–378

Ellman R, Angeli N, Christians A, Moss S, Chamberlain J, Maguire P 1989 Psychiatric morbidity associated with screening for breast cancer. British Journal of Cancer 60: 781–784

Hallissey M T, Allum W H, Jewkes A J, Ellis D J, Fielding J W L 1990 Early detection of gastric cancer. British Medical Journal 301: 513–515

Hardcastle J D, Chamberlain J, Sheffield J et al 1989 Randomised controlled trial of faecal occult blood screening for colorectal cancer: results from the first 107,349 patients. Lancet i: 1160–1164

Hisamichi S, Sugawara N 1984 Mass screening for gastric cancer by X-ray examination. Japanese Journal of Clinical Oncology 14: 211–223

Klemi P J, Joensuu H, Toikkanen S et al 1992 Aggressiveness of breast cancers found with and without screening. British Medical Journal 304: 467–469

Office of Population Censuses & Surveys 1994 Series DH2 No. 19. Mortality statistics for 1992. Cause. HMSO, London

Shapiro S 1981 Evidence on screening for breast cancer from a randomised trial. Cancer 39: 618–627

Tabar L, Fagerberg F, Duffy S W, Day N E 1989 The Swedish two counties trial of mammographic screening for breast cancer: recent results and calculation of benefit. Journal of Epidemiology and Community Health 43: 107–114

Wald N, Frost C, Cuckle H 1991 Breast cancer screening: the current position. British Medical Journal 302: 845–846

Williams C 1992 Ovarian & cervical cancer. British Medical Journal 304: 1501–1504

Woodman C B J, Threlfall A G, Boggis C R M, Prior P 1995 Is the three year breast screening interval too long? Occurrence of interval cancers in NHS breast screening programme's north western region. British Medical Journal 310: 224–226

39. Genetic aspects of surgery

K. D. MacDermot   M. C. Winslet

RELEVANCE OF CLINICAL GENETICS TO SURGERY

In certain genetic disorders, life-threatening complications may occur during surgery and anaesthesia. The recognition of clinical signs or family history suggestive of these genetic disorders is important for diagnosis so that appropriate perioperative management of the patient is undertaken. Furthermore, the study of the molecular basis of genetic disorders, human development, carcinogenesis and many other biological events is now possible, due to exciting advances in laboratory techniques for the analysis of human genome.

Genes involved in the control of cell proliferation and transcription of genetic information have been shown to cause increased susceptibility to cancer if their function is defective. Thus, genetic analysis and the development of new methods for clinical diagnosis, monitoring of cancer progression and treatment are being reported in medical literature and incorporated in clinical medicine. These advances clearly illustrate the link between basic sciences and clinical practice and an understanding of basic genetic concepts is now required to keep abreast of new developments.

BASIC GENETICS CONCEPTS AND TERMINOLOGY

Genes are units of genetic information which are passed on from generation to generation. Biochemically, genes are stretches of *DNA* (deoxyribonucleic acid) which direct the synthesis of a specific protein. DNA is tightly coiled and packaged in *chromosomes*, which are visible under the light microscope in the nucleus of dividing cells. *Somatic cells* (non-germ-line tissue) have 23 pairs of chromosomes (*diploid* number 46), one chromosome from each pair is inherited from each parent. Chromosome pairs 1–22 are called *autosomes*, whilst the 23rd

pair are the *sex chromosomes* (XX in females and XY in males). In the ovum or sperm (*germ cells* or gonadal tissue cells) one set of autosomes and a sex chromosome are present (*haploid* set), so on fertilization a diploid set of chromosomes is restored. It can be seen that males determine the sex of the offspring. When viewed under the microscope, each chromosome has a visible constriction (*centromere*). The part of the chromosome above the centromere is usually shorter and is referred to by standard nomenclature as the short arm or *p* (from *petite*), the long arm is termed *q*. Each arm of the chromosome is further divided into bands for easy reference. Thus, 5q21 is the position of the adenomatous polyposis coli gene on the long arm of chromosome 5. *Mutation* is a change in the gene function which either results in activation (more protein is produced) or, more often, inactivation of the gene with reduction or loss of function.

Mendelian inheritance refers to the mode of transmission of genetic information from generation to generation as proposed by Mendel. *Dominant inheritance* (autosomal or X linked) is clinically expressed when only one copy of the mutated gene is present. In *recessive inheritance* the signs of the disease are only clinically evident when both copies of the gene have the mutation. *Oncogenes* are genes, present in normal cells, which promote cell growth and proliferation. *Tumour suppressor genes* (or antioncogenes) have the opposite function.

An essential aid for establishing the diagnosis of genetic disorder is, of course, a *family history* of the same disease or clinical signs in relatives. The drawing of a family tree (*pedigree*) is straightforward and shows in graphic form the mode of genetic transmission (Fig 1). When a complex of symptoms and signs occur together in a particular disorder, this is referred to as a *syndrome*, usually named after the author(s) of the first report (e.g. Li Fraumeni syndrome) or by an acronym which describes the clinical signs (e.g. HNPCC, hereditary non-polyposis colon cancer).

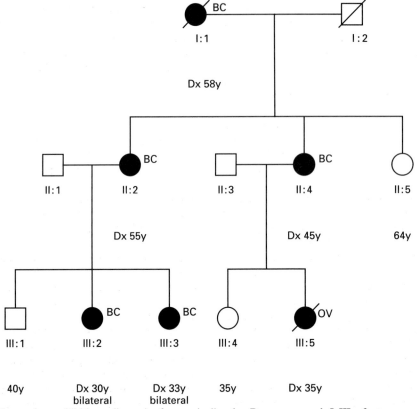

Fig. 39.1 A family tree for establishing a diagnosis of a genetic disorder. Roman numerals I–III refer to generations; arabic numerals refer to the individual (e.g. III:5, fifth individual from the third generation shown on the pedigree). (O) Female; (□) male; filled symbols, affected; crossed symbols, dead; BC, breast cancer; OV, ovarian cancer; Dx, diagnosed; y, years (present age or age at diagnosis in affected individuals).

GENETIC DIAGNOSIS FOR PREOPERATIVE ASSESSMENT AND PERIOPERATIVE MANAGEMENT OF SURGICAL PATIENTS

In this section we concentrate on those genetic disorders which the trainee surgeon should be familiar with since they may result in serious complications during surgery and anaesthesia. These genetic disorders can be divided into four groups: defects of haemoglobin and haemostasis; defects of muscle; connective tissue defects; and skeletal dysplasias.

Defects of haemoglobin and haemostasis

Enquire about history of anaemia, bleeding tendency or recurrent venous thrombosis in the patient or their relatives. The development of sickle cell crisis due to hypoxia during surgery and the need for factor VIII infusion in haemophilia A are well known. Most rare defects of other clotting factors will be diagnosed on a routine screen, when a suggestive history is obtained. For example, in Noonan syndrome with a birth frequency of 1 in 2000, factor XI and XII deficiency and thrombocytopenia occur in 60% of patients. The clinical signs include short stature, neck webbing and congenital heart defects.

Patients with thromboembolic disease due to inherited protein C or S deficiency may give a history of superficial and deep vein thrombosis, thrombosis of the mesenteric, cerebral, renal, axillary and portal veins and pulmonary embolism.

Muscle defects

Enquire about the development of hyperthermia, acute renal failure and tonic spasms during previous surgery or anaesthetic death in relatives. Malignant hyperthermia is the most serious genetic disorder of muscle presenting in the operating theatre. It consists of acute onset of skeletal muscle rigidity, metabolic acidosis and malignant hyperpyrexia. If not immediately reversed, these episodes can lead to tissue damage and death. The mainstay of treatment is dantrolene, given either prophylactically or immediately a hyperthermic episode is suspected. Malignant hyperthermia is estimate to affect approximately 1 in 15 000 paediatric patients and 1 in 40 000 adult patients. It is triggered by halogenated anaesthetic agents with or without depolarizing muscle relaxants. The inheritance is autosomal dominant or recessive, and approximately 50% of families have a mutation in the calcium release channel gene on chromosome 19.

Hand-grip weakness and difficulty in walking are symptoms of myotonic dystrophy and a positive family history is usually present. Myotonic dystrophy affects approximately 1 in 10 000 individuals and the clinical expression is very variable. Myotonic dystrophy and the other less common myotonias are due to defects in the chloride and sodium channels of the muscle membrane. Patients show undue sensitivity to various anaesthetics and sedative agents, including opioids, barbiturates and benzodiazepines. Tonic spasms during operation, prolonged recovery from anaesthetic and depression of the respiratory centre necessitating prolonged ventilation have been reported. Cold and shivering also induces myotonia. Myotonic dystrophy usually presents between the ages of 15 and 35 years. The most noticeable clinical signs are facial and neck weakness with ptosis. Patients usually notice weakness of hand grip, inability to open clenched fist and difficulty in walking due to weakness of foot dorsiflexion. This is a multisystem disorder; heart block frequently develops in adults and patients should be fully evaluated before surgery. Anaesthetic management may be difficult and regional anaesthesia should be used whenever possible.

Connective tissue defects

Enquire about poor wound healing, paper-thin scar tissue, joint dislocations and the diagnosis of aortic aneurysm in relatives.

Connective tissue abnormalities may cause difficulty during suturing, resulting in a high incidence of anastomoses and wound dehiscence. In Marfan's syndrome, the clinical signs are usually obvious: the patient has tall thin stature, long slim fingers, chest deformity, scoliosis and dislocated optic lens. Preoperative cardiac assessment is mandatory, as there is high incidence of dissecting aortic aneurysm with aortic valve insufficiency at a young age.

Ehrles Danlos syndrome, particularly the arterial type IV, is characterized by friable arteries and veins, and spontaneous arterial rupture has been reported. Paper-thin scars, joint dislocations and spontaneous colonic perforation may also occur. Arteriography and vascular surgery is particularly hazardous; varicose vein surgery, if absolutely necessary, should be performed with the utmost care!

Skeletal dysplasias

Patients with such disorders may have odontoid dysplasia or C1–C2 subluxation due to ligamentous laxity. The patient is of short stature, with some body disproportion. The most commonly encountered conditions are achondroplasia and Down's syndrome, which are easily recognized. Skeletal dysplasia due to mucopolysaccharidosis, an inborn metabolic storage disorder (such as Hurler's syndrome), are characterized by 'coarse' looking face and mental retardation. During surgery, head and neck manipulation should be limited, as cervical medullary compression has been reported. In certain cases, elective cervical vertebral fusion may be required.

Congenital malformations and genetic disorders may indicate the presence of unsuspected anatomical abnormalities of obvious importance to the surgeon. Patients with Sturge–Weber syndrome have a port wine stain on the skin which, if present over the face or cranium, is associated with epilepsy or mental retardation. Multiple arteriovenous malformations may be encountered during surgical manipulation of tissues beneath the port wine stain. Similarly, hypoplasia of the lesser wing of the sphenoid bone is a developmental abnormality associated with peripheral neurofibromatosis type 1. The operative reduction of raised intracranial pressure in such patients may be associated with enophthalmos.

GENETIC MECHANISM OF CANCER DEVELOPMENT

Cancer development is the result of an accumulation of mutations in a number of genes (4–5 in colorectal cancer), over time, in somatic tissues. Each mutation results in step-wise clonal proliferation of cells, with the next mutation giving rise to further expansion. The mutations are present in two types of gene which regulate cell growth. There is a mutational activation of oncogenes and mutational inactivation of tumour suppressor genes. A genetic model for colorectal tumorigenesis has been particularly well studied (Fearon & Vogelstein 1990). Early mutations in the bowel epithelium in the oncogene ras and the tumour suppressor genes on 5q and 18q give rise to a colon adenoma. Additional mutation of the tumour suppressor gene p53 (localized at 17p) results in progression to carcinoma. Further tumour growth results from the accumulated loss of suppressor genes on additional chromosomes. This correlates with the ability of the carcinomas to metastasize and cause death.

GENETIC SUSCEPTIBILITY TO CANCER

The great majority of malignant tumours are sporadic (in one individual in the family) and develop in old age. Cancer is a common cause of death in the population, but cancer occurring in successive generations in a family is rare.

As molecular genetic analysis methods have become available, attention has focused over the last 10 years on unusual families where a particular type of cancer (breast, ovary, colorectal) has developed in many relatives, over several generations and at a young age. Significantly, the tumours were often bilateral or multifocal. This clinical presentation could be explained by an inherited mutation of a tumour suppressor gene (which is present in all tissues). Subsequent mutations of further genes results frequently in multiple tumours at a young age of onset. This mechanism of genetic susceptibility to cancer was initially proposed by Knudson in 1986 (Knudson hypothesis), and has recently been confirmed. Among the first genes to be localized were those causing clinically well-characterized disorders such as familial retinoblastoma, Wilms' tumour and adenomatous polyposis coli (APC). Table 39.1 shows the gene localization and clinical presentation of some of the more common cancer susceptibility genetic disorders. One disorder is described here in more detail in order to illustrate the clinical presentation, surgical management and impact of diagnosis on a family.

Adenomatous polyposis coli (APC) is a serious autosomal dominant disorder presenting in late childhood/early teens with abdominal pain or bleeding per rectum due to multiple large bowel polyps. At colonoscopy, numerous polyps, almost replacing the bowel mucosa will be identified. Polyps may also be present in the rest of the gastrointestinal tract. The frequency of progression of such polyps to the adenoma–carcinoma sequence is high. Proctocolectomy with ileoanal pouch formation or, in the young, initial total colectomy with ileorectal anastomosis and surveillance of the rectal stump to minimize psychosexual sequelae, are the procedures of choice. Another serious complication occurring in approximately 10% of patients with APC are desmoid tumours arising mainly from the peritoneum or abdominal wall, which are highly vascular and difficult to resect in their entirety. When the clinical diagnosis of APC is made, the patient's close relatives have to be informed and counselled about their increased cancer risk. They will have to make a decision of whether or not to have regular colonoscopy, as in some gene carriers the polyps appear later, or to opt for a predictive genetic test. Such potentially predictive tests may carry social stigma and be potentially misused by insurance and employment agencies, while the knowledge of future risk for cancer and subsequent need for major surgery is stressful to the patients and their families alike. Mutation analysis in the APC gene has to be performed on a sample from the affected family member, as many different mutations from different families may be found spanning the whole length of the gene. When the mutation is identified in a family, prenatal diagnosis is also possible. The decision to terminate the pregnancy is difficult to make because of the relatively late onset of the disease.

Recently, the cloning of a breast/ovarian cancer susceptibility gene (BRCA1) has been accomplished (Miki et al 1994). This constitutes a major advance in the study of these common cancers. Mutations have been identified in all areas of this large gene. For practical clinical application, a less expensive and less laborious method of gene analysis will have to be developed. Genetic susceptibility to breast and ovarian cancer is impossible to diagnose clinically in the absence of convincing pedigree suggestive of autosomal dominant inheritance. The population risk for breast cancer in a woman aged 30–39 years is 4 in 1000. Whilst the number of cases analysed to date has been relatively small, and with only preliminary data available, the percentage of breast cancer due to BRCA1 within that age range has been estimated at 5%.

A number of cancer syndromes have been described, showing a characteristic combination of cancers (Table 39.1). As the gene mutations responsible for these syndromes have only been described recently, it is likely that a more accurate clinical spectrum will be available in the future.

The study of families with a high frequency of site-specific colorectal cancer and colorectal cancer associated with malignant tumours of the genitourinary tract, uterus, breast cancer and other malignancies has facilitated the recent discovery of several new genes. These syndromes were initially described by Lynch et al (1988), but have subsequently been termed 'hereditary non-polyposis colon cancer' and 'cancer family syndrome'. The colorectal cancer is of early onset, with a proclivity to the proximal colon and an excess of synchronous/metachronous lesions. It is often, but not always, preceded by colonic polyps. Colonoscopy is advocated every 3–5 years, with an increasing frequency in the presence of polyps. The surveillance for the associ-

Table 39.1 Gene localization and clinical presentation of common disorders with genetic susceptibility to cancer

Disorder	Mode of inheritance	Gene localization	Tumour susceptibility
Retinoblastoma	Autosomal dominant	13q14	Retinoblastoma, osteogenic sarcoma
Wilms's tumour	Autosomal dominant	11p13	Nephroblastoma
Adenomatous polyposis coli	Autosomal dominant	5q21	Colorectal, gastrointestinal tract
Li Fraumeni S	Autosomal dominant	17p12	Rhabdomyosarcoma, leukaemia, glioma, breast cancer
Breast and ovarian cancer	Autosomal dominant	BRCA1 – 17q21 BRCA2 – 13q21	Breast and ovarian, prostate, pancreas
Hereditary non-polyposis colon cancer	Autosomal dominant	hMSH2 – 2p12 hMLH1 – 3p21 hPMS1 – 2q31 hPMS – 7p22	Colorectal and gastrointestinal, ureteric, endometrial ovarian cancer
Neurofibromatosis 1	Autosomal dominant	17q11	Benign schwanoma, brain tumours (rare)
Neurofibromatosis 2	Autosomal dominant	22q13	Optic neuroma, acoustic neuroma, meningioma, glioma
von Hippel Lindau S	Autosomal dominant	3p25	Meningioma, renal
Peutz–Jaegher S	Autosomal dominant	Unknown	Hamartoma, gastrointestinal tract

ated cancers is problematic as, again, clinical diagnosis is difficult. Genetic diagnosis is now possible, but methodological problems will have to be overcome for potential clinical application, as is the case with the BRCA1 gene.

It has been noted that tumours from affected individuals contain a large number of DNA replication errors. The normal function of these newly discovered genes is to survey the fidelity of DNA replication and repair. Mistakes are frequently introduced during normal DNA replication and DNA repair has to take place, especially when the cell is exposed to carcinogens, ionizing radiation or alkylating agents. The clinical expression of mutations in these genes is compatible with their function as tumour suppressor genes. The frequency of these gene mutations in the population is unknown, but in patients with colorectal cancer, genetic susceptibility has been estimated to account for 5–10% of cases.

Advances in molecular genetics continue at a rapid pace. With the current application of oncogene amplification to tumour stage and ultimately prognosis, the further development of tumour drug targeting and gene therapy, and major practical advances in cancer prediction, detection and therapy should be forthcoming in the foreseeable future.

REFERENCES

Fearon E R, Vogelstein B 1990. A genetic model for colorectal tumourogenesis. Cell 61: 759–767
Lynch H T, Lanspa S J, Bonan B M, Smyth T, Walson P, Lynch J F 1988 Hereditary non-polyposis colorectal cancer Lynch syndromes I & II. Gastroenterology Clinics of North America 174: 679–715
Miki Y, Swensen J, Shattuck-Eidens D et al 1994. A strong candidate for the breast and ovarian susceptibility gene BRCA1. Science 266: 66–71

40. Economic aspects of surgery

R. W. Hoile

This is probably a subject which, up to now in your surgical career, you have not needed to think about or understand. Before you progress much further you will undoubtedly be exposed to economic considerations and the consequences of your actions, so it is worthwhile discussing some of the principles used when addressing this topic.

The National Health Service was developed on the principle of fairness and that health care was free to the patient at the point of delivery, but with the rising costs of health care, limited resources and the heightened expectations of our patients it is inevitable that a debate about costs will occur. Will the economic arguments take over and conflict with good patient care, or can good economic strategies mean better patient care? At all times the outcome for the patient must be central to this debate.

WHERE DO SURGEONS GO WRONG?

Looked at from the standpoint of health-care economics (and accepting the conflict between caring for an individual and considering the wise use of resources for the good of all), we make mistakes. These include:

- Using resources inefficiently or inappropriately
- Using investigative or operative techniques which are outdated
- Not acting in the patient's interests but perhaps in the interest of academia or research
- High complication rates
- The poorly considered introduction of new techniques which demand expensive technological back-up or instrumentation for an unproved gain.

How can we address these issues?

THE MEASUREMENT OF COST-EFFECTIVENESS

The cost of surgery is not just monetary but also personal

and social. For the patient there is pain, suffering, time spent in hospital and the economic consequences of the disease, hospitalization and time off work. Whilst we should be striving to deliver a cost-effective health-care system, we should not lose sight of these personal costs. Measuring cost-effectiveness is an unfamiliar process to clinicians, but it is important in evaluating and practising modern surgery. Before the cost-effectiveness of any surgical management is understood, it is necessary to understand some of the principles, definitions and accounting practices which are applied to problems of health-care and the way in which they may affect clinical decision-making.

WHAT DOES COST-EFFECTIVENESS MEAN?

There are four ways of interpreting cost-effectiveness in clinical practice:

- Cost savings
- Effectiveness in improving health care
- Cost savings with an equal (or better) health outcome
- Having an additional benefit worth the additional cost.

It is the last two of these four which are used most in evaluating surgical practice. It should be noted that the third option requires no compromise by accountants or clinicians, i.e. it is a 'win-win' situation. Both of the last two categories in the list require judgement to decide whether additional cost is worth the anticipated benefit and to select the course of action with the least cost at the most probable benefit.

MEASURING COSTS AND BENEFITS

Cost–benefit and cost-effective analyses measure and compare the significant gains and losses associated with different methods of patient management. One could try to equate the value, in financial terms, of a year of healthy life. One such method is the calculation of quality-life-years (QUALYs). The benefits used in any calculation might include:

- Cure
- Increase in life expectancy
- Increased quality of life.

Some of the costs to be considered might include:

- Medical and surgical risks
- Operative or hospital mortality
- Disability
- Pain and suffering
- Financial cost.

Imagination and a critical attitude often result in an improvement in cost effectiveness. The intensive care unit (ICU) is a good example of a high-cost-benefit area where carefully thought through policy changes can result in proven cost savings without changes in the quality of care.

CLINICAL 'PROFIT'

This is what primarily interests the patient because it could be described as the gain to be expected from a clinical decision once the patient has paid the price of pain, disability and financial loss whilst under treatment. Similarly, a consultation or clinic visit should be of benefit to the patient and/or clinicians. Consultations are often expensive, worthless and overused (e.g. follow-up appointments after routine surgical procedures).

CLINICAL RELEVANCE

Clinical decisions and the tests that support those decisions will be relevant in terms of cost-effectiveness depending upon their potential for clinical benefit. For instance, a test which, with great accuracy, confirms a diagnosis of extensive pancreatic cancer is less relevant than a test which would confirm gallstones with the same accuracy. One test has a small potential for prolonged benefit. The other will probably result in cure.

Benefit to patients should be proven for high-cost supportive treatments and services (e.g. nutritional support is of proven benefit). Minimal evidence of benefit requires a re-evaluation of the therapy in question.

HOW CAN SURGEONS INFLUENCE HOSPITAL COSTS?

The introduction of day surgery as a low-cost/high-throughput service reduces the cost of procedures without increased morbidity. Similarly, short stay, 5-day wards and low-dependency units (or hotels) also reduce costs without detriment (or even with advantage) to the patient. Preadmission clinics, which may avoid last minute cancellations, are also proven to be cost-effective.

Laboratory tests

'Routine' investigations for all admissions are an example of uncritical and inefficient use of laboratory tests. Costs of laboratory tests constitute a significant part of the cost of health care. The effectiveness of a test is a measure of how the test findings influence the subsequent diagnostic or surgical strategy. Many tests are expensive and overlap others and, while being prestigious and impressive, may constitute poor medical practice. The best surgeon orders the fewest tests, in an appropriate order, that will provide the speediest diagnosis. Try to become familiar with the sensitivity, specificity and broad costs of the tests which are commonly used in your practice.

New technologies

Advances always emerge with benefits and limitations. Following evaluation, appropriate use of these new techniques will allow replacement of some costly procedures; for example, fine needle aspiration biopsies of the breast and aspiration of abscesses may, under some circumstances, replace open procedures. Some new techniques, although being considered as high-cost/high-yield procedures, are adopted because they revolutionize the management of certain conditions; for example, if successful, pouch surgery for ulcerative colitis and angioplasty for peripheral or coronary arterial disease can have immense gains in terms of quality of life for the patient. The danger is in accepting new glamorous ideas without adequate evaluation. For instance, laparoscopic cholecystectomy is associated with a significantly reduced length of hospital stay, shorter recovery and a significantly shorter back-to-work time than the open counterpart. The hospital costs are also lower. However, when laparoscopic hernia repair is investigated from the economic point of view the costs are, at best, comparable to the open approach and, in some hospitals, higher. There may be considerable cost reductions if clinicians could agree 'best practices' for procedures, develop local protocols and adhere to them.

Complications

Postoperative complications are expensive and can spoil any attempt to improve the cost effectiveness of surgery. The impact can be minimized by the use of clinical audit, specialization, abandoning out-dated unproved procedures, prophylactic regimes (e.g. antibiotics and thromboembolic prophylaxis), cautiously adopting new proven techniques and recognizing individual performance limitations. A single postoperative complication can completely wipe out the advantages and savings of careful, well thought out preoperative diagnosis and operative surgery. The main burden of a complication falls, of course, on the patient, but inevitably the knock-on effect will have consequences for your departmental budget. A wound infection, reoperation for infection, bleeding or anastomotic breakdown, pulmonary embolus and cardiac or renal failure are but a few of the complications which we could all list and which happen within our practice and have implications for labour and resources. If you think of the prolonged hospitalization and expensive investigations involved and translate these into monetary terms, it will demonstrate to you how the overall costs of surgery within your department will rise in the presence of complications; this could eventually double or triple the costs of uncomplicated surgery. Obviously, a certain level of complications should be built in when costs are calculated, but this will usually assume fairly minimal rates of incidence of complications. We all have complications sooner or later and they are all detrimental to the patient, the hospital and the budget! Your objective should be to minimize the incidence of such complications and, when they occur, to limit their duration, extent and cost (in all senses of the word).

Even as a trainee surgeon you should appreciate the economic consequences of your own behaviour; careful clinical decision-making and operative technique will help you to reduce your own personal complication rates. This will be for the good of the patient (which is, after all, your first concern), your reputation and also for the good of the department within which you work, as it will reduce the expense of surgery. This expense is something which not only you should be concerned about; it will also be of concern to your managers and those who must eventually foot the bill for health care, (i.e. the public at large).

The detection of metastases

The detection of metastases in malignant disease must be analysed carefully and the value of commonly performed clinical procedures questioned. Is there a proven benefit? Similarly, playing 'hunt the primary' may be of no value to the patient in terms of palliation or survival, while having a considerable cost implication for the health care organization (i.e. your hospital).

Diagnosis

Staging for ovarian malignancy involves inherently high costs but has great clinical value when properly performed. It is inappropriate if done routinely or when the attempt at staging is poorly designed. In situations with a high cost and low yield, especially if there may be disabling side-effects, then ethical considerations may also come into play. Consider projectile vomiting in infancy. A clinical finding of hypertrophic pyloric stenosis would be a low-cost/high-yield diagnosis, whereas duodenal atresia might be a high-cost/low-yield condition.

Screening

There is much discussion about screening. Does the expense of setting up population screening (e.g. for breast cancer, colonic cancer and aortic aneurysms) produce better survival figures and quality of life for the patients? Can the health services cope with the increased elective workload? Is the subsequent treatment cheaper? Certainly for abdominal aortic aneurysm the outcome is better for elective surgery and the treatment is cheaper. Many of these issues are for society to decide; discrimination with regard to sex and age and the influence of pressure groups all play their part in decisions about the provision of health care.

Operations

Some procedures are of low benefit with a slight chance of cure (e.g. surgery for oesophageal carcinoma). However, the palliative benefits may be high; this is an area where careful clinical judgement is required. The open surgery of adult inguinal hernia is an example of a relatively well accepted low-cost/high-yield treatment with an accumulative economic importance in view of the disease frequency. Laparoscopic surgery may not have the same benefits. Similarly, total hip replacement is a high-cost/high-yield procedure. In emergency surgery (e.g. appendicitis) costs can be minimized by attempting to avoid negative laparotomies and complications.

CONCLUSIONS

Thinking about the economics of health care raises questions which are sometimes uncomfortable. Questions about waste, the inappropriateness of investigations and operations, rationing, cost-containment, ethics, etc. The response to these questions needs to be well thought out and workable. It is possible to set professional standards and deliver appropriate care whilst eliminating the unwarranted use of medical resources. It is easy to 'do something', particularly when faced with an individual patient, but perhaps we should stand back, take a broader view and consider whether an action for the individual patient is appropriate and/or cost-effective. A multitude of tests and procedures does not necessarily produce an accurate or speedy diagnosis, a lower morbidity or mortality, or 'better' health care. Professional guidelines and clinical audit may sometimes help us when it is necessary to say 'no'.

We have not found all the answers yet but you must begin to address these difficult questions.

FURTHER READING

Eiseman B, Stahlgren L 1987 Cost-effective surgical management. W B Saunders, Philadelphia

Hicks N R 1994 Some observations on attempts to measure appropriateness of care. British Medical Journal 309: 730–733

O'Brien B 1986 'What are my chances doctor?' A review of clinical risks. Health Economics Research Group, Brunel University

41. Revising for the MRCS examination

R. Carpenter

The MRCS is a new diploma to signify completion of basic surgical training. The new examination will not separately examine the applied basic sciences, but instead examines the science with clinical surgery in an integrated fashion. New regulations for basic surgical training (the MRCS Regulations) will come into effect on 1 August 1996 and will apply to all those who start training on or after that date in surgical posts approved for entry into the examination. The examination is undertaken in three stages. Firstly, there are two multiple-choice question (MCQ) papers. One is based on the core modules and one on systems modules (see syllabus below), which may be taken together or separately at least 8 months after starting basic surgical training. Secondly, there will be a clinical short case section taken at least 20 months after starting training and after successful completion of the MCQ exam. Thirdly, there will be a viva voce section taken at least 22 months after starting training and having acquired a certificate of competence on an approved Basic Surgical Skills course.

THE MRCS SYLLABUS

Core Module 1: Perioperative management 1

Unit 1   Preoperative management

- Assessment of fitness for anaesthesia and surgery
- Tests of respiratory, cardiac and renal function.
- Management of associated medical conditions (e.g. diabetes; respiratory disease, cardiovascular disease; psychiatric disorders; malnutrition; anaemia; steroid, anticoagulant, immunosuppressant and other drug therapy).

Unit 2   Infection

- Pathophysiology of the body's response to infection
- The sources of surgical infection – prevention and control

- Surgically important microorganisms
- Principles of asepsis and antisepsis
- Surgical sepsis and its prevention
- Aseptic techniques
- Skin preparation
- Antibiotic prophylaxis
- Sterilization.

Unit 3   Investigative and operative procedures

- Excision of cysts and benign tumours of skin and subcutaneous tissue
- Principles of techniques of biopsy
- Suture and ligature materials
- Drainage of superficial abscesses
- Basic principles of anastomosis.

Unit 4   Anaesthesia

- Principles of anaesthesia
- Premedication and sedation
- Local and regional anaesthesia
- Care and monitoring of the anaesthetized patient.

Unit 5   Theatre problems

- Surgical technique and technology
- Diathermy – principles and precautions
- Lasers – principles and precautions
- Explosion hazards relating to general anaesthesia and endoscopic surgery
- Tourniquets – uses and precautions
- Prevention of nerve and other injuries in the anaesthetized patient
- Surgery in hepatitis and HIV carriers – special precautions
- Disorders of coagulation and haemostasis – prophylaxis of thromboembolic disease

Core Module 2: Perioperative management 2

Unit 1   Skin and wounds

- Pathophysiology of wound healing
- Classification of surgical wounds
- Principles of wound management
- Incisions and their closure
- Suture and ligature materials
- Scars and contracture
- Wound dehiscence
- Dressings.

Unit 2   Fluid balance

- Assessment and maintenance of fluid and electrolyte balance
- Techniques of venous access
- Nutritional support – indications, techniques, total parenteral nutrition.

Unit 3   Blood

- Disorders of coagulation and haemostasis
- Blood transfusion – indications, hazards, complications, plasma substitutes
- Haemolytic disorders of surgical importance
- Haemorrhagic disorders; disorders of coagulation.

Unit 4   Postoperative complications

- Postoperative complications – prevention, monitoring, recognition, management
- Ventilatory support – indications.

Unit 5   Postoperative sequelae

- Pain control
- Immune response to trauma, infections and tissue transplantation
- Pathophysiology of the body's response to trauma
- Surgery in the immunocompromised patient.

Core Module 3: Trauma

Unit 1   Initial assessment and resuscitation after trauma

- Clinical assessment of the injured patient
- Maintenance of airway and ventilation
- Haemorrhage and shock.

Unit 2   Chest, abdomen and pelvis

- Cardiorespiratory physiology as applies to trauma
- Penetrating chest injuries and pneumothorax
- Rib fractures and flail chest
- Abdominal and pelvic injuries.

Unit 3   Central nervous system trauma

- Central nervous system – anatomy and physiology relevant to clinical examination of the central nervous system; the understanding of its functional disorders, particularly those caused by cranial or spinal trauma; interpretation of special investigations
- Intracranial haemorrhage
- Head injuries – general principles of management
- Surgical aspects of meningitis
- Spinal cord injury and compression
- Paraplegia and quadriplegia – principles of management.

Unit 4   Special problems

- Prehospital care
- Triage
- Trauma scoring systems
- Traumatic wounds – principles of management
- Gunshot and blast wounds
- Skin loss – grafts and flaps
- Burns
- Facial and orbital injuries.

Unit 5   Principles of limb injury

- Peripheral nervous system – anatomy and physiology
- Fractures – pathophysiology of fracture healing
- Non-union, delayed union, complications
- Principles of bone grafting
- Traumatic oedema, compartment and crush syndrome, fat embolism
- Brachial plexus injury.

Core Module 4: Intensive care

Unit 1   Cardiovascular

- The surgical anatomy and applied physiology of the heart relevant to clinical cases
- Physiology and pharmacological control of cardiac output, blood flow, blood pressure, coronary circulation
- Cardiac arrest, resuscitation
- Monitoring of cardiac function in the critically ill patient, central venous pressure, pulmonary wedge

pressure, tamponade, cardiac O/P measurements

- The interpretation of special investigations
- The management of haemorrhage and shock
- Pulmonary oedema
- Cardiopulmonary bypass – general principles, cardiac support.

Unit 2   Respiratory

- The surgical anatomy of the airways, chest wall, diaphragm and thoracic viscera
- The mechanics and control of respiration
- The interpretation of special investigations – lung function tests, arterial blood gases, radiology
- The understanding of disorders of respiratory function caused by trauma, acute surgical illness and surgical intervention
- Respiratory failure
- Adult respiratory distress syndrome
- Endotracheal intubation, laryngotomy, tracheostomy
- Artificial ventilation.

Unit 3   Multisystem failure

- Multisystem failure
- Renal failure – diagnosis complications
- Gastrointestinal tract, hepatic
- Nutrition.

Unit 4   Problems in intensive care

- Sepsis, predisposing factors, organisms causing septicaemia
- Complications of thoracic operations
- Localized sepsis, pneumonia, lung abscess, bronchiectasis, empyema, mediastinitis.

Unit 5   Principles of the ICU

- Indications for admission
- Organization and staffing
- Scoring
- Costs.

Core Module 5: Neoplasia. Techniques and outcome of surgery

Unit 1   Principles of oncology

- Epidemiology of common neoplasms and tumour-like conditions; role of cancer registries
- Clinicopathological staging of cancer
- Pathology, clinical features, diagnosis and principles

of management of common cancers in each of the surgical specialities

- Principles of cancer treatment by surgery, radiotherapy, chemotherapy, immunotherapy and hormone therapy
- The principles of carcinogenesis and the pathogenesis of cancer relevant to the clinical features, special investigations, staging and the principles of treatment of the common cancers
- Principles of molecular biology of cancer – carcinogenesis, genetic factors, mechanisms of metastasis.

Unit 2   Cancer screening and treatment

- The surgical anatomy and applied physiology of the breast relevant to clinical examinations, the interpretation of special investigations, the understanding of disordered function and the principles of the surgical treatment of common disorders of the breast
- The breast – acute infections, benign breast disorders, nipple discharge, mastalgia
- Carcinoma of breast – mammography, investigation and treatment
- Screening programmes.

Unit 3   Techniques of management

- Terminal care of cancer patients; pain relief
- Rehabilitation
- Psychological effects of surgery and bereavement.

Unit 4   Ethics and the law

- Medical/legal ethics and medicolegal aspects of surgery
- Communication with patients, relatives and colleagues.

Unit 5   Outcome of surgery

- The evaluation of surgery and general topics
- Decision-making in surgery
- Clinical audit
- Statistics and computing in surgery
- Principles of research and design and analysis of clinical trials
- Critical evaluation of innovations – technical and pharmaceutical
- Health-service management and economic aspects of surgical care.

System Module A: Locomotor system

Musculoskeletal anatomy and physiology relevant to clinical examination of the locomotor system and to the understanding of disordered locomotor function, with emphasis on the effects of acute musculoskeletal trauma.

Unit 1   Effects of trauma and lower limb

- Effects of acute musculoskeletal trauma
- Common fractures and joint injuries
- Degenerative and rheumatoid arthritis (including principles of joint replacement)
- Common disorders of the foot
- Amputations.

Unit 2   Infections and upper limb

- Common soft tissue injuries and disorders
- Infections of bones and joints (including implants and prostheses)
- Pain in the neck, shoulder and arm
- Common disorders of the hand, including hand injuries and infections.

Unit 3   Bone disease and spine

- Common disorders of infancy and childhood
- Low back pain and sciatica
- Metabolic bone disease (osteoporosis, osteomalacia)
- Surgical aspects of paralytic disorders and nerve injuries.

System Module B: Vascular

The surgical anatomy and applied physiology of blood vessels relevant to clinical examination, the interpretation of special investigations and the understanding of the role of surgery in the management of cardiovascular disease.

Unit 1   Arterial diseases

- Chronic obliterative arterial disease
- Amputations
- Aneurysms
- Carotid disease
- Special techniques used in the investigation of vascular disease
- Limb ischaemia – acute and chronic, clinical features, gangrene, amputations for vascular disease
- Principles of reconstructive arterial surgery.

Unit 2   Venous diseases

- Vascular trauma and peripheral veins
- Varicose veins
- Venous hypertension, postphlebitic leg, venous ulceration
- Disorders of the veins in the lower limb
- Deep venous thrombosis and its complications
- Chronic ulceration of the leg
- Thrombosis and embolism.

Unit 3   Lymphatics and spleen

- Thromboembolic disease
- Spleen – splenectomy, hypersplenism
- Lymph nodes, lymphoedema
- Surgical aspects of autoimmune disease
- The anatomy and physiology of the haemopoeitic and lymphoreticular systems
- Surgical aspects of disordered haemopoiesis.

System Module C: Head, neck, endocrine and paediatric

The surgical anatomy and applied physiology of the head and neck relevant to clinical examination, the interpretation of special investigations, the understanding of disorders of function, and the treatment of disease and injury involving the head and neck.

Unit 1   The head

- Acute and chronic inflammatory disorders of the ear, nose, sinuses and throat
- Intracranial complications
- Foreign bodies in ear, nose and throat
- Epistaxis
- Salivary gland disease
- The eye – trauma, common infections.

Unit 2   Neck and endocrine glands

- The surgical anatomy and applied physiology of the endocrine glands relevant to clinical examination, the interpretation of special investigations, the understanding of disordered function and the principles of the surgical treatment of common disorders of the endocrine glands
- Common neck swellings
- Thyroid – role of surgery in diseases of the thyroid, complications of thyroidectomy, the solitary thyroid nodule

- Parathyroid, hyperparathyroidism, hypercalcaemia
- Secondary hypertension.

Unit 3   Paediatric disorders

- Neonatal physiology – special problems of anaesthesia and surgery in the newborn; principles of neonatal fluid and electrolyte balance
- Correctable congenital abnormalities
- Common paediatric surgical disorders – cleft lip and palate, pyloric stenosis, intussusception, hernia, maldescent of testis, torsion, diseases of the foreskin.

System Module D: Abdomen

The surgical anatomy of the abdomen and its viscera and the applied physiology of the alimentary system relevant to clinical examination, the interpretation of common special investigations, the understanding of disorders of function, and the treatment of abdominal disease and injury.

Unit 1   Abdominal wall

- Anatomy of the groin, groin hernias, acute and elective, clinical features of hernias, complications of hernias
- Anterior abdominal wall, anatomy, incisions, laparoscopic access.

Unit 2   Acute abdominal conditions

- Peritonitis, intra-abdominal abscesses
- Common acute abdominal emergencies
- Intestinal obstruction, paralytic ileus
- Intestinal fistulae
- Investigation of abdominal pain
- Investigation of abdominal masses
- Gynaecological causes of acute abdominal pain
- Pelvic inflammatory disease
- Abdominal injury.

Unit 3   Elective abdominal conditions

- Common anal and perianal disorders
- Jaundice – differential diagnosis and management
- Portal hypertension
- Gallstones
- Gastrostomy, ileostomy, colostomy and other stomata.

System Module E: Urinary system and renal transplantation

The surgical anatomy and applied physiology of the genitourinary system relevant to clinical examination, special investigations, understanding of disordered function, and the principles of the surgical treatment of genitourinary disease and injury.

Unit 1   Urinary tract 1

- Urinary tract infection
- Haematuria
- Trauma to the urinary tract
- Urinary calculi.

Unit 2   Urinary tract 2

- Retention of urine
- Disorders of prostate
- Pain and swelling in the scrotum; torsion.

Unit 3   Renal failure and transplantation

- Principles of transplantation
- Renal failure, dialysis.

TIMETABLE AND DISTANCE LEARNING

A timetable for sitting the examination can be suggested by the Royal College of Surgeons of England.

The Royal College of Surgeons of England also recommends that trainees should enrol for and follow its MRCS distance-learning course in parallel with the training posts. This is a 20-month course comprising five 10-week core modules and five 6-week systems modules which cover the syllabus. This should allow study, assimilation of new material and preparation for the examinations to occur from the start of Basic Surgical Training.

PREPARATION FOR THE MCQs

The core modules form the 'bread and butter' of the knowledge base for basic surgical training and therefore require a proportionately long period of study prior to attempting the MCQ exam. The systems modules may more conveniently and enjoyably be studied during the appropriate clinical specialty training period. If the MRCS distance-learning course is not used it is strongly advised that preparation and study for the MRCS commences at the start of clinical training. Who knows, this might make the clinical work more enjoyable!

It is likely that the MCQs will be of a variable type and include extended matching questions with which you may be unfamiliar. Examples are included in the MRCS distance learning course.

PREPARATION FOR THE CLINICAL EXAM

The clinical exam will probably take the form of multiple short cases, possibly in the objective structured clinical examination (OSCE) format. Revision for this exam is along conventional lines and most will have experience of OSCE-type examinations prior to sitting the clinical part of the MRCS examination. Most undergraduate examinations now include an OSCE assessment and, if unfamiliar with this type of examination, helping with or observing such an examination might be useful prior to sitting the clinical exam. It is likely that revision courses for the clinical parts of the exam will be available to provide invaluable practice in examination technique.

PREPARATION FOR THE VIVA VOCE EXAM

This is the final part of the examination and in principle any aspect of the syllabus may be examined at this stage. Clearly last-minute preparation for this exam will be of limited value and this again reinforces the need to spread learning and revision over the whole period of clinical training. The log book may be inspected and used as a means of raising questions on many aspects of basic surgical training. Having attended an Advanced Trauma Life Support and Critical Care course the candidate may feel more confident in handling many clinically orientated questions in a viva examination.

42. The MRCS examination

R. M. Kirk

The examination replaces the Applied Basic Sciences and Clinical Surgery in General examinations (see Ch. 41). It is intended to demonstrate that successful candidates have the required basic knowledge and training to proceed to Higher Surgical Training.

Ideally, examinations should test objectively whether candidates have all the aptitudes required of a surgeon. Unfortunately, most of the required qualities can be assessed only by seeing surgeons in practice and evaluating their results.

Tests of cognition, factual knowledge (What does the candidate know?) can be assessed with fair objectivity. How that knowledge is used to make accurate diagnoses, sensible decisions and effective management is more difficult to determine. To assess psychomotor skills (What can the candidate do?) usually requires observation of the taking of a history and examination of a patient, and this is very subjective. Even greater difficulty is encountered in assessing the affective characteristics (What sort of person is this?), which include integrity, 'common sense', motivation, determination, perfection-seeking and interpersonal qualities. Even if we were able to assess all these aptitudes individually, we could not be sure we had a good or bad surgeon. The German Gestalt (= form, pattern) school of psychology averred that it is useless to try and assess the whole by looking only at the parts, since the whole is greater than the sum of the parts. We all have deficiencies but we compensate for them, or overcompensate, with our strengths. It is, therefore, tragic if a potentially excellent surgeon fails to pass the examination, not because of a deficiency in the required qualities or knowledge, but because of failure as an examination candidate.

Too many examination candidates spend all their energies taking in facts. The prospect of an examination has a valuable function in stimulating candidates to complete their knowledge. But you do not pass examinations with facts alone. It is what you do with those facts that gains marks. Now you must organize the knowledge you have acquired and practise using it in order to display it suc-cessfully to the examiners and subsequently use it clinically for the benefit of your patients.

Apply your knowledge in the way it will be tested in the examination. It is well recognized that practice improves performance in examinations. This explains why those who fail usually pass eventually, if they persist.

MULTIPLE-CHOICE QUESTIONS

Multiple-choice questions (MCQs) are well known to most trainees. What is not always appreciated is that there are variations in the format and marking system. The simplest form is a 'stem' or statement inviting the candidate to select the most appropriate answer to a proposal or question from five possibilities. Four of the proffered answers may be 'distractors', the remaining one being the correct answer. In order to make the candidate positively select the best answer, the four distracters must be possible, though unlikely.

The marking system may vary. Marks are gained for correct answers. As a rule, marks are deducted for wrong selections, while unmarked selections do not score or lose marks, but this is not invariable.

Perhaps the most common variation is the independent true–false format. One, some, all, or none of the proffered answers can be correct. This requires candidates to make a decision about each of the answers, not merely select the correct one and discard the remainder. As a rule there are three choices for each of the five proffered answers: true, false, don't know. A correct answer usually gains a mark, an incorrect answer loses a mark and 'don't know' neither gains nor loses a mark.

Another variation is to provide a stem in the form, perhaps, of a case history. Five possible diagnoses are offered for selection. On the basis of the same stem, further series of answers can be offered for selection, related to investigation or management of the condition.

You must read the preliminary instructions that explain what you should do. To plunge into answering the questions without so doing is like starting to treat patients before you have found out what is wrong with them.

Do not destroy your chances of success by doggedly worrying over an insoluble problem. Move on and complete those that you can complete. Only then can you return to the difficult questions.

MCQs have the merit that they can test knowledge over a wide area in a fairly objective manner. However, because the correct answer must be present, the candidate does not need to develop it from the given information, as happens in clinical practice. It is a format that encourages the setting of 'small print' problems. Unless the modifiers in the stem are selected carefully, knowledgeable candidates may fail. For example, if the absolute words 'never', 'invariably', etc., are used they may mislead an experienced candidate who has seen the rare exception. Because absolutes are so rare in medicine, candidates often sense that when these terms are used, the statement is usually false.

Extended-matching items

This is a format that breaks with standard MCQ tests. A list of options is provided and this may be used for a number of questions.

As an example, the option list may include 14 or 15 causes of abdominal pain. A lead-in statement then asks for the selection of the likeliest diagnosis for one or more patients. A stem is provided for each patient, describing the age, gender, specific features and perhaps the results of simple investigations. Further lists of investigations or treatment options can be offered for selection.

An option list may look like this:

(A) Ureteric colic
(B) Abdominal muscle strain
(C) Mesenteric adenitis
(D) Herpes zoster
(E) Torn inferior epigastric vessels
(F) 'Mittelschmerz'
(G) Appendicitis
(H) Intraperitoneal hernia
(I) Ruptured ectopic pregnancy
(J) Perforated peptic ulcer
(K) Spinal nerve compression
(L) Meckel's diverticulitis
(M) Small intestinal obstruction
(N) Terminal ileitis.

The 'Lead in' may read:

For each patient with acute pain in the right iliac fossa, select the most likely diagnosis. Each option may be used once, more than once, or not at all.

A number of 'stems' may be used, such as:

1. A 26-year-old man sent by the general practitioner with a letter stating that the patient had sudden intense epigastric pain with tenderness and guarding. Bowel sounds were normal, pulse 85 per minute, temperature 38.2°C. The patient now complains only of pain in the right iliac fossa. The abdomen is soft but there is tenderness in the right iliac fossa. Bowel sounds are still present. Pulse is 110 per minute, temperature 39°C.

2. A 15-year-old girl complains of sudden, excruciating right iliac fossa pain, now more diffuse in the lower abdomen. She had previously been well but is slightly constipated. Soon after the pain developed she had an urgent desire to pass urine. Her periods were regular, the last one had started 15 days ago. You find no abnormal physical signs apart from a little tenderness in the lower abdomen and in the rectovaginal pouch on rectal examination. Bowel sounds are normal. Pulse is 85 per minute, temperature 38.6°C.

This method of examination may be unfamiliar to you, so endeavour to practise answering such questions.

OBJECTIVE STRUCTURED CLINICAL EXAMINATION (OSCE)

This is a versatile method of examining and allows a group of candidates to be tested in a single session. A number of 'stations' are arranged. At each station the candidate is tested in some way. The same number of candidates can be admitted as there are stations, so that one stands at each station. After a fixed period, usually $4\frac{1}{2}$ minutes, a signal is given and the candidates move to the next station, taking 30 seconds. The moves continue until each candidate has passed through every station.

A series of questions are asked and skills are demonstrated. The tests are selected so that they will all take approximately the same time to perform. Some of the stations need to be manned when the candidates are performing a task which needs to be evaluated by watching or listening. At such stations the observer is normally given a checklist to tick off the steps of the task as being performed correctly. At others the candidates can record their responses to tests, which are marked later.

Suitable tests include:

1. A patient (or simulated patient) with a clinical history or physical signs that need to be diagnosed. Such a station must be supervised by an examiner who awards marks. This has some advantages over ordinary clinical 'cases'. Preagreed points can be looked for and evaluated, giving the tests objectivity. Simulated patients can appear to have conditions that are difficult to display, such as acute abdominal emergencies.

2. An X-ray, clinical photograph, pathology specimen,

biochemical or other investigation result can be displayed for interpretation. A clinical background may be given to the candidate who can be asked to offer a diagnosis, and suggest relevant investigations or management. This station need not be supervised; the candidate records the answer for subsequent marking.

3. A simulation can be provided on which the candidate demonstrates a skill such as passing a urinary catheter, setting up an intravenous infusion or suturing an incision. At these supervised stations, marks are awarded for preagreed correct actions.

The possibilities are extensive. Many aspects of knowledge and skill can be tested. Your best chance of success is to ensure that you take every opportunity to practise your clinical skills. Reading about them is not the same as practising them.

CLINICAL EXAMINATION

The examiners have the opportunity to evaluate your psychomotor skills in handling patients, extracting an accurate history and carrying out a careful examination to elicit and evaluate relevant physical signs. It allows you to display your ability to select discriminant features, put them together to make a diagnosis and use this as a basis for making decisions about management. Importantly, it allows the examiners to assess your interpersonal and communicating skills when dealing with patients.

The 'clinical' is a vital part of the examination. Examiners are unforgiving of incompetence. After all, this tests one of the fundamental skills required of a surgeon.

You will see a series of 'short cases' not preceded by a 'long case'. You may be asked to take a history from a patient while the examiner listens, or asked to examine a part or a specific lesion (see Ch. 1). Make sure you know what is expected of you. If you would like to carry out a specific test, or ask the patient to cooperate by, for instance, standing up, ask the examiner if you are in doubt. In some cases it is obvious that you cannot do so, but make a mental note to state that in normal circumstances you would do so.

Introduce yourself to the patient and ask permission to perform the examination. Unless you are forbidden to do so, ask about the history of any lesion and any other relevant information.

Carry out a systematic examination, after making sure there are no tender regions. 'Spot diagnoses' are dangerous. Anyway, the examiner may demand that you justify your spot diagnosis. You may not be able to make a diagnosis, but the examiner will expect you to state accurately the physical signs. If you give a good account

the examiner usually helps you to reach a diagnosis – or admits that no one knows it.

Do not obsessively carry out repeated examinations. Determine to carry out each examination once only, concentrating on the findings.

Even though you may be asked to concentrate on a single area, do not fail to take in the general appearance of the patient. Their age, gender and general condition will influence treatment decisions. Ask yourself if you should specifically look elsewhere. For example, if you find an enlarged lymph node, you should examine the whole reticuloendothelial system. If you find localized vascular disease, you should examine the whole cardiovascular system. If you find joint disease you should examine the other joints. You may be barred from extending the examination, but make sure you inform the examiner that you would normally do so.

Do not raise your head or signal to the examiner that you have completed the examination until you have answered the following questions:

- Have you completed it in a systematic manner?
- Is there any question you should have asked?
- Is there anywhere you should look?
- Have you prepared what you will say to the examiner?
- Have you a diagnosis? How would you confirm it and assess the severity of the condition?
- Is there a differential diagnosis? How will you elucidate it?
- What are the treatment options and how will you decide on the best choice?
- What will you say to the patient?
- What is the examiner likely to ask you as a supplementary question – and have you prepared the answer?

When you are sure you have answers to the questions, thank the patient and indicate to the examiner that you are ready. Do not necessarily wait for the examiner to ask you a question. If you are confident, state the findings and diagnosis – and what is your evidence. Continue by stating what actions you would take and what you would say to the patient, unless the examiner interrupts you to ask a specific question, or guides you to the next patient.

If you are unsure of the diagnosis, state in order the relevant findings. For example, state where a lump is both in area and depth, its attachments, tenderness, size, shape, surface, consistency, fluctuation and any other features.

Do not start re-examining the patient at this stage. If there is anything you realize that you have missed, declare it. Honesty and willingness to admit error are valuable qualities, and the examiner will be more sympathetic than if you try to cover up your omission.

It is likely that you will be asked to discuss with a patient or simulated patient the sort of problems you encounter in clinical practice. These include the choices of treatment for particular conditions, and the risks of complications and how you will anticipate and try to avoid them. You may also be asked to explain what the patient will experience in discomfort, pain, aftercare and recovery. If short-stay or day-case surgery is contemplated, you may be asked to explain the selection process and what the patient will need to arrange. Your communication and interpersonal skills can be assessed in this manner.

Practise for the clinical examination by examining patients as often as possible. After each examination have someone question you so that you practise presenting your findings.

VIVA VOCE EXAMINATIONS

These are wide-ranging face-to-face question and answer encounters. The task of the examiners is to find out not how little you know, but how much you know. For this reason, as soon as the examiner realizes that you know the subject he or she should explore some other topic. If you do not know an answer, the examiner may help you, or change the subject, to allow you to display your knowledge in another area. For this reason, do not be upset when the examiner interpolates a change of subject.

If you do not know the answer to an important question, it is better to admit it than try to bluff your way out of difficulty. We all have our 'blind spots' and the examiner will not trust you if you are dishonest. However, you may sometimes be able to state that, although you are not sure of the answer, on logical grounds you would expect the answer to be such and such.

Equally, if you make a statement and subsequently realize it was incorrect, do not hesitate to admit it and correct it. If you make a mistake, do not feel that you have failed. If you do make a single mistake the examiner will judge it in the context of the other answers you have given. Often, you fail because of the effect the failure has had on your self-confidence. Take a deep breath and determine to 'dig yourself out of the hole'. Do not give up. The examiners appreciate a candidate who does not give up in the face of disaster.

Have your logbook available, since the examiners may consult it to see what experience you have had, before questioning you on operative surgery.

There are certain important surgical procedures you are expected to know, for instance life-saving operations. For example, you must be able to describe the surgical management of traumatically sustained wounds, or describe the competent accomplishment of a small intestinal anastomosis (see Ch. 41).

MARKING

MCQ answers can be marked by computers. The examiners decide what will be a pass mark and thereafter candidates either pass or fail, although the pass mark may be adjusted from time to time.

Clinical and viva voce examiners work in pairs. In order to ensure that the standard remains steady, newly appointed examiners work with senior, experienced colleagues. One discusses with the candidate and the other listens. As a rule the examiners take it in turns to question each candidate. They each take notes of the cases seen, questions asked and answers received. They subsequently agree on a mark. At the end of the day, some candidates have obviously passed, some have obviously failed. Those on the borderline are discussed to ensure that the fairest level is achieved. Each examiner declares before the Court what happened in the clinical examination and what discussion took place in the viva voce examination, and why a particular mark was given. When all the examiners have completed their reports, the Chairman sums up in as neutral a fashion as possible. The Court then votes whether the candidate should pass or fail, with the Chairman having the casting vote. In this way each candidate is assured that the difficulties of clinical cases and questions asked are taken into account. It is doubtful if a fairer method of examining complex qualities and skills can be constructed.

The Court does not have, as some candidates believe, a 'ration' of passes. As far as is humanly possible the examinations are criterion referred – that is, there are agreed standards of performance required for a pass mark. Inevitably, the standard in, for example, the MCQ may need to be adjusted if almost no one is passing, or no one is failing; to this extent the examination is peer referred – you are in competition with your fellow candidates. The examiners do not know how candidates have performed with other examiners until the end of the examination.

CONCLUSIONS

Multiple choice questions test only your cognitive (factual) capabilities. Clinical examinations test your psychomotor and interpersonal skills. Viva voce examinations display your affective skills to the examiners. In the clinical and viva voce examinations your decision-making skills can be tested. The only objective test is that of your factual knowledge. Most of the qualities that are amenable to objective measurement are of limited importance. The really important qualities – integrity, commitment, common sense, leadership, etc. – can be evaluated subjectively only. The fact that these other qualities cannot be assessed objectively does not absolve examiners from trying to evaluate them.

THE FUTURE

Throughout the world efforts are being made to improve our selection and assessment of surgeons. The educators and examiners are constantly reviewing new methods.

Some of the qualities required of a clinical surgeon can be tested by interactive computer programs that assess your knowledge and decision-making capabilities. It is likely that the examination format will change. Be assured, though, that fairness of the selection is considered paramount. The examiners are under great pressure to protect the public from incompetent surgeons. However, the cost of training a surgeon is very high. It would be wasteful to undertake training of surgeons, only to reject them for no good reason.

Index